Dermatology Cyberderm WebBook

Günter Burg
Editor-in-Chief

Harald Gollnick • Martine Bagot
Jonathan M. White
Editors

Dermatology Cyberderm WebBook

Second Edition

Springer

Editor-in-Chief
Günter Burg
Dermatology
Zurich, Switzerland

Editors
Harald Gollnick
Department of Dermatology & Venereology
Otto-von-Guericke University
Magdeburg, Germany

Martine Bagot
Service de Dermatologie
Université Paris Cité, Hôpital Saint-Louis
Paris, France

Jonathan M. White
Ecole de Santé Publique
Université libre de Bruxelles
Brussels, Belgium

ISBN 978-3-031-78493-4 ISBN 978-3-031-78491-0 (eBook)
https://doi.org/10.1007/978-3-031-78491-0

Original English edition published by ABW-Wissenschaftsverlag, Berlin, 2017.

This Springer imprint is published by the registered company Springer Nature Switzerland AG
The registered company address is: Gewerbestrasse 11, 6330 Cham, Switzerland

For our patients, medical students, and employees in the health care services

Foreword

A major challenge for our universities is how to provide the highest quality education in science and medicine for students and finally for the patients. The best solution for the dilemma of expanding knowledge and increasing number of students, where there are limited resources, is "blended learning", which combines classical teaching and learning modules (e.g. campus-based lectures) and self-guided autonomous learning with print or electronic media, which allows students to learn at their own pace, tailored to the individual capacities and needs of each student.

This second edition of the *Cyberderm WebBook* builds on the strengths of the first edition and the excellent feedback from users. Drs Burg, Gollnick, Bagot and White have developed an outstanding and flexible educational programme which will be of great benefit to dermatology trainees internationally.

Professor of Dermatology
Cardiff University
Cardiff, UK

Andrew Y. Finlay

Preface

Dear Students

Our skin is an amazing complex organ. Around 100 billion readily renewable cells combine to form a 2 m^2 covering that generates the protective layer of the body. Skin provides a mechanical barrier against the external environment, but has further roles in thermoregulation, metabolism, and the regulation of fluid balance, as well as being socially important in contributing to physical and emotional attraction between individuals.

There are more than 2000 different skin diseases; also, some skin conditions can reflect a general medical problem such as a systemic infection or a cutaneous manifestation of internal disease.

Less than 2% of medical students after their exam go into specialization in Dermatology. However, knowledge in Dermatology is helpful in 20–25% of patients in a general practitioner's and non-dermatology office. Therefore, the skills perceived as undergraduate student may be the only source of knowledge when dealing with patients after graduation.

As part of an Erasmus+ project, 30 authors from 11 European countries have compiled the most important information in a short and concise style in 10 main chapters and 34 subchapters, comprising 190 dermatological or venerological diagnoses, illustrated by more than 500 full color pictures: (1) Inflammatory Dermatoses; (2) Infectious Diseases; (3) Nevi, Tumors, and Cysts; (4) Diseases of the Appendages and of the Mucous Membranes; (5) Diseases of Blood and Lymph Vessels, Ulcers, and Panniculitis; (6) Genodermatoses, Metabolic Diseases, and Pigmentary Disorders; (7) Proctologic Disorders and Psychodermatoses; (8) Special Conditions, Symptoms, and Syndromes; (9) General Dermatology; (10) Neglected Tropical Dermatoses (NTDs) including traveler's dermatoses.

Each diagnosis is strictly structured, describing Synonyms; Epidemiology; Definition; Aetiology and Pathogenesis; Signs and Symptoms; Localization; Classification; Laboratory and other Workups; Dermatopathology; Course; Complications; Diagnostic Hallmarks; Differential Diagnosis; Prevention and Therapy.

The latest ICD-11 key of the International Classifications of Diagnoses (WHO-FIC) is given for each of the diagnoses, which are assigned to categories A, B, or C. Category A: Know and care; corresponds to common diseases that the General Practitioner (GP) must be able to diagnose and to treat. Category B: Know and care with guidance; corresponds to diseases which should be referred to the dermatologist, but still within the capacity of the GP to evaluate the emergency and to make the first intervention/management step. The GP must be guided to follow the patient in cooperation with the dermatovenerologist. Category C: Know and refer; corresponds to diseases which the GP must know just enough to recognize and understand and to refer to the dermatovenerologist.

Over 300 multiple-choice questions (FlashCards) comprising all dermatological and venereological specialties are the highlights of this book and make it the most valuable interactive learning aid.

The owners of this WebBook may be interested in visiting the following URLs on YouTube, which are part of the educational project complementary to the Springer book, but independent and not coupled or related to Springer Nature.

- https://www.youtube.com/watch?v=iFCQnM2JKEM (Demo of the online teaching and learning platform for Dermatology and Venerology. www.cyberderm.net; awarded the Medida-price 2009)
- https://www.youtube.com/watch?v=Z3qdogG2mlw&t=180s (movie "From Hippokrates to E-Learning")

Magdeburg, Germany — Harald Gollnick
Paris, France — Martine Bagot
Brussels, Belgium — Jonathan M. White
Zürich, Switzerland — Günter Burg

Acknowledgment

Text and pictures of this WebBook are based on the lectures on "Dermatology and Dermatovenerology" presented at the University School of Dermatology in Zürich/Switzerland by G. Burg and collaborators (1991–2006). The start was sponsored by the Swiss Virtual Campus and the Swiss Universities, followed by the kind support of the European Dermatology Forum (EDF) and the Erasmus^{+} Project hEduLearnIt (2018–2022). This WebBook is the fourth updated revision, to which 30 specialists of Dermatology from 11 countries have contributed.

Concept and Coordination and technical support by Vahid Djamei and Anna Darzina from Swiss4ward, Zürich, and Alicante.

We acknowledge the kind support of Springer Nature publisher and its co-workers Juliette Kleemann and Pinky Sathishkumar.

Disclaimer

This WebBook is for teaching and learning purposes of students and workers in the health care sciences only. The WebBook accepts no liability whatsoever for any errors or incompleteness in the content or misuse of this.

Prof & Chairm. emer., Dermatology Guenter Burg
Former Dean of the Faculty of Medicine
University of Zürich
Zürich, Switzerland
g.burg@access.uzh.ch

Contents

Part I

Inflammatory Dermatoses

They comprise a broad spectrum of non-infectious dermatoses, including allergic and non-allergic, i.e. toxic or physically induced intolerance reactions of the skin, autoimmune, bullous, granulomatous and papulosquamous dermatoses, the most common of which is psoriasis vulgaris.

Allergic/Non-allergic and Other Immunologic Reactions

1

Ramon María Pujol Vallverdú, Martine Bagot, Veronique del Marmol, Evelyn Gaffal, Ana María Giménez-Arnau, Giampiero Girolomoni, Paolo Gisondi, Harald Gollnick, and Jonathan M. White

Contents

R. M. Pujol Vallverdú (✉) · A. M. Giménez-Arnau
Dermatology and Venereology, Universitat Autònoma de Barcelona, Hospital del Mar. IMIM, Barcelona, Spain
e-mail: rpujol@psmar.cat

M. Bagot
Service de Dermatologie, Université Paris Cité, Hôpital Saint-Louis, Paris, France
e-mail: martine.bagot@gmail.com

V. del Marmol
Département of Dermatology, Hôpital Erasme-HUB, Université Libre de Bruxelles, Brussels, Belgium
e-mail: veronique.delmarmol@hubruxelles.be

E. Gaffal
Department of Dermatology, University of Lübeck, Lübeck, Germany
e-mail: evelyn.gaffal@med.ovgu.de

G. Girolomoni · P. Gisondi
Department of Medicine, Università degli Studi di Verona, Verona, Italy
e-mail: giampiero.girolomoni@univr.it; paolo.gisondi@univr.it

H. Gollnick
Department of Dermatology & Venereology, Otto-von-Guericke University, Magdeburg, Germany
e-mail: Harald.Gollnick@med.ovgu.de

J. M. White
Ecole de Santé Publique, Université libre de Bruxelles, Brussels, Belgium
e-mail: Jonathan.White@ulb.be

H. Gollnick et al. (eds.), *Dermatology Cyberderm WebBook*,
https://doi.org/10.1007/978-3-031-78491-0_1

Test your learning and check your understanding of this book's contents: use the "Springer Nature Flashcards" app to access questions.

To use the app, please follow the instructions below:

1. Go to https://flashcards.springernature.com/login
2. Create a user account by entering your e-mail address and assigning a password.
3. Use the following link to access your SN Flashcards set: ▶ https://sn.pub/1rhh6k

If the link is missing or does not work, please send an e-mail with the subject "SN Flashcards" and the book title to customerservice@springernature.com

Urticaria and Angioedema

Urticaria [3]

Figures 1.1, 1.2, 1.3 and 1.4

Grading of Importance
A

Level
Advanced

ICD-11
Chronic Spontaneous Urticaria EB00.1;
Acute Urticaria: EB00.0;
Inducible Chronic Urticaria: EB01

Synonyms
Hives, wheals, weals.

Fig. 1.1 Urticaria

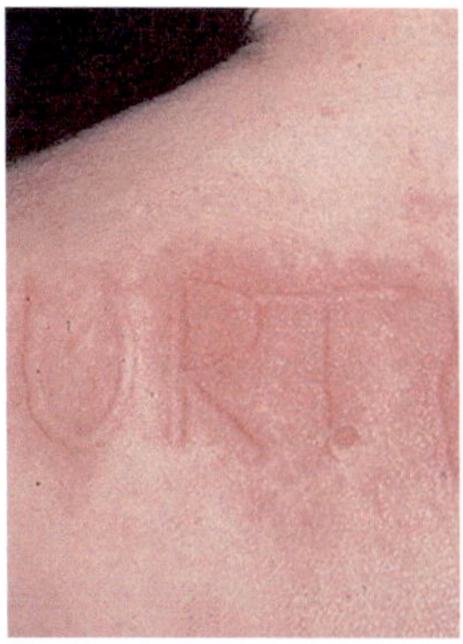

Fig. 1.2 Urticaria

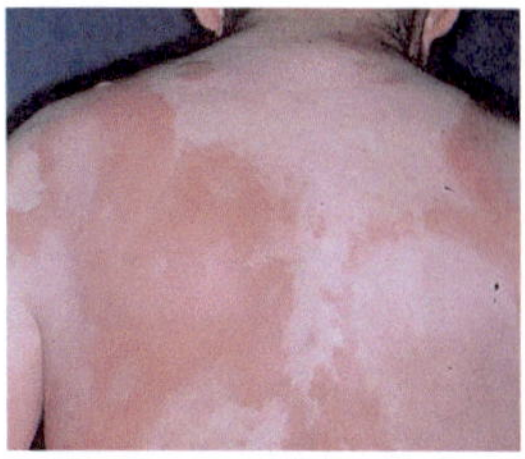

Fig. 1.3 Urticaria

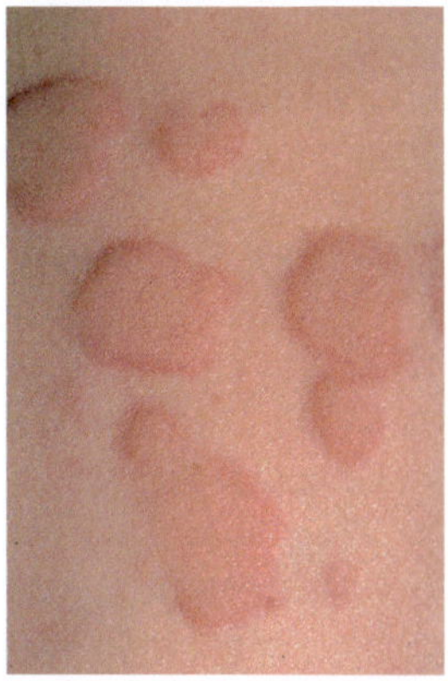

Fig. 1.4 Urticaria

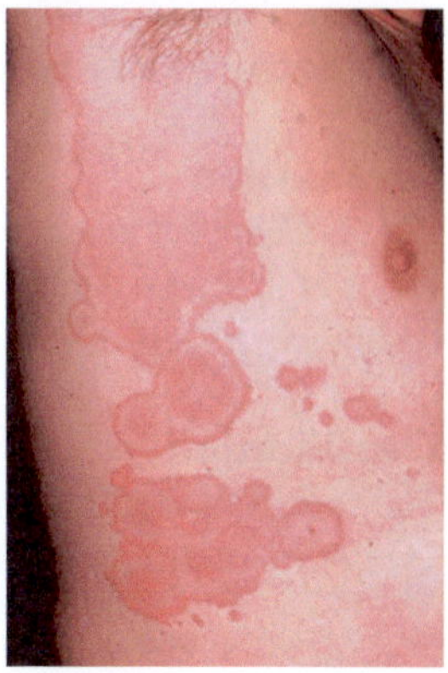

Epidemiology

Acute urticaria: Life prevalence around 2–8%. For non-acute urticaria, around 0.1–0.6% in the general population.

Definition

Urticaria is a group of diseases characterised by the development of wheals (hives), angioedema (see section "Eczematous Dermatoses" in Chap. 1) or both. Hives are defined as pruritic transient swellings of the upper dermis with multiple causes, usually mediated mainly by histamine release.

Urticaria needs to be differentiated from other medical conditions where wheals, angioedema or both can occur, e.g. anaphylaxis, auto-inflammatory syndromes, urticarial vasculitis or bradykinin-mediated angioedema including hereditary angioedema (HAE).

Aetiology and Pathogenesis

Urticaria is a mast cell-driven disease. Release of histamine and other mediators such as platelet-activating factor (PAF) and cytokines released from activated skin mast cells result in vasodilatation and plasma extravasation as well as sensory nerve activation and cell recruitment to urticarial lesions.

The mast cell-activating signals in urticaria are ill-defined and likely to be heterogeneous and diverse (IgE-mediated type I reaction, non-specific histamine liberators, activation of complement, autoimmune-mediated urticaria—IgG against IgE or against high-affinity IgE receptor and IgE against autoantigens, as well as other poorly understood mechanisms).

Signs and Symptoms

- Central swelling of variable size surrounded by reflex erythema and a fleeting nature, with the skin returning to its normal appearance, usually within 30 minutes to 24 h. Itching or sometimes burning sensation.
- Urticaria may be associated with angioedema: Pronounced erythematous or skin-coloured swelling of the lower dermis and subcutis or mucous membranes. Sometimes pain, rather than itch.
- Sudden appearance of erythematous lesions and hives whose appearance varies over the course of a few hours. Marked pruritus. If individual hives persist for more than 24 hours, the possibility of urticarial vasculitis must be considered (skin biopsy may be useful).

Localisation

Hives can appear in any part of the skin, showing variable size and extension. In some forms of urticaria, the lesions may be papular (e.g. cholinergic urticaria). Angioedema commonly affects mucous membranes, eyelids and lips and hands and feet.

Classification

The spectrum of clinical manifestations of different urticaria subtypes is very wide. Two or more different subtypes of urticaria can coexist in any given patient:

- Acute spontaneous urticaria: Occurrence of spontaneous wheals, angioedema or both for less than 6 weeks.
- Chronic spontaneous urticaria: appearance of wheals, angioedema or both for more than 6 weeks due to known or unknown causes.
- Acute or chronic inducible urticaria include symptomatic dermographism, cold urticaria, delayed pressure urticaria, solar urticaria, heat urticaria, vibratory angioedema, cholinergic urticaria, contact urticaria and aquagenic urticaria.

Based on Aetiology

- Immunological:
  1. IgE-mediated (type I reaction) foods, medications, bee or wasp toxins, foreign proteins and other exogenous materials such as latex or plant products (contact urticaria).
  2. Immune complex-mediated (type III reaction).
  3. Autoimmune (autoantibodies against IgE or the FcE receptor or IgE against autoantigens).
- Non-immunologic:
  1. Direct mediator release from mast cells: caused by foods/food additives/ medications.
  2. Physical forms (pressure, heat, vibration).
  3. Intolerance of NSAID (non-steroidal anti-inflammatory drugs).
- Underlying diseases such as intestinal parasites, foci of infection, thyroid disease, liver disease (viral hepatitis), other viral infections, connective tissue disorders.
- Idiopathic

Laboratory and Other Workups

Acute urticaria: Does not require a diagnostic workup, as it is usually self-limiting. Choice based on history and clinical findings, could include prick testing for medications and foods, if relevant.

Chronic Spontaneous Urticaria: Limited investigations are recommended. Full blood count (FBC), CRP and/or ESR. In patients with long-standing and/or uncontrolled disease, further diagnostic procedures based on the patient history and examinations are recommended.

Standardised provocation testing to diagnose chronic inducible urticaria is required for an accurate diagnosis.

Dermatopathology

Oedema of the upper and mid dermis is the prevalent histological feature; perivascular inflammatory infiltrate of variable intensity depends on different subtypes, consisting mainly of eosinophils and lymphocytes and occasional neutrophils with or without basophils. No vascular damage.

Course

Acute urticaria: Self-limiting.

Chronic spontaneous Urticaria: Unpredictable. Spontaneous remissions. Variable remission rates (45% at 5 years).

Several factors have been associated with a long duration in chronic spontaneous urticaria: 1.disease activity, 2. angioedema, 3. combination of chronic spontaneous urticaria with inducible urticaria and 4. autoreactivity (positivity in the autologous serum skin test).

Complications

Anaphylactic shock should be considered in some type of urticaria as allergic acute urticaria, acquired cold urticaria or cholinergic urticaria. Not common in chronic spontaneous urticaria.

Diagnosis

Clinical.

Differential Diagnosis

Urticarial vasculitis (individual hives persist for more than 24 hours), maculopapular exanthems, maculopapular cutaneous mastocytosis (formerly called urticaria pigmentosa), urticaria syndromes (see section "Urticarial Syndromes" in Chap. 25), auto-inflammatory syndromes (e.g. cryopyrin-associated periodic syndromes or Schnitzler's syndrome), non-mast cell mediator-mediated angioedema (e.g. bradykinin-mediated angioedema), Sweet's syndrome, erythema multiforme.

Prevention and Therapy

- Acute urticaria—systemic: non-sedating H1-antihistamines. If severe, consider short course of systemic corticosteroids.
- Chronic spontaneous urticaria:
  - To identify and eliminate underlying cause(s) and/or eliciting trigger(s).
  - Non-sedating second-generation H1-antihistamines at licenced doses and at higher dose. In refractory cases, the recommendation is to add anti-IgE therapy, nowadays omalizumab. Ciclosporin could be recommended if omalizumab fails partially or completely. A good number of alternative treatments can be considered, e.g. methotrexate or some special diets.

Angioedema [6]

Figures 1.5 and 1.6

Grading of Importance

B

Level

Advanced

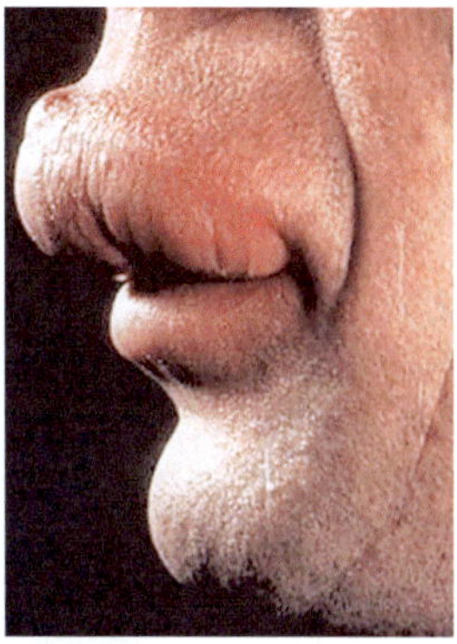

Fig. 1.5 Angioedema

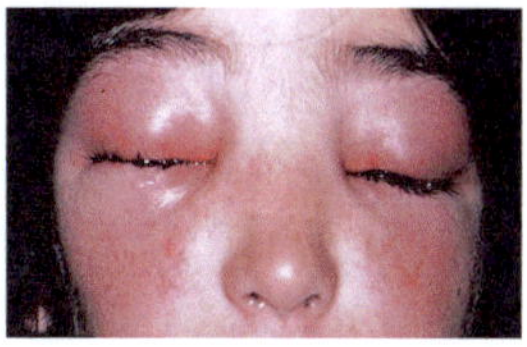

Fig. 1.6 Angioedema

ICD-11

Idiopathic: EB04

Synonyms

Quincke oedema, angioneurotic/heriditary oedema.

Epidemiology

Frequent but no statistical data available for spontaneous angioedema; prevalence heriditary angioedema 1:50,000 for types I and II, type III rare, females more commonly.

Definition

Acute or slowly progressing dermal and subdermal persistent swellings over several hours to days involving subcutis, mucosa and submucosal tissue. It may occur either as a solitary finding localised or disseminated and following or in parallel with urticaria.

Aetiology and Pathogenesis

Most of the pathogenic causes are histamine related allergic or pseudoallergic following the course of different types of urticaria. Additionally, there are forms without urticaria such as bradykinin-related HAE types I and II (INH-activity partial deficient), III (INH-activity normal). C1-esterase inhibitor deficiency types I and II: renin-angiotensin system-related drugs (ACE and dipeptidylpeptidase inhibitors) or paraneoplastic causes.

Signs and Symptoms

Subcutaneous and mucosal oedema (upper and lower airways, oesophageal-gastrointestinal tract) with the sensation of tightness or swelling, sometimes itchy or painful.

Localisation

Sites of predilection: face (eyelids, lips), mucosal (tongue, larynx, genitalia).

Classification

Spontaneous and urticaria-related; acquired bradykinin driven without C1-INH deficiency; types I–II hereditary C1-INH deficiency and type III bradykinin driven without C1-INH deficiency.

Laboratory and Other Workups

See urticaria for diagnostics. Allergic: IgE, specific IgE, histamine, diaminooxidase. In addition: C1-esterase inhibitor analysis and complement C4 (both concentration + activity). C1-INH and C1q autoantibodies.

Dermatopathology

Oedema of the dermal, subcutaneous, submucosal and mucosal tissue without inflammatory infiltrate. Mast cell degranulation.

Clinical Presentation

See symptoms

Course

Acute onset or progressive development. In allergic and hereditary types: chronic relapsing course.

Complications

Airway obstruction, laryngeal oedema, birth delivery complications (be aware of hereditary C1-esterase inhibitor deficiency).

Diagnosis

Clinical, laboratory.

Differential Diagnosis

Physical urticaria (pressure, vibration), autoimmune diseases (e.g. lupus erythematosus), lymphedema, acute phase of herpes zoster and erysipelas. Acute contact dermatitis.

Prevention and Therapy

Acute: depending on localisation and acuity, systemic antihistamines; systemic corticosteroids and adrenaline. For C1-esterase inhibitor deficiency: replacement of C1-esterase inhibitor (if not available, fresh frozen plasma); concentrated C1-inhibitor infusion; bradykinin-B2-receptor antagonist infusion (lanadelumab); recombinant C1 inhibitor (danazol or tranexamic acid for long-term prophylaxis only).

Eczematous Dermatoses

Atopic Dermatitis [4, 15]

Figures 1.7, 1.8, 1.9, 1.10, 1.11, 1.12 and 1.13

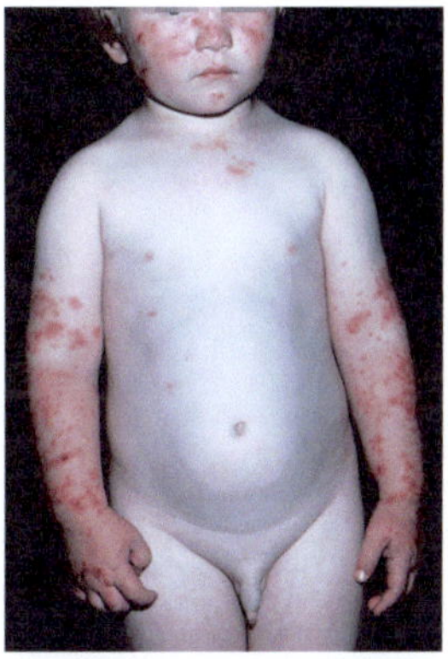

Fig. 1.7 Atopic dermatitis in a child

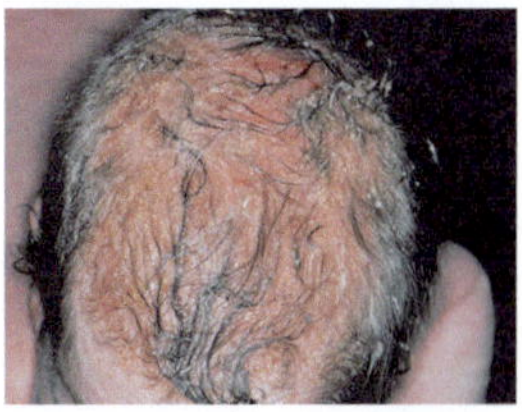

Fig. 1.8 Atopic dermatitis of the head (crusta lacteal)

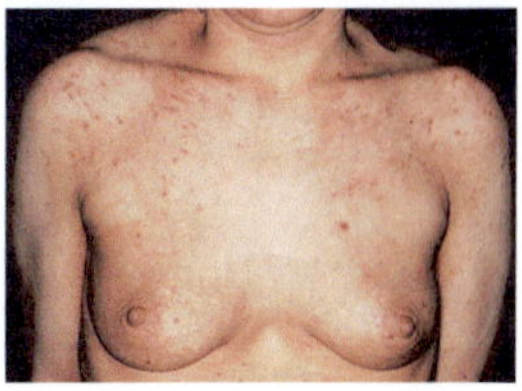

Fig. 1.9 Atopic dermatitis in an adult

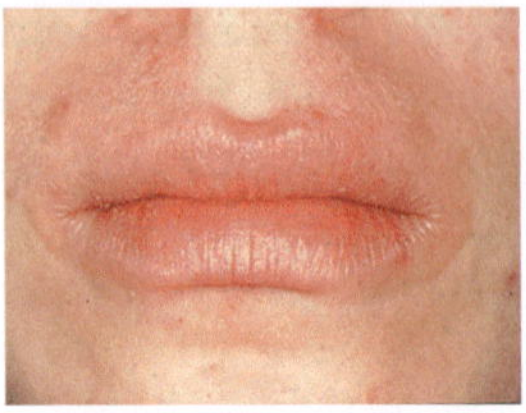

Fig. 1.10 Atopic dermatitis periorally

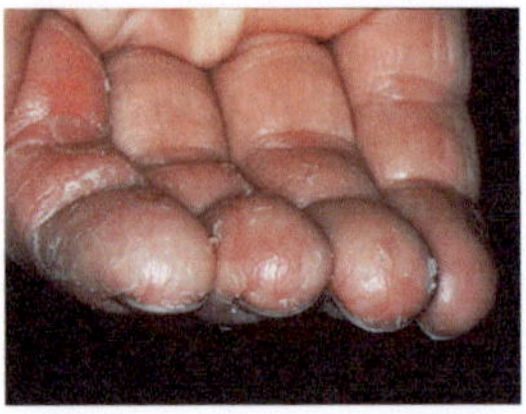

Fig. 1.11 Atopic dermatitis: pulepite sèche

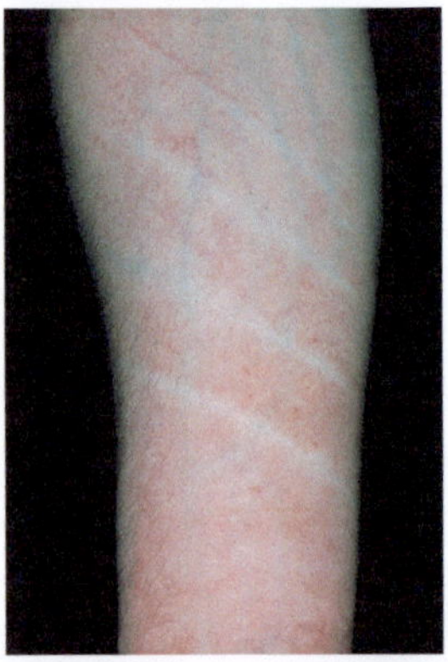

Fig. 1.12 Atopic dermatitis: white dermographism

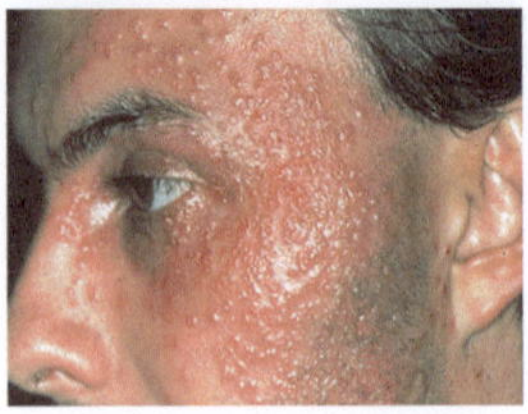

Fig. 1.13 Atopic dermatitis: eczema herpeticum

Grading of Importance

B

Level

Advanced

ICD-11

EA80

Synonyms

Atopic eczema, endogenous eczema, neurodermatitis.

Epidemiology

Highly prevalent in infants and children (10–20%) and adults (2–4%).

Definition

Dermatitis in patients with atopic diathesis with a chronic-recurrent course, characterised by classical findings of dry skin, pruritus and textural change.

Aetiology and Pathogenesis

1. Genetically determined or acquired epidermal barrier defects (in some parts of the population mutation in profilaggrin gene and other structural epidermal proteins, alterations in the desquamation process), xerosis
2. Genetically determined immune reaction pattern (excessive IgE production possible, disturbance in helper T-cell balance with Th2 favoured over Th1)
3. Common triggers: environmental factors (humidity, water hardness, pollution), house dust mites, psychological stimuli

Signs and Symptoms

Eczema appearance with erythema and vesiculation in the acute phase and erythema, scaling and lichenification in the chronic phases. Another clinical feature is prurigo. Pruritus is always present; it can be devastating and interfere with sleeping and work productivity.

Additional signs:

- Dry skin (xerosis).
- An atopy score (SCORAD, EASI, POEM) can be used to quantify diagnosis.

Localisation

All parts of the body can be affected, even extending to erythroderma.

Localisation may be age dependent

Preferential localisations:

- Face and neck
- Flexures (antecubital, popliteal, flexor aspect of wrist)
- Hands

Classification

Intrinsic and extrinsic atopic dermatitis.

- Extrinsic: also defined allergic type, characterised by high total serum IgE levels and the presence of IgE to allergens; associated with asthma and/or rhino-conjunctivitis.
- Intrinsic: non-allergic, normal total serum IgE levels and the absence of specific IgE.

Laboratory and Other Workups

Total serum IgE >100 kU/l, sometimes blood eosinophilia, often multiple positive skin prick tests, consider patch testing against airborne allergens after tape stripping of stratum corneum (atopy patch test).

Dermatopathology

Acute: spongiosis, perivascular lymphohistiocytic infiltrates in upper dermis.

Chronic: parakeratosis, acanthosis, perivascular lymphohistiocytic infiltrates in upper dermis.

Clinical Presentation

See symptoms

Course

Chronic-relapsing course. Cradle cap after 3 months of age; weeping dermatitis in childhood; dry, itchy skin in adolescents and adults.

Complications

Tendency to superinfection by bacteria (*S. aureus*: impetiginisation) and viruses (eczema herpeticum; molluscum contagiosum).

Diagnosis

Typical personal and family history, characteristic clinical picture, relevant laboratory tests, often coexisting atopic disorders (allergic rhinitis, conjunctivitis, asthma or type I food allergies).

Differential Diagnosis

Seborrhoeic dermatitis, psoriasis, allergic contact dermatitis, tinea, scabies, early patch stage mycosis fungoides.

Prevention and Therapy

1. General measures:
   - Counselling regarding skin care, avoidance of aggravating factors. Patient handouts and educational material or links are valuable.
   - Moisturising, preferentially with emollients containing urea.
   - Gentle cleansing (use of soap substitutes).
2. Mild forms:
   - Topical corticosteroids, perhaps combination products also containing antimicrobial agents (short-term to avoid bacterial resistance)V
   - Topical immune modulators (tacrolimus, pimecrolimus, crisaborole)
3. Severe forms:
   - Ciclosporin or other immunosuppressants (methotrexate, azathioprine, mycophenolate mofetil)
   - Short-term systemic corticosteroids

- Biological therapy: Dupilumab, a human monoclonal antibody directed against IL-4/IL-13 receptor-α
- Several new treatments under development

Allergic Contact Dermatitis [11]

Figures 1.14, 1.15, and 1.16

Grading of Importance

B

Level

Advanced

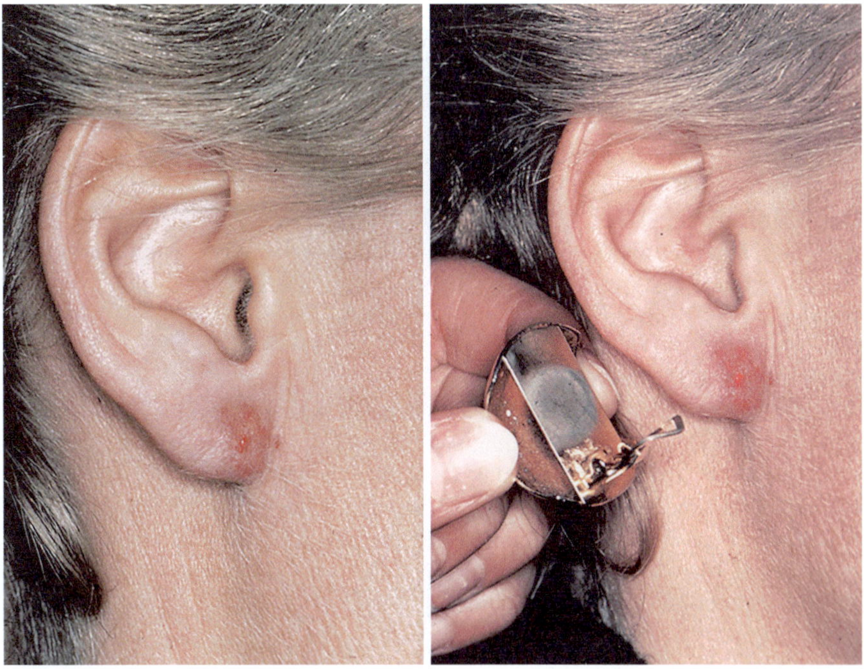

Fig. 1.14 Allergic contact dermatitis due to nickel

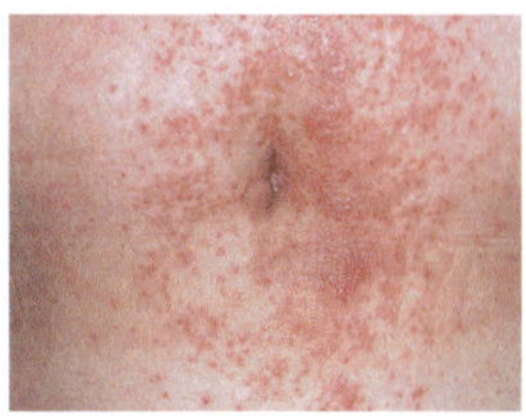

Fig. 1.15 Allergic contact dermatitis due to nickel in belt buckle

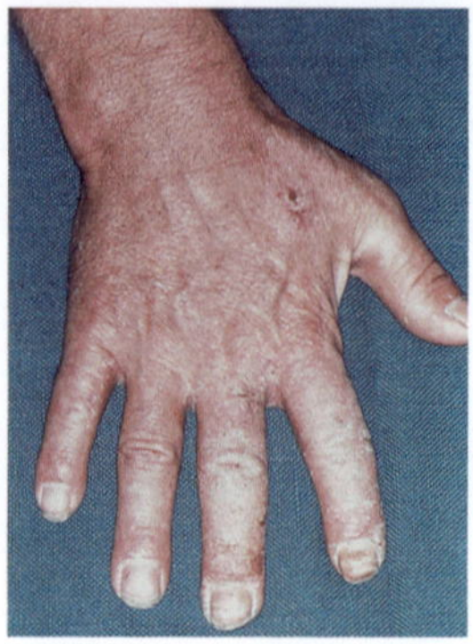

Fig. 1.16 Allergic contact dermatitis due to chromium in cement

ICD-11

EK00

Synonyms

Allergic contact eczema, contact dermatitis.

Epidemiology

An estimated 15–20% of the general population suffers from contact allergy.

Definition

Allergic contact dermatitis is a common type of dermatitis caused by delayed hypersensitivity reaction (type IV) to exogenous (contact-) allergens (haptens) in contact with the skin.

Aetiology and Pathogenesis

Allergic contact dermatitis is mediated by allergen-specific sensitised T cells and is a form of type IV reaction, according to Gell and Coombs. Immunological sensitisation time is at least 5–10 days; clinical symptoms may first develop after months to years. The dermatitis appears in sensitised individuals after a latency period of 8–24 hours, occasionally longer. Individual allergens have varying degrees of allergic potential. Most frequent contact allergens are metals, rubber ingredients, preservatives and occupational substances.

Signs and Symptoms

- The reaction starts at the site of allergen exposure as an acute papulo-vesicular eruption which soon becomes eroded and forms an exudate. It is accompanied by intense pruritus. The lesions present with irregular border, spreading outside area of contact. Later, scaling and crusting can occur.
- In chronic forms, lichenification and fissuring dominate. Sometimes, allergic contact dermatitis may present as a chronic disease without an acute clinical phase.

Localisation

The localisation depends on the type of exposure. Extensive (haematogenous) contact dermatitis may be caused by systemic exposure (ingestion, inhalation) of contact allergens. The affected site is a clue to the possible culprit allergen:

- Face: cosmetics, airborne allergens (paint vapours or pollens)
- Ears: jewellery, glasses, hearing aids. Lips: cosmetics, herpes simplex medications
- Forehead/neck: shampoos, hair dyes
- Neck/fingers/wrist: jewellery
- Hands: occupational and recreational contact allergens
- Axillae: deodorants
- Feet: shoes, antifungals
- Mouth: dentures, other dental products
- Lower leg: elastic stockings, medications for leg ulcers

Laboratory and Other Workups

The allergen causing contact dermatitis may be determined by patch testing. Several series of patch tests can be used: standard series of most frequent allergens; special series for peculiar occupational diseases; own substances brought by the patient. ROAT (repeated open application test) may be useful for low allergenic substances.

Dermatopathology

Cutaneous histology of the lesions shows parakeratosis, spongiosis, acanthosis and an inflammatory lymphohistiocytic infiltrate with exocytosis of lymphocytes into the epidermis.

Clinical Presentation

See symptoms

Course

The clinical features usually subside after 1–2 weeks of allergen avoidance; contact sensitivity usually persists indefinitely.

Complications

Allergic contact dermatitis can be complicated by impetiginisation; the disease can become chronic (even after allergen avoidance). The lesions can disseminate and cause erythroderma.

Diagnosis

It is mandatory to seek the causative allergen by performing detective work (detailed history—profession, hobbies, habits) and patch testing guided by the history.

Differential Diagnosis

Other inflammatory diseases such as psoriasis and dermatophyte infection in case of foot and hand involvement. It must also be differentiated from therapy-resistant localised dermatoses: Bowen's disease, Paget's disease of the nipple and lupus vulgaris. Reaction to latex can cause an IgE-mediated immediate-type allergy in addition to a type IV allergic reaction to rubber accelerators.

Prevention and Therapy

It is very important to avoid contact with the causative allergens and also with concomitant irritants (e.g. by using soap substitutes). Topical therapy consists of wet dressings or baths and mainly corticosteroids in the appropriate vehicle (ointment, cream, lotion) chosen according to the nature of skin lesions. Phototherapy may be indicated in some cases. Alitretinoin (retinoid) can be used in severe refractory hand dermatitis.

Irritant Contact Dermatitis [4]

Figures 1.17, 1.18, 1.19, 1.20 and 1.21

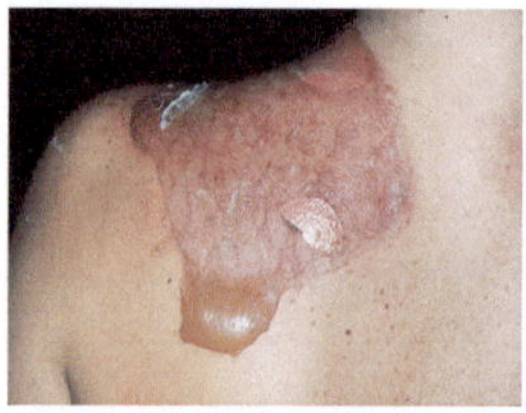

Fig. 1.17 Irritant contact dermatitis from band aid with undiluted ingredient

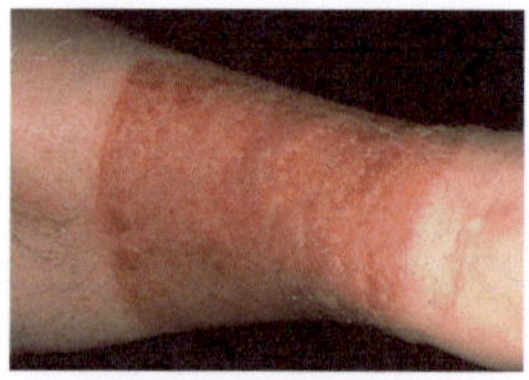

Fig. 1.18 Irritant contact dermatitis from toxic solution under occlusive dressing

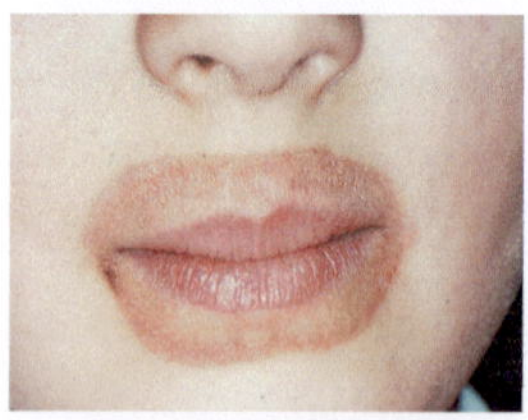

Fig. 1.19 Irritant contact dermatitis from chronic lip licking

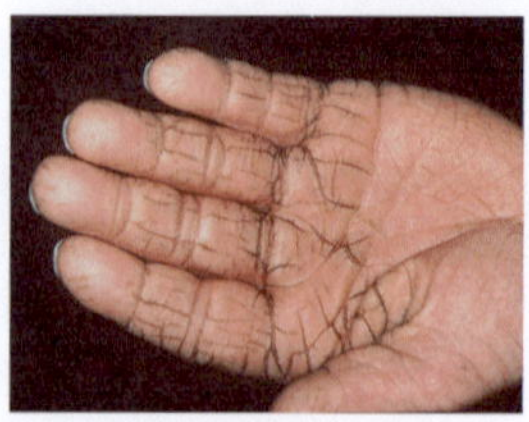

Fig. 1.20 Irritant contact dermatitis in a farmer

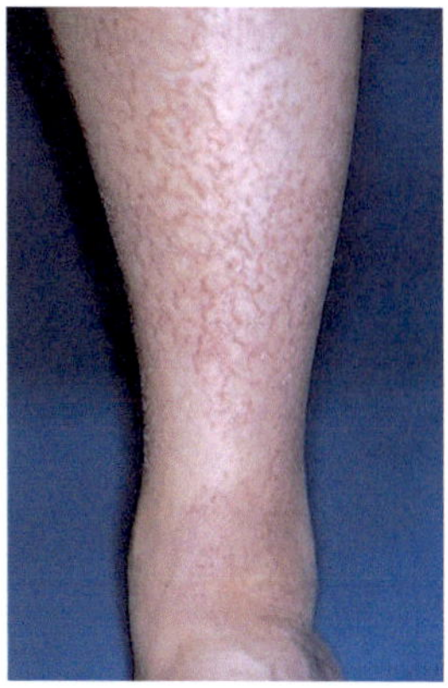

Fig. 1.21 Irritant contact dermatitis: eczema craquelé due to excessive washing

Grading of Importance
B

Level
Advanced

ICD-11
EK0

Synonyms
Irritant contact dermatitis (ICD), cutaneous irritation, irritant dermatitis, irritant contact eczema, toxic dermatitis, "wear and tear" dermatitis, friction dermatitis.

Epidemiology
In general, ICD is more frequent than allergic contact dermatitis.

Definition
Non-allergic eczematous inflammatory reaction of the skin secondary to an external agent, not requiring sensitisation.

Aetiology and Pathogenesis
ICD is caused by chemicals, which damage skin structures in a direct non-allergic way. It is strictly dose-dependent. The most frequent chemical irritative factors are long lasting and repetitive contact with water ("wet work"), detergents, solvents or a combination of these factors.

Skin barrier perturbation leads to ICD. Once an irritant has penetrated the stratum corneum, the ICD reaction is initiated.

Signs and Symptoms
The morphology of cutaneous irritation varies widely and depends on the type and intensity of the irritant(s). There may be just simple erythema but also blister

formation, blennorrhoea and crusts. All symptoms are strictly confined to the area of exposure.

Localisation

ICD can involve any area of the body surface in contact with the irritant. The most common location for chronic ICD is the hands, often having occupational relevance.

Classification

Clinical classification of ICD is based on both morphology and mode of onset (acute, recurrent or chronic): Asteatotic irritant eczema is due to excessively dry skin.

Laboratory and Other Workups

Patch testing is mandatory when ICD lasts longer than 3 months. Patch test results differentiate an allergic reaction from an irritative reaction. Longer or repeated contacts with irritants may induce sensitisation with an allergic reaction as well.

Clinical Presentation

See symptoms

Dermatopathology

Irritants produce a diversity of histopathological changes (epidermal necrosis, spongiotic dermatitis) depending on the concentration of the irritant, type, duration of exposure, site and individual reactivity of the skin.

Course

The course can be acute, recurrent or chronic depending on the concentration and length of exposure to the exogenous irritant.

Complications

ICD increases the risk of allergic contact sensitisation. Superinfection of irritated skin by bacteria can occur (impetiginisation).

Diagnosis

The diagnosis is based on the history, clinical features and localisation usually limited to areas of contact. It is necessary to rule out allergic contact sensitisation using patch testing.

Differential Diagnosis

Allergic contact dermatitis, psoriasis.

Prevention and Therapy

Education and information about the causative irritative background and prevention of irritants, especially in the professional environment of the workplace, which may need to be changed.

Mild forms may be controlled by the regular use of emollients. Severe relapsing forms require topical or for a short boost even oral corticosteroids; topical calcineurin inhibitors; ultraviolet light.

Nummular Dermatitis [8, 18]

Figures 1.22, 1.23 and 1.24

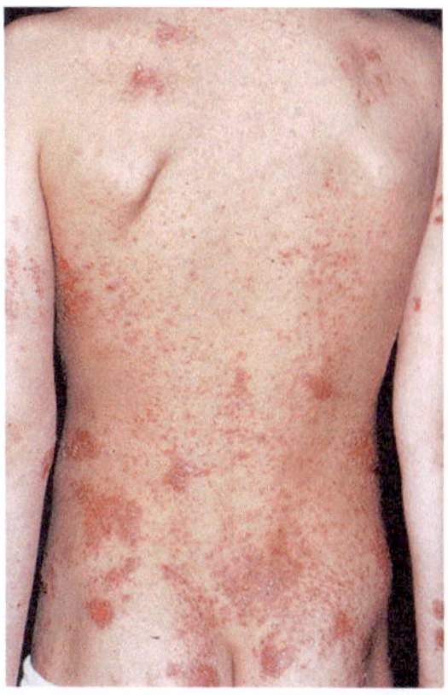

Fig. 1.22 Nummular dermatitis on the trunk

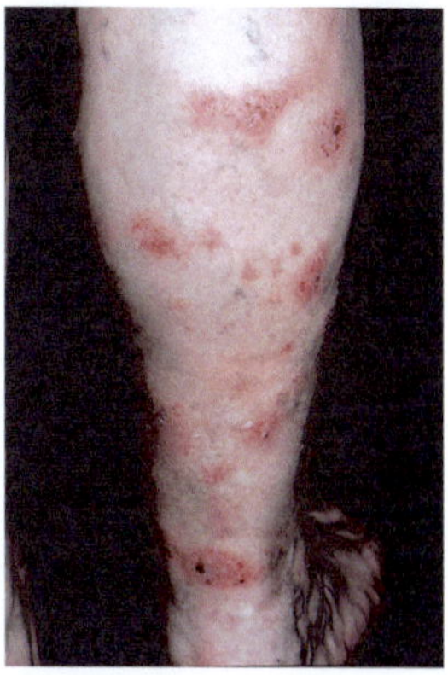

Fig. 1.23 Nummular dermatitis on the leg

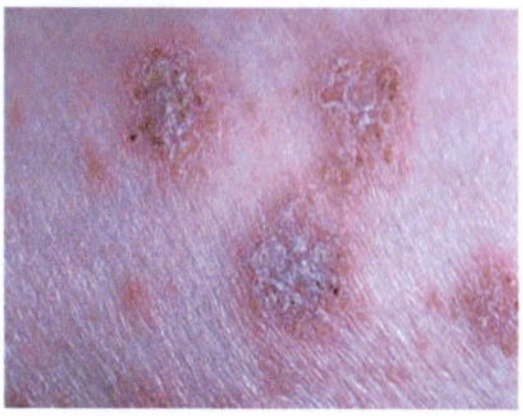

Fig. 1.24 Nummular dermatitis close up view of nummular lesions

Grading of Importance
B

Level
Advanced

ICD-11
EA82

Synonyms
Discoid eczema; nummular eczema

Epidemiology
The prevalence of nummular eczema in total populations depends on geographic area and is between 0.1–0.2%.

Definition
Dermatitis with sharply bordered, coin-shaped patches or plaques.

Aetiology and Pathogenesis
Mostly unknown. Microbial colonisation, local superficial trauma. Sometimes associated with dry skin and stasis dermatitis. In many patients, particularly children, it is a manifestation of atopic dermatitis.

Signs and Symptoms
Nummular (circular or oval = coin-shaped), exudative patches and plaques, often with crusts. Pruritus and sometimes excoriations.

Localisation
Sites of predilection: Extremities (lower legs, hands, forearms), trunk occasionally in a symmetrical distribution.

Classification
Different patterns: Discoid eczema of the hands and forearms. Discoid eczema of the limbs and trunk. "Dry" discoid eczema.

Laboratory and Other Workups
Scales: Direct microscopic examination to exclude fungal infection.

Clinical Presentation
See symptoms

Dermatopathology
Typical histology for dermatitis reflecting acute/subacute nature of lesion, usually few eosinophils (see Atopic Dermatitis).

Course
Chronic, with recurrent flares, may be somewhat resistant to therapy. Waxing and waning dependent on climate conditions.

Complications
Secondary bacterial infection.

Diagnosis
Clinical features, histopathological examination in some cases for confirmation and for exclusion of differential diagnoses or of fungal infection.

Differential Diagnosis
Tinea corporis, psoriasis, irritant and allergic contact dermatitis, cutaneous T-cell lymphoma, impetigo.

Prevention and Therapy
Topical corticosteroids or combinations of corticosteroids with antimicrobials.

Acute lesions: Local astringent measures and antiseptics.

Disseminated forms: Occasionally oral antibiotics and systemic corticosteroids.

Prevention: Emollients and avoidance of irritants.

Seborrhoeic Dermatitis [16]

Figures 1.25, 1.26 and 1.27

Grading of Importance
B

Level
Advanced

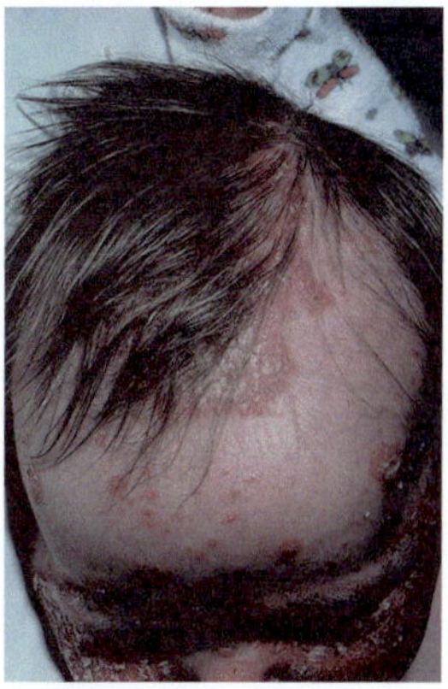

Fig. 1.25 Seborrhoeic dermatitis of the scalp of a baby

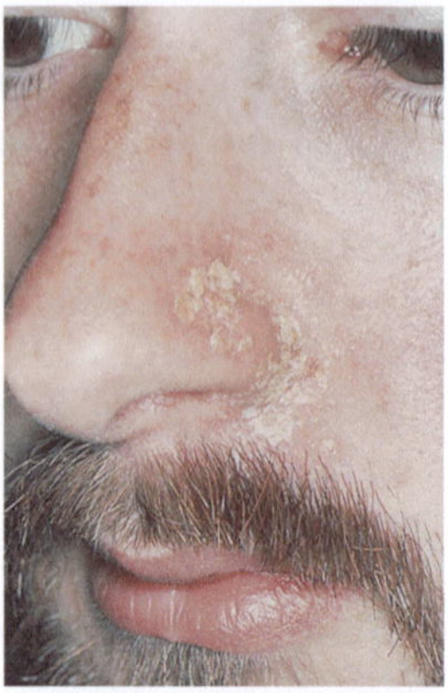

Fig. 1.26 Seborrhoeic dermatitis in the nasolabial fold

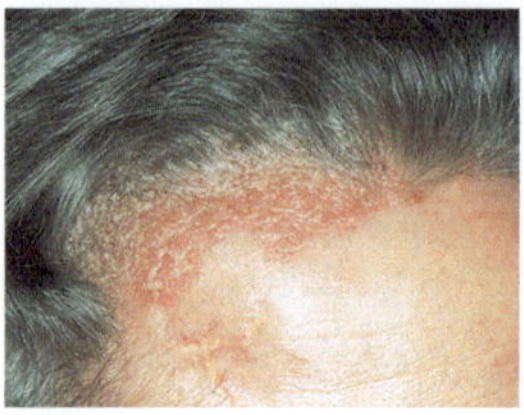

Fig. 1.27 Seborrhoeic dermatitis on the border of the hair, simulating psoriasis

ICD-11

EA81

Synonyms

Seborrhoeic otitis externa; malassezia folliculitis; seborrhoeic eczema; cradle cap (in infants).

Epidemiology

Very common in different ages. Infants first 3 months, and in the 4th decade of life. All ethnic groups.

Definition

Chronic recurrent inflammatory dermatitis with yellow-white scaling on an erythematous background involving seborrhoeic areas.

Aetiology and Pathogenesis

Seborrhoea (oily skin), increased colonisation of seborrhoeic areas by commensal lipophilic yeast *Malassezia* spp. (formerly called *Pityrosporum ovale*). Often as HIV/AIDS-related dermatosis. Often seen in Parkinson's disease.

Signs and Symptoms

Scale; itch; irritation.

Localisation
Seborrhoeic areas: scalp, glabella, eyebrows, submental, retroauricular, mid-face, presternal, nasolabial folds and rarely intrascapular.

Classification
- Seborrhoeic dermatitis of infants during the first 3 months of life: scalp and intertriginous areas
- Seborrhoeic dermatitis of adults: Seborrheic areas; overlapping with psoriasis ("seborrhiasis"); may be indication for HIV infection

Laboratory and Other Workups
Not necessary.

Dermatopathology
Hyper- and parakeratosis, crusts, serum and spongiosis, no Munro abscesses.

Course
Worsens with stress, inflammatory and infectious diseases (HIV). UV light reported may improve or worsen.

Complications
Overlap with psoriasis ("seborrhiasis"). Sometimes superinfection with *S. aureus*.

Diagnosis
Oily skin, typical clinical features and distribution.

Differential Diagnosis
Atopic dermatitis in childhood, psoriasis, tinea.

Prevention and Therapy
Reduction of Malassezia colonisation with topical imidazoles, keratolytic agents, topical zinc pyrithione or topical zinc oil, especially in newborns. Short-term mild topical corticosteroids combined with clotrimazol.

Napkin Dermatitis (Classical) [5]

Figure 1.28

Grading of Importance
B

Level
Advanced

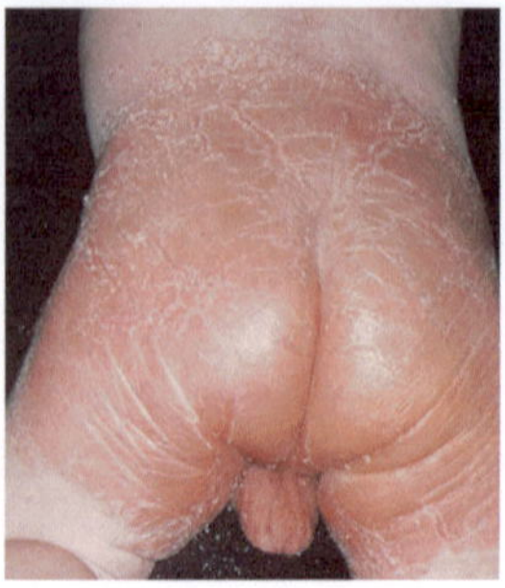

Fig. 1.28 Napkin dermatitis in the gluteal region of a child

ICD-11
EH40.10

Synonyms
Diaper dermatitis; nappy rash; diaper rash.

Definition
Irritant contact dermatitis in diaper region.

Aetiology and Pathogenesis
Disturbance of the epidermal barrier by lipases and proteases from urine and faeces. Skin maceration through moisture and prolonged exposure to alkaline urine and faeces under occlusion.

Diaper area particularly prone to suffer disruption from damage (friction), irritation and secondary bacterial or fungal (*Candida*) infection.

Signs and Symptoms
Acute to subacute dermatitis. Well-demarcated, confluent erythema confined to the diaper area. Skin folds often spared.

Localisation
Area covered by nappies (diapers), typically flexural areas. May involve the inner (frictional) or convex (irritant) surfaces or may be present as a diffuse red erythema on the thighs, genitalia, buttocks and lower abdomen.

Classification
Depending on etiologic factors, such as frictional (chafing) dermatitis, irritant contact dermatitis, allergic contact dermatitis and diaper candidiasis.

Laboratory and Other Workups
Clinical diagnosis. In refractory cases, swabs may useful in detecting a superimposed bacterial or fungal infection.

Dermatopathology
Not necessary.

Course
Diaper dermatitis responds well to treatment. Recurrences may occur if preventive measures are not undertaken.

Complications
Superinfection (*Candida*, streptococci), allergic contact dermatitis.

Diagnosis
History, clinical features. KOH examination to exclude candidiasis and microbial swab for streptococci.

Differential Diagnosis
Atopic dermatitis, seborrheic dermatitis, candidiasis, perianal streptococcal dermatitis, allergic contact dermatitis and psoriasis should be considered. Rarely Langerhans cell histiocytosis and nutritional deficiency (acrodermatitis enteropathica).

Prevention and Therapy
Preventive measures (parental advice on napkin care):

- Frequent diaper changes and optimise the size of the diaper. Keep the skin clean and dry under the diaper
- Protect infant skin from irritants. Avoid potential skin irritants (soaps, detergents perfumed products and alcohol/fragrance-containing products)
- Advise to wash with an emollient soap-free, fragrance-free liquid cleanser, or warm water
- Use good-quality super-absorbent napkins and apply barrier compounds (creams, ointments or pastes) which protect skin from exposure to moisture
- Treat secondary infections
- Short-term mild topical corticosteroids

Dyshidrotic Dermatitis [19]

Figures 1.29, 1.30, 1.31 and 1.32

Grading of Importance
B

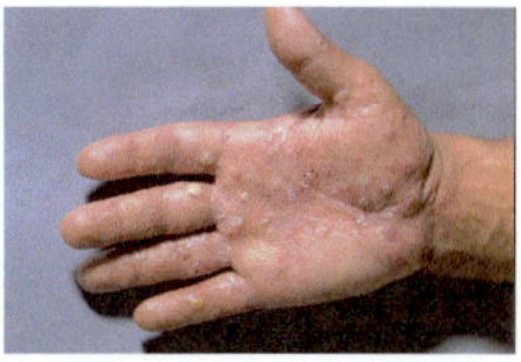

Fig. 1.29 Dyshidrotic dermatitis showing small vesicles on the palm

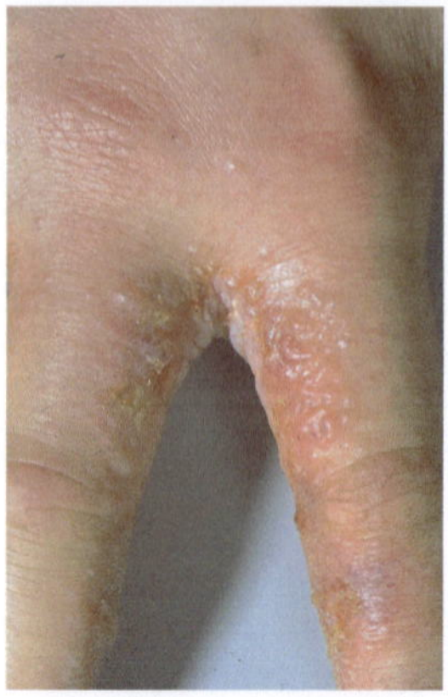

Fig. 1.30 Dyshidrotic dermatitis: vesicles between fingers

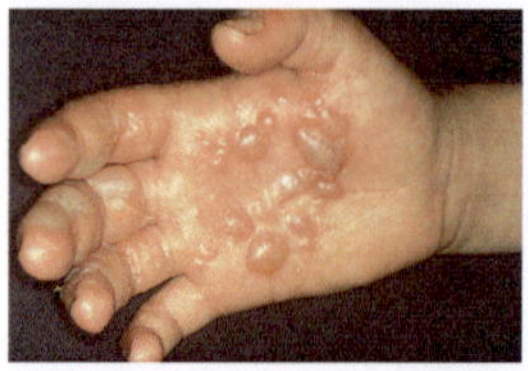

Fig. 1.31 Dyshidrotic dermatitis: bullae (chairopompholyx) on the palm

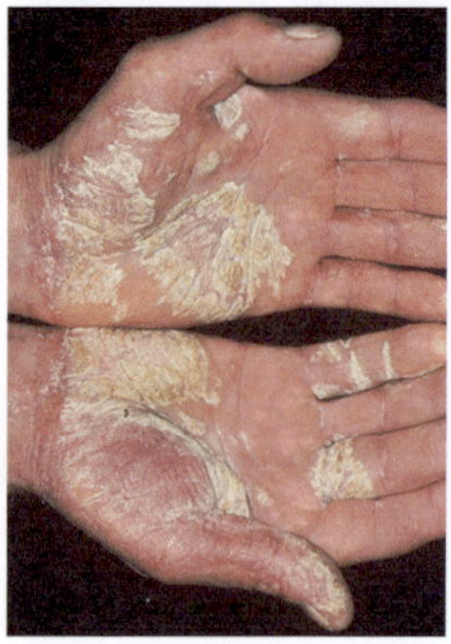

Fig. 1.32 Dyshidrotic dermatitis: chronic hyperkeratotic

Level
Advanced

ICD-11
EA85.0

Synonyms
Dyshidrosis; cheiro-podo-pompholyx; vesicular dermatitis of hands and feet.

Definition
Vesicular to bullous palmoplantar dermatitis.

Aetiology and Pathogenesis
Idiopathic, allergic contact reactions, atopy, eczematous reaction to infections such as tinea (so-called id reaction) or bacterial infections. No connection with eccrine sweat gland activity or malfunction.

Signs and Symptoms
Tiny pruritic, fluid-filled vesicles or bullae on palms and soles. Patients often report pruritus as the first symptom; then tiny vesicles become visible, later followed by erythema and scaling.

Localisation
Hands and feet, palmar and plantar and on lateral areas of the fingers and toes.

Classification
Acute, subacute and chronic types.

Laboratory and Other Workups
When associated fungal or bacterial infection is suspected, microbiological cultures may be useful. Patch test to rule out a concomitant allergic contact dermatitis.

Dermatopathology
Intraepidermal spongiotic vesicles with consecutive closure of acrosyringia and subepidermal accumulation of eccrine gland fluid. The image of the dyshidrotic vesicles is that of any eczema with large spongiotic vesicles and discrete dermal inflammatory reaction.

Course
Idiopathic and atopic forms are often chronic and recurrent.

Complications
Superinfection with gram negative bacteria, allergic contact dermatitis.

Diagnosis
Typical clinical features. To distinguish from atopic dermatitis: check for atopic stigmata. Patch test is useful to exclude allergic contact dermatitis.

Differential Diagnosis
Tinea pedis, early stages of palmoplantar pustulosis, pustular psoriasis, atopic dermatitis and allergic contact dermatitis.

Prevention and Therapy
Topical non-occlusive galenic formulations of corticosteroids; on occasions, short courses of systemic corticosteroids; wet dressings with antiseptic solutions, topical calcineurin antagonists. Sedative antihistamines are sometimes useful in cases of intense pruritus.

Drug Reactions [1, 10]

Figures 1.33, 1.34 and 1.35

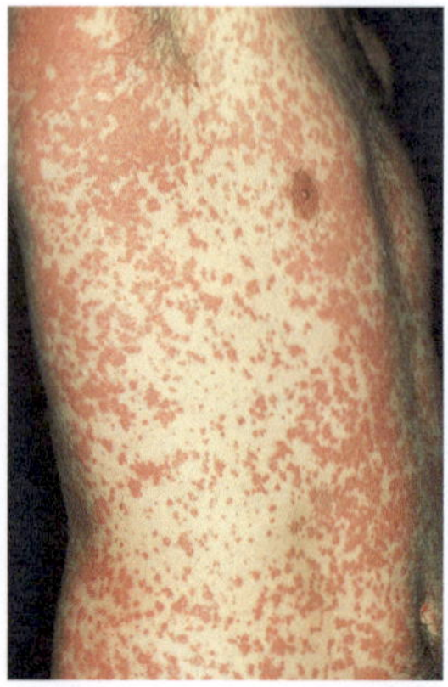

Fig. 1.33 Drug reactions: exanthematous reaction on the trunk

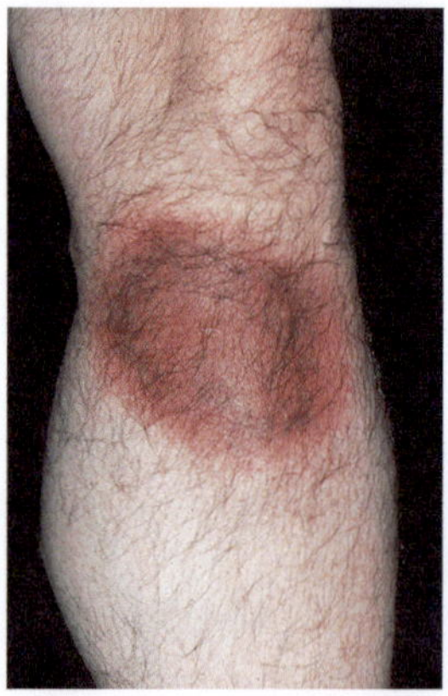

Fig. 1.34 Drug reactions: localized fixed drug reaction

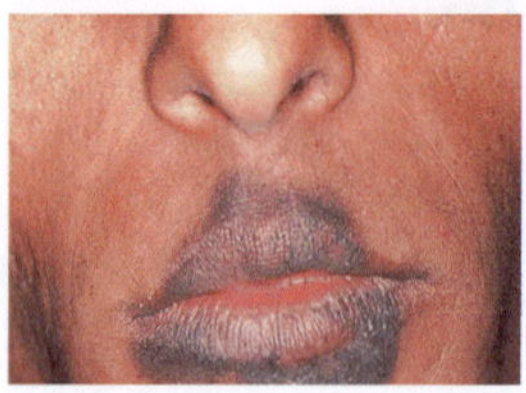

Fig. 1.35 Drug reactions: localized fixed drug reaction

Grading of Importance

A

Level

Advanced

ICD-11

NE60

Synonyms

Drug rash, drug exanthema

Epidemiology

Cutaneous drug reactions are the most frequently occurring adverse reactions to drugs. Among hospitalised patients, their incidence ranges from 0.1 to 5%. Predisposing factors include advanced age, gender (more frequent in women), underlying diseases, genetic factors and the use of multiple drugs.

Definition

Undesirable (not pharmacological, not toxic) side effect of systemic medication affecting the skin.

Aetiology and Pathogenesis

Various mechanisms:

- Immunological (types I, III and IV reactions, sometimes combined)
- Non-immunological (pseudoallergenic, overdose, cumulative toxicity)
  Common causes:
- Antibiotics (sulphonamides, ampicillin, penicillins, cephalosporins)
- Non-steroidal anti-inflammatory drugs (NSAIDs)
- Anticonvulsant medications (phenytoin, barbiturates)
- Diuretics
- Contrast media

Signs and Symptoms

Extensive number of clinicopathological presentations. Usually involving large areas, often pruritic. Drug reactions may appear immediately (urticaria/angio-oedema) or delayed 5–15 days after the drug administration.

The most common reactions produced by drugs are exanthematous/morbilliform rashes (30%), followed by urticaria and angioedema (27%).

Other less common clinicopathological patterns: Fixed drug eruption (16%), erythema multiforme, vesicular and bullous eruptions, purpuric lesions, photosensitivity eruptions, acute exanthematous pustulosis, neutrophilic dermatoses, erythema nodosum, vesiculo-bullous eruptions, acneiform eruptions, vasculitis, lichenoid eruptions, sclerodermoid lesions, pseudolymphomatous reactions, panniculitis, granulomatous eruptions, erythroderma, hypertrichosis, alopecia. Mucosal and internal organ (liver, kidneys) involvement possible.

The most severe drug reactions are exfoliative dermatitis, drug-related rash with eosinophilia and systemic symptoms (DRESS) syndrome, Stevens-Johnson syndrome and toxic epidermal necrolysis (TEN). Severe cutaneous drug eruptions may be accompanied by fever, chills, lymphadenopathy, arthralgias and wheezing.

Localisation

Highly variable, usually symmetrical. May be generalised including mucosae.

Classification

Common:

- Exanthematous maculopapular drug reaction
- Urticarial drug reaction. Angioedema
- Fixed drug reaction
- Erythema multiforme

Less common:

- Acneiform, pustular, lichenoid lesions
- Vasculitis
- Erythema nodosum
- Phototoxic dermatitis
- Acute generalised exanthematous pustulosis
- Drug-related rash with eosinophilia and systemic symptoms (DRESS)
- Erythroderma
- Toxic epidermal necrolysis (TEN)

Laboratory and Other Workups

Peripheral eosinophilia in a subset of patients. Hepatic and renal screening to exclude systemic involvement. After healing, try to identify causative agent with skin tests and in vitro tests (only for selected medications with standardised tests, such as IgE-mediated penicillin allergy). Rarely: provocation test (Cave: precipitation of severe skin reaction is possible with re-challenge).

Dermatopathology

Highly variable. Morphologic findings depending on the different clinical patterns.

Course

Cutaneous lesions generally resolve after drug discontinuation. Recurrences are common when the patient is re-challenged with the drug.

Complications

Liver, renal and haematologic abnormalities (in a subset of patients) depending on aetiological factors.

Diagnosis

Careful history (time course fits with drug exposure), clinical features, histology and laboratory studies. Resolving of lesions after cessation of the suspected drug.

If possible identification of the culprit drug—check drug database. No completely reliable specific confirmatory tests.

Differential Diagnosis

Other generalized exanthema, depending on lesion morphology, such as viral exanthema, secondary syphilis and lupus erythematosus.

Prevention and Therapy

Discontinue the suspected medication in discussion with the prescriber, antihistamines, topical and even systemic corticosteroids. In severe drug eruptions, hospitalisation and specific treatments. Avoid poly-pharmacy and potential drug interactions when possible.

Erythema Multiforme [7, 14]

Figures 1.36, 1.37, 1.38 and 1.39

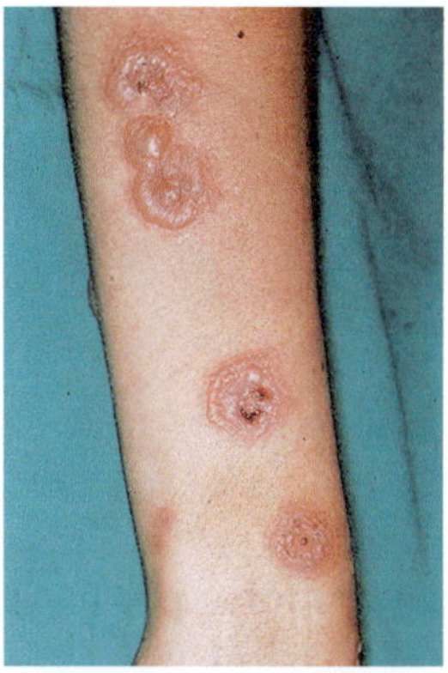

Fig. 1.36 Erythema multiforme: target lesions on the arm

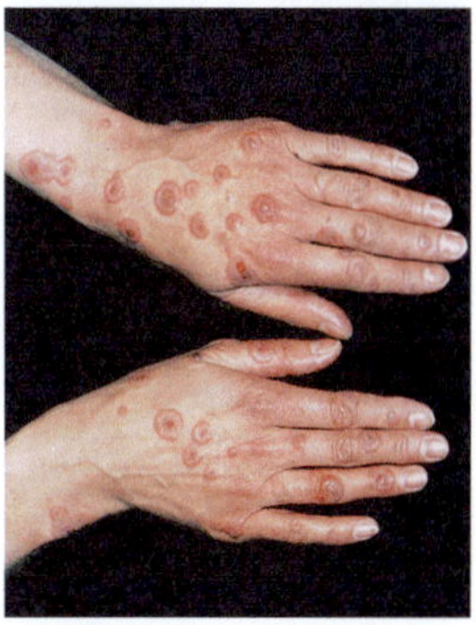

Fig. 1.37 Erythema multiforme: Back of the hands

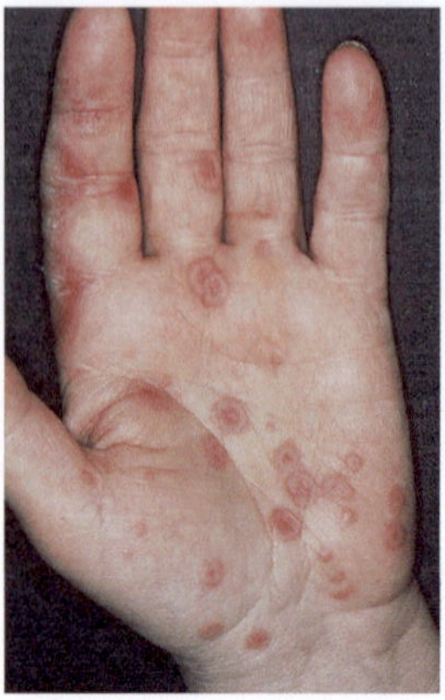

Fig. 1.38 Erythema multiforme: Palms

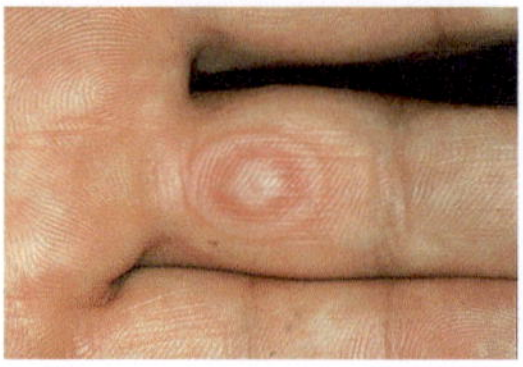

Fig. 1.39 Erythema multiforme: typical target lesion on the finger

Grading of Importance
A

Level
Advanced

ICD-11
EB12

Synonyms
Erythema exsudativum multiforme.

Definition
Acute, self-limited disease with typical target or iris like lesions and frequent mucosal blisters and erosions.

Aetiology and Pathogenesis
Many causes, mostly infectious: herpes simplex (HSV), *Mycoplasma pneumoniae*, streptococci; less common are medications (antibiotics, anti-epileptics, protease inhibitors, pyrazolone), connective tissue diseases (systemic lupus erythematosus); often (>50%) no cause found. A skin-directed immune reaction appears to play a pathogenetic role.

Signs and Symptoms

Frequently observed in young adults. Acral exanthem with formation of typical target lesions with multiple concentric rings of varying colour tones occasionally with a central bulla. Mucosal involvement (lips, mouth, genitalia) with erosions and crusts.

Localisation

Symmetrically distributed on the distal extremities: backs of the hands and palms, forearms as well as on knees, elbows, nape; on mucosae: vesiculo-bullous lesions leading to erosions involving the lips, mouth, eyes, nose, trachea and genitalia.

Classification

Divided into minor (80%) and major forms (depending on the absence or presence of mucosal involvement and systemic symptoms).

Dermatopathology

Strong lymphocytic epidermotropism followed by vacuolar alteration of the basal layer, apoptosis of individual keratinocytes. Oedema of papillary dermis sometimes with blistering. Prominent superficial polymorphous inflammatory infiltrate with mononuclear cells and neutrophils.

Course

Abrupt onset (24–72 hours). Resolution in 2–3 weeks. In cases associated with HSV infection and certain drugs recurrences are frequent.

Complications

No sequelae, except in cases with ocular involvement.

Diagnosis

Clinical features. In atypical lesions, histopathological examination may be useful.

Differential Diagnosis

Typical target lesions are diagnostic. The differential diagnostic possibilities include acute urticaria, subacute cutaneous lupus erythematosus, urticarial vasculitis, and erythema annulare centrifugum. For the mucosal lesions: Stevens-Johnson syndrome, erosive lichen planus, autoimmune bullous diseases, and viral diseases (especially herpes simplex).

Prevention and Therapy

Elimination and treatment of underlying causes. Corticosteroids topically and in severe cases systemically. In cases with mucosal disease, topical corticosteroids in appropriate vehicle along with antimicrobial solutions to prevent superinfection. In cases with eye involvement ophthalmologic consultation is mandatory (risk of permanent scarring and visual impairment). Prophylactic oral antiviral treatment in cases of HSV association with frequent recurrences.

Drug-Related Rash with Eosinophilia and Systemic Symptoms (DRESS)

No pictures

Grading of Importance
C

Level
Advanced

ICD-11
EH65

Synonyms
DRESS syndrome; drug-induced hypersensitivity syndrome; drug-induced delayed multi-organ hypersensitivity syndrome.

Epidemiology
Incidence 10/million/year

Male/female ratio 0.8; median age at diagnosis 53 years

Definition
Drug-induced rash with blood eosinophilia and involvement of internal organs.

Aetiology and Pathogenesis
Examples for medications that may cause a DRESS are:

- Antiarrhythmics: Mexiletine
- Anticonvulsants: Carbamazepine, phenytoin, lamotrigine, phenobarbital, zonisamide
- Anti-retrovirals: Abacavir, nevirapine
- Antibacterials: Amoxicillin, levofloxacin, minocycline
- Other: Dapsone, sulfonamides, allopurinol, vemurafenib, cobimetinib

A possible association with reactivation of HHV-6 infections as well as genetic factors possible.

Laboratory and Other Workups
- Eosinophilia (>1500/μl)
- Leukocytosis (> 11 × 109/L)
- Circulating atypical lymphocytes

Depending on the affected organ increase of transaminases, creatinine kinase, creatinine, amylase and lipase.

Dermatopathology

The histological picture can be very diverse, including spongiosis, apoptotic keratinocytes, a superficial perivascular lymphocytic infiltrate and few dermal eosinophils.

Course

Depends on elimination of eliciting drug.

Clinical Presentation

- Acute or delayed (up to 6 weeks after taking the drug) onset of symptoms.
- Reduced general condition
- Generalised maculopapular rash, in the course of disease possible development of an exfoliative dermatitis or erythroderma
- Eventually mucosal enanthema
- Facial oedema
- Fever >38.5 °C
- Lymphadenopathy
- Involvement of minimum one internal organ (liver > kidney > lung, heart, pancreas)

Complications

Permanent damage of involved organs. Mortality up to 10%.

Diagnosis

Clinical picture, blood tests, histology.

Differential Diagnosis

Stevens-Johnson syndrome/toxic epidermal necrolysis (SJS/TEN)
Acute generalized exanthematous pustulosis (AGEP)
Hypereosinophilic syndromes
Acute cutaneous lupus erythematosus

Prevention and Therapy

Drug withdrawal. Systemic glucocorticoids for several weeks.

Stevens-Johnson Syndrome [13]

Figures 1.40, 1.41 and 1.42

Grading of Importance

C

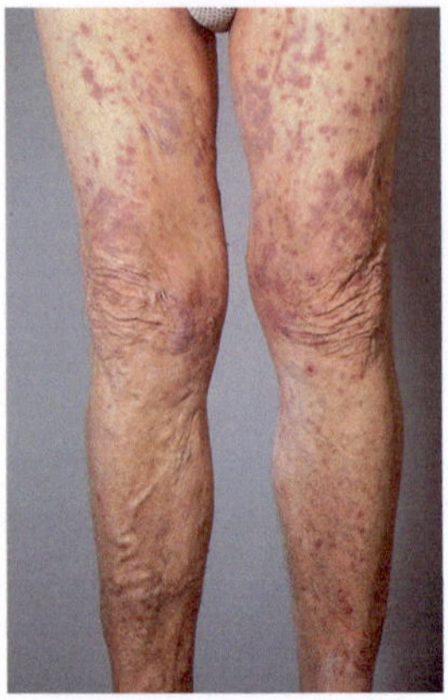

Fig. 1.40 Stevens-Johnson syndrome: early red-grey macular exanthema on the legs

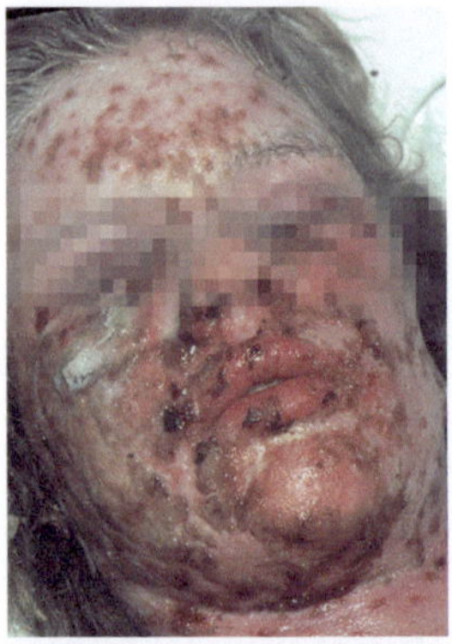

Fig. 1.41 Stevens-Johnson syndrome: laminar erosions in the face

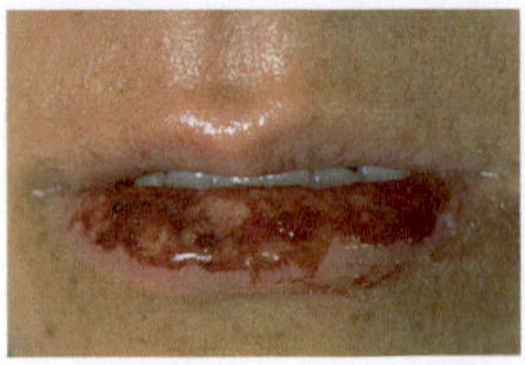

Fig. 1.42 Stevens-Johnson syndrome: involvement of mucosae

Level
Advanced

ICD-11
EB13

Synonyms
SJS

Epidemiology
Rare disease 1–2 per 1 million. Higher risk in HIV/AIDS.

Definition
Part of a spectrum of skin and mucosal disease, which ranges from SJS, where 30% of the body surface (BS) shows loss of the epidermis. Involvement of 10% to 30% of the BS is referred to as SJS-TEN (Toxic Epidermal Necrolysis)-overlap syndrome.

Aetiology and Pathogenesis
Many causes, most often medications, less often infections (viruses, mycoplasma). Hereditary predisposition to severe cutaneous drug reactions. Chinese and Thai HLA-B*1502 related, in Europeans HLA-A*3101. In both groups HLA-B*5801 related to allopurinol.

Signs and Symptoms
Macular exanthema, usually on trunk, often becoming confluent, with formation of atypical target lesions. Mucosal involvement is mandatory and erosions present around and inside mucosal orifice. Fever, conjunctivitis, throat pain, balanitis, later upper respiratory and gastrointestinal tract involved. Nikolski sign positive.

Localisation
Skin and mucosa.

Classification
Part of the erythema multiforme—SJS/TEN complex.

Laboratory and Other Workups
Check electrolytes, kidney and liver parameters, cardiac function.

Dermatopathology
Cytotoxic T-lymphocytes attacking the epidermal keratinocytes, but also mucous epithelia. Apoptosis and necrosis of cells. Disruption of epidermal/dermal connection. Bulla formation.

Course
Depends on age, comorbidity, body function status.

Complications
Mortality 1–5%. Scarring of blepharon, ectropium, phimosis, vaginal synechia.

Diagnosis
Typical clinical features and histology. SCORTEN (score of TEN) score recommended.

Differential Diagnosis
Disseminated herpes simplex infection (primary course), drug reaction, pemphigus vulgaris, DRESS.

Prevention and Therapy

Therapy has to be adapted to course of the development of body surface and mucosal involvement. Patient should be directly referred to a dermatologic centre.

Decision on systemic corticosteroids, IV immunoglobulins, TNF alpha blockers and symptomatic topical measures will be done according to course (see TEN).

Toxic Epidermal Necrolysis [12]

Figures 1.43, 1.44 and 1.45

Fig. 1.43 Toxic epidermal necrolysis: erythroderma and loss of sheets of epidermis on the trunk

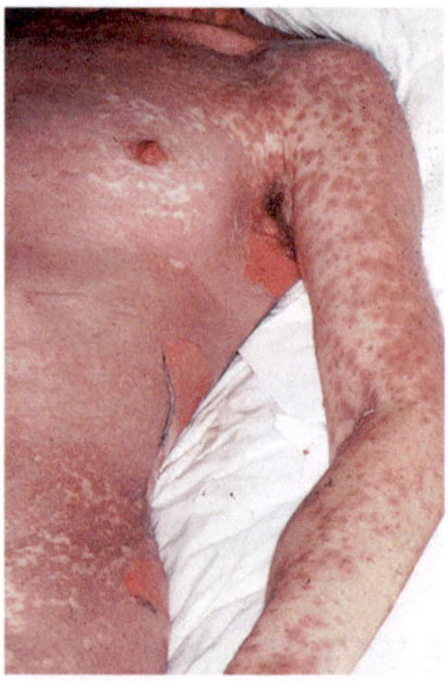

Fig. 1.44 Toxic epidermal necrolysis: loss of sheets of epidermis on the trunk

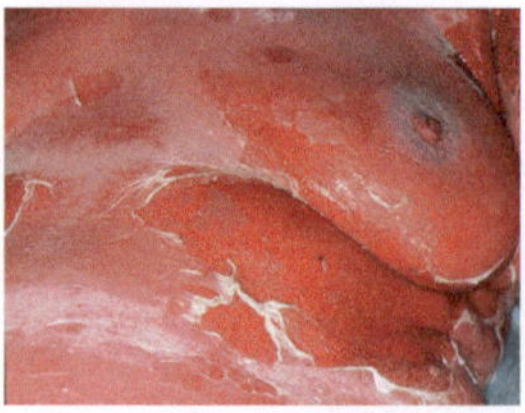

Fig. 1.45 Toxic epidermal necrolysis: superficial epidermal necrolysis on the hands

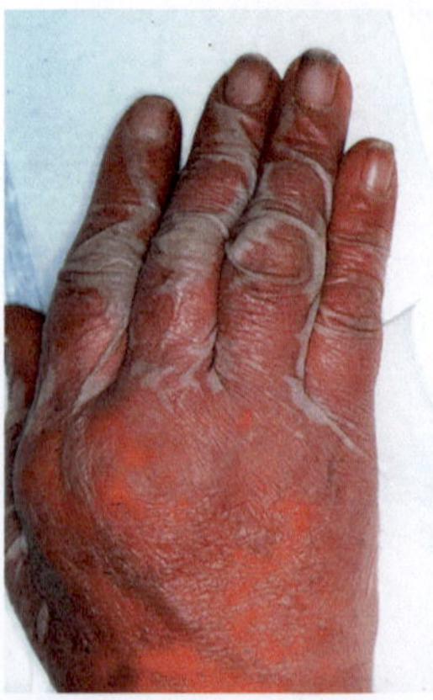

Grading of Importance
C

Level
Advanced

ICD-11
EB13

Synonyms
Lyell syndrome

Epidemiology
Rare disease 1–2 per 1 million. Higher risk in HIV/AIDS.

Definition
Severe drug-induced skin reaction characterized by necrosis of epidermal keratinocyte and marked mucosal erosions. Part of a spectrum, which ranges from SJS, where 30% of the body surface is affected to as SJS-TEN-overlap syndrome.

Aetiology and Pathogenesis
Triggers are medications (typically antibiotics and antiepileptic drugs). Immunologically induced apoptosis of keratinocytes evolving into massive epidermal destruction. Necrolysis by TNF alpha and gamma IFN. AnnexinA 1 promotes apotosis of keratinocyes.

Signs and Symptoms
Starting with a confluent maculopapular exanthema without the classical erythema multiforme like lesions, haemorrhagic blisters, epidermal necrosis followed by loss of sheets of epidermis; positive Nikolsky sign; usually severe periorificial mucosal erosions.

Localisation
Skin and mucosa.

Classification
Maximal variant of the erythema multiforme –SJS/TEN complex.

Laboratory and Other Workups
Check electrolytes, kidney and liver parameters, cardiac function.

Dermatopathology
Cytotoxic CD8 T-lymphocytes attacking the epidermal keratinocytes, but also mucous epithelia. Apoptosis and necrosis of cells. Disruption of epidermal/dermal

connection. Bulla formation because of severe epidermal necrosis. Epidermal remnants separated from dermis with only sparse inflammatory infiltrate.

Course

More than 40% complications. 30% mortality rate. More than 50% of TEN patients suffer from long-term sequelae.

Complications

Infection, electrolyte and fluid disturbances. Ophthalmic involvement including ectropium and synechia, phimosis, vaginal synechia. Scarring in esophagus and mouth mucosa.

SCORTEN (score of TEN) evaluation essential.

Diagnosis

Clinical features and histology, showing necrolysis throughout all epidermal layers.

Differential Diagnosis

Staphylococcal scalded skin syndrome, burns, erythema multiforme, disseminated fixed drug eruption, pemphigus and pemphigoid variants and linear IgA disease.

Prevention and Therapy

Immediate referral to special dermatologic and intensive care centre. Aggressive burn therapy (fluid and electrolyte management, appropriate antibiotic coverage). According to course and body surface and mucosal involvement. Intravenous immunoglobulins, TNF alpha blockers. High-dose ciclosporine and/or systemic corticosteroids.

Special

Ophthalmologic consultation.

Erythema Nodosum (EN) [7]

Figures 1.46 and 1.47

Grading of Importance

B

Level

Advanced

ICD-11

EB31

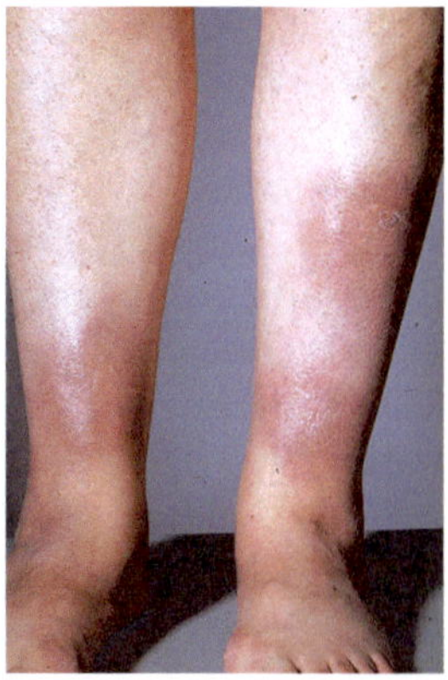

Fig. 1.46 Erythema nodosum: painful contusiform lesions on the legs

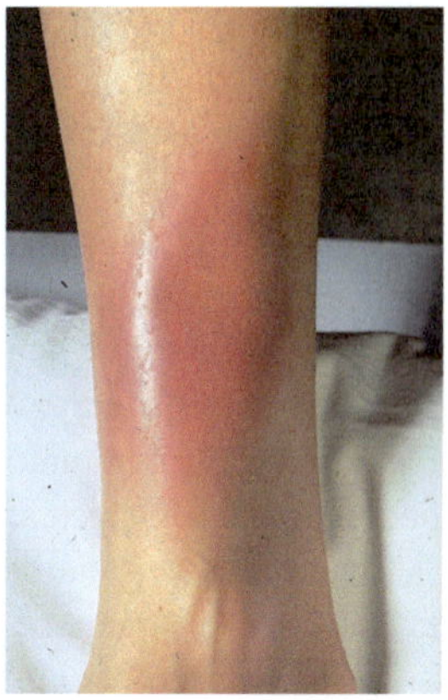

Fig. 1.47 Erythema nodosum: contusiform lesion on the leg

Synonyms

Subacute nodular migratory panniculitis

Epidemiology

2.4/1000 population/year, mostly in spring and autumn (due to streptococcal infections). F:M = 3–6:1. Especially children and adults (20–40 years).

Definition

Tissue-reaction pattern with many causes, characterised by painful subcutaneous nodules on the shins, most commonly in women.

Pathogenesis

Specific common causes include:

- Streptococcal infections
- Hepatitis B
- Sarcoidosis

- Bowel infections (e.g. *Yersinia*)
- Medicaments (e.g. penicillins, sulphonamides, oral contraceptives)
- Crohn's disease
- Tuberculosis

Signs and Symptoms

Often prodrome with malaise, fever, joint pain followed by tender, poorly defined subcutaneous erythematous, warm nodules. Over time, colour changes from bright red to finally light grey.

Localisation

Shins, occasionally thighs, buttocks or arms

Classification

None.

Laboratory and Other Workups

Blood tests with several serologic markers (rheumatism, streptococci, tuberculosis, yersiniosis, angiotensin converting enzyme, pancreatic enzymes, antinuclear antibodies), stool culture and radiographic studies.

Dermatopathology

Early phase: inflammatory infiltrate of neutrophils in the subcutaneous fat septae, oedema, macrophages and foam cells.

Later phase: granulomatous reaction and finally fibrous septae with scarring of fat tissue. It is in general a septal panniculitis.

Course

EN usually heals spontaneously without scarring within 3–6 weeks.

Complications

Depends on the underlying cause. There are long-standing and migrating subtypes of EN.

Diagnosis

Clinical feature. Occasionally biopsy may be required. A careful search for the underlying disease is needed. Despite investigations, in 25–50% of cases no cause is identified.

Differential Diagnosis

Erythema nodosum leprosum; erysipelas; urticaria.

Prevention and Therapy

Depends on underlying cause. The underlying disease(s) should be treated. Systemic NSAIDs may be helpful. If the clinical symptoms are severe, short-term systemic corticosteroids may be given. Supportive measures: bed rest, heparinoid creams, and compression stockings.

Pyoderma Gangrenosum (PG) [2]

Figures 1.48, 1.49 and 1.50

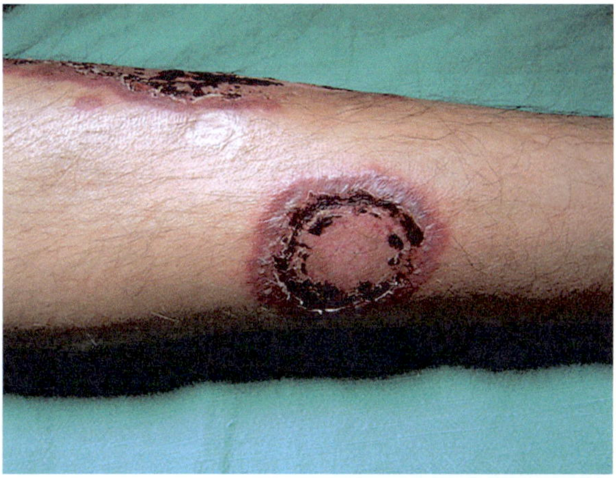

Fig. 1.48 Pyoderma gangrenosum: early target lesion on the leg

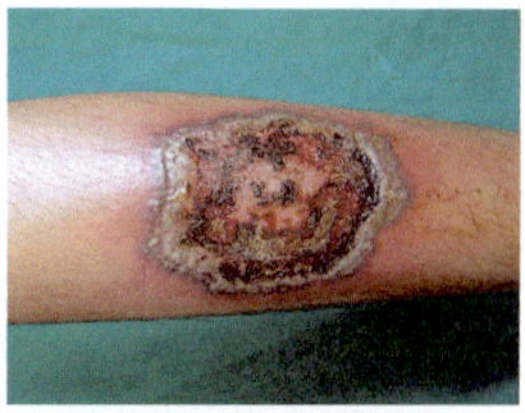

Fig. 1.49 Pyoderma gangrenosum: advanced lesion showing typical violaceous borders

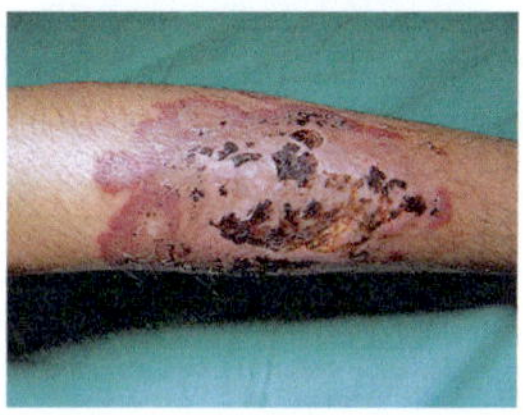

Fig. 1.50 Pyoderma gangrenosum: cribriform scar following healing from the center to the periphery

Grading of Importance
C

Level
Basic

ICD-11
EB-21

Synonyms
Dermatitis ulcerosa; phagedenic ulcer.

Epidemiology
Incidence: 3–10 per million per year. Age peak between 20 and 50 years. Women slightly more often affected than men. Men are more commonly affected in malignancy-associated PG.

Definition
Pyoderma gangrenosum (PG) is a rare, chronic and painful neutrophilic dermatosis that presents with rapidly developing, painful skin ulcers presenting with violaceous undermined borders and peripheral erythema.

Aetiology and Pathogenesis
More than 50% of patients with PG have an associated systemic disease, including:

- Inflammatory bowel disease (IBD) (40%). No correlation within the severity of IBD.
- Arthritis (12%): Seronegative. Rheumatoid arthritis and ankylosing spondylitis.
- Hematologic malignancies (7%). Most commonly acute myeloic leukaemia and a broad spectrum of lymphoproliferative disorders.
- Drugs: Interferon-α2b, G-CSF.
- Auto-inflammatory diseases:
  - PAPA syndrome characterised by destructive polyarthritis, severe nodulocystic acne and PG.
- PASH syndrome (PG, acne and hidradenitis suppurativa)
  - PAPASH syndrome (pyogenic arthritis, PG, acne and hidradenitis suppurativa)

Overlap between PG and Sweet's syndrome: Usually observed in patients with myeloproliferative disorders.

Signs and Symptoms
Tender nodule, plaque, or sterile pustule that enlarges progressing to sharply marginated painful ulcer with central necrosis, undermined violaceous borders and surrounding erythema and/or bullous lesions. The ulcer usually increases in size and depth (phagedenism).

Solitary lesion or multiple simultaneous recurrent lesions. Tends to develop at areas of previous trauma including surgery (pathergy phenomenon) (25–50%). As the lesions heal, cribriform or wrinkled (cigarette paper-like) scars often persist.

Localisation

The pretibial area (shins) is most commonly affected, but other parts of the skin and mucous membranes also can be affected.

Classification

Different clinical variants of PG have been defined:

- Ulcerative (classical) PG: Most commonly occurs at sites of trauma. Associated disorders: IBD, haematological malignancies, rheumatoid and seronegative arthritis and monoclonal gammopathy.
- Bullous PG: Painful bulla(e) that can progress to erosion and/or ulcer. Associations: myeloproliferative disorders (70%) and IBD.
- Pustular PG: Pustules with erythematous borders. Association: IBD.
- Vegetating PG: low-growing, non-purulent, superficial ulcer; borders are not undermined. No associated disorders.
- Peristomal PG: Papules that erode into ulcers adjacent to the stoma. Associations: IBD, enteric malignancy, connective tissue disease and monoclonal gammopathy.
- Postoperative PG: Erythema at the surgical site, wound dehiscence or painful ulcerations that coalesce. Abdominal and breast surgery.

Laboratory and Other Workups

Depends on the cause of the disease.

PG diagnostic workup includes a complete blood count with peripheral blood smear, biochemical survey, serum and urine protein electrophoresis, syphilis serologic tests and immunological tests (pANCA, cANCA). Skin biopsy for microbiological studies (bacterial, fungal and mycobacterial) should be obtained.

Additional tests may be indicated in cases with concomitant joint or gastrointestinal symptoms or suspicion of underlying hematologic malignancies. Age-appropriate cancer screening in selected cases.

Dermatopathology

The histopathology of PG is non-specific and depends on the stage of the lesion. Dermal oedema, suppurative inflammation and sterile abscess formation. The initial lesions show a deep suppurative folliculitis like pattern with a dense neutrophilic infiltrate.

Course

Variable. Chronic, relapsing or self-limiting disease. From mild to aggressive with intense morbidity.

Complications

Secondary infection, tissue destruction, intractable pain. Impact on quality of life (depression). Complications secondary to long-term immunosuppressive therapy.

Diagnosis

Diagnosis of PG is based on history of an underlying disease, typical clinical presentation, and exclusion of other diseases that would lead to persistent painful ulcers.

Differential Diagnosis

The differential diagnosis should include a wide range of diseases manifested as chronic and persistent cutaneous ulcers:

Vascular occlusive or venous disease, vasculitis (rheumatoid arthritis, ANCA-related vasculitis, Behçet's disease etc.), hypercoagulable states (anti-phospholipid syndrome), malignant neoplasms (leukemia), infectious diseases (ecthyma, deep mycoses, atypical mycobacterial infections, late, necrotizing cellulitis), exogenous tissue injuries (facticial panniculitis), insect or spider bites, and pustular drug reactions. Pemphigus vegetans.

Prevention and Therapy

High-dose oral corticosteroids (0.5–1 mg/kg/day) are the mainstay of treatment for rapid control of the disease, and, in other cases, ciclosporin may be used as a steroid-sparing agent either alone or in combination with corticosteroids.

In refractory cases, the combination of steroids with different immunosuppressants or steroid-sparing agents such as dapsone, colchicine, azathioprine, mycophenolate mofetil, methotrexate, cyclophosphamide, clofazimine, thalidomide, tacrolimus, sulfasalazine and minocycline have been proposed.

Anti-tumour necrosis alpha (TNF) therapy (infliximab, etanercept, adalimumab, certolizumab) could be prescribed in cases of PG associated with IBD. Other systemic treatments include high doses of intravenous immunoglobulins (IVIG); IL-1 and IL-23 inhibitors (ustekinumab); anti-IL-23 (tildrakizumab), anti-IL-17 (secukinumab) and IL-1 antagonists (anakinra, canakinumab, gevokizumab); and small molecules (JAK–STAT inhibitors).

Appropriate wound dressings of different types according to stage of ulcer. Topical and intralesional treatments (corticosteroids, calcineurin inhibitors) may be used as adjuvant therapies.

Prognosis

Unpredictable clinical course: from a precipitous onset with rapid spread to a more indolent pattern. Frequent relapses. Potentially life-threatening disease.

Special

PG is included within the spectrum of neutrophilic dermatoses.

Neutrophilic dermatoses are a heterogeneous group of inflammatory skin disorders characterised histologically by a neutrophilic infiltrate with no evidence of underlying infection or vasculitis.

Sweet's Syndrome (Acute Neutrophilic Dermatosis) [9, 17]

Figures 1.51, 1.52 and 1.53

Grading of Importance
C

Level
Basic

ICD-11
EB20

Synonyms
Acute febrile neutrophilic dermatosis.

Epidemiology
Worldwide distribution. Usually presenting in middle age women (30–60 years) with a 4:1 female to male ratio. No racial predilection.

Definition
Sweet's syndrome is a disorder characterized by a variety of symptoms, clinical and histological findings, which include fever, neutrophilia, erythematous, pressure-sensitive plaques or nodules and a diffuse dermal neutrophilic infiltrate.

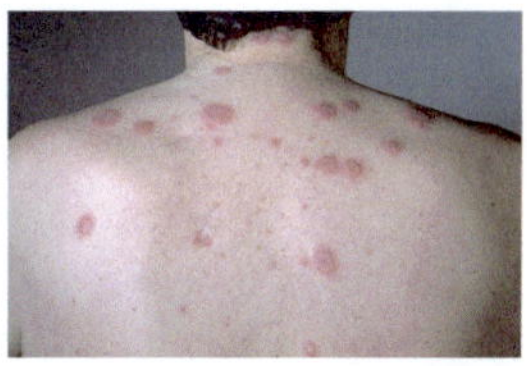

Fig. 1.51 Sweet's syndrome: disseminated lesions on the back

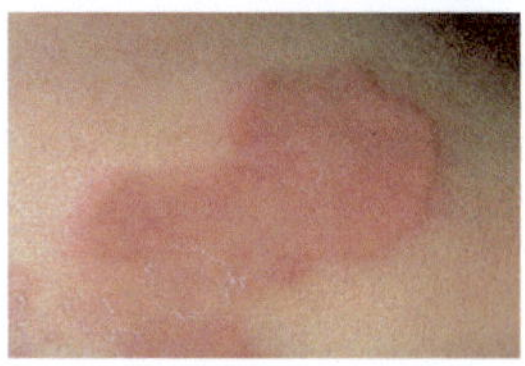

Fig. 1.52 Sweet's syndrome: urticarial lesion with elevated borders

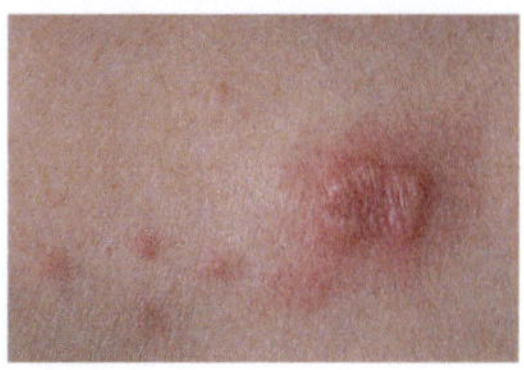

Fig. 1.53 Sweet's syndrome: urticarial papular lesion with bullous reaction

Aetiology and Pathogenesis

Most cases of Sweet's syndrome are considered to be idiopathic, but could also be associated with different disorders:

- Malignancy (10–20%): Myeloproliferative disorders; rarely with solid tumours
- Inflammatory and autoimmune disorders: Inflammatory bowel disease (ulcerative colitis or Crohn's disease), rheumatoid arthritis, systemic lupus erythematosus, Sjögren syndrome, thyroid disease (Graves disease and Hashimoto thyroiditis)
- Infectious diseases: HIV, viral hepatitis, tuberculosis, chlamydia infection
- Drugs: antibiotics, antihypertensives, NSAIDs, immunosuppressives, antiepileptics, anti-neoplastic, tyrosine-kinase inhibitors, antipsychotics, anti-thyroidals
- Pregnancy

Pathogenesis unknown. Possible hypersensitivity reaction to a variety of eliciting bacterial, viral or tumour antigens that may trigger neutrophil activation and infiltration. Possible role of activating cytokines and chemokines.

Some genetic factors and chromosomal abnormalities have been observed in patients with Sweet's syndrome.

Signs and Symptoms

Acute febrile episode associated with well-defined cutaneous eruptions accompanied by fever and constitutional symptoms (myalgia, fatigue, headache).

The lesions appear as solitary or multiple 0.5 to 12 cm, tender (leading symptom), oedematous, erythematous plaques or nodules with a pseudovesicular appearance. They may also have an urticaria-like pattern. The classical (idiopathic) form is often preceded by an upper respiratory or gastrointestinal tract infection.

In patients with malignancy-associated Sweet's syndrome, the lesions may adopt atypical clinical patterns (bullous, ulcerated or mimicking pyoderma gangrenosum).

Sweet's syndrome lesions can be associated with extracutaneous systemic manifestations (especially in the setting of an underlying malignancy) including arthralgias and arthritis (30–60%), ocular inflammation (conjunctivitis, episcleritis, uveitis), myocarditis, alveolitis, hepatitis and aseptic meningitis.

Localisation

The eruption is often distributed asymmetrically. The most frequent locations are at the upper extremities, face and neck; trunk and lower extremities also may be involved.

Classification

Sweet's syndrome may occur in the following clinical settings:

- Classical (idiopathic) Sweet's syndrome (50%). It may be associated with infection (upper respiratory tract or gastrointestinal tract), inflammatory bowel disease or pregnancy.
- Malignancy-associated Sweet's syndrome (< 35%). In patients with an established cancer or in individuals with a previous diagnosis of a malignant

haematological or solid neoplasm. The dermatosis can precede, follow or appear concurrent with the diagnosis of the patient's cancer.
- Drug-induced Sweet's syndrome.

Laboratory and Other Workups

Workup shall include determining the underlying cause if present. Complete blood cell count with leukocyte differentiation. Acute phase reactants (including the erythrocyte sedimentation rate or C-reactive protein), hepatic and renal function tests and urine analysis. Serologic evaluation for antistreptolysin-O antibody, rheumatoid factor and thyroid function. Additional tests if extracutaneous involvement is clinically suspected.

Age-appropriate cancer screening, including colonoscopy, mammography and PAP smears, should be pursued.

Dermatopathology

Diffuse dense dermal neutrophilic infiltrates in the upper dermis and marked oedema of the papillary dermis. Leukocytoclasia may be present. No primary vasculitic changes.

Course

The individual Sweet's syndrome lesions enlarge and may coalesce over a period of days to weeks. Subsequently, either spontaneously or after treatment, the lesions usually resolve without scarring. Recurrences may occur in up to 50% of patients, usually in cases associated with an underlying inflammatory disease or hematologic malignancy.

Complications

Depending on the presence of associated disorders or extracutaneous systemic diseases.

Diagnosis

The diagnosis is established on the basis of characteristic clinical, blood cell profile and histopathological findings. Histopathology is required for the diagnosis of Sweet's syndrome.

Diagnostic criteria for Sweet's syndrome have been proposed. Diagnosis may be based on fulfilling of both major criteria and two of the four minor criteria.

- Major criteria:
  - Sudden onset eruption of tender, painful plaques or nodules.
  - Neutrophilic infiltrate in the dermis without vasculitis.
- Minor clinical criteria:
  - Fever >38C
  - Illness preceded by an upper respiratory or gastrointestinal infection or associated with an underlying inflammatory disorder, malignancy or pregnancy

- Elevated white cell count with neutrophil predominance and elevated inflammatory serum markers
- Positive response to systemic glucocorticosteroids

Differential Diagnosis

Febrile infectious disorders (viral, bacterial, fungal and mycobacterial) with urticaria-like pattern.

Prevention and Therapy

Systemic glucocorticosteroids are the treatment of choice often achieving a rapid response. Other oral systemic agents are dapsone and colchicine. If glucocorticosteroids are contraindicated or a recurrence develops after tapering, a detailed work-up of the diagnoses has to be made. If no underlying diseases are found, several steroid-sparing agents such as methotrexate, doxycycline, indomethacin and cyclosporine could be prescribed.

Topical high potency or intralesional glucocorticosteroids may be used for localised lesions.

Prognosis

Sweet's syndrome typically follows a benign course and can resolve spontaneously without scarring in 5–12 weeks. Prognosis varies depending on the underlying associated disorder.

Special

Sweet's syndrome is the most representative entity of febrile neutrophilic dermatoses. See also chapter Pyoderma gangrenosum. Neutrophilic dermatoses are a heterogeneous group of inflammatory cutaneous disorders characterised histologically by a neutrophilic infiltrate with no evidence of underlying infection or vasculitis.

References

1. Abdollahi M, Radfar M (2003) A review of drug-induced oral reactions. J Contemp Dent Pract 4(1):10–31
2. Alavi A, French L, Davis M, Brassard A, Kirsner R (2017) Pyoderma Gangrenosum: an update on pathophysiology, diagnosis and treatment. Am J Clin Dermatol 18:355–372
3. Antia C, Baquerizo K, Korman A, Bernstein JA, Alikhan A (2018) Urticaria: a comprehensive review: epidemiology, diagnosis, and work-up. J Am Acad Dermatol 79(4):599–614
4. Bains SN, Nash P, Fonacier L (2019) Irritant contact dermatitis. Clin Rev Allergy Immunol 56(1):99–109
5. Benitez Ojeda AB, Mendez MD (2020) Diaper dermatitis. StatPearls, Treasure Island (FL)
6. Busse PJ, Christiansen SC (2020) Hereditary angioedema. N Engl J Med 382(12):1136–1148
7. Hafsi W, Badri T (2020) Erythema nodosum. StatPearls, Treasure Island, FL
8. Hardin CA, Love LW, Farci F (2020) Nummular dermatitis. StatPearls – NCBI Bookshelf
9. Heath M, Ortega-Loayza A (2019) Insights into the pathogenesis of sweet's syndrome. Front Immunol 10:414

10. Hoetzenecker W, Nägeli M, Mehra ET, Jensen AN, ISaulite I, Schmid-Grendelmeier P, Guenova E, Cozzio A, French LE (2016) Adverse cutaneous drug eruptions: current understanding. Semin Immunopathol 38:75–86
11. Nassau S, Fonacier L (2020) Allergic contact dermatitis. Med Clin North Am 104(1):61–76
12. Nowsheen S, Lehman JS, El-Azhary RA (2021) Differences between Stevens-Johnson syndrome versus toxic epidermal necrolysis. Int J Dermatol 60(1):53–59
13. Oakley A, Krishnamurthy K (2020) Stevens Johnson Syndrome. StatPearls – NCBI Bookshelf
14. Samim F, Auluck A, Zed C, Williams PM (2013) Erythema multiforme: a review of epidemiology, pathogenesis, clinical features, and treatment. Dent Clin N Am 57(4):583–596
15. Sidbury R, Kodama S (2018) Atopic dermatitis guidelines: diagnosis, systemic therapy, and adjunctive care. Clin Dermatol 36(5):648–652
16. Tucker D, Masood S (2020) Seborrheic dermatitis. StatPearls – NCBI Bookshelf
17. Villarreal-Villarreal C, Ocampo-Candiani J, Villarreal-Martínez A (2016) Sweet syndrome: a review and update. Actas Dermosifiliogr 107(5):369–378
18. Weidman AI, Sawicky HH (1956) Nummular eczema; review of the literature: survey of 516 case records and follow-up of 125 patients. AMA Arch Derm 73(1):58–65
19. Wollina U (2010) Pompholyx: a review of clinical features, differential diagnosis, and management. Am J Clin Dermatol 11(5):305–314

Autoimmune and Bullous Dermatoses

2

Giampiero Girolomoni, Paolo Gisondi,
and Martina Maurelli

Contents

G. Girolomoni (✉) · P. Gisondi · M. Maurelli
Department of Medicine, Università degli Studi di Verona, Verona, Italy
e-mail: giampiero.girolomoni@univr.it; paolo.gisondi@univr.it

H. Gollnick et al. (eds.), *Dermatology Cyberderm WebBook*,
https://doi.org/10.1007/978-3-031-78491-0_2

Test your learning and check your understanding of this book's contents: use the "Springer Nature Flashcards" app to access questions using ▶ https://sn.pub/1rhh6k.

To use the app, please follow the instructions in Chap. 1.

Lupus Erythematosus (LE) [5, 6]

Figures 2.1, 2.2, 2.3, 2.4, 2.5, 2.6, 2.7 and 2.8

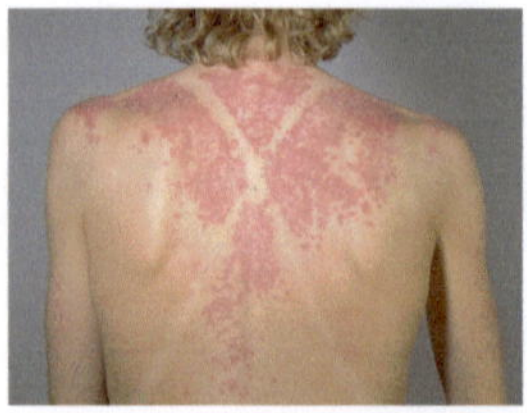

Fig. 2.1 Lupus erythematosus: systemic LE in sun exposed areas

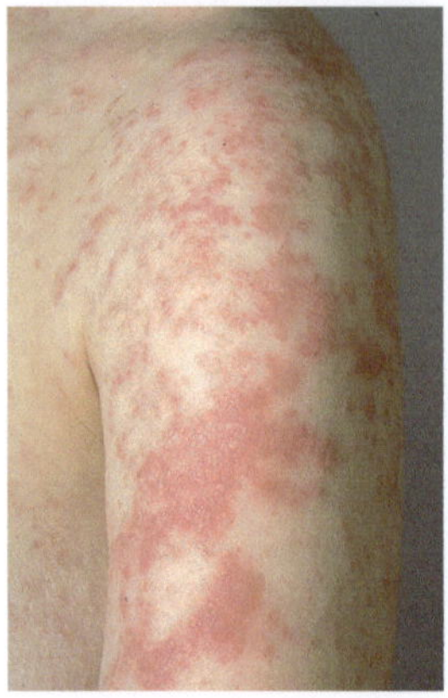

Fig. 2.2 Lupus erythematosus: macular lesions on the upper arm in systemic LE

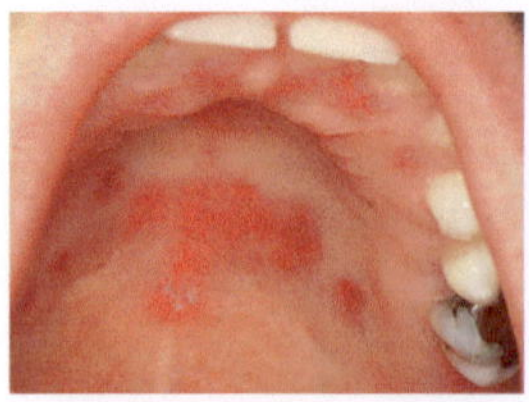

Fig. 2.3 Lupus erythematosus: involvement of palate in systemic LE

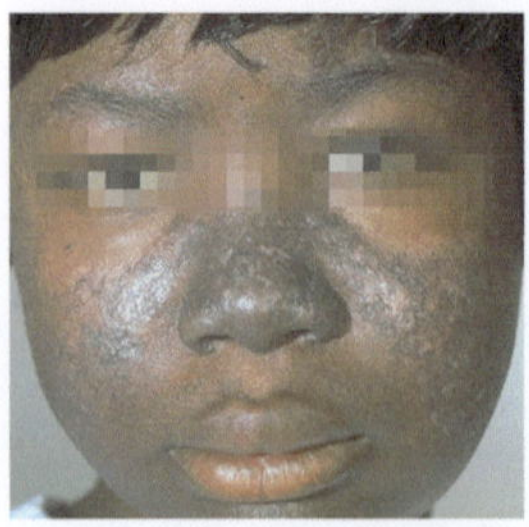

Fig. 2.4 Lupus erythematosus: butterfly rash in systemic LE on colored skin

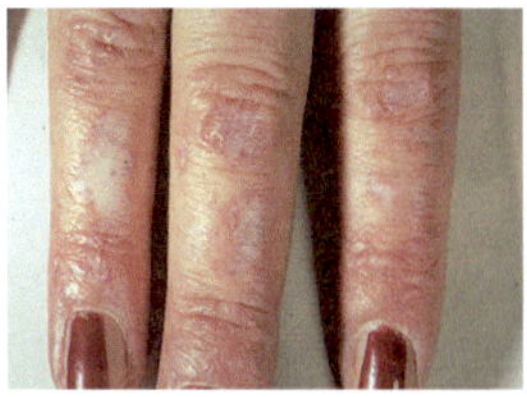

Fig. 2.5 Lupus erythematosus: erythema of fingers in systemic LE (chilblain LE)

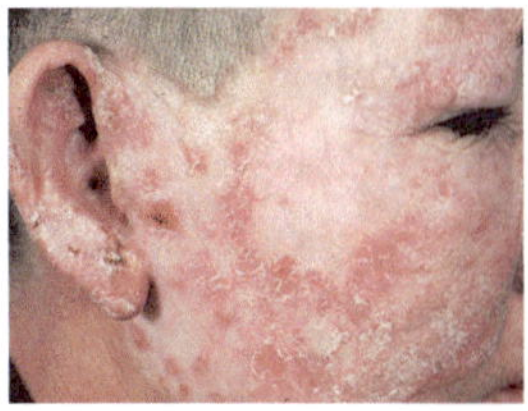

Fig. 2.6 Lupus erythematosus: erythema, follicular keratotic plugs, and atrophy in discoid LE

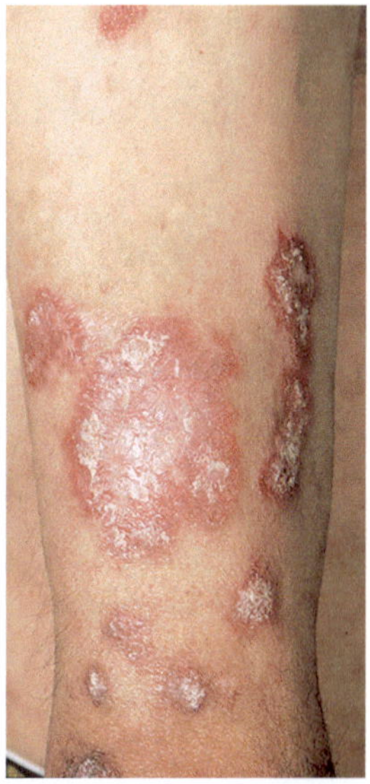

Fig. 2.7 Lupus erythematosus: erythema, follicular keratotic plugs, and atrophy in discoid LE

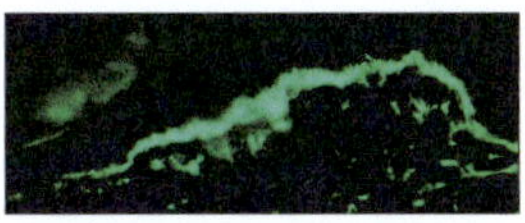

Fig. 2.8 Lupus erythematosus: DIF (direct immunofluorescence) showing granular band of C3- and IgG along the epidermal-dermal junction

Grading of Importance

C

Level

Advanced

ICD-11

4A40

Synonyms

Discoid LE, systemic LE.

Epidemiology

Usually affects young adults 20–40 years of age; F:M = 3:1, in systemic lupus erythematosus 8:1.

Definition

Chronic inflammatory autoimmune disease with marked immunogenetic component which involves the skin and/or other organs.

Aetiology and Pathogenesis

Immunogenetic susceptibility: HLA associations.

Polyclonal B-cell activation with autoantibody formation: direct pathogenic antibodies (autoimmune haemolytic anaemia), circulating immune complexes (vasculitis, nephritis), antibody-mediated cytotoxicity (skin lesions).

Precipitating factors: UV, medications, oestrogens (oral contraceptives, pregnancy), possibly some viruses, trauma (Koebner phenomenon).

Signs and Symptoms

- In discoid LE persistent several mm to cm sharply bordered, sometimes confluent, and painful lesions with triad of erythema, follicular keratotic plugs, and atrophy (each of which can dominate clinical picture).
- In systemic LE butterfly rash. Non-specific changes include erythematous maculopapular exanthema, diffuse hair loss, Raynaud syndrome and livedo racemosa (anticardiolipin antibodies and others) as a sign of cutaneous vasculitis, which can all be present.

Localisation

Usually light-exposed areas, especially face, nose, ears, cheeks (butterfly rash), scalp.

Classification

Chronic cutaneous lupus erythematosus (chronic cutaneous discoid LE (CCLE))

Coin or disk-shaped erythematous plaques with follicular hyperkeratosis and a tendency to heal with scarring, usually on light-exposed areas or scalp (acquired, circumscribed scarring alopecia).

Variants

- Hypertrophic LE (verrucosus LE)
- Disseminated DLE
- Chilblain LE (acral involvement)
- Lupus profundus/lupus panniculitis (deeper involvement)

Subacute Cutaneous LE (SCLE)

Non-scarring, polycyclic-annular or papulosquamous (psoriasiform) plaques which usually involve the upper half of the body and are photosensitive. Systemic symptoms (arthritis, fever, malaise) are milder than in SLE.

Systemic LE (SLE)

ACR (American College of Rheumatology) criteria:

1. Butterfly rash (acute cutaneous LE)
2. Discoid lesions
3. Photosensitivity
4. Oral ulcerations
5. Non-erosive arthritis

6. Serositis: pleuritis; pericarditis
7. Neurologic disease: seizures; psychosis
8. Renal disease (proteinuria >0.5 g/d, cellular casts)
9. Hematologic abnormalities (haemolytic anaemia, leukopenia)
10. Antinuclear antibodies (ANA)
11. Anti-dsDNS, anti-Sm, false-positive syphilis serology >6 months (e.g. with anticardiolipin antibodies)

Most of the skin findings of DLE and SCLE can be found in SLE.

The diagnosis is based on > = 4 ACR criteria being fulfilled. Other non-specific skin changes: Raynaud's syndrome, diffuse alopecia, vasculitis/vasculopathy, maculopapular and other exanthems.

Laboratory and Other Workups

CCLE: ANA in 25–60% (often low titres); anti-dsDNA negative; complement factors C3, C4 normal.

SCLE: With active disease erythrocyte sedimentation rate elevated, anti-SSA (Ro) 70–90%, anti-dsDNA 30–40%, rheumatoid factor (RF) 20%, leukopenia (lymphopenia).

SLE: Normo-hypochromic anaemia, leukopenia, thrombocytopenia, C-reactive protein and sedimentation rate elevated, anti-native-DNA (40–90%), anti-U1-RNP (40–60%), anti-SSA (Ro) (40–60%), anti-histone (70%), RF 30%, anti-cardiolipin antibodies (false-positive syphilis serology).

Dermatopathology

CCLE: Epidermal atrophy, hyperkeratosis (primarily follicular), vacuolar degeneration of basal keratinocytes, thickened basement membrane zone (PAS stain), oedema, dense lymphocytic perivascular and periadnexal infiltrate at all levels, including subcutaneous fat in lupus profundus.

In SCLE and SLE milder and less characteristic histologic changes, but lymphomononuclear infiltrate surrounding the capillaries. Vacuolar change of the dermal-epidermal junction (interface). Incontinence of melanin pigment.

Direct immunofluorescence examination: identification of granular band of C3- and IgG along the epidermal-dermal junction in lesional skin; in SLE also in sun-exposed normal skin (lupus band test).

Course

Pure cutaneous disease usually chronic with hypopigmentation and scarring, especially when discoid. Systemic disease takes highly variable course, ranging from mild disease to acute, life-threatening disease, especially with renal, cardiac or central nervous system involvement.

Complications

Depends on systemic involvement (CNS lupus, lupus nephritis).

Rarely squamous cell carcinoma (lupus carcinoma) develops in old DLE scars.

Diagnosis

Clinical features (using ACR criteria); immune serology (autoantibody profile); histology; direct immunofluorescence.

Differential Diagnosis

CCLE: psoriasis, tinea,other photodermatoses.

SCLE: psoriasis, tinea,pityriasis rosea, syphilis, other photodermatoses.

SLE: depending on pattern of systemic involvement, other multisystem diseases, such as rheumatoid arthritis, dermatomyositis or mixed connective tissue diseases.

Prevention and Therapy

CCLE and SCLE: antimalarials (hydroxychloroquine, chloroquine) can be combined with low-dose corticosteroids, light protection; in SCLE: thalidomide off-label.

SLE: multidisciplinary management adjusted to organ involvement (antimalarials, systemic immunosuppression with corticosteroids and immunosuppressive agents such as azathioprine, cyclophosphamide, biologicals: belimumab and ustekinumab).

Systemic Scleroderma (SSc) [9]

Figures 2.9, 2.10, 2.11, 2.12 and 2.13

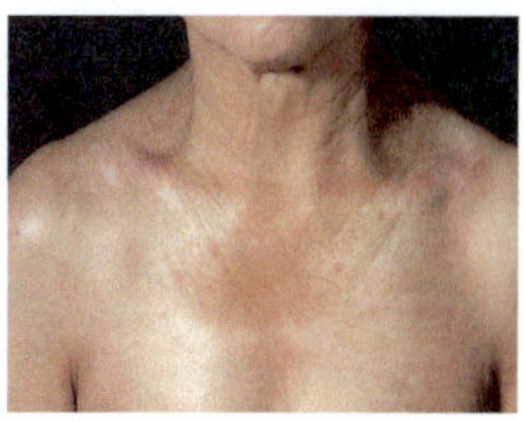

Fig. 2.9 Systemic scleroderma: tight, yellowish skin on the breast

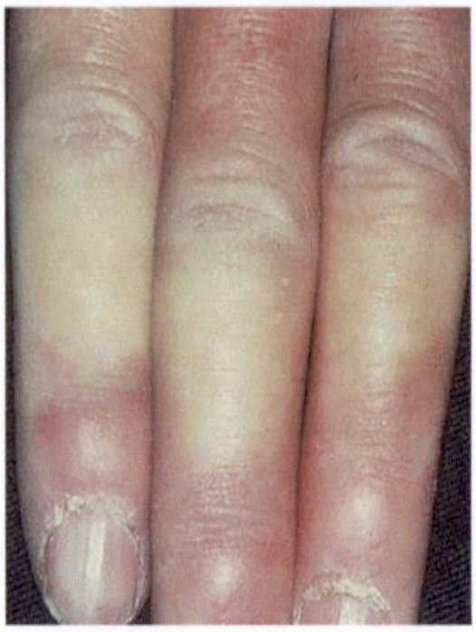

Fig. 2.10 Systemic scleroderma: Raynaud's syndrome of the fingers

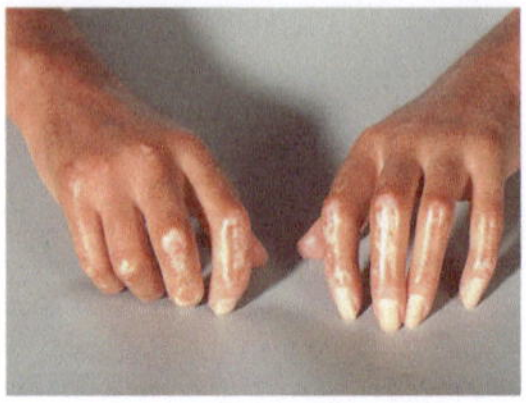

Fig. 2.11 Systemic scleroderma: sclerodactyly

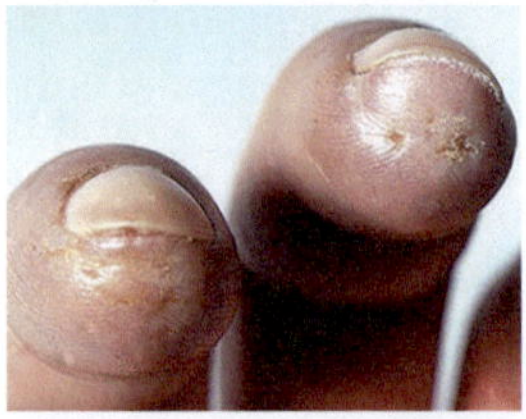

Fig. 2.12 Systemic scleroderma: painful fingertip ulcers

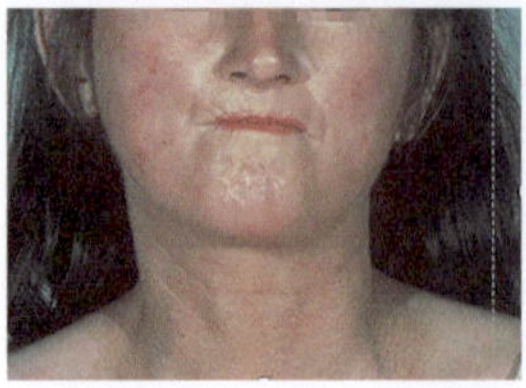

Fig. 2.13 Systemic scleroderma: microstomia

Grading of Importance

C

Level

Advanced

ICD-11

4A42

Synonyms

Progressive systemic sclerosis.

Epidemiology

Incidence varies between 0.1 and 4.3/100000; F:M = 4:1.

Definition

Chronic progressive multi-systemic disease involving skin, vessels and internal organs (lung, heart, gastrointestinal tract, kidney).

Aetiology and Pathogenesis

Multi-factorial: immunogenetic predisposition (HLA association), disturbed vascular regulation, humoral and cellular immune phenomena, altered collagen synthesis. Some chemical triggers identified (polyvinyl chloride, organic solvents, epoxy resins, silica).

Signs and Symptoms

Cutaneous

- Hands: sclerodactyly, painful fingertip ulcers, fingers initially puffy, later atrophic with distal thinning
- Face: microstomia, perioral radial folds (purse string mouth), telangiectases
- Entire skin: increasing thickness
- Vessels: Raynaud's syndrome, often primary symptom

Internal Organs

- Gastrointestinal tract: sclerosis of frenulum of tongue, disturbed swallowing, constipation, diarrhoea
- Lungs: pulmonary fibrosis, pulmonal artery hypertension (PAH)
- Kidneys: proteinuria, haematuria, renal crisis due to nephrosclerosis
- Heart: myocardial fibrosis, right heart failure secondary to PAH

- Liver: primary biliary cirrhosis
- Joints: pain, swelling, arthralgias, arthritis, dermatogenic contractures
- Bones: osteolysis, osteomyelitis possible due to digital ulcerations
- Muscles: muscle weakness from myositis

Localisation

See Classification.

Classification

- Limited SSc (43%): Raynaud's phenomenon precedes skin changes by years. Limited cutaneous sclerosis distal to knees and elbows, involvement of the face. Oesophageal disease, telangiectases, increased risk of developing PAH. Anti-centromere antibodies usually positive.
- Diffuse SSc (32%): Raynaud's phenomenon usually appears shortly before.
- Overlap syndrome (10%): Patients simultaneously show typical signs of SSC and other rheumatologic diseases.
- Others (undifferentiated forms, sclerosis sine scleroderma).

Laboratory and Other Workups

Immune serology: antinuclear antibodies (ANAs)/extractable nuclear antibodies (ENAs), anti-centromere antibodies (acral type), anti-Scl70 antibodies (diffuse type). Nail fold capillary microscopy (giant capillaries). Depending on clinical pattern, organ-specific studies.

CAVE: Clinically silent pulmonary or renal involvement.

Dermatopathology

Early lesions: dense superficial and deep perivascular and periadnexal lymphocytic infiltrate.

Late lesions: increased collagen (sclerosis) with loss of adnexal structures (alopecia, impaired sweating).

Course

Chronic and progressive.

Complications

Contractures, trophic ulcers, oesophageal stenosis, Barrett (narrow) oesophagus, pulmonary fibrosis (pulmonary hypertension), renal failure (renal hypertension, renal crisis), cardiac failure, cardiac rhythm disorders, right heart overload.

Diagnosis

Clinical features, histology, immune serology.

- Provocation testing for Raynaud's phenomenon: immerse hands in ice water for 10–20 minutes
- Capillary microscopy: early stage: ectasia of capillaries; active stage: mega-capillaries, haemorrhages; late stage: rarefaction and tufting of capillaries

In case of respiratory problems:

- Pulmonary function test, high-resolution CT (if pulmonary fibrosis is suspected)
- EKG, echocardiogram, 6-minute walking test to assess right heart overload

In case of gastrointestinal problems:

- Scintigraphy or dynamometry of oesophagus, gastroscopy, (dysphagia, reflux oesophagitis), colonoscopy

In case of renal involvement:

- Blood pressure monitoring, renal function tests, 24 hour urine, ultrasound, kidney biopsy in selected cases

In case of musculoskeletal problems:

- Muscles: CK, myositis-specific antibodies, EMG, MRI, muscle biopsy
- Joints: x-ray, sonography, rheumatoid factor, anti-CCP antibodies

Differential Diagnosis

(Pseudosclerodermas)

Eosinophilic fasciitis, chronic graft-vs-host disease, genodermatoses (Werner syndrome), porphyria cutanea tarda, amyloidoses, mucinoses, gadolinium-induced sclerosis.

Chemically induced scleroderma (polyvinyl chloride, silica, organic solvents, epoxy resins), drug-induced sclerosis (bleomycin, pentazocine, L-tryptophan).

Prevention and Therapy

No causal therapy available. Interdisciplinary treatment and guidance.

Localised Scleroderma [3]

Figures 2.14, 2.15 and 2.16

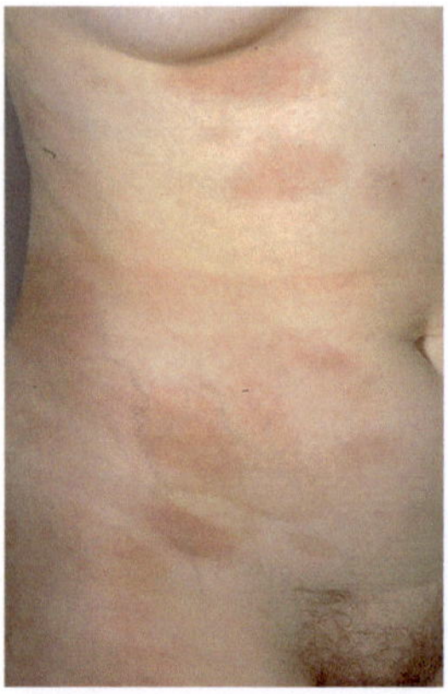

Fig. 2.14 Localized scleroderma: superficial form of Pierini-Pasini

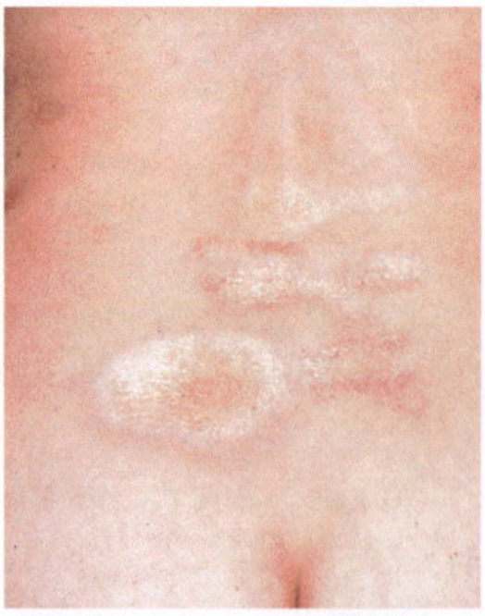

Fig. 2.15 Localized scleroderma: circumscribed lesion with lilac ring

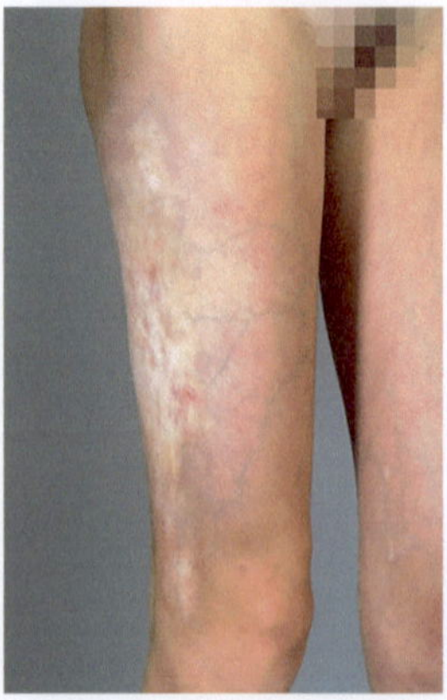

Fig. 2.16 Localized scleroderma: linear scleroderma of the leg with atrophy

Grading of Importance

C

Level

Advanced

ICD-11

EB61.0

Synonyms

Morphea, scleroderma circumscriptum.

Epidemiology

Age 20–40 years in15% of patients.

Definition

Uncommon localised connective tissue disease with inflammatory border (lilac ring).

Aetiology and Pathogenesis

Unknown. In some cases tick bite in patient's history.

Signs and Symptoms

Centrifugally spreading erythema with progressive central white-yellow induration and loss of adnexal structures. Border often with purple tones (lilac ring) as sign of disease activity.

Severe course with involvement of deeper structures possible, especially in cases with linear scleroderma ("en coup de sabre" on scalp), facial hemiatrophy.

Localisation

Varies with classification.

Classification

- Limited forms: plaque-type morphea, guttate morphea, atrophoderma of Pierini-Pasini
- Generalised forms: generalised circumscribed scleroderma, disabling pansclerotic morphea, eosinophilic fasciitis
- Linear forms: linear circumscribed scleroderma including type "en coup de sabre," Parry-Romberg syndrome
- Deep morphea

Laboratory and Other Workups

Routine laboratory tests; Borrelia serology; ANA. In children with severe linear forms: rheumatoid factor.

Dermatopathology

Interface dermatitis in early phases with varying intensity of inflammatory cellular infiltrates and changes of collagen structure depending on time of the disease course. Identical to progressive systemic sclerosis.

Course

Plaque-type morphea: usually self-limited within years leaving sclerotic, pigmented scars. Linear circumscribed scleroderma and haemifacial atrophy: chronic with significant impairment of growth and function.

Complications

Depends on localisation (face, overlying joints), depth and extension (pansclerotic morphea).

Generally, no systemic involvement, in contrast to progressive systemic sclerosis. In patients with linear type "en coup de sabre" or Parry-Romberg syndrome, possible underlying bone and CNS involvement.

Diagnosis

Clinical features, histology. In patients with linear type "en coup de sabre" or Parry-Romberg syndrome, cranial magnetic resonance imaging (MRI) and high-resolution CT scan should be performed to document bone involvement and exclude CNS involvement.

Differential Diagnosis

Lichen sclerosus (et atrophicus), acrodermatitis chronica atrophicans (borreliosis), dermatosclerosis associated to severe chronic venous insufficiency, progressive systemic sclerosis, eosinophilic fasciitis.

Prevention and Therapy

No causal therapy available.

- Topical therapy: corticosteroids; calcipotriol
- Intralesional corticosteroids
- Systemic therapy: methotrexate; corticosteroids; hydroxychloroquine, in severe refractory cases only
- Phototherapy: PUVA; bath PUVA; UVA-1
- Physical therapy: range of motion exercises; manual lymphatic drainage

Dermatomyositis [2, 10]

Figures 2.17, 2.18, 2.19 and 2.20

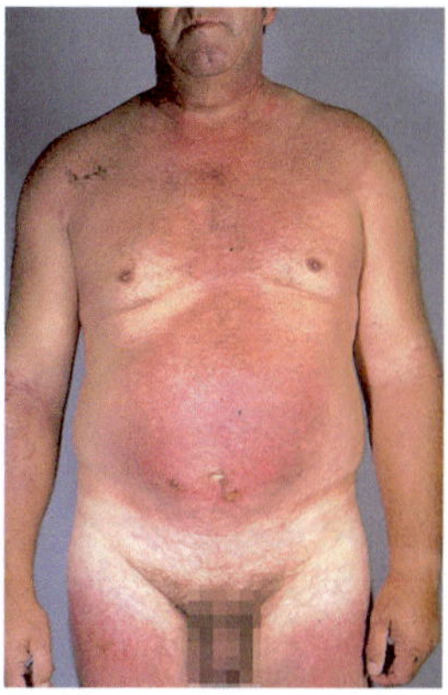

Fig. 2.17 Dermatomyositis: poikilodermtous discoloration of the bally and upper legs

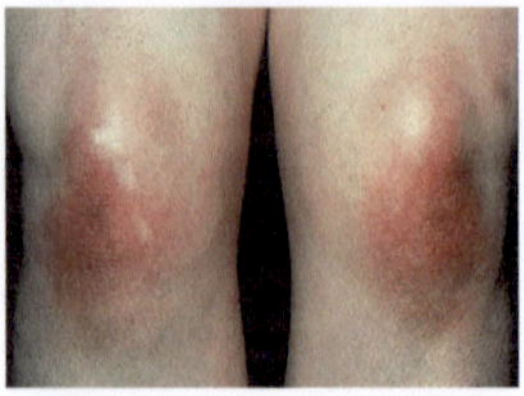

Fig. 2.18
Dermatomyositis: colored patches over knees

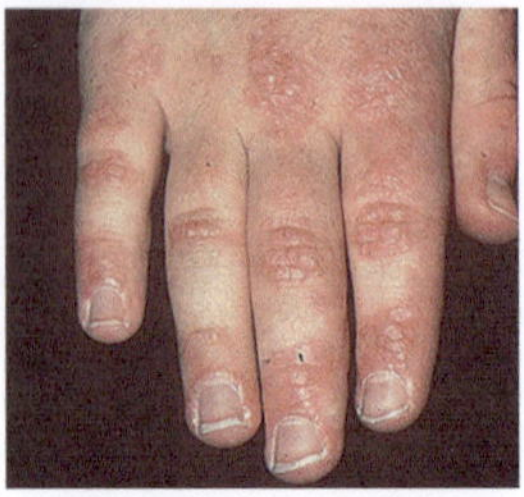

Fig. 2.19
Dermatomyositis: violaceous lichenoid papules on dorsal surface of the fingers (Gottron's papules)

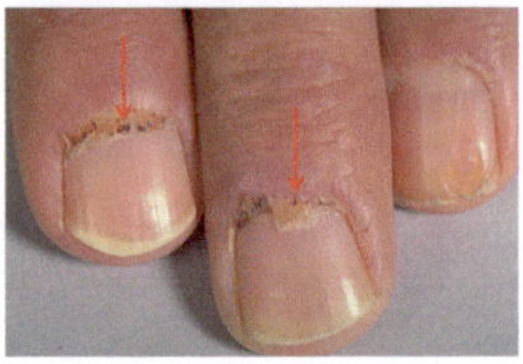

Fig. 2.20
Dermatomyositis: hyperkeratosis of the eponychium

Grading of Importance

C

Level

Advanced

ICD-11

4A41.0

Synonyms

None.

Epidemiology

The incidence of dermatomyositis ranges from 2 to 9 per million with a F:M = 3:1. It is characterised by a bimodal age distribution, with two peaks of incidence in <10 years and from 30 to 60 years.

Definition

Rare inflammatory systemic autoimmune disease involving skin and muscle.

Aetiology and Pathogenesis

Autoimmune disease, in adults, 15% paraneoplastic (carcinomas: GI tract, lungs, breast, reproductive organs).

Signs and Symptoms

- Skin: violaceous lichenoid papules on dorsal surface of the fingers (Gottron's papules), similarly coloured patches over knees, elbows and malleoli (Gottron's sign), heliotrope periorbital oedema, periungual telangiectasesiae, poikiloderma, vasculitis with necrosis
- Muscles: necrosis of proximal muscle groups (hips, shoulders) with weakness and pain, dysphagia, dyspnoea; in children often calcinosis
- Systemic: acute severe form with vasculitis and visceral involvement

Localisation

Dorsal aspects of fingers, knees, elbows, malleoli, face.

Classification

- Dermatomyositis
- Polymyositis (no skin involvement)
- Dermatomyositis sine myositis (no muscle involvement within 2 years of rash developing)
- Paraneoplastic dermatomyositis
- Juvenile dermatomyositis
- Dermatomyositis overlap syndromes, most commonly with progressive systemic sclerosis

Laboratory and Other Workups

- ESR rate elevated, ALT, AST, LDH and muscle enzymes, especially CPK, elevated
- ANA (40–60%), specific anti-myositis antibodies including anti-synthetase antibodies including anti-Jo-1 antibodies (may indicate a severe course with pulmonary fibrosis), ant—PL7, and others (anti-TIF1-gamma, anti-NPX2, anti-MDA-5 pulmonary interstitial disease, anti-Mi-2)
- Electromyography (EMG): polyphasic potentials
- Directed muscle biopsy (when EMG abnormal)

Dermatopathology

Similar to lupus erythematosus, often non-specific. Muscle biopsy: muscle degeneration with lymphocytic infiltrates and obliterative vasculopathy.

Course

Chronic. Remission in those cases where an associated malignant tumour is successfully treated.

Complications

Respiratory failure, progressive loss of muscle function, renal impairment secondary to muscle damage, calcinosis (children), vasculitis.

Diagnosis

Clinical features (distinctive skin findings and muscle involvement), laboratory (muscle enzymes), EMG (polyphasic potentials), MRI, muscle biopsy.

Differential Diagnosis

MCTD (mixed connective tissue disease = Sharp syndrome); dermatomyositis overlap with progressive systemic sclerosis and/or lupus erythematosus; trichinosis; thyrotoxic myopathy. If skin findings are not clear, wide range of myopathies.

Prevention and Therapy

Systemic corticosteroids, immunosuppression (cyclophosphamide, methotrexate, ciclosporin), high-dose intravenous immunoglobulins, bed rest, passive physiotherapy, photoprotection.

Pemphigus Vulgaris [8]

Figures 2.21 and 2.22

Grading of Importance

C

Level

Advanced

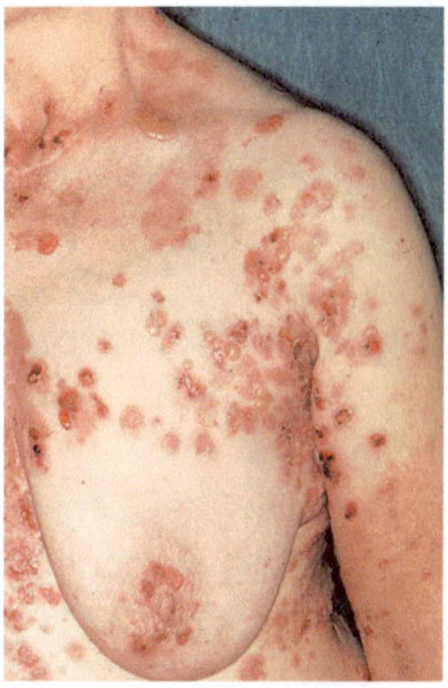

Fig. 2.21 Pemphigus vulgaris: blistering lesions on the shoulder

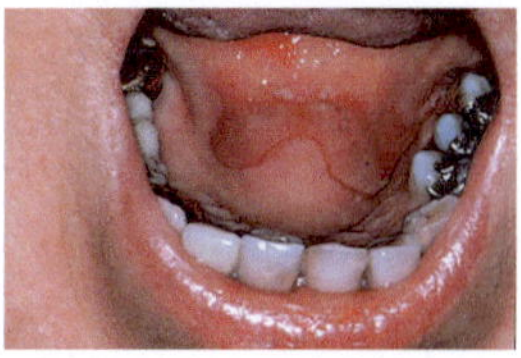

Fig. 2.22 Pemphigus vulgaris: sublingual erosion

ICD-11

EB40.0

Synonyms

None.

Epidemiology

Incidence of 2–7 new cases per million per year. F = M, 30–60 years. Ethnic variations.

Definition

Autoimmune disease with intraepidermal blister formation.

Aetiology and Pathogenesis

Loss of cell adhesion within epidermis (acantholysis) and blister formation by circulating autoantibodies against desmosomal proteins (desmogleins 1 and 3).

Signs and Symptoms

Pemphigus vulgaris: onset with oral erosions in more than 50% of cases, later superficial, fragile blisters with rapid transition to crusted erosions. The lesions usually develop in non-inflamed skin. Nikolski's signs positive (Nikolski I, blisters induced by rubbing normal skin; Nikolski II, existing blisters extend with lateral pressure).

Pemphigus foliaceus: It manifests with impetigo-like crusted erosions usually on an erythematous base and usually starts in seborrheic areas. Mucosae are usually spared.

Localisation

Oral mucosae and entire skin surface, especially head, neck and trunk.

Classification

- Pemphigus vulgaris: target antigens desmoglein 3 and desmoglein 1, suprabasal blister formation. Rare variants include neonatal pemphigus, pemphigus vegetans
- Pemphigus foliaceus: target antigen desmoglein 1, subcorneal blister formation:
  - Fogo selvagem (Brazilian pemphigus): endemic form of pemphigus foliaceus in Brazil; black flies (Simulium) may be vectors.
  - Pemphigus erythematosus: pemphigus foliaceus with positive ANA and photosensitivity.
- Paraneoplastic pemphigus: autoantibodies against both intraepidermal and sub-epidermal attachment proteins. Intraepidermal and sub-epidermal blister formation
- IgA pemphigus
- Pemphigus herpetiformis

Laboratory and Other Workups

Direct immunofluorescence (DIF): identification of in vivo bound intraepidermal, intercellular autoantibodies in the skin biopsy.

Indirect immunofluorescence (IIF): identification in patient's serum of circulating autoantibodies against stratified squamous epithelium.

ELISA for detection of anti-desmoglein 1 and 3 and autoantibodies in serum.

Dermatopathology

Intraepidermal clefts secondary to acantholysis.

Course

Chronic, progressive. If untreated may be fatal.

Complications

Before the introduction of systemic corticosteroids, high mortality rate (skin-related sepsis, marasmus secondary to fluid and protein loss, difficulty in eating). Today complications secondary to high-dose corticosteroids and other immunosuppressive therapy.

Diagnosis

Tzanck test: direct identification of acantholytic cells in smear of blister content (smear, Giemsa stain). Histology (acantholysis). DIF, intraepidermal intercellular IgG deposits. IIF, circulating IgG, which binds to stratified squamous epithelium in intercellular pattern. Immunoblot/ELISA, antibodies anti-desmoglein 1 and 3 autoantibodies in serum.

Differential Diagnosis

- Mucosal and erosive oral lesions: acute herpetic stomatitis, aphthous stomatitis, erosive lichen planus, erythema multiforme major/Stevens-Johnson syndrome.
- Skin lesions: other autoimmune bullous diseases, erythema multiforme, Hailey-Hailey disease, staphylococcal scalded skin syndrome (SSSS), toxic epidermal necrolysis (TEN).

Prevention and Therapy

Systemic: rituximab, long-term immunosuppressive therapy (corticosteroids, azathioprine, methotrexate, dapsone, cyclophosphamide). In refractory cases: High-dose intravenous immunoglobulins. Topical: general wound care.

Pemphigoid Group [1]

Figures 2.23, 2.24 and 2.25

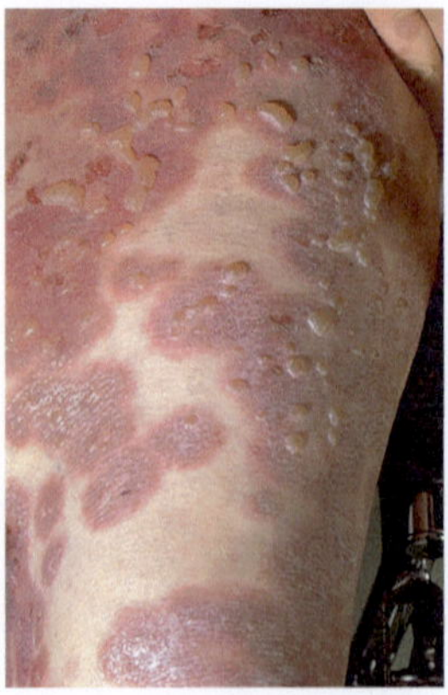

Fig. 2.23 Pemphigoid group: violaceous erythema and bullae on the upper leg

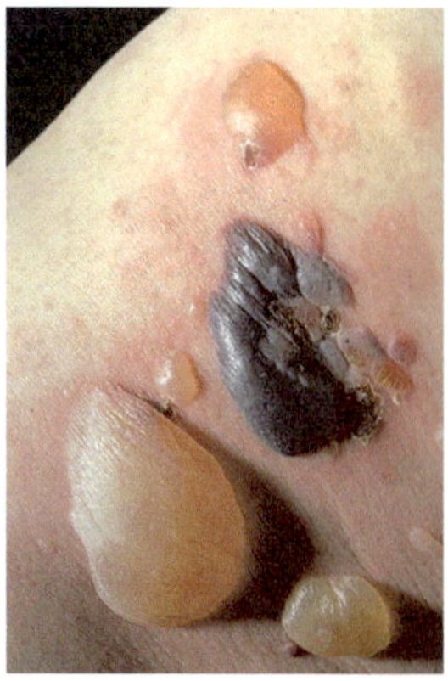

Fig. 2.24 Pemphigoid group: tense bullae some with hemorrhage

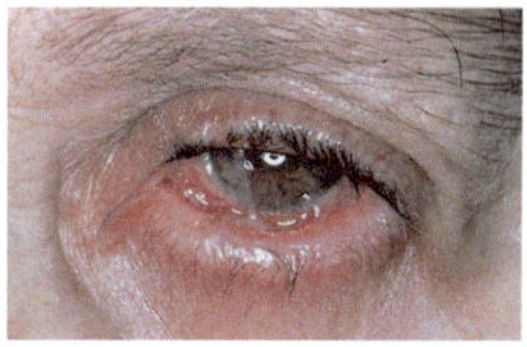

Fig. 2.25 Pemphigoid group: involvement of eye

Grading of Importance

C

Level

Advanced

ICD-11

EB41.0

Synonyms

None.

Epidemiology

Bullous pemphigoid is the most common type: typically present in older adults (>60–70 years). Annual incidence: 6–30 new cases per million population. M = F.

Definition

Autoimmune diseases with sub-epidermal blister formation.

Aetiology and Pathogenesis

Sub-epidermal separation caused by circulating auto-antibodies directed against hemi-desmosomal adhesion proteins of the cutaneous basement membrane (bullous pemphigoid antigens, BP180 and BP230). Triggered in some cases by drugs (gliptins, diuretics).

Signs and Symptoms

- Bullous pemphigoid: initially erythematous and urticarial patches and plaques and marked pruritus, followed by tense, sometimes haemorrhagic blisters. Mucosal involvement is uncommon. M = F, >60–70 years.
- Pemphigoid gestationis: pemphigoid-like clinical picture but occurring in second-third trimesters of pregnancy. Disease usually starts around the umbilicus and heals spontaneously after delivery.

Localisation

Skin and sometimes mucous membranes.

Classification

- Bullous pemphigoid
- Pemphigoid gestationis = pemphigoid of pregnancy (formerly known as herpes gestationis)
- Mucous membrane pemphigoid (former cicatricial pemphigoid)
- Linear IgA disease (chronic bullous dermatosis of childhood)
- Epidermolysis bullosa acquisita

Laboratory and Other Workups

Direct and indirect immunofluorescence: demonstration of antibodies directed against basement membrane zone (linear deposits of C3 and IgG). Hypereosinophilia is common; ELISA for detection of BP180 and BP230 specific auto-antibodies in serum.

Dermatopathology

Sub-epidermal blister with tissue eosinophilia.

Course

Chronic, progressive.

Complications

Skin-related sepsis, fluid and protein loss. High mortality among elderly patients. Permanent mucosal scars in mucous membrane pemphigoid.

Diagnosis

Tzanck test negative. Histology (sub-epidermal blister formation, tissue eosinophilia). Direct immnunofluorescence: linear deposits of C3 and IgG along the dermo-epidermal junction. Indirect inmmunofluorescence: circulating IgG which binds to the dermo-epidermal junction of normal skin and to the roof of human sodium chloride split skin. ELISA for detection of BP180 and BP230 specific autoantibodies in serum.

Differential Diagnosis

With other autoimmune bullous dermatoses, especially epidermolysis bullosa acquisita, which is caused by antibodies against collagen VII. Linear IgA dermatosis is characterised by linear deposits of IgA rather than IgG along the basement membrane zone (this is the most common autoimmune bullous disease in childhood). Bullous arthropod bites, allergic contact dermatitis, Steven-Johnson syndrome, erythema multiforme, porphyria cutanea tarda/pseudoporphyria.

Prevention and Therapy

Topical treatments: High potency topical corticosteroids (e.g. clobetasol propionate), anti-septics, general wound care. Systemic: corticosteroids (first-line therapy), azathioprine, mycophenolate mofetil, dapsone, methotrexate, nicotinamide/tetracycline, rituximab and high-dose intravenous immunoglobulins.

Dermatitis Herpetiformis [4, 7]

Figures 2.26, 2.27 and 2.28

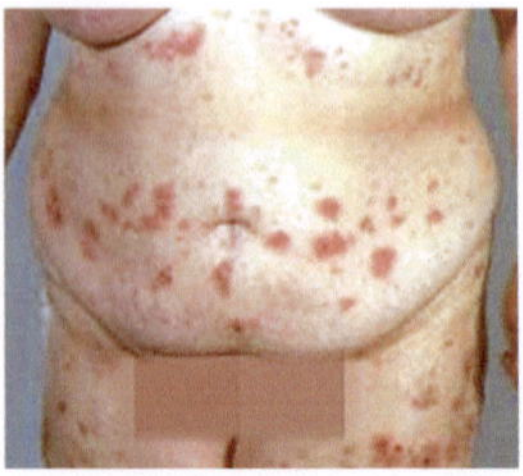

Fig. 2.26 Dermatitis herpetiformis: papulo-vesicles on an erythematous base on the trunk

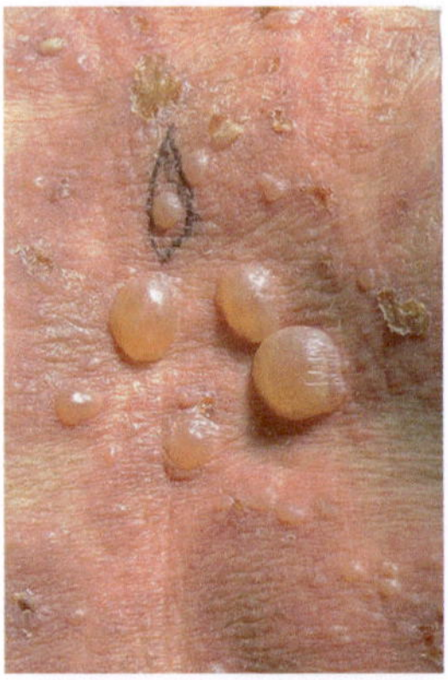

Fig. 2.27 Dermatitis herpetiformis: bullae on an erythematous base

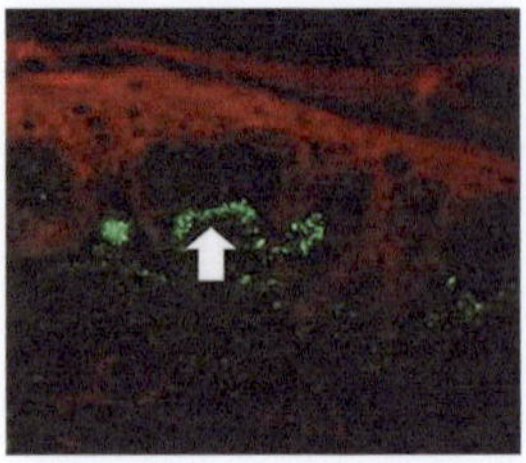

Fig. 2.28 Dermatitis herpetiformis: DIF showing granular IgA deposition in papillary dermis

Grading of Importance

C

Level

Advanced

ICD-11

EB44

Synonyms

None.

Epidemiology

Prevalence: 10.4 per 100′000 individuals. Annual incidence: 1.3 per 100′000 persons. M > F, 20–70 years.

Definition

Chronic recurrent polymorphic blistering dermatosis with intense pruritus, associated with gluten-sensitive enteropathy (coeliac disease, with IgA autoantibodies against tissue transglutaminase).

Aetiology and Pathogenesis

Gluten complexes precipitate with IgA in the dermal papillae and lead to subepidermal blister formation. The anti-transglutaminase IgA autoantibodies are triggered by the gluten-sensitive enteropathy.

Signs and Symptoms

Marked burning and pruritus, usually small tense grouped (herpetiform) papulovesicles on an erythematous base, sometimes eczematous, often with secondary excoriations.

Localisation

Shoulders, buttocks, extensor surfaces of extremities with a symmetrical distribution, especially knees and elbows.

Classification

None.

Laboratory and Other Workups

Direct immunofluorescence: granular IgA deposits in the tips of the dermal papillae.

Serum: IgA anti-transglutaminase antibodies.

Dermatopathology

Sub-epidermal blister formation with papillary abscesses (accumulation of neutrophils and occasionally eosinophils).

Course

Chronic, recurrent.

Complications

Related to enteropathy and malabsorption. Augmented incidence of enteropathy-associated T-cell lymphoma, but it is rare.

Diagnosis

Serum anti-transglutaminase antibodies, histology and DIF (granular IgA deposition in papillary dermis), small bowel biopsy (optional). Gluten-sensitive enteropathy can be confirmed in over 90% (symptomatic in only 15%).

Differential Diagnosis

Other autoimmune bullous dermatoses, especially linear IgA disease (no gluten-sensitive enteropathy), *arthropod bites*, scabies.

Prevention and Therapy

Dapsone (rapid relief from pruritus), gluten-free diet. Prior to starting dapsone measure G-6-P-dehydrogenase. While on dapsone monitor for side effects: agranulocytosis, anaemia, methaemoglobinaemia, hepatitis.

References

1. Bernard P, Antonicelli F (2017) Bullous pemphigoid: a review of its diagnosis, associations and treatment. Am J Clin Dermatol 18(4):513–528
2. DeWane ME, Waldman R, Lu J (2020) Dermatomyositis: clinical features and pathogenesis. J Am Acad Dermatol 82(2):267–281
3. Distler O, Cozzio A (2016) Systemic sclerosis and localized scleroderma—current concepts and novel targets for therapy. Semin Immunopathol 38(1):87–95
4. Mirza HA, Gharbi A, Bhutta BS (2020) Dermatitis herpetiformis. StatPearls, Treasure Island, FL
5. Okon L, Werth V (2013) Cutaneous lupus erythematosus: diagnosis and treatment. Best Pract Res: Clin Rheumatol 27(3):391–404
6. Patel P, Werth V (2002) Cutaneous lupus erythematosus: a review. Dermatol Clin 20(3):373–385. v
7. Salmi TT (2019) Dermatitis herpetiformis. Clin Exp Dermatol 44(7):728–731
8. Schmidt E, Kasperkiewicz M, Joly P (2019) Pemphigus. Lancet 394(10201):882–894
9. Sticherling M (2019) Systemic sclerosis – the dermatological perspective. J Dtsch Dermatol Ges 17(7):716–728
10. Waldman R, DeWane ME, Lu J (2020) Dermatomyositis: diagnosis and treatment. J Am Acad Dermatol 82(2):283–296

Physically Induced Dermatoses

3

Harald Gollnick, Günter Burg,
and Ramon María Pujol Vallverdú

Contents

H. Gollnick (✉)
Department of Dermatology & Venereology, Otto-von-Guericke University, Magdeburg, Germany
e-mail: Harald.Gollnick@med.ovgu.de

G. Burg
Dermatology, Zurich, Switzerland
e-mail: g.burg@access.uzh.ch

R. M. Pujol Vallverdú
Dermatology and Venereology, Universitat Autònoma de Barcelona, Hospital del Mar. IMIM, Barcelona, Spain
e-mail: rpujol@psmar.cat

H. Gollnick et al. (eds.), *Dermatology Cyberderm WebBook*,
https://doi.org/10.1007/978-3-031-78491-0_3

Test your learning and check your understanding of this book's contents: use the "Springer Nature Flashcards" app to access questions using ▶ https://sn.pub/1rhh6k.

To use the app, please follow the instructions in Chap. 1.

Thermal Injury [4, 5]

Figures 3.1, 3.2 and 3.3

Grading of Importance

A

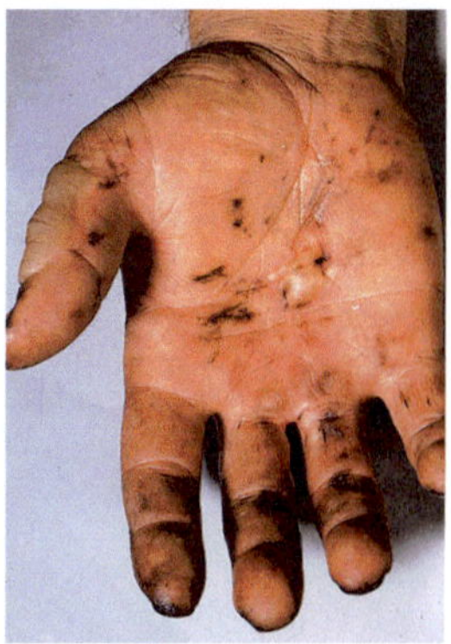

Fig. 3.1 Thermal injury: blisters and necrosis due to fire injury

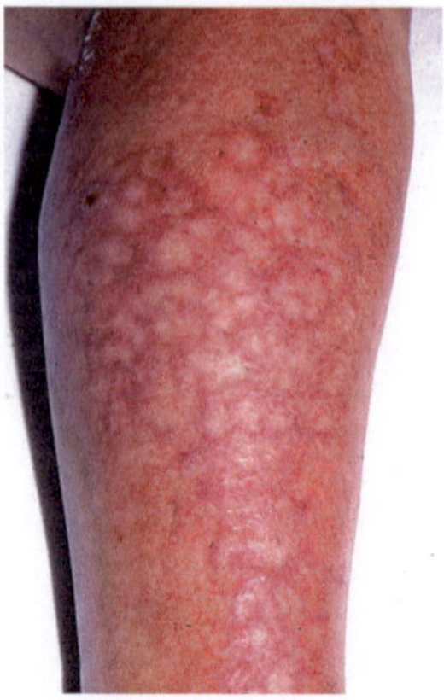

Fig. 3.2 Thermal injury: retiform skin reaction from chronic heat exposure (Buschke melanosis)

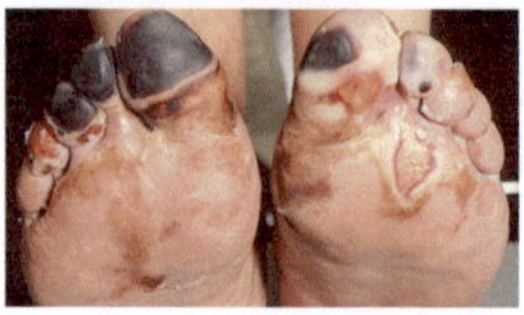

Fig. 3.3 Thermal injury: necrosis of toes from freezing

Level

Advanced

ICD-11

NE2Z

Synonyms

Burns; combustio, ambustio.

Epidemiology

Most frequent accidents in household and leisure.

Definition

Physical damage to the skin with tissue destruction of varying degrees caused by thermal energy.

Aetiology and Pathogenesis

Direct tissue damage from exogenous thermal energy of different origin.

Signs and Symptoms

Cascade of erythema, blistering and necrosis depending on severity and length of exposure.

Localisation

Area of exposure with strongest damage is related to the site of highest exposure.

Classification

Burns are divided into three degrees:

- First degree characterised by erythema and pain.
- Second degree characterised by:
  - grade 2 a: superficial with epidermal and dermal blistering
  - grade 2 b: deep dermal blistering and destruction of hair
- Third degree characterised by involvement of all layers and all adnexae, with extension to the subcutis and muscles.

Laboratory and Other Workups

Grade 2b and grade 3: monitoring of electrolyte and protein balance.

Dermatopathology

Depending on the degree of tissue damage, varying from little papillary oedema with initial subepidermal blistering and dilatation of blood vessels, vacuolated or necrotic keratinocytes without inflammatory infiltrate to complete tissue necrosis.

Course

Varies with degree of severity and extent. More extensive burns treated in specialised burn centres with intensive care. Burns involving >40% of skin surface area are often fatal.

Complications

Shock in severe cases and super-infections. Children with >5% and adults with >10% surface involvement have to be admitted to the hospital.

Diagnosis

History and clinical features.

Differential Diagnosis

Scalds, chemical burns.

Prevention and Therapy

Must be adjusted to extent and severity. Minor burns should be cooled, local corticoid emulsions; prevention of superinfection. With more severe burns, temperature control is a problem. Management involves wound care, electrolyte and protein replacement, pain control and systemic antibiotics and referral to regional burn centre for intensive care. Skin transplantation can be considered. Preservation of normal skin for in vitro growth and cell culture.

Special

Critical body surface involvement >10% children and > 20% adults.

Pernio

Figures 3.4 and 3.5

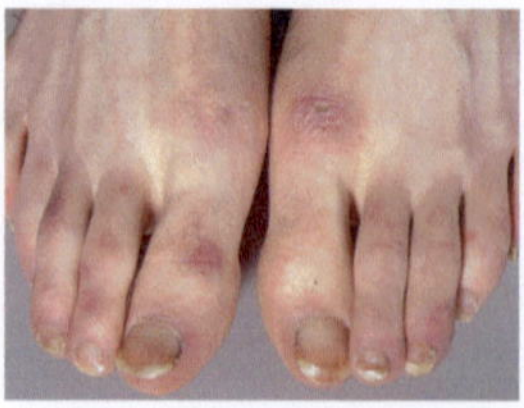

Fig. 3.4 Pernio: violaceous frostbites on the feet

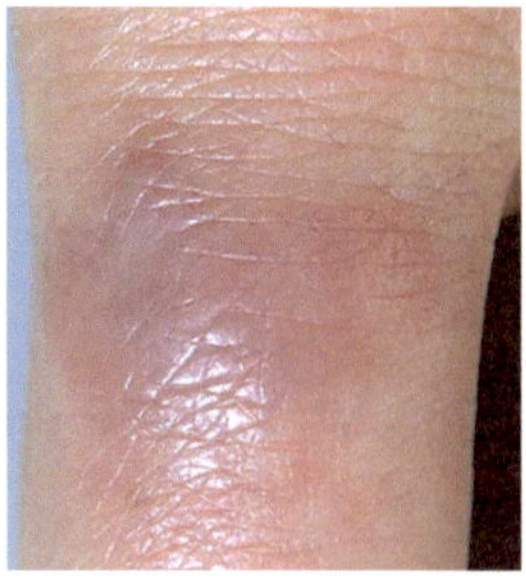

Fig. 3.5 Pernio: acral violaceous frostbites on the knee

Grading of Importance

A

Level

Advanced

ICD-11

NF03.0

Synonyms

Dermatitis congelatio escharotica; chilblains; perniosis

Epidemiology

Congelatio quite frequent in winter sport activities, mountain tracking; perniones mostly appear in spring and autumn around 0 °C. Often in adolescents with acrocyanosis (horse riding, long time cycling, inappropriate shoes, wet socks).

Definition

Congelatio: first to third degree with maximum of irreversible necrosis or death.

Perniones: cold-induced blue-red indurated papules or nodules, usually on legs or feet. F > M.

Aetiology and Pathogenesis

Congelatio dependent on temperature grade and exposure time. Persistent exposure to cold, damp conditions predisposes to development of pernio over days to weeks.

Signs and Symptoms

In congelatio in grade 1 erythematous lesions, in grade 2 bullous lesions and grade 3 necrosis with irreversible sequelae.

In perniones blue-red oedematous papules or nodules, sometimes quite tender or painful.

Localisation

Typically occur at acral sites and in areas which are easily cooled (especially the shins, fingers, toes and other thighs in equestrians). Dampness is also important, and some professions are at increased risk, such as butchers and farmers. In congelatio depending if local or full body cold exposure.

Classification

Congelatio: Grades 1–3.

Laboratory and Other Workups

None.

Dermatopathology

Congelatio: depending on degree vessel narrowing, blistering, apoptosis and necrosis.

Perniones: severe courses show blistering, oedema, hyperemic vessels and lymphocytic vasculitis.

Course

Congelatio: depending on length of injury in part reversible or irreversible.

Perniones: Recurrent, more common in spring and autumn (cool, moist climatic conditions).

Complications

Congelatio: long-term downcooling leads to death.
Perniones: Rarely ulceration.

Diagnosis

History, localisation, clinical features.

Differential Diagnosis

Lupus pernio (sarcoidosis), chilblain lupus (lupus erythematosus).

Prevention and Therapy

Congelatio: slow warming up of central temperature, no direct warming of involved lesions. Hyperbaric oxygenation to avoid amputation, prostaglandin infusions.

Perniones: warm, water-resistant protective clothing, topical or oral vasodilators (e.g. calcium channel blockers).

Special

Severe congelatio must be referred to special centres for intensive care.

Sunburn

Figure 3.6

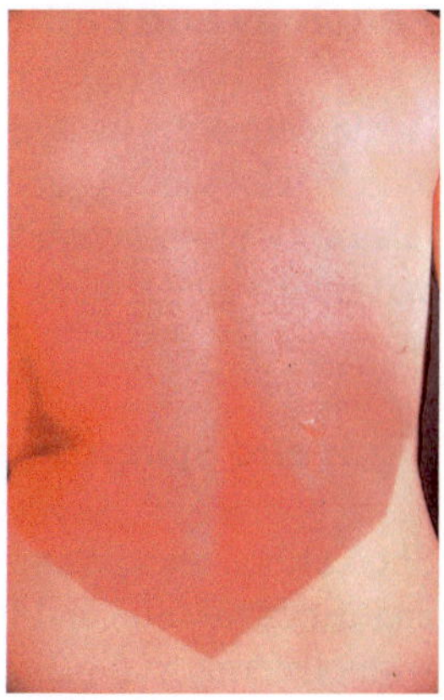

Fig. 3.6 Sunburn: erythema following unprotected sun exposure

Grading of Importance

A

Level

Advanced

ICD-11

EJ40

Synonyms

Solar dermatitis.

Epidemiology

Very often to be observed during leisure time and vacation in sun rich areas, i.e. when no or inappropriate sun protection is available or used.

Definition

Acute toxic photo-dermatitis caused by electromagnetic radiation in UVB range (290–320 nm). Unphysiologically high UVA (320–400 nm) doses can elicit an erythema too.

Aetiology and Pathogenesis

Acute dermatitis caused by erythematogenic doses of UVB radiation, more common in fair-skinned patients (Fitzpatrick skin types I-II). More severe cases result in release of proinflammatory cytokines (IL-6), prostaglandins (PGE2), leucotrienes and isoprostans leading to systemic symptoms.

Signs and Symptoms

Short after overexposure to UVB prickling, itching and burning. Depending on dose and exposure time and latitude within 12 to 24 hours erythema. In severe courses with blistering and pain. Fever.

Localisation

In areas exposed to light.

Classification

First degree: burning, erythema, desquamation.

Second degree: blisters, weeping, crusts.

Rarely third degree: necrosis.

Laboratory and Other Workups

CRP may be increased.

Dermatopathology

Apoptosis and necrosis of epidermal keratinocytes. Langerhans cell dysfunction and decrease in numbers. Oedema. Submicroscopically mutations by cyclobutan dimers.

Course

Highly variable clinical appearance (just as in acute dermatitis): erythema, vesicles or blisters, weeping, crusts, scales. When severe, fever and malaise. Complete spontaneous healing.

Complications

Frequent sunburns, especially in childhood, lead to increased numbers of melanocytic naevi and an increased risk of malignant melanoma as well as non-melanoma skin cancer later in life.

Diagnosis

By case history and clinical picture.

Differential Diagnosis

Acute contact dermatitis, photoallergic or phototoxic reactions, diseases provoked by light, lupus erythematosus.

Prevention and Therapy

Within the first 12 hours nonsteroidal anti-inflammatory drugs and class 3 antihistamines with effects on leucotrienes combined. Cooling topical agents (lotions, cold creams), wet dressings, later topical or systemic corticosteroids. Oral fluid.

Special

Solar injury to brain with complications and oedema need hospitalisation especially in children.

Photodermatoses [6, 2]

Figures 3.7, 3.8, 3.9 and 3.10

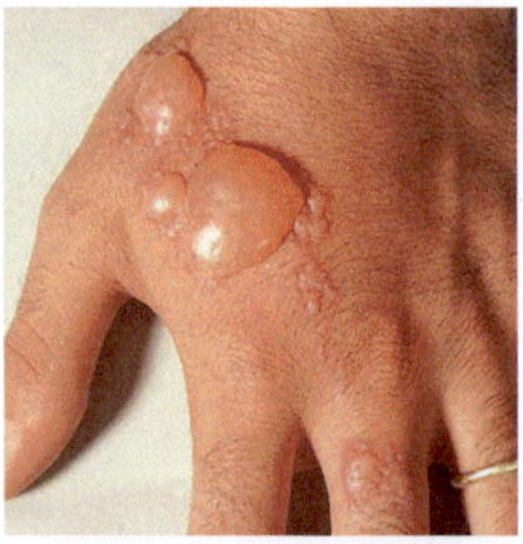

Fig. 3.7 Photodermatoses: blister formation due to furocoumarin contact from meadow

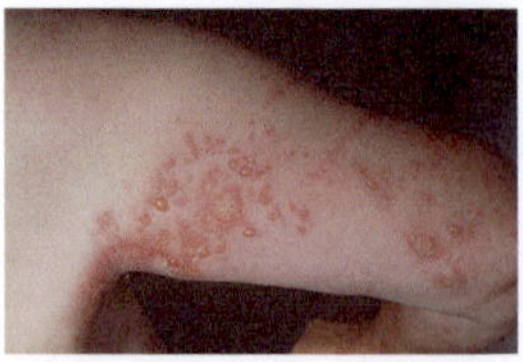

Fig. 3.8 Photodermatoses: polymorphic light eruption of the upper arm

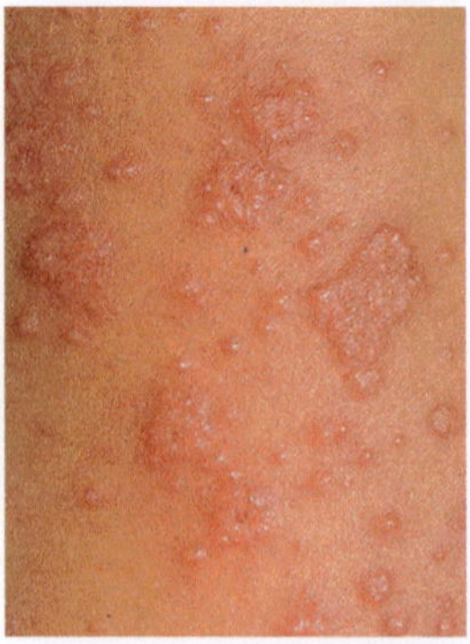

Fig. 3.9 Photodermatoses: closeup view of polymorphic light eruption

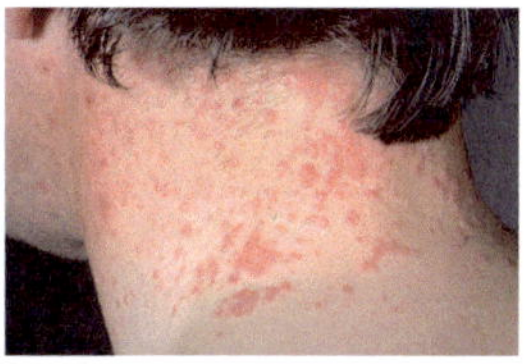

Fig. 3.10 Photodermatoses: polymorphic light eruption of the neck

Grading of Importance

C

Level

Advanced

ICD-11

EJ30

Synonyms

Photodermatitis.

Epidemiology

Polymorphous light eruption (PMLE) is the most common photodermatosis (prevalence 10% to 20%), followed in decreasing order of frequency by photoaggravated dermatoses, drug-induced photosensitivity, chronic actinic dermatitis (CAD), porphyrias and solar urticaria (SU).

Definition

Dermatoses caused by electromagnetic radiation in the ultraviolet (UV) or visible light spectrum with or without other enhancing co-factors.

Aetiology and Pathogenesis

UV light can cause dermatitis as a single agent (sunburn; see section "Sunburn" in Chap. 3) or in combination with phototoxic (furocoumarins such as psoralens) or photoallergic substances (medications such as sulphones, promethazine). Ultraviolet B (UVB) is the main spectrum responsible for skin erythema, whereas ultraviolet A (UVA) is mostly involved in the drug-induced photosensitivity reactions. In all instances, oxygen-free radicals trigger the release of pro-inflammatory cytokines (acute dermatitis) or cause permanent skin damage (chronic actinic damage). In addition, some skin disorders are negatively influenced by light; e.g. lupus erythematosus and herpes simplex.

Signs and Symptoms

The most relevant idiopathic immune-mediated or drug-induced photodermatoses is polymorphic light eruption (PMLE) exhibiting itching in exposed skin (occasionally sparing the face). It develops minutes to hours after sun exposure and tends to resolve within hours, days or rarely weeks.

Chronic actinic dermatitis (CAD) is a rare, persistent chronic, usually lichenified (UV- and rarely visible) light-induced dermatosis. CAD occurs most commonly in elderly men. Tends to persist over many years.

Solar urticaria (SU). UVB, UVA and chronic visible light inducible urticaria. Wheals confined to sunlight-exposed skin appear a few minutes after visible radiation exposure.

Drug- and exogenous chemical-induced photosensitivity include:

- **Phototoxic** (non-immunologically mediated) reactions are the result of direct tissue injury caused by a phototoxic agent and radiation. Clinically may resemble acute sunburn. May be induced by either topical or systemic medications, as well as systemic/topical agents (e.g. food ingredients)
- **Photoallergic** reactions are type IV delayed hypersensitivity responses that occur only in pre-sensitised individuals and require only a minimal concentration of the photoallergen. Clinically resembles eczematous dermatitis. Induced mostly by systemic medications

Localisation

In phototoxic reactions usually are restricted to area(s) of light exposure. Photoallergic reactions may show distant spread.

Classification

Photosensitive cutaneous disorders can be classified into four main categories:

- Idiopathic photodermatoses, immunologically mediated where light alone triggers the disease, e.g. polymorphic light eruption, solar urticaria, hydroa vacciniforme

- Drug- and chemical-induced photosensibility, including a subgroup of phototoxic or photoallergic dermatoses triggered by exogenous topical or systemic substances, and a second subgroup of metabolic disorders in which there is endogenous accumulation of phototoxic substances because of enzymatic defects, e.g. cutaneous porphyrias
- Genodermatoses characterised by a defective DNA repair, in which there is increased sensitivity to light, e.g. xeroderma pigmentosum secondary to a defect in DNA-repair enzymes
- Photoaggravated dermatoses. Include a heterogeneous group of disorders

Laboratory and Other Workups

In cases of photodistributed eruption of unknown aetiology, consider a complete blood cell count, biochemical evaluation (liver function tests) and autoantibody screening (ANA, anti-dsDNA, anti-Ro) to exclude connective tissue diseases, and porphyrins in blood, urine and stool may be useful for a definite diagnosis. Genetic testing in rare situations.

Dermatopathology

Histological changes are often non-specific. May be helpful in some cases of PMLE or CAD to rule out other possible diagnoses.

Course

Variable. Depending on the different subtypes.

Complications

In severe SU, anaphylactic shock may occur after whole-body exposure.

Diagnosis

History is often most helpful. Questioning regarding possible exposure to various photosensitisers, such as topical and systemic medications, cosmetics and fragrances, and plant extracts may suggest a diagnosis of phototoxicity or photoallergy. Light testing: monochromatic UVA and UVB sensitivity testing, photo patch testing, provocation challenge with UV and/or visible light. In some cases patch testing should be recommended to rule out associated allergic contact dermatitis.

Differential Diagnosis

Depending on the different entities. In PMLE the differential diagnosis should be established with photoallergic eczemas, solar urticaria, erythema multiforme, even lupus erythematosus (LE), malabsorption, etc. SU lesions should be distinguished from erythropoietic protoporphyria, urticarial phototoxic reactions, other forms of physical urticaria and PMLE (urticarial lesions), whereas in patients with CAD, the diagnoses of photoallergic reaction, airborne contact dermatitis, mycosis fungoides, and chronic atopic eczema should be ruled out.

Prevention and Therapy

Light protection: Appropriate clothing; appropriate environmental UV exposure modification (e.g. at workplace). Appropriate sunscreens with SPF 50/UVA filters. Treatment of any underlying disorder.

Topical steroids and antihistamines can be used for symptomatic relief. Possible systemic treatments for chronic, refractory cases: antimalarials or immunosuppressive drugs (azathioprine, ciclosporin, mycophenolate mofetil) or thalidomide. Avoid potential photosensitising agents.

Radiation Dermatitis [1]

Figures 3.11 and 3.12

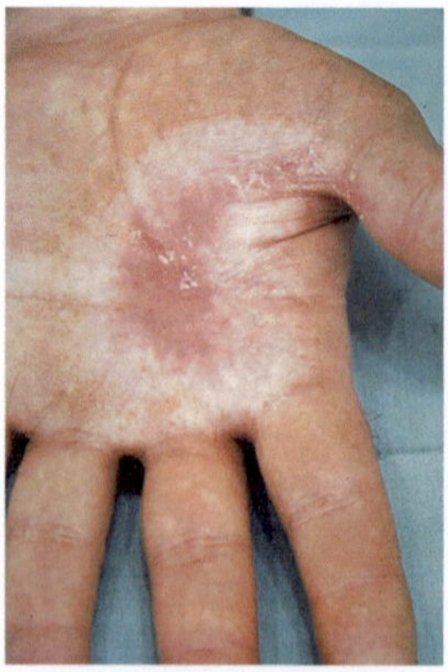

Fig. 3.11 Radiation dermatitis: atrophy following radiation of malignant tumor

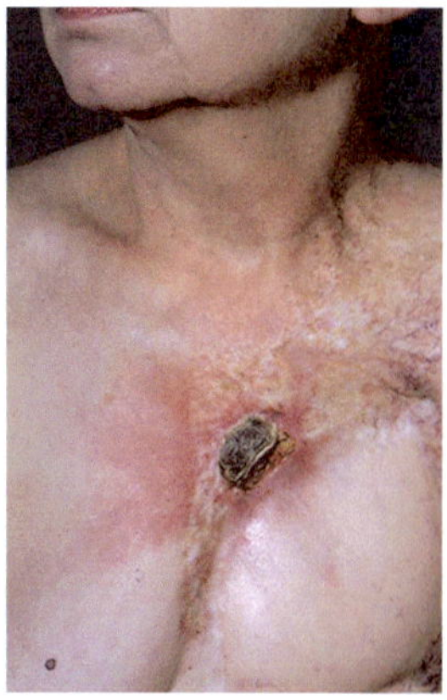

Fig. 3.12 Radiation dermatitis: ulceration and chronic radiodermatitis following radiation on breast tumor. Development of non-melanoma skin cancer to be ruled out

Grading of Importance

B

Level

Advanced

Definition

Acute or chronic skin damage caused by short wavelength electromagnetic radiation (x-rays or gamma rays).

ICD-11

EL61

Aetiology and Pathogenesis

DNA damage from high energy radiation.

Signs and Symptoms

Varies with acuity:

- Acute radiation dermatitis: erythema 10 days after exposure.
- Chronic radiation dermatitis: poikiloderma (hypo- and hyperpigmentation, atrophy and telangiectasia) occurring more than 2 years after exposure.

Localisation

Irradiated area.

Classification

Acute and chronic radiation dermatitis.

Course

Most acute radiation dermatitis heals completely; chronic radiation dermatitis leads to atrophy of skin, scarring and thus permanent changes.

Complications

In chronic radiation dermatitis, there is a risk of developing radiation ulcers and radiation keratosis and, rarely, squamous cell carcinomas or other radiation-induced non-melanoma skin cancer and other skin tumours.

Diagnosis

History, clinical features.

Differential Diagnosis

Burn, scars.

Prevention and Therapy

Acute radiation dermatitis: topical corticosteroids, sometimes systemic corticosteroids for their anti-inflammatory action.

Chronic radiation dermatitis: light protection, protection from physical or chemical irritation, topical retinoids.

References

1. Bhangoo R, Cheng T, Petersen M, Thorpe C, DeWees T, Anderson J, Vargas C, Patel S, Halyard M, Schild S, Wong W (2022) Radiation recall dermatitis: a review of the literature. Semin Oncol 49:152–159
2. Furukawa JY, Martinez RM, Morocho-Jacome AL, Castillo-Gomez TS, Pereda-Contreras VJ, Rosado C, Velasco MVR, Baby AR (2021) Skin impacts from exposure to ultraviolet, visible, infrared, and artificial lights – a review. J Cosmet Laser Ther 23(1–2):1–7
3. Wollina U (2022) Disorders Caused by Physical and Chemical Damage in Braun-Falco´s Dermatology pp 775–793.
4. Handford C, Thomas O, Imray CHE (2017) Frostbite. Emerg Med Clin North Am 35(2):281–299
5. Cappel JA, Wetter DA. Clinical characteristics, etiologic associations, laboratory findings, treatment, and proposal of diagnostic criteria of pernio (chilblains) in a series of 104 patients at Mayo Clinic, 2000 to 2011. Mayo Clin Proc. 2014;89(2):207–15. https://doi.org/10.1016/j.mayocp.2013.09.020. PMID: 24485134
6. Burfield L, Rutter KJ, Thompson B, Marjanovic EJ, Neale RE, Rhodes LE. Systematic review of the prevalence and incidence of the photodermatoses with metaanalysis of the prevalence of polymorphic light eruption. J Eur Acad Dermatol Venereol. 2023;37(3):511–520. https://doi.org/10.1111/jdv.18772. Epub 2022 Dec 3. PMID: 36433668.
7. Neale RE, Lucas RM, Byrne SN, Hollestein L, Rhodes LE, Yazar S, Young AR, Berwick M, Ireland RA, Olsen CM. The effects of exposure to solar radiation on human health. Photochem Photobiol Sci. 2023;22(5):1011–1047. https://doi.org/10.1007/s43630-023-00375-8. Epub 2023 Mar 1. PMID: 36856971; PMCID: PMC9976694

Granulomatous Dermatoses

4

Martine Bagot and Christos C. Zouboulis

Contents

M. Bagot (✉)
Service de Dermatologie, Université Paris Cité, Hôpital Saint-Louis, Paris, France
e-mail: martine.bagot@gmail.com

C. C. Zouboulis
Departments of Dermatology, Venereology, Allergology and Immunology, Staedtisches Klinikum Dessau, Brandenburg Medical School Theodor Fontane and Faculty of Health Sciences Brandenburg, Dessau, Germany
e-mail: christos.zouboulis@mhb-fontane.de

H. Gollnick et al. (eds.), *Dermatology Cyberderm WebBook*,
https://doi.org/10.1007/978-3-031-78491-0_4

Test your learning and check your understanding of this book's contents: use the "Springer Nature Flashcards" app to access questions using ▶ https://sn.pub/1rhh6k.
To use the app, please follow the instructions in Chap. 1.

Sarcoidosis [1–3]

Figures 4.1, 4.2 and 4.3

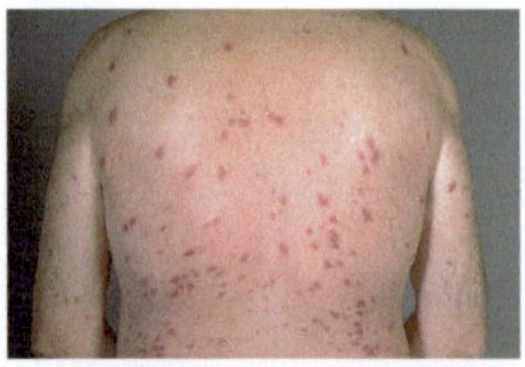

Fig. 4.1 Sarcoidosis: dermal papules, plaques and nodules on the back

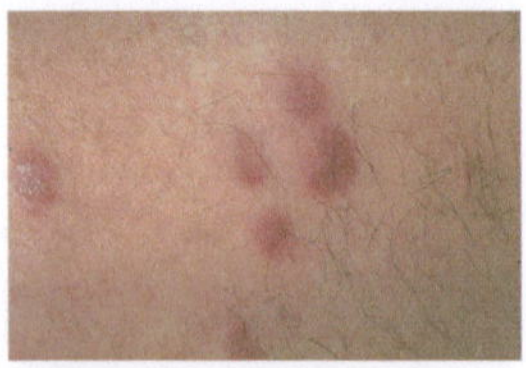

Fig. 4.2 Sarcoidosis: closeup view of brown-violaceous lesions

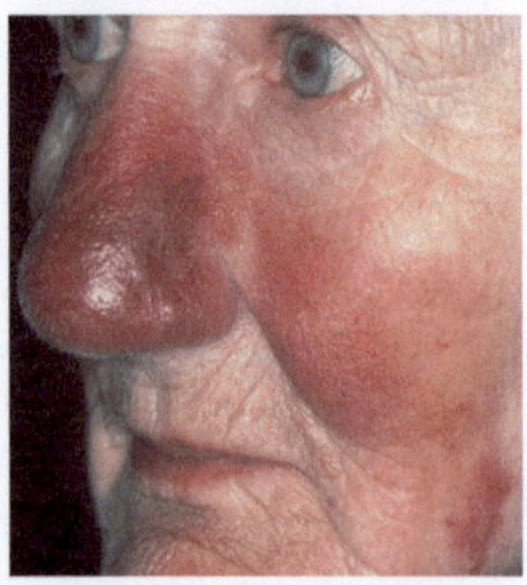

Fig. 4.3 Sarcoidosis: Lupus pernio (centrofacial skin involvement)

Grading of Importance

B

Level

Advanced

ICD-11

4B20

Synonyms

Boeck disease, Besnier-Boeck-Schaumann disease, benign lymphogranulomatosis.

Epidemiology

Rare disease. Skin involvement in 20–35% of cases; in 11% skin as first manifestation. The estimated prevalence in Europe is around 10/100,000 inhabitants; significantly higher in northern countries.

Definition

Systemic granulomatous disease with skin involvement.

Aetiology and Pathogenesis

Unclear, found worldwide, female > male. It occurs most commonly in young and middle-aged individuals of all races. Afro-Caribbeans and African-Americans more commonly involved.

Signs and Symptoms

Many possible skin findings: brown-violaceous dermal papules, plaques or nodules. Often associated with erythema nodosum. Systemic disease involve lymph nodes in 90% of patients, mostly intrathoracic, lungs (90%), eyes (30%), kidneys, bones, neural system, liver and GI tract.

Localisation

All skin areas can be involved.

Classification

Special forms:

- Löfgren's syndrome (acute onset of fever, bilateral hilar lymphadenopathy and erythema nodosum)
- Lupus pernio (centrofacial skin involvement)
- Scar and tattoo sarcoidosis

Laboratory and Other Workups

- Angiotensin converting enzyme (ACE; indicating cumulative involvement) and interleukin 2 receptor (IL2R; indicating disease activity) in serum sometimes elevated
- Hypercalcaemia
- Lymphopenia
- ESR elevated
- Impaired delayed (type IV) hypersensitivity
- Tuberculin skin test (negative)
- Chest x-ray (may show bilateral hilar lymphadenopathy or interstitial changes)

Dermatopathology

Epithelioid cell granulomas without caseation, few CD4+ T lymphocytes (naked granulomas).

Course

Chronic; spontaneous remission in about 25%.

Complications

Restrictive lung disease, immune suppression (lymphopenia), osteoporosis (in corticosteroid-treated patients; calcium supplementation contraindicated). Cutaneous calcification (calcinosis cutis).

Diagnosis

Clinical features, histology, laboratory findings.

Differential Diagnosis

Tuberculosis, leprosy, granuloma annulare, necrobiosis lipoidica, lymphoma, leishmaniasis, amyloidosis, rosacea (lupus pernio).

Prevention and Therapy

Prevention of occupational and individual chronic small particle inhalation:

- Skin involvement: Corticosteroids (topical, intralesional, systemic; first line), methotrexate (second line), chloroquine/hydroxychloroquine, PUVA.
- Systemic involvement: Corticosteroids (systemic; first line), methotrexate (second line), azathioprine, (leflunomide, mycophenolate mofetil, cyclophosphamide, TNF antagonists. Biologics may induce sarcoidosis.

Granuloma Annulare (GA) [4, 5, 6]

Figures 4.4 and 4.5

Grading of Importance

C

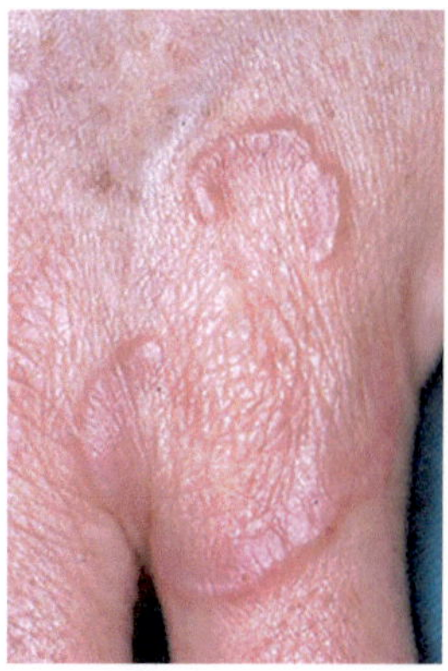

Fig. 4.4 Granuloma annulare: ringlike arrangement of small papules on the dorsum of the hand

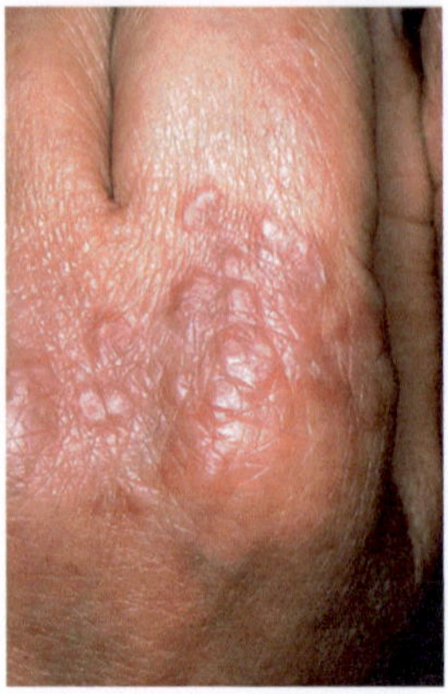

Fig. 4.5 Granuloma annulare: papules over the finger joint

Level

Advanced

ICD-11

EE80.0

Synonyms

None.

Epidemiology

Granuloma annulare is a common skin disorder. Prevalence is 0.1% to 0.4%, annual incidences 0.1% to 0.4%, women more frequently affected than men, and 2/3 of the patients are less than 30 years old.

Definition

Granuloma annulare is a granulomatous dermal or subcutaneous disorder characterised by infiltrating mononuclear cells that presents with skin-coloured or reddish, annular or papular lesions related to different aetiologic background.

Aetiology and Pathogenesis

The cause of granuloma annulare is unclear, but it can be associated with autoimmune diseases, diabetes mellitus, HIV infection or malignancies.

Signs and Symptoms

Granuloma annulare consists of localized or disseminated firm, small, skin-coloured or reddish papules arranged in rings or arcs or hard, mobile, dermal and subcutaneous nodules.

Localisation

Granuloma annulare typically appears on the extensor surfaces of the extremities, in a disseminated form also on the trunk.

Classification

Localized, disseminated, subcutaneous and perforating types.

Laboratory and Other Workups

In isolated granuloma annulare, no laboratory testing is needed. In disseminated granuloma annulare, HIV serology, complete blood count, glycaemia and lipid profile may be tested. Unusual courses of the disease and clinical pictures need histological confirmation.

Dermatopathology

Granuloma annulare is characterized by loose, degenerative collagen bundles (necrobiosis) with a peripheral cuff of lymphocytes and histiocytes and palisading of the granuloma.

Course

Spontaneous remission, recurrences, or a chronic evolution are possible. The treatment of disseminated chronic forms is difficult.

Complications

None, except possibly underlying associated disease.

Diagnosis

The diagnosis is obtained by clinico-pathological correlation.

Differential Diagnosis

Sarcoidosis, necrobiosis lipoidica, foreign body granuloma, rheumatoid nodules, interstitial granulomatous dermatitis, tuberculoid leprosy and syphilis.

Prevention and Therapy

Therapeutic abstention except detection of underlying disease or psychoreactive reactions, topical corticosteroids or cryotherapy are possible in limited forms. Phototherapy, dapsone, retinoids, hydroxychloroquine and TNF alpha blockers can be considered in disseminated forms. Strong regulation of diabetic metabolism. Appropriate medication in rheumatic diseases.Preventive measures are not possible.

References

1. Haimovic A, Sanchez M, Judson MA, Prystowsky S (2012a) Sarcoidosis: a comprehensive review and update for the dermatologist: part I. Cutaneous disease. J Am Acad Dermatol 66(5):699 e691–699 e618; quiz 717–698
2. Haimovic A, Sanchez M, Judson MA, Prystowsky S (2012b) Sarcoidosis: a comprehensive review and update for the dermatologist: part II. Extracutaneous disease. J Am Acad Dermatol 66(5):719 e711–719 e710; quiz 729–730
3. Iannuzzi MC, Rybicki BA, Teirstein AS (2007) Sarcoidosis. N Engl J Med 357(21):2153–2165
4. Piette EW, Rosenbach M (2016a) Granuloma annulare: clinical and histologic variants, epidemiology, and genetics. J Am Acad Dermatol 75(3):457–465
5. Piette EW, Rosenbach M (2016b) Granuloma annulare: pathogenesis, disease associations and triggers, and therapeutic options. J Am Acad Dermatol 75(3):467–479
6. Schmieder SJ, Harper CD, Schmieder GJ (2020) Granuloma Annulare. StatPearls, Treasure Island, FL

Papulosquamous Disorders

5

Christos C. Zouboulis, Günter Burg, and Harald Gollnick

Contents

C. C. Zouboulis (✉)
Departments of Dermatology, Venereology, Allergology and Immunology, Staedtisches Klinikum Dessau, Brandenburg Medical School Theodor Fontane and Faculty of Health Sciences Brandenburg, Dessau, Germany
e-mail: christos.zouboulis@mhb-fontane.de

G. Burg
Dermatology, Zurich, Switzerland
e-mail: g.burg@access.uzh.ch

H. Gollnick
Department of Dermatology & Venereology, Otto-von-Guericke University, Magdeburg, Germany
e-mail: Harald.Gollnick@med.ovgu.de

H. Gollnick et al. (eds.), *Dermatology Cyberderm WebBook*,
https://doi.org/10.1007/978-3-031-78491-0_5

Test your learning and check your understanding of this book's contents: use the "Springer Nature Flashcards" app to access questions using ▶ https://sn.pub/1rhh6k.

To use the app, please follow the instructions in Chap. 1.

Psoriasis [1, 2]

Figures 5.1, 5.2, 5.3, 5.4, 5.5, 5.6, 5.7, 5.8, 5.9 and 5.10

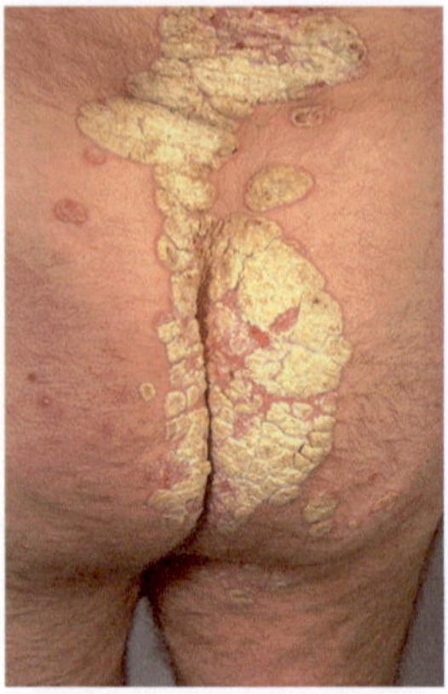

Fig. 5.1 Psoriasis: thick, hyperkeratotic plaques on the buttocks

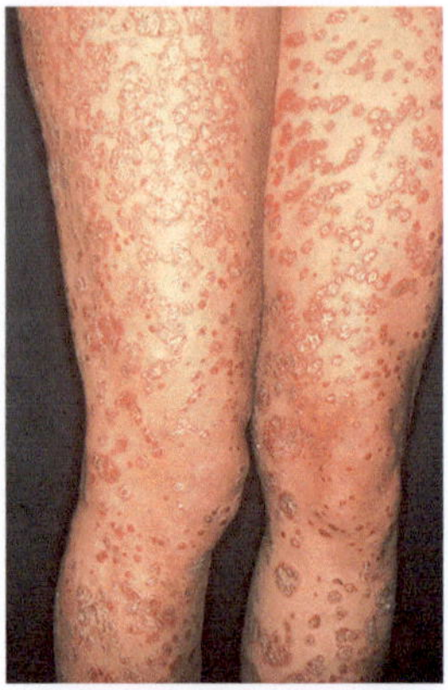

Fig. 5.2 Psoriasis: guttate type psoriasis

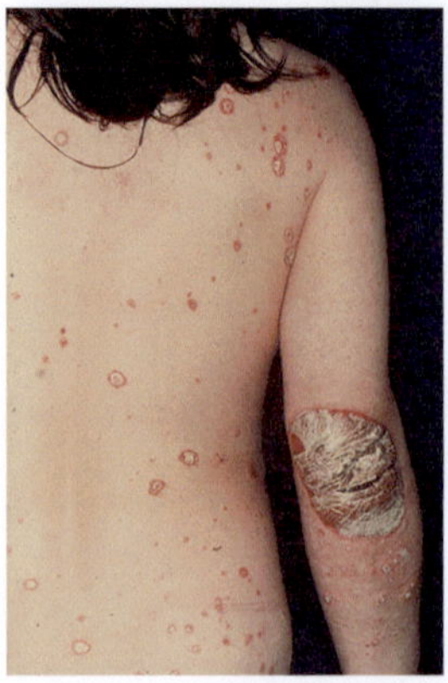

Fig. 5.3 Psoriasis: thick hyperkeratotic plaque with fissures on the elbow

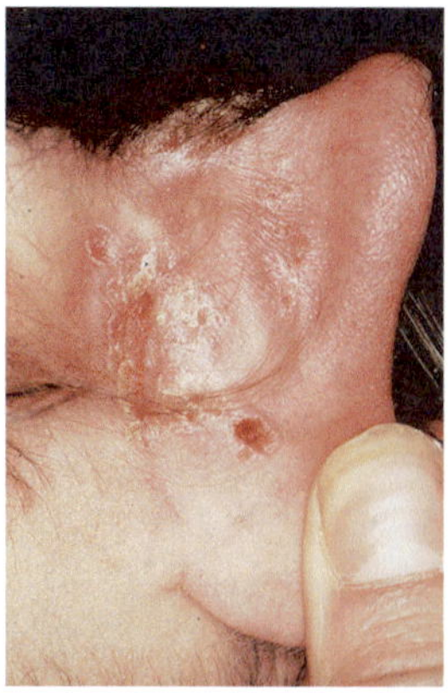

Fig. 5.4 Psoriasis: retro auricular scaly lesion

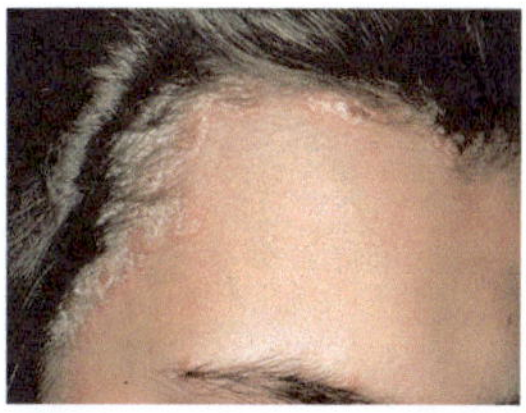

Fig. 5.5 Psoriasis: scalp involvement

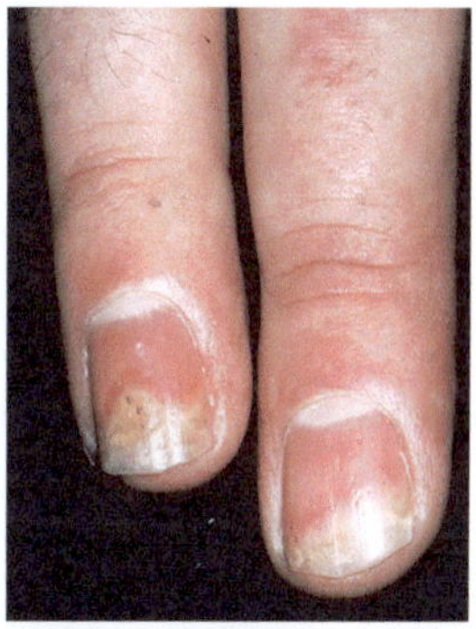

Fig. 5.6 Psoriasis: nail involvement with pits and oil spot

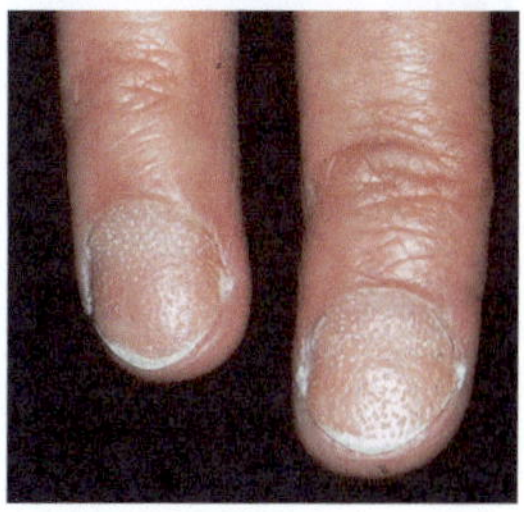

Fig. 5.7 Psoriasis: nail pits

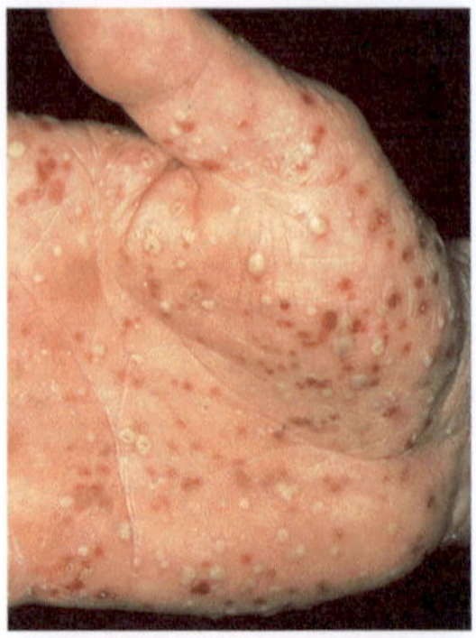

Fig. 5.8 Psoriasis: palmar pustulosis

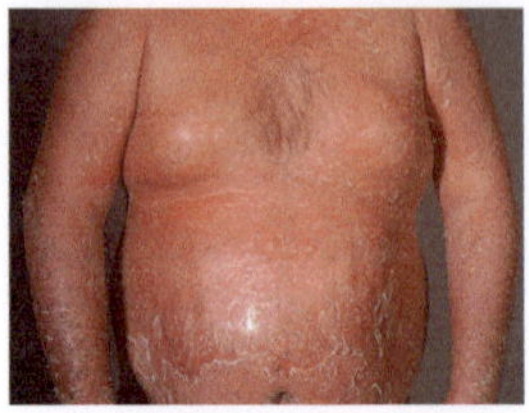

Fig. 5.9 Psoriasis: psoriatic erythroderma

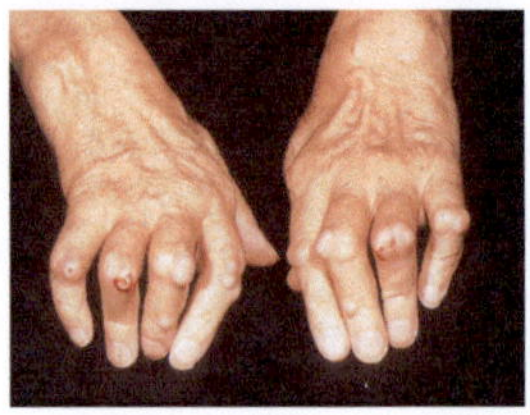

Fig. 5.10 Psoriasis: psoriatic arthritis

Grading of Importance

B

Level

Advanced

ICD-11

EA90

Synonyms

"Schuppenflechte" (German); "leprosy" in former times (nowadays wrong term)

Epidemiology

- About 125 million people worldwide affected (2%–4% of the population in Western countries)
- Different degrees of clinical manifestation depending on genetic background, age and geographic as well as environmental factors
- Adults (from 0.9% to 8.5%) more frequently affected than children (from 0% to 2.1%)
- Dual peak of incidence: 30–39 years (type 1) and > 40 years of age (type 2)
- About 20% of psoriatic patients develop sero-negative arthritis
- Many co-morbidities (see below)

Definition

- Systemic, chronic auto-inflammatory and auto-immune, hyperkeratotic skin disease with a spectrum of clinical phenotypes, frequently associated with co-morbidities (psychological, metabolic, arthritic and cardiovascular co-morbidities)
- Interplay of genetic, epigenetic, environmental and immunological factors.

Aetiology and Pathogenesis

Susceptibility to psoriasis involving both adaptive and innate immune system. While adaptive immune responses predominate in chronic plaque psoriasis, innate and auto-inflammatory responses dominate in pustular forms of psoriasis.

- Psoriasis shows polygenic inheritance. Genome-wide association studies report that the histocompatibility complex HLA-C*06:02 (previously known as HLA-Cw6) is associated with early-onset psoriasis and guttate psoriasis.
- Genotype and exogenous factors (e.g. local effects like Köbner's phenomenon or systemic ones) are responsible for phenotypic expression.
- Psoriasis is multifactorial and an immune-mediated inflammatory disease (IMID). Pathological mechanisms: Th17 cells play a key role with interleukin IL-23 mainly produced by dendritic cells. Null-Th17 cells produce various cytokines, including IL-17A, IL-17F and IL-22. IL-17A and IL-22 induce not only keratinocyte proliferation but also tumour necrosis factor (TNF)-a. TNF-a accelerates the infiltration of inflammatory cells, including lymphocytes, monocytes and neutrophils.
- Provocation and maintaining factors: physical, chemical, metabolic, certain inflammatory diseases (dermatoses), drugs (lithium, chloroquine, beta-blockers, interferon-alpha), infections (streptococci, HIV), alcohol, nicotine, fatty food and stress.

Signs and Symptoms

- Circumscribed erythematous-squamous plaques bordering silvery scales of different sizes and thickness ranging from guttate to large "geographic" plaque lesions.
- Never vesicles or blisters.
- Pustules may appear on site of lesions or primarily (pustular psoriasis).
- Dystrophic or pitted nails or yellowish discolouring (oil patch).
- Palmo-plantar hyperkeratosis.
- Occasionally gyrate pattern on the mucosa (tongue, lips or glans penis/labiae).
- When scales are very thick: intense itch, pain and scaly skin lesions that can crack and bleed.
- Koebner's sign; candle sign: production of candle grease-like scale when scraping a plaque with curette.
- Auspitz sign: punctate bleeding when psoriasis scales are scraped away, due to a thin layer of suprapapillary epidermis.

Localisation

- Sites of predilection: extensor surfaces (knees, elbows), scalp, retroauricular, sacral, gluteal cleft, umbilicus, genital, intertriginous (psoriasis inversa type with involvement of scalp, axillae, genitalia, groins, rima ani), palmo-plantar, nails.

Classification

The recent last classifications of the acute and chronic types proposed by the International Psoriasis Council identifies the following main forms of psoriasis:

- Plaque-type
- Guttate
- General pustular psoriasis (GPP)
- Erythroderma
- In addition several further subphenotypes may be differentiated according to distribution (localised vs. widespread), anatomical localisation (flexural, scalp, palms/soles/nail, inversal areas), size (large vs. small) and thickness (thick vs. thin) of plaques and scales, onset (early vs. late) and disease activity (active vs. stable)
- Psoriatic arthritis (HLA-B27): different subphenotypes with localisation at vertebrae, cervical, iliosacral, distal joints or fingers

Laboratory and Other Workups

No specific blood test for psoriasis, sometimes HLA- C6 can help in differentiating type 1 from type 2.

- Laboratory workup for co-morbidities (CRP, blood count, kidney, liver and lipid values can be examined).
- A skin biopsy should be taken if uncertain type of lesions occur or other differential diagnoses have to be excluded.

Dermatopathology

- Confluent hyperkeratosis and parakeratosis.
- Intracorneal neutrophils (Munro microabscesses).
- Acanthosis is thickening of the rete ridges or reduced layers above papilla.
- Elongation and widening of the papillary spiral-like formed capillaries.
- A strong lympho-mononuclear inflammatory infiltrate mixed with neutrophilic granulocytes in the dermis.

Course

In general, the course is chronic-recurrent or chronic-persistent. Acute eruptions such as the guttate forms sometimes clear with complete resolution (streptococcal infection, drug cessation). Chronic plaque-like types may suddenly show exacerbations with disseminated guttate lesions or becoming more inflammatory and growing in size.

Complications

- Co-morbidities (see above).
- Reduced quality of life and reduced life span.
- Disabling features (nails, joints).
- Superinfections (staphylococci, streptococci, Malassezia furfur).
- Non-melanoma skin cancer in patients with long-term photo- or photochemotherapy or therapy with cytotoxic agents.
- Incidence of lung cancer and CTCL type of lymphoma may be increased, but not colon, breast or prostate cancer.

Diagnosis

Clinical features and histopathology in unclear cases.

Differential Diagnosis

- Pityriasiform or guttate like lesions such as in secondary syphilis, pityriasis rosea, in those of the parapsoriasis group, in pityriasis rubra pilaris and in cutaneous T-cell lymphoma (mycosis fungoides)
- Chronic nummular eczema
- Hypertrophic lichen planus
- Tinea corporis, pemphigus foliaceus, glucagonoma syndrome
- Discoid and subacute cutaneous lupus erythematosus
- Seborrhoeic dermatitis, especially on the head and neck area (combined type seborrhiasis with M. furfur pityriasis capillitii and psoriasis of scalp and face)

Prevention and Therapy

Prevention

Avoidance of provocation factors (see above).

Therapy

In general, the type of psoriasis, acute or non-acute, localisation, age and professional activities, adherence and quality of life, co-morbidities and additional arthritis have in each patient individually to be considered.

Topical Therapy

Topical therapy is indicated when less than 10% of body surface is involved or PASI score is <10. Certain localisations such as face, scalp, nails and hands need combined therapies.

- Salicylic acid in varying concentrations (5–10%) depending on localisation and age (cave: resorption in childhood)
- Dithranol 0.03–2% in vaseline or zinc paste (overnight or minute therapy)
- Topical corticosteroids, especially higher potency (short term)
- Vitamin D3 and its analogues (calcipotriol, tacalcitol)
- Combination of betamethasone and calcipotriol
- Vitamin A acid derivatives (tazarotene gel)
- Crisaborole (PDE 4 inhibitor)
- UV light therapy regimen such as photo bath therapy 15% NaCl + UVB Phototherapy (UVA +) UVB/narrow band UVB 311 nm.

Photochemotherapy: 8-(5-) MOP + UVA (PUVA) via local cream, via full skin surface bathing (bath PUVA) or systemic oral application.

Systemic Therapy

To qualify for systemic therapy, the following criteria according to the International Psoriasis Council are recommended:

- Psoriasis lesions on 10% or more of the body surface, PASI score > 10 and quality of life >10
- Psoriasis lesions on sensitive areas of the body (i.e., hands/feet, face, genitals, scalp)
- Topical therapy failed to control symptoms
  Options for systemic therapy:
- Methotrexate oral or subcutaneous
- Retinoids, i.e. acitretin
- Cyclosporine
- Fumarates
- Biologics
- YAK/TYK inhibitors
- PDE 4 inhibitors

Special

The disease basically needs in certain courses with involvement of joints or metabolic syndrome or cardial tachy**arrhythmia** an interdisciplinary approach.

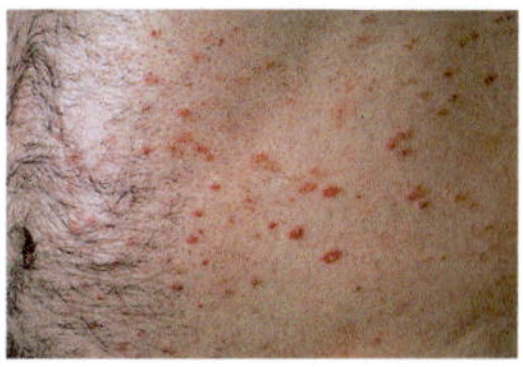

Fig. 5.11 Pityriasis lichenoides: disseminated erythematous papules on the trunk

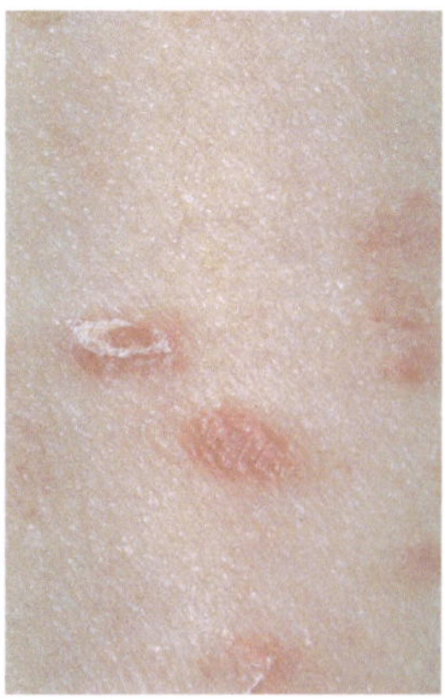

Fig. 5.12 Pityriasis lichenoides: lenticular, erythematous lesion with a scaling lid

Pityriasis Lichenoides [3]

Figures 5.11 and 5.12

Grading of Importance

B

Level

Basic

ICD-11

EA93

Pityriasis lichenoides chronica (Parapsoriasis guttata) (PLC): LB161.
Pityriasis lichenoides et varioliformis acuta (PLEVA): LB160.

Synonyms

PLEVA: Mucha-Habermann disease.

Epidemiology

PLEVA: Children and adolescents.
PLC: young adults M > F.

Definition

Acute (PLEVA), subacute or chronic erythemato-squamous or papulo-necrotising (PLEVA) or ulcero-necrotic types; nosologic relationship to vasculitis and to lymphomatoid papulosis (LyP; spontaneously regressive papular-necrotic form of CTCL).

Aetiology and Pathogenesis

Unknown. Viral (Epstein-Barr and other viruses) and other infectious agents (upper respiratory tract) discussed as trigger factors.

Signs and Symptoms

PLC: Lenticular, erythematous, macular or papular or ulcero-necrotic lesions with scaling.

PLEVA: Disseminated, small papules and plaques with scaling or superficial crust, sometimes haemorrhagic. Development to necrotic lesions and healing with varioliform scarring.

Localisation

Predominantly trunk > extremities

Classification

Variable: acute (PLEVA), subacute or chronic.

Laboratory and Other Workups

Looking for infections (upper respiratory tract), blood picture, biopsy.

Dermatopathology

Depending on acuity

- PLEVA: Focal hyperparakeratosis; apoptosis of single keratinocytes; interface-dermatitis (oedema in the epidermal-dermal junction with vacuolisation of basal keratinocytes); lymphocytic (wedge shaped) infiltrate in the dermis and extravasation of erythrocytes.
- PLC: Like in PLEVA, but less prominent.

Course

Weeks or months; maximum 2 years.

Complications

Fever and superinfection

Diagnosis

Clinical and histologic findings.

Differential Diagnosis

Psoriasis guttata, secondary *syphilis*, necrotising vasculitis.

Prevention and Therapy

No prevention. Skin care, prevention of superinfection; erosive lesions may be treated topically with combined anti-microbial-glucocorticosteroid (grade I) cream.

Pityriasis Rubra Pilaris (Prp) [10]

Figures 5.13 and 5.14

Grading of Importance

C

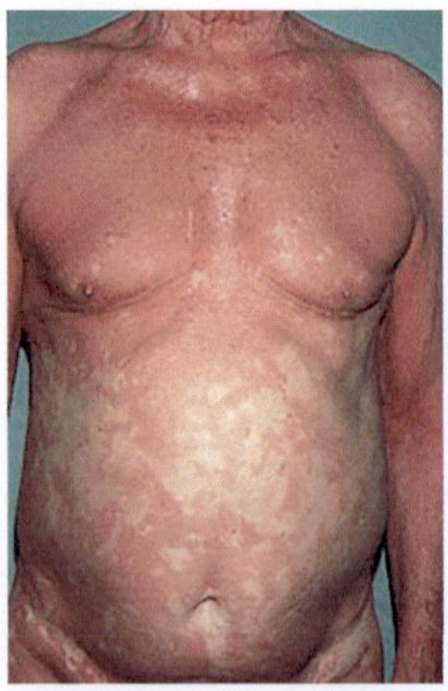

Fig. 5.13 Pityriasis rubra pilaris: reddish-orange tiny pinpoint papules, forming sharply demarcated patches

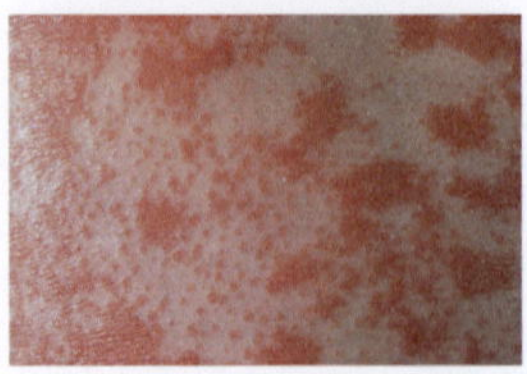

Fig. 5.14 Pityriasis rubra pilaris: closeup view of follicular bound papules

Level

Basic

ICD-11

EA94; ORPHA: 2897

Synonyms

Lichen accuminatus; Morbus Divergie.

Epidemiology

Rare papulo-squamous disease. 1: 3500–5000 in the USA and UK. Prevalence of 2.5 million cases in all totalling on average 1 case per 400,000 of the population. Any ethnic group. F = M.

Definition

Chronic inflammatory papulo-squamous skin disease with a spectrum of several clinical phenotypes.

Aetiology and Pathogenesis

No clear genetic background. In familial cases, mutations in the caspase recruitment domain family. It is occasionally precipitated and aggravated or even maintained by infections or drugs such as sorafenib, insulin, imatinib, telaprevir and vaccinations.

Signs and Symptoms

Psoriasiform reddish-orange tiny pinpoint elevated and follicular bound scaling, forming small and large sharply demarcated patches, sometimes burning and evolving into erythroderma; uninvolved skin in-between (nappes claires). Involvement of palms and soles, mimicking psoriasis, chronic eczema or keratoderma.

Localisation

Localised on trunk, elbows, knees, palms and soles or total body (erythroderma).

Classification

A recent classification identifies six main forms of pityriasis rubra pilaris:

- Type 1: classical adult-onset
- Type 2: atypical adult-onset
- Type 3: classical juvenile-onset
- Type 4: circumscribed juvenile
- Type 5: atypical juvenile-onset
- Type 6: HIV-associated

Laboratory and Other Workups

No specific tests; biopsy.

Dermatopathology

Plump acanthosis and papillomatosis with broad rete ridges, horizontally and vertically alternating hyper-ortho- and hyper-parakeratosis (checkerboard sign); follicular hyperkeratotic plugs. No or rather sparse lymphocytic infiltrate.

Course

Disease duration in most of the patients <1 year.

Complications

None except erythrodermic courses and type 1 associated underlying malignancy disorder.

Diagnosis

Clinical features and histopathology.

Differential Diagnosis

Psoriasis, secondary syphilis, pityriasis rosea, parapsoriasis, nummular eczema, hypertrophic lichen planus, chronic palmo-plantar eczema, keratosis follicularis, Darier disease.

Prevention and Therapy

Avoiding aggravating factors:

- ***Topical therapy*** depending on lesion type and amount of body surface area
  - Topical corticosteroids, especially mid to higher potency
  - Vitamin D3 and its analogues (calcipotriol, tacalcitol)
  - Vitamin A acid derivatives (tazarotene gel)
  - UV light therapy regimen such as bath-photo therapy 15% NaCl + UVB. Phototherapy (UVA +) UVB/narrow band UVB 311 nm. Photochemotherapy: 8-(5-) methoxypsoralen (MOP) + UVA (PUVA)
- ***Systemic treatment*** in widespread PRP: methotrexate, azathioprine, retinoids (acitretin, isotretinoin, alitretinoin), cyclosporine, fumarates, biologics (**anti-tumour necrosis factor, anti-interleukin (IL) 12/IL-23, and anti-IL-17 agents)**

Lichen Planus [5, 8, 9]

Figures 5.15, 5.16, 5.17, 5.18 and 5.19

Grading and Level of Importance

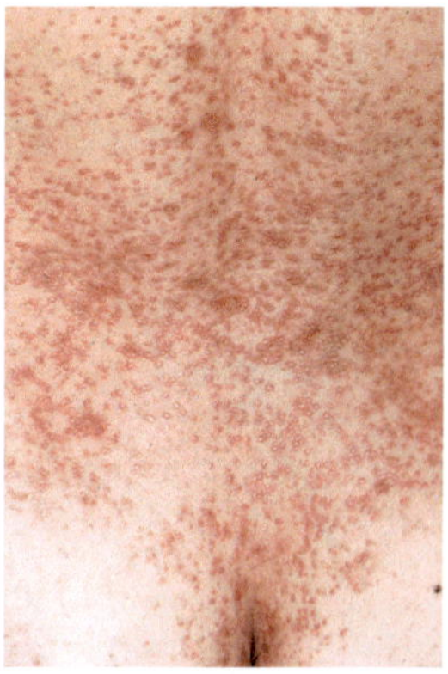

Fig. 5.15 Lichen planus: exanthematous eruption

B

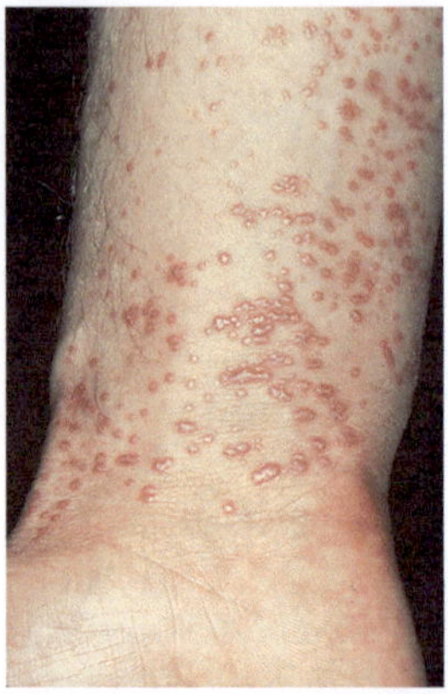

Fig. 5.16 Lichen planus: lichenoid papules on the lower arm

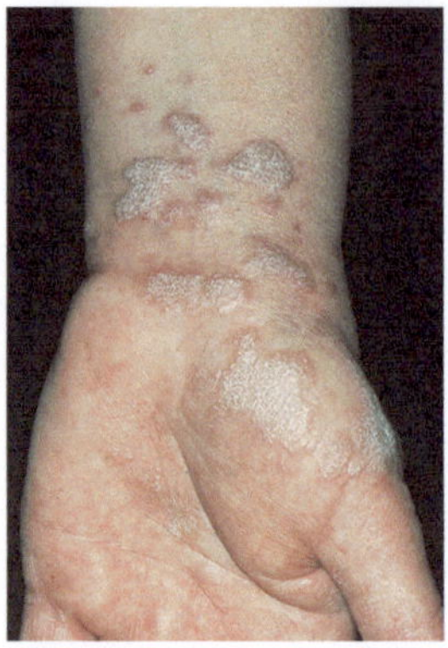

Fig. 5.17 Lichen planus: hyperkeratotic plaques on the wrist

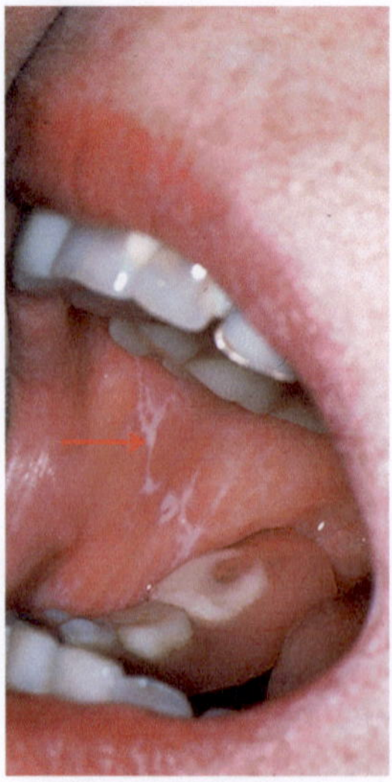

Fig. 5.18 Lichen planus: netlike lesion on the buccal mucosa

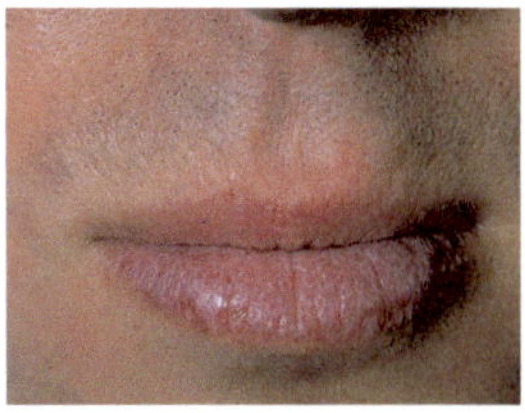

Fig. 5.19 Lichen planus: fine lichenoid net on the lips

ICD-11

EA91

Synonyms

Lichen ruber planus.

Epidemiology

Prevalence between 0.1 and 4%, with most cases occurring between 30 and 60 years of age, and with a slight predominance in perimenopausal women.

Definition

Idiopathic subacute to chronic inflammatory dermatosis involving the skin, mucosae, nails and/or hair.

Aetiology and Pathogenesis

Very likely to be an autoimmune disorder, associations with collagen-vascular diseases, vitiligo and diabetes mellitus. Graft-versus-host-disease (GvHD) has similar morphology. Hepatitis B and C, stress and various drugs may also play a role in its induction.

Signs and Symptoms

- Skin: polygonal violaceous papules, white net-like superficial markings (Wickham's striae), marked pruritus; Köbner phenomenon
- Mucosae: lips, tongue, cheeks, genital and anal areas (annular, bullous, erosive, atrophic), net-like white, non-removable pattern

- Nails: nonspecific changes (longitudinal stripes), nail dystrophy, nail matrix destruction
- Scalp: lichen planopilaris, atrophic scarring alopecia
- Palmoplantar: hyperkeratosis and fissures

Localisation

More commonly flexor aspects of wrists, nails, oral and genital mucosae; can be disseminated.

Classification

Various types: localised, exanthematous, mucosal.

Laboratory and Other Workups

None specific.

Dermatopathology

Acanthosis, saw-toothed dermal-epidermal junction profile, hypergranulosis, subepidermal interface band-like infiltrate of T lymphocytes, pigment incontinence.

Course

Lichen planus of the skin often resolves after a few months or years, although it may recur. If caused by medication or tooth fillings, lichen planus will clear after the treatment is stopped or the fillings removed. Lichen planus of the mucosa, nails and scalp rarely clears by itself and can cause permanent scarring.

Complications

Erosive lichen planus of the mucosae can lead to squamous cell carcinoma, making follow-up mandatory.

Diagnosis

Clinical features, histology, Köbner phenomenon.

Differential Diagnosis

Lichenoid drug reactions: Skin eruptions caused by commonly used medications can resemble lichen planus. Quinine in tonic water and over-the-counter leg cramp medicines can cause a lichen planus-like condition. In the mouth, allergy to the metals in fillings and oral appliances can cause sores that look like oral lichen planus.

Prevention and Therapy

Prevention: Avoid/control predisposing factors:

- Topical: high potency corticosteroids, calcineurin inhibitors (mucosal involvement), tazarotene, calcipotriol, UVA/B, PUVA, UVA1.
- Systemic: corticosteroids, systemic PUVA, dapsone, hydroxychloroquine, methotrexate, mycophenolate mofetil, acitretin, alitretinoin, cyclosporine, azathioprine, apremilast, sedatives.

Special

TNF blockers exhibit fairly controversial effects in lichen planus, since they can trigger proinflammatory reactions.

Pityriasis Rosea [6]

Figures 5.20, 5.21 and 5.22

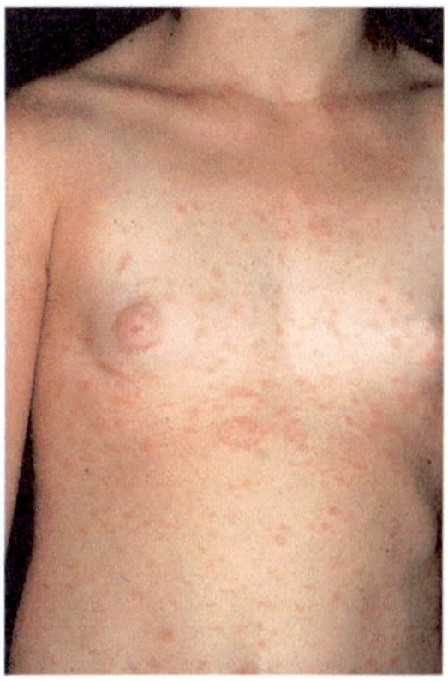

Fig. 5.20 Pityriasis rosea: erythematous papules and plaques on the trunk

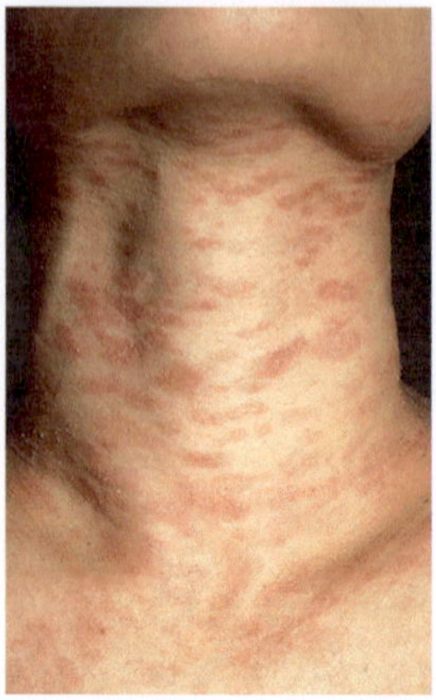

Fig. 5.21 Pityriasis rosea: lesions on the neck, following skin lines

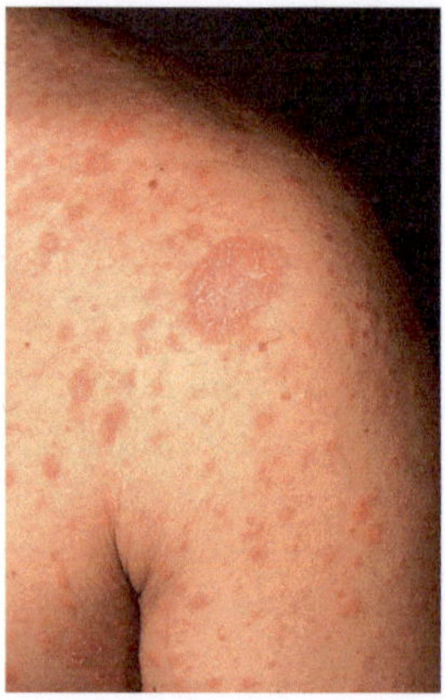

Fig. 5.22 Pityriasis rosea: herald patch with collarette scale

Grading of Importance

B

Level

Advanced

ICD-11

EA10

Synonyms

Pityriasis circinata; Gibert pityriasis; pityriasis rosea Gibert.

Epidemiology

Common disease (incidence 0.68/100 dermatology patients, prevalence 0.5–2%). Affects adolescents and young adults (aged 10 to 35 years).

Definition

Acute, disseminated, symmetrical exanthema with collarette scale.

Aetiology and Pathogenesis

Probably viral induction (human herpes virus 6 or 7).

Signs and Symptoms

The initial lesion is a large, flat erythematous (salmon coloured) plaque (herald patch (medallion, up to 5 cm in diameter), followed by multiple smaller lesions frequently following skin lines (e.g. Christmas tree distribution around ribs) with a typical collarette scale. Pruritus can occur (50%) and is variable in intensity, especially when the skin is irritated by intense washing and sweating or with simultaneous concurrent dermatitis. Prodromal symptoms (fever, headache, arthralgia, cough, vomiting or lymphadenopathy) have been reported in up to 60% of the patients.

Localisation

Typically, on trunk (occasionally neck and proximal extremities).

Classification

Atypical variants can occur.

Laboratory and Other Workups

Not necessary.

Dermatopathology

Not required. Corresponds to eczematous dermatitis; patchy lymphocytic infiltrate in the dermis and a few intraepidermal erythrocytes.

Course

Self-limiting with spontaneous resolution after 4–8 weeks or sometimes longer. May leave hyperpigmentation but no scarring.

Complications

Relapse rate up to 26% in 4 years.

Diagnosis

Clinical criteria:

- Herald patch
- Peripheral collarette scales
- Predominant truncal and proximal limb distribution of the lesions
- Orientation of lesions along the lines of cleavage

Differential Diagnosis

Secondary syphilis, drug reaction, tinea, psoriasis parapsoriasis, nummular eczema.

Prevention and Therapy

No preventive measurements or effective treatment. Mild skin care and avoidance of irritating factors. If pruritic, topical antipruritic agents: weak corticosteroids or emollients. In selected cases narrow band UVB.

Special

Relapses can especially occur in pregnancy. If in the first 15 weeks, close follow-up is required due to reported miscarriages.

Prurigo Simplex [4, 7]

Figures 5.23 and 5.24

Grading of Importance

B

Level

Advanced

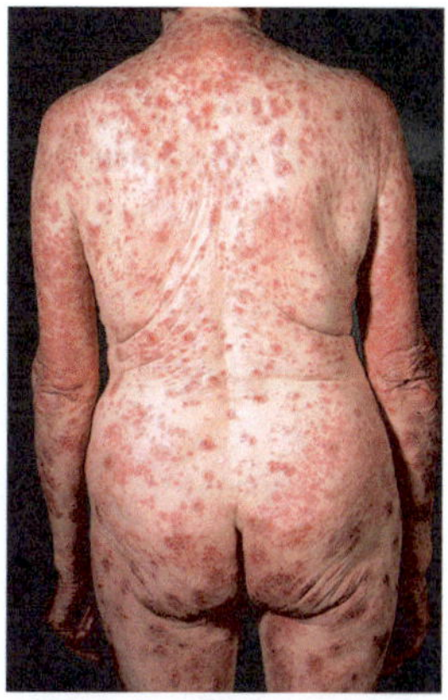

Fig. 5.23 Prurigo Simplex: widespread itching, dome shaped papules

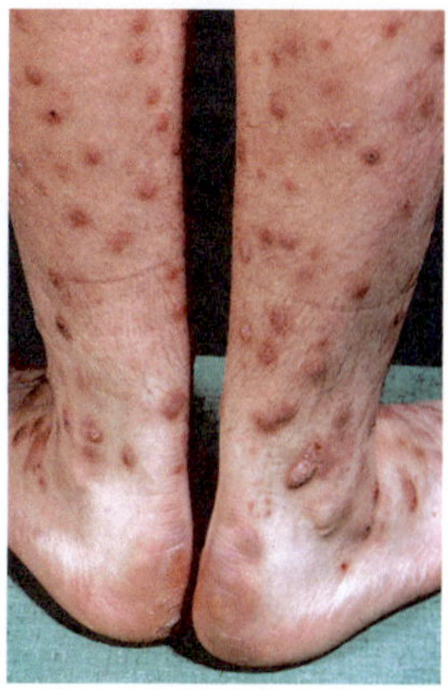

Fig. 5.24 Prurigo Simplex: nodular lesions on the legs

ICD-11

EC91

Synonyms

Prurigo simplex acuta et chronica.

Epidemiology

Rather common disease, standing alone or associated with atopic dermatitis.

Definition

Group of dermatoses with many causes, all featuring intense pruritus followed by reactive crusted papules (prurigo = itchy crust).

Aetiology and Pathogenesis

Prurigo seems to develop in individuals, who overreact to pruritus (itch) inducing factors.

Causes: systemic and local triggers of pruritus, idiopathic, atopic constitution. Sometimes acute, more chronic, persistent disease with proliferation of peripheral sensory nerves of the skin.

Prurigo simplex and prurigo nodularis seem to be different stages of a common disease.

Signs and Symptoms

Pruritus, small sero-papules (beginning) and excoriations with symmetrical distribution of secondary prurigo lesions on the extensor surfaces of the extremities, neck, lower trunk, and buttocks. Typically, patients present with widespread dome shaped papules, which are intensely itchy leading to sleep deprivation.

Localisation

Extremities, trunk (interscapular area is usually spared!).

Classification

Acute, subacute and chronic forms.

Laboratory and Other Workups

Exclude underlying metabolic diseases, malfunctions of kidneys and liver, hematologic disorders and parasitic infestations. Blood: Eosinophils, IgE (DD: prurigo type of atopic dermatitis). Psychological/psychiatric consultation recommended (67% abnormal).

Dermatopathology

Acute to chronic dermatitis with epidermal acanthosis and spongiosis, strong inflammatory cell infiltrate. Sensory nerve proliferation.

Course

Chronic, symptoms often persist for months to years.

Complications

Superinfections of excoriated lesions.

Diagnosis

Clinical features.

Differential Diagnosis

Atopic dermatitis (prurigo variant), folliculitis and perifolliculitis in cutem penetrans, scabies, dermatitis herpetiformis and bullous pemphigoid (prurigo variant).

Prevention and Therapy

Secondary prevention: Exclude underlying disorders and avoid scratching.

- Topical: corticosteroids, capsaicin cream, narrow band UVB, PUVA
- Systemic: sedative antihistamines. In prurigo type of atopic dermatitis: dupilumab

References

1. Armstrong AW, Read C (2020) Pathophysiology, clinical presentation, and treatment of psoriasis: a review. JAMA 323(19):1945–1960
2. Boehncke WH, Schon MP (2015) Psoriasis. Lancet 386(9997):983–994
3. Bowers S, Warshaw EM (2006) Pityriasis lichenoides and its subtypes. J Am Acad Dermatol 55(4):557–572; quiz 573–556
4. Jorizzo JL, Gatti S, Smith EB (1981) Prurigo: a clinical review. J Am Acad Dermatol 4(6):723–728
5. Le Cleach L, Chosidow O (2012) Clinical practice. Lichen planus. N Engl J Med 366(8):723–732
6. Litchman G, Nair PA, Le JK (2020) Pityriasis Rosea. StatPearls, Treasure Island, FL
7. Pereira MP, Steinke S, Zeidler C, Forner C, Riepe C, Augustin M, Bobko S, Dalgard F, Elberling J, Garcovich S, Gieler U, Goncalo M, Halvorsen JA, Leslie TA, Metz M, Reich A, Savk E, Schneider G, Serra-Baldrich E, Stander HF, Streit M, Wallengren J, Weller K, Wollenberg A, Bruland P, Soto-Rey I, Storck M, Dugas M, Weisshaar E, Szepietowski JC, Legat FJ, Stander S, E. T. F. P. g. members (2018) European academy of dermatology and venereology European prurigo project: expert consensus on the definition, classification and terminology of chronic prurigo. J Eur Acad Dermatol Venereol 32(7):1059–1065
8. Tziotzios C, Brier T, Lee JYW, Saito R, Hsu CK, Bhargava K, Stefanato CM, Fenton DA, McGrath JA (2018a) Lichen planus and lichenoid dermatoses: conventional and emerging therapeutic strategies. J Am Acad Dermatol 79(5):807–818
9. Tziotzios C, Lee JYW, Brier T, Saito R, Hsu CK, Bhargava K, Stefanato CM, Fenton DA, McGrath JA (2018b) Lichen planus and lichenoid dermatoses: clinical overview and molecular basis. J Am Acad Dermatol 79(5):789–804
10. Wang D, Chong VC, Chong WS, Oon HH (2018) A review on pityriasis rubra pilaris. Am J Clin Dermatol 19(3):377–390

Part II

Infectious Diseases

They include viral, mycotic, parasitic and bacterial infections which also comprise the socioeconomically important group of sexually transmitted infections (STI). Neglected tropical dermatoses (NTD's) with an infectious pathogenetic background will be dealt with in a separate chapter (Chap. 10).

Viral Infections

6

Jonathan M. White, Farrah Bakr, Günter Burg, Veronique del Marmol, Evelyn Gaffal, Su Lwin, and John A. McGrath

Contents

J. M. White (✉)
Ecole de Santé Publique, Université libre de Bruxelles, Brussels, Belgium
e-mail: Jonathan.White@ulb.be

F. Bakr · S. Lwin
Department of Dermatology, King's College, London, UK
e-mail: farrahbakr@doctors.org.uk; su.m.lwin@kcl.ac.uk

G. Burg
Dermatology, Zurich, Switzerland
e-mail: g.burg@access.uzh.ch

V. del Marmol
Département of Dermatology, Hôpital Erasme-HUB, Université Libre de Bruxelles, Brussels, Belgium
e-mail: veronique.delmarmol@hubruxelles.be

E. Gaffal
Department of Dermatology, University of Lübeck, Lübeck, Germany
e-mail: evelyn.gaffal@med.ovgu.de

J. A. McGrath
St John's Institute of Dermatology, King's College London, London, UK
e-mail: john.mcgrath@kcl.ac.uk

H. Gollnick et al. (eds.), *Dermatology Cyberderm WebBook*,
https://doi.org/10.1007/978-3-031-78491-0_6

Test your learning and check your understanding of this book's contents: use the "Springer Nature Flashcards" app to access questions using ▶ https://sn.pub/1rhh6k.

To use the app, please follow the instructions in Chap. 1.

Varicella and Herpes Zoster [6]

Figures 6.1, 6.2, 6.3 and 6.4

Grading of Importance

A

Fig. 6.1 Varicella and Herpes Zoster: varicella in an adult

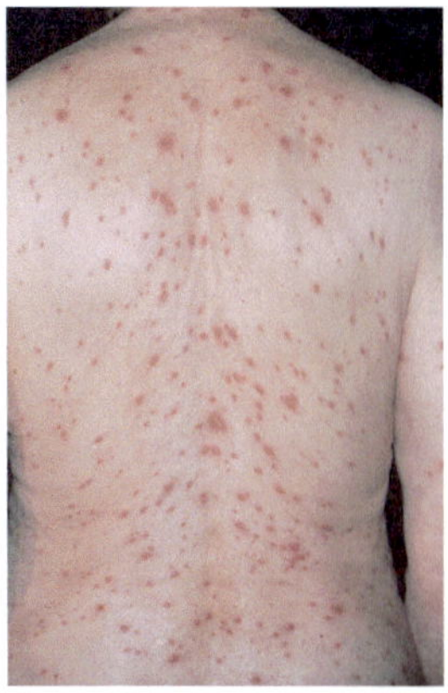

Fig. 6.2 Varicella and Herpes Zoster: zoster, segmental erythema and vesicles

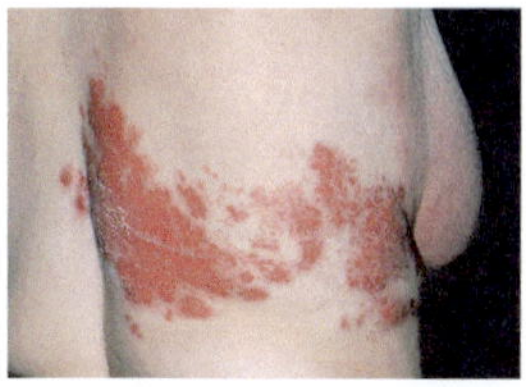

Fig. 6.3 Varicella and Herpes Zoster: zoster with aberrant vesicles

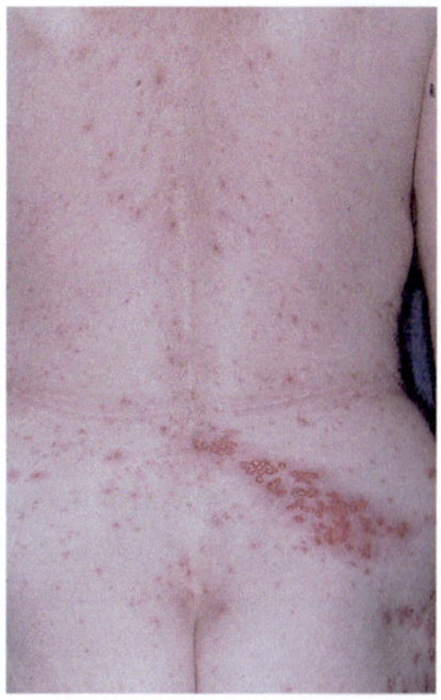

Fig. 6.4 Varicella and Herpes Zoster: ballooned keratinocytes from blister bottom (Tzanck smear)

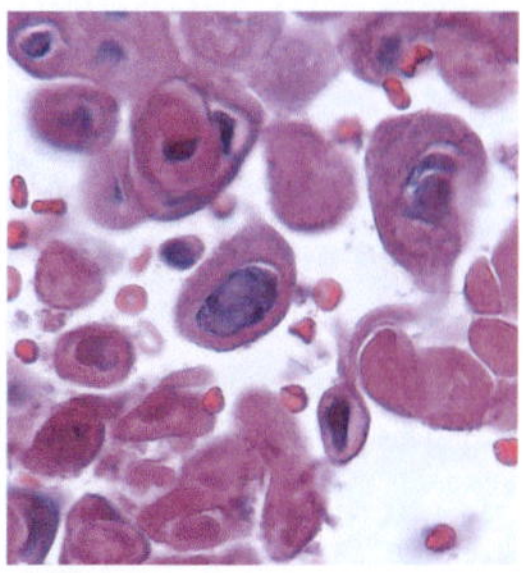

Level

Advanced

ICD-11

1E90

Synonyms

Chickenpox; shingles.

Definition

Varicella-zoster virus (VZV) causes a primary infection usually in childhood (varicella, chickenpox) and may later be reactivated in a nerve (herpes zoster, shingles).

Epidemiology

Disease of childhood. Primary infection in adults may show a severe course.

Aetiology and Pathogenesis

Infection by varicella-zoster virus (VZV).

Primary infection leads to varicella; reinfection or reactivation of viruses persisting in the spinal and cranial ganglia (Gasserian ganglion, geniculate ganglion) sometimes in conjunction with exacerbating factors (immunosuppression, trauma, sunlight, severe illnesses) leads to herpes zoster.

Signs and Symptoms

Varicella: incubation period, 2–3 weeks, highly contagious. Clinical features: generalised papulo-vesiculo-pustular exanthema with lesions in varying stages of development (stary sky-pattern), in contrast to smallpox, in which all lesions are in the same stage of development.

Herpes zoster: segmental lesion not crossing the midline with burning, pain, erythema, blisters, necrosis, scars, post-herpetic neuralgia. Look for aberrant vesicles, which always exist in varying number apart from the involved nerve segment. Herpes zoster haemorrhagicus, gangrenosus, more severe forms; generalised, widespread, resembles varicella with aberrant blisters.

Localisation

Varicella: head and mouth (gums) are often involved but palms and soles are usually spared.

Zoster: in affected dermatome. Aberrant vesicles are always present in varying number apart from the involved nerve segment.

Variants: ophthalmic herpes zoster, first trigeminal branch (V1 nerve) sometimes with nasociliary branch; be aware of need for urgent opthalmology review, keratitis. Herpes zoster second or third trigeminal branch. Aural herpes zoster (VIIIth nerve); acoustic nerve and potential facial paralysis.

Classification

Herpes zoster: according to dermatome.

Laboratory and Other Workups

Only required if severe involvement or other relevant clinical question. Viral swabs may confirm the diagnosis days later. Immediate confirmation when required via Tzanck smear, PCR of vesicle fluid or antigen test.

Dermatopathology

Usually not required.

The histopathologic changes in herpes simplex and in varizella/zoster eruptions are basically the same. Differentiation can be achieved by immunohistochemistry or PCR:

- Inter- and intracellular oedema of the epidermis with intraepidermal acantholytic blister formation
- Ballooning degeneration of keratinocytes (swollen pyknotic ("steel-grey") nuclei)
- Syncytial multinucleated epithelial giant cells (positive Tzanck smear)
- Dermal oedema with predominantly lymphocytic, mixed cellular infiltrate in the dermis with many eosinophils

Course

Usually a self-limiting disease. Varicella is commonly mild in young children but may be disseminated and severe in adults (especially in pregnancy), rarely leading to multi-organ failure.

Complications

Varicella: fever, malaise, pneumonia, scarring, especially when lesions display secondary infection. Foetal malformations may occur after infection in the first trimester; neonatal varicella when infection occurs in the third trimester.

Herpes zoster: dissemination, superadded infection, keratitis and painful postherpetic neuralgia.

Diagnosis

Usually clinical.

Differential Diagnosis

- Varicella: insect bites, coxsackie virus infection, generalised herpes zoster, eczema herpeticum and other viral exanthems
- Herpes zoster: insect bites; herpes simplex; pain from other causes

Prevention and Therapy

Prevention of herpes zoster reactivation: immunisation.

Topical: antiseptics (e.g. chlorhexidine 1% lotion).

Systemic: antiviral agents (e.g. aciclovir). Indications for systemic treatment: patients>50 years, disease present less than 3 days, tendency toward generalisation, eye involvement (first branch of trigeminal nerve), immunodeficiency. Analgesics as required (NSAIDs, but acetyl salicylic acid contraindicated in children, risking Reyes syndrome causing swelling in the liver and brain.) and, in special cases, corticosteroids.

Special

Ask about contacts of the index patient (pregnant individuals, children, immunocompromised).

Herpes Simplex [4]

Figures 6.5, 6.6, 6.7, 6.8, 6.9, 6.10 and 6.11

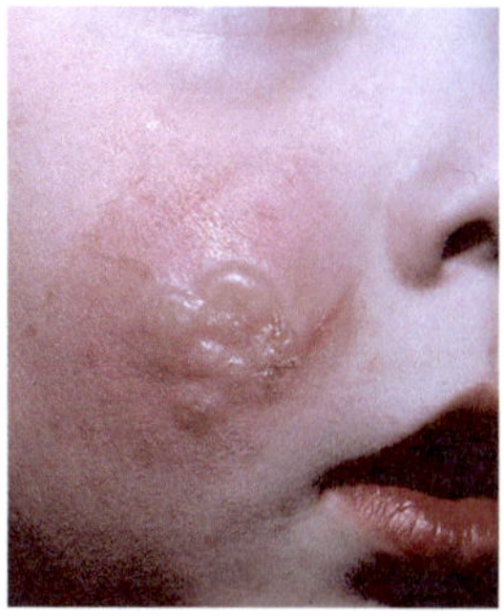

Fig. 6.5 Herpes simplex: primary infection in a child

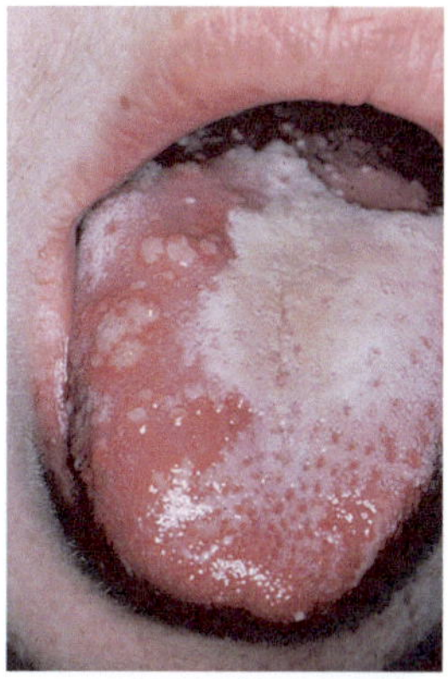

Fig. 6.6 Herpes simplex: herpetic gingivostomatitis

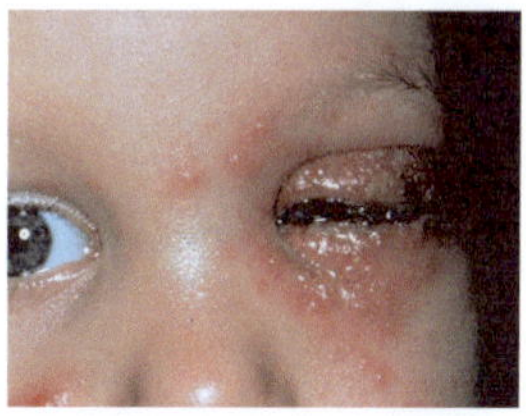

Fig. 6.7 Herpes simplex: eye involvement

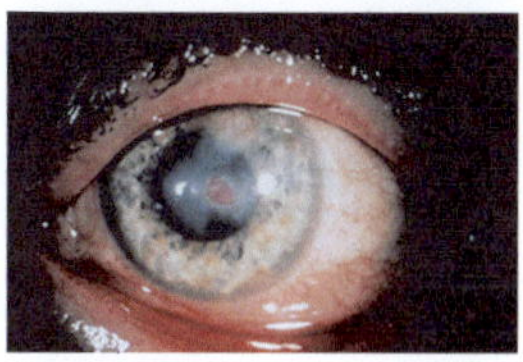

Fig. 6.8 Herpes simplex: keratitis lenticularis (complication)

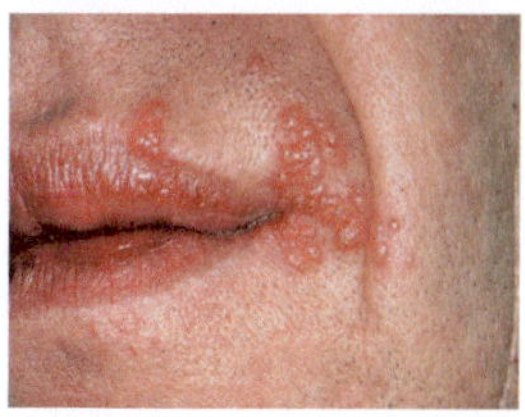

Fig. 6.9 Herpes simplex: recurrent grouped vesicles (herpetiform) on an erythematous base

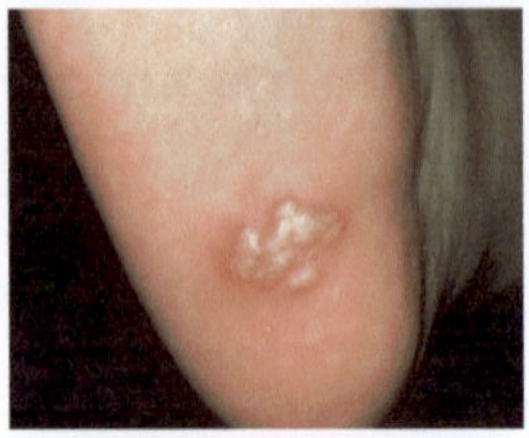

Fig. 6.10 Herpes simplex: unusual localization on the heel

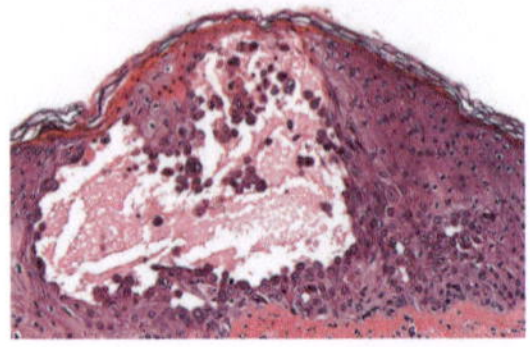

Fig. 6.11 Herpes simplex: balloon degeneration of keratinocytes in blister

Grading of Importance

A

Level

Advanced

ICD-11

1F00.0

Synonyms

Cold sore; fever spot; herpes; (herpetic) whitlow.

Epidemiology

About 90% of adult population have evidence of previous infection.

Definition

Viral infection with herpes simplex virus Types 1 and 2.

Aetiology and Pathogenesis

Primary or secondary infection with the more common herpes simplex virus; Type 1 (H. labialis) or less frequently; Type 2 (H. genitalis). These DNA viruses are epidermotropic and neurotropic. Transmission: fomites (contaminated surfaces) or direct contact. Reservoir: humans. Incubation period: 2–7 days.

Signs and Symptoms

Painful, grouped vesicles (herpetiform) on an erythematous base which quickly evolve into pustules.

Primary Infection

- Herpetic gingivostomatitis
- Herpes genitalis (including herpetic vulvovaginitis)
- Herpes neonatorum

Secondary Infections

- Recurrent herpes simplex labialis (Type 1) or genitalis (Type 2), herpetic keratitis, eczema herpeticatum.
- Aetiology: endogenous re-infection, usually at the same site, triggered by UV light, stress, hormonal changes and other factors.

Localisation

Lips, mouth, fingers, ano-genital skin, buttocks or potentially any part of the skin or intermediate epithelium/mucous membranes.

Classification

Viral Subtypes 1 and 2.

Laboratory and Other Workups

Usually not required. Antigen test or PCR to differentiate Type 1 from Type 2. Tzanck smear test: Multinucleate keratinocytes (giant cells with viral inclusion bodies).

Dermatopathology

Not usually required. Balloon degeneration of keratinocytes in blister.

See also section "Varicella and Herpes Zoster".

Course

Usually self-limiting. Individual periodicity of reactivation.

Complications

Persistent ulceration, eczema herpeticatum, secondary bacterial infection, keratitis lenticularis potentially leading to blindness, viral encephalitis, erythema multiforme.

Diagnosis

Clinical. Laboratory tests only in cases of diagnostic difficulty.

Differential Diagnosis

Impetigo, sexually transmitted infections (STI), aphthous ulcers.

Prevention and Therapy

Topical: astringents, antiseptics, virostatics.

Systemic: virostatics (e.g. aciclovir).

Indications:

- Herpes vulvitis and stomatitis
- Herpes neonatorum
- Herpes labialis with erythema multiforme
- Herpes genitalis
- Treatment of recurrent disease either at first sign of disease or as long-term prophylactic therapy

Special

Beware of disseminated infection in those with atopic dermatitis (eczema herpeticatum) or those who are immunocompromised. All ano-genital HSV needs investigation for other sexually transmitted diseases.

Eczema Herpeticatum [10]

Figures 6.12 and 6.13

Grading of Importance

C

Level

Advanced

ICD-11

1F00.03

Synonyms

Disseminated virus infection, Kaposi varicelliform eruption.

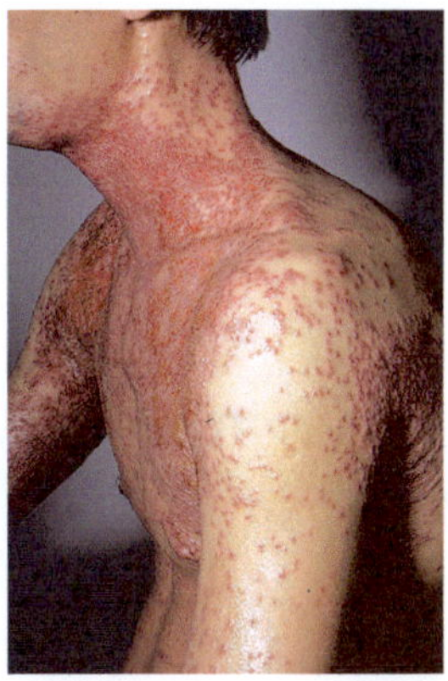

Fig. 6.12 Eczema herpeticatum: disseminated lesions in a patient with atopic eczema

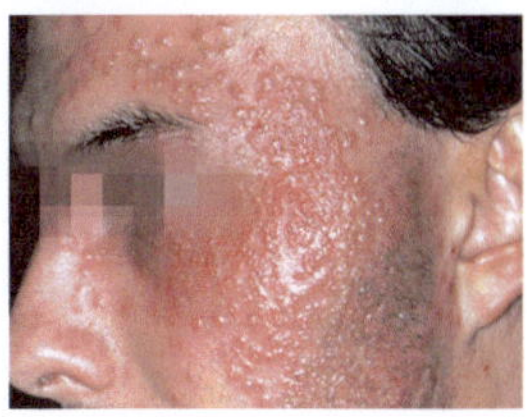

Fig. 6.13 Eczema herpeticatum: facial involvement

Definition

Severe cutaneous infection mostly with herpes simplex virus Type I (HSV- 1). Infections with HSV-2, varicella zoster virus, or vaccinia adverse event have also been described.

Aetiology and Pathogenesis

Due to local and systemic immune dysfunction and impaired skin barrier function, patients with atopic dermatitis are at highest risk to develop eczema herpeticatum. Infection occurs either by auto-inoculation (e.g. herpes labialis) or through contact with infected individuals.

Signs and Symptoms

Eruption of vesicles primarily in areas of severe dermatitis (face, neck, flexures), later developing into pustules, erosions and crusts. Generalised symptoms including high fever, marked pruritus, sometimes pain and lymphadenopathy.

Localisation

Usually face, neck and flexures. Rapid spreading all over the body.

Classification

None.

Laboratory and Other Workups

Non-specific, depending on the underlying disease, PCR confirmation.

Dermatopathology

Intraepidermal vesicles containing acantholytic cells, involvement of sebaceous glands, moderate dermal lymphocytic infiltration and oedema.

Course

Massive eruption of vesicles and high fever in the beginning. Later vesicles become pustular and erosive. After 4–5 days general symptoms improve, scarring is possible.

Complications

Ocular involvement, secondary bacterial infections, pneumonia, herpetic encephalitis, viral sepsis.

Diagnosis

History of atopic dermatitis, identification of the virus by PCR.

Differential Diagnosis

Bacterial infection, pre-existing bullous disease, other viral exanthemas (e.g. coxsackie), drug eruptions.

Prevention and Therapy

Limited disease can be treated with oral aciclovir, famciclovir or valacyclovir. Disseminated disease requires i.v. aciclovir. Secondary infections should be treated with culture-directed antibiotic therapy. Topical therapy includes wet dressings and antiseptics.

Warts [3, 8]

Figures 6.14, 6.15, 6.16, 6.17 and 6.18

Grading of Importance

A

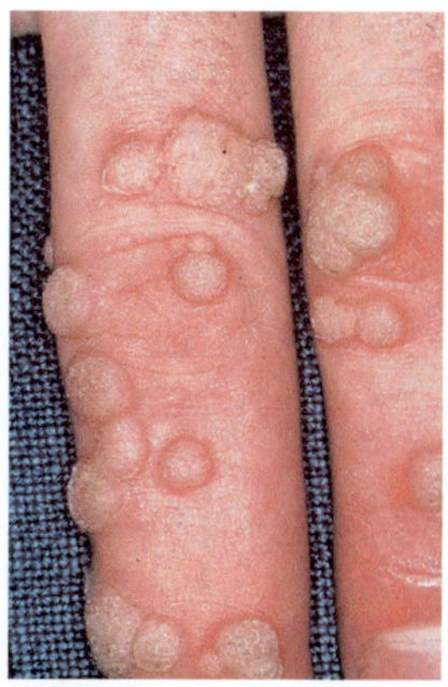

Fig. 6.14 Warts: verrucous lesions with erythematous border in a butcher

Fig. 6.15 Warts: nail dystrophy due to subungual warts

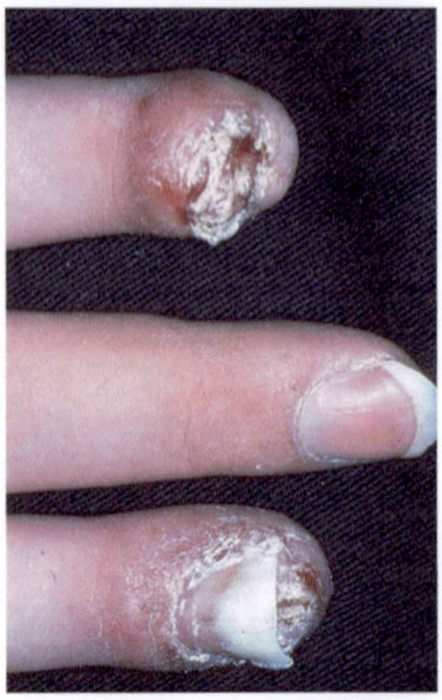

Fig. 6.16 Warts: plantar warts

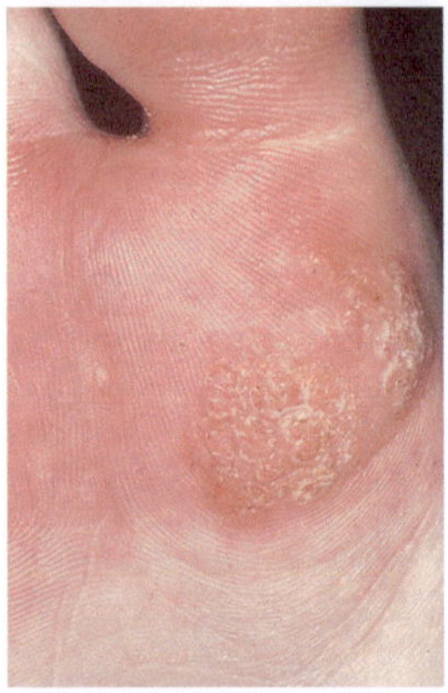

Fig. 6.17 Warts: verrucae planae juveniles

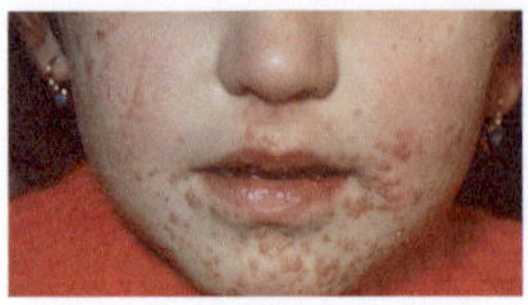

Fig. 6.18 Warts: typical histology, showing church-spire like hyperkeratosis

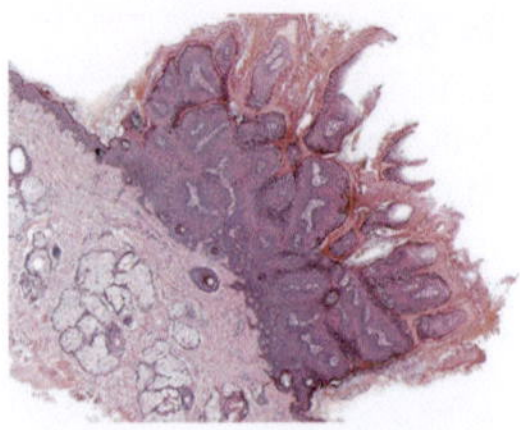

Level

Advanced

ICD-11

1E80

Synonyms

Common warts; verruca vulgaris; filiform warts; digitate warts; verruca.

Epidemiology

Affects 7–10% of the population, most commonly in first three decades of life.

Definition

Infection caused by human papilloma viruses (HPV), a DNA virus with more than 100 types, karyotropic. Transmission: human to human or animal to human. Incubation period: weeks to months. Predisposing factors: impaired skin barrier, immunosuppression, hyperhidrosis, impaired peripheral circulation, occupation (e.g. butchers).

Aetiology and Pathogenesis

Superficial keratinocyte infection by human papilloma virus.

Signs and Symptoms

Dome-shaped, firm papules with a papillomatous, hyperkeratotic (verruciform) surface, along with typical dark punctae (capillary thrombi). Plantar warts are flat (mosaic or thorn-like) with pressure-induced inward growth. Warts may be pigmented and painful.

Localisation

Any part of the body, particularly hands and feet.

Classification

According to HPV subtype, e.g. verruca vulgaris, common wart (HPV 1, 2); v. plantaris, mosaic warts (HPV 2, 4); v. plana, (HPV 1, 3).

Laboratory and Other Workups

Usually not required.

Dermatopathology

Usually not required. Acanthotic epidermis with vacuolation of keratinocytes and parakeratotic plug (church-spire feature).

Course

Usually self-limiting.

Complications

May persist and become disseminated in immunocompromised individuals. Rarely may lead to fingernail destruction. Some HPV subtypes may lead to neoplasia including squamous cell carcinoma.

Diagnosis

Clinical.

Differential Diagnosis

Corns, macrocomedones, *lichen planus*, Darier's disease, condylomata lata (Lues II), squamous cell carcinoma.

Prevention and Therapy

Spontaneous resolution in 95% within 2 years. Therefore aggressive therapy should be avoided. Beware scarring from over- treatment (no surgery). Cryosurgery, keratolytics (e.g. salicylic acid), topical retinoids (for facial involvement), 5-fluoro-uracil (5-FU), diphenylcyclopropenone immunotherapy (DCP), imiquimod.

Special

Consider underlying immunosuppression in extensive or treatment-resistant warts.

Condylomata Acuminata [7]

Figures 6.19, 6.20 and 6.21

Grading of Importance

C

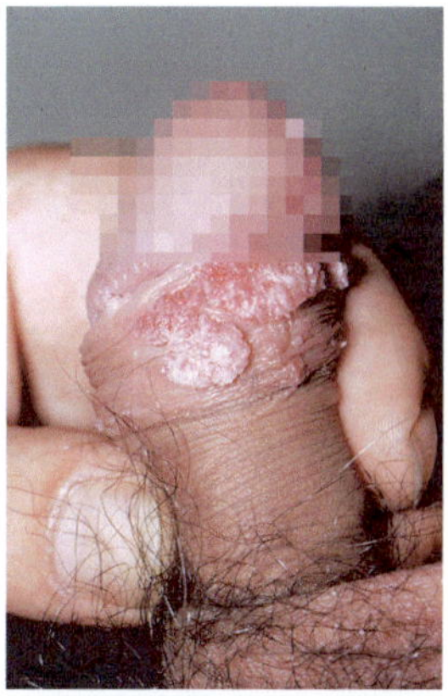

Fig. 6.19 Condylomata acuminata: penile lesions

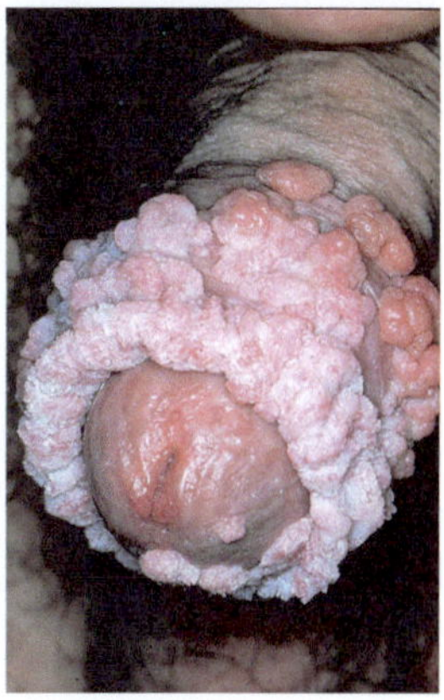

Fig. 6.20 Condylomata acuminata: giant condylomata Buschke-Löwenstein

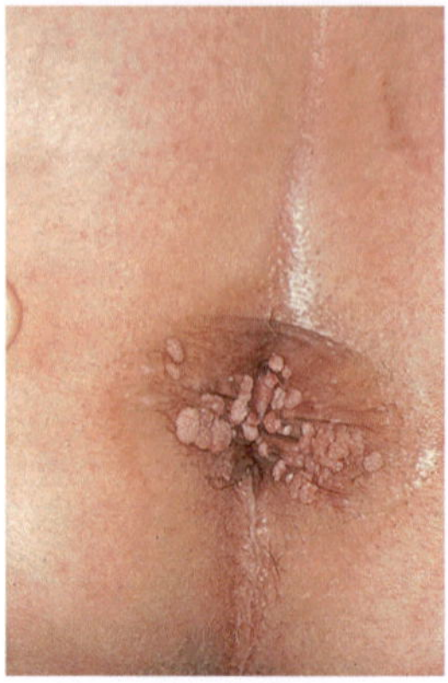

Fig. 6.21 Condylomata acuminata: perianal lesions

Level

Advanced

ICD-11

1A95

Synonyms

Ano-genital warts; venereal warts; verrucae ano-genitales; genital warts; verruca acuminata.

Epidemiology

Probably under-reported with a high annual incidence between 100 and 300 per 100,000. 4% have sub-clinical infection, and 10% have positive DNA tests. Higher incidence in those with high numbers of sexual partners.

Definition

Hyperplastic epidermal and mucosal lesions caused by HPV 6 and 11 and oncogenic HPV subtypes i.p.16/18 or 31, 33, 45, 52 and 58 cause more than 15% cervical cancer but larynx cancer,too.

Aetiology and Pathogenesis

Sexual transmission of virus via micro-trauma to the skin or mucous epithelia; 50% of partners are infected after 6 months. Non-sexual transmission is also possible. Incubation time weeks to months.

Cave: In children presenting with genital warts, the possibility of sexual abuse should be considered.

Signs and Symptoms

Pale to livid, sometimes hyperpigmented, narrow-based accuminated papules with a papillomatous surface. Lesions start as tiny papules, usually asymptomatic, which may be initially overlooked and can develop into large "cauliflower" tumours.

Localisation

Peri-/intra-anal, glans penis, prepuce, labia, introitus vulvae, urethral meatus, oral cavity. Note: some genital HPV types (16, 18, 31 and 33) cause bowenoid papulosis (clinically benign) as well as precancerous lesions and carcinomas of the cervix, vulva, penis and anus, sometimes in combination with co-factors such as HIV infection and immunosuppression.

Classification

According to HPV subtype.

Laboratory and Other Workups

Pap smear test in females potentially including PCR for oncogenic subtypes.

Dermatopathology

Indistinguishable histologically from common warts.

Course

Most are self-limiting; some persist and some evolve.

Complications

Development of carcinoma in oncogenic subtypes. May cause sexual, mechanical and psychologic dysfunction.

Diagnosis

Usually clinical. Exclusion of different STIs by blood tests and smears. Sometimes a skin biopsy is required to exclude other diagnoses.

Differential Diagnosis

Condylomata lata, squamous cell carcinoma, aggregated molluscum contagiosum.

Prevention and Therapy

Prevention and treatment: consider immunisation before puberty. Barrier methods of contraception do not always prevent infection.

Electro- or laser coagulation, cryosurgery in non-mucosal lesions, podophyllotoxin, imiquimod. Do not forget to treat contact(s) if infected. Beware over-treatment of exophytic lesions and the possibility of peri-meatal scarring.

Molluscum Contagiosum [5]

Figures 6.22 and 6.23

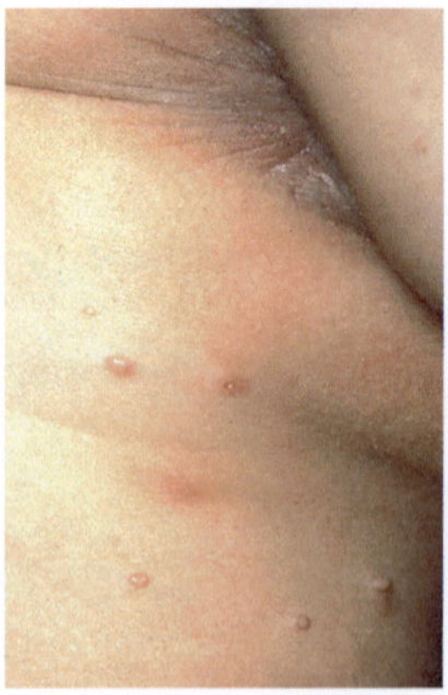

Fig. 6.22 Molluscum Contagiosum: disseminated dell warts in a child

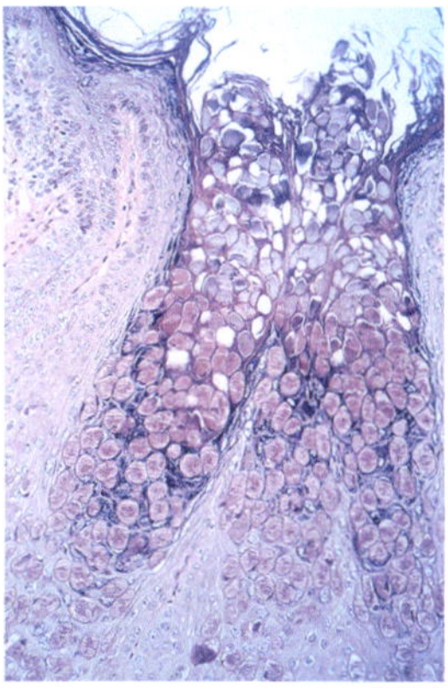

Fig. 6.23 Molluscum Contagiosum: histology showing degenerated keratinocytes like nuts in a sack (molluscum bodies)

Grading of Importance

A

Level

Advanced

ICD-11

1E76

Synonyms

Water warts; molluscum verrucosum; dell wart.

Definition

Superficial viral infection of the skin.

Aetiology and Pathogenesis

Causative agent: molluscum contagiosum (epidermotropic pox) virus, transferred between humans by direct contact, usually in children or sexual partners.

Signs and Symptoms

Single or multiple dome-shaped papules with a central dell, usually skin-coloured, often translucent, may be red. Typically not itchy or painful.

Localisation

Normally clustered; may be linear along excoriations. Children: usually extragenital. Sometimes solitary, disseminated and giant in adults.

Laboratory and Other Workups

Not required.

Dermatopathology

Only required in cases of diagnostic difficulty. Lobulated endophytic hyperplasia. Basophilic intracytoplasmic inclusions in keratinocytes.

Course

May spread, particularly in the setting of atopic dermatitis or immunosuppression/HIV infection. Spontaneous resolution may occur within weeks to 18 months.

Complications

Secondary bacterial infection; scarring (usually from treatments rather than the disease itself); rarely conjunctivitis or keratitis.

Diagnosis

Usually clinical; expelling of molluscum bodies.

Differential Diagnosis

Plane warts; condylomata accuminata in ano-genital area, basal cell carcinoma in solitary lesions in adults.

Prevention and Therapy

Despite spontaneous regression, therapeutic approaches such as 5% potassium hydroxide solution; destruction with curettage; cryosurgery for single or giant lesions; antiseptics if secondary infection.

Ecthyma Contagiosum [2]

Figures 6.24 and 6.25

Grading of Importance

A

Level

Null

ICD-11

1E75

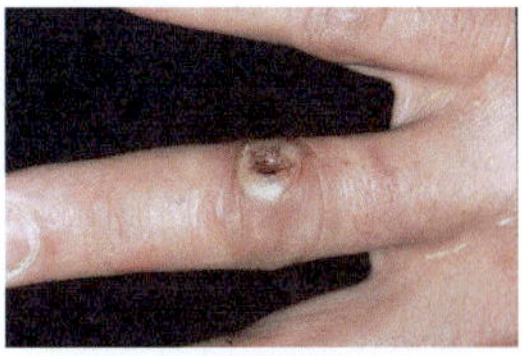

Fig. 6.24 Ecthyma contagiosum: inflamed pustular lesion with central necrosis on the finger of a farmer

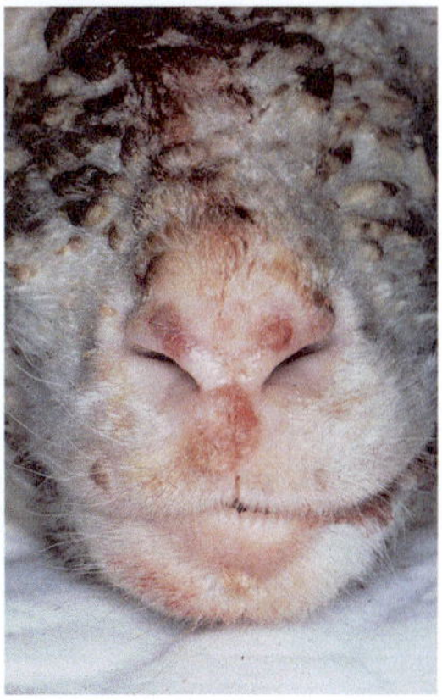

Fig. 6.25 Ecthyma contagiosum: sheep with lesions on nose and mouth

Synonyms

Orf, bovine pustular stomatitis. Orf and milker's nodule are caused by two closely related parapoxviruses; they are clinically very similar, and transfer in both cases is from an infected animal to a human.

Epidemiology

Worldwide. Prevalence of the disease in 15% of sheep, especially in young lambs. Persons at risk are farmers, vetenarians, shearers, sheepherders and butchers. Poxviruses are endemic in large parts of Africa (Democratic Republic of the Congo).

Definition

Zoonotic infection of the skin caused by the parapoxvirus, *Orfviridae*, contracted from sheep, lambs and goats.

Aetiology and Pathogenesis

By direct or indirect contact with diseased animals the highly contagious zoonotic virus *Parapoxvirus ovis* is transmitted. It stimulates angiogenesis by viral vascular endothelial growth factor E (VEGF-E). No human-to-human transfer.

Signs and Symptoms

Single lesion, developing through several stages after inoculation: erythematous macule, inflamed pustular lesion with central necrosis and peripheral red halo; regression after 4–6 weeks and healing, mostly without scar. In addition, there may be fever, malaise and regional lymphadenopathy. In immunocompromised patients autoinoculation and multiple "giant" lesions may occur.

Localisation

They occur most commonly on the fingers, hands or forearms but can appear on the face or mucous membranes as well.

Classification

Poxviruses

- Orthopoxviruses
  - Smallpox
  - Vaccinia
  - Cowpox
  - Monkey pox
- Parapoxviruses
  - Ecthyma contagiosum (orf)
  - Milker's nodule
- Molluscum contagiosum

Laboratory and Other Workups

The relatively large virus can be identified by electron microscopy, by special culture or by PCR.

Dermatopathology

- Prominent reticular degeneration and necrosis of the epidermis.
- Ballooning and necrosis of keratinocytes.
- Blister formation may be minimal. Multinucleated giant cells usually are absent.

Accompanying papillary oedema with erythrocyte extravasation and inflammatory infiltrate.

Course

Spontaneous healing without scar within 6–8 weeks.

Complications

Secondary bacterial infection with lymphangitis and erysipelas. Development of erythema multiforme in 10–20% of patients 3–4 weeks after inoculation or of other immunological reactions like Stevens-Johnson syndrome or blistering disorders.

Diagnosis

History (animal contacts); typical clinical feature.

Differential Diagnosis

Poxvirus infections; variola vera; monkey pox; milker's nodule; pyogenic granuloma; bacillary angiomatosis; impetigo contagiosa; dermatitis due to mites; varicella; pustula maligna (anthrax).

Prevention and Therapy

Prevention of contacts with infected animals. The lesions are self-limiting in immunocompetent patients.

Topical: drying measures and topical antiseptics usually are sufficient. In immunocompromised patients topical cidofovir or imiquimod along with mechanical eradication (i.e. cryotherapy, surgical excision) may be applied.

Smallpox [9]

Figures 6.26, 6.27 and 6.28

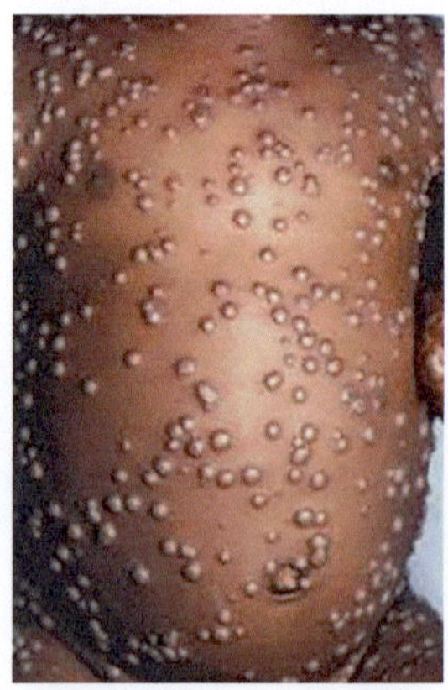

Fig. 6.26 Smallpox: simultaneous eruption of pustules in an African child

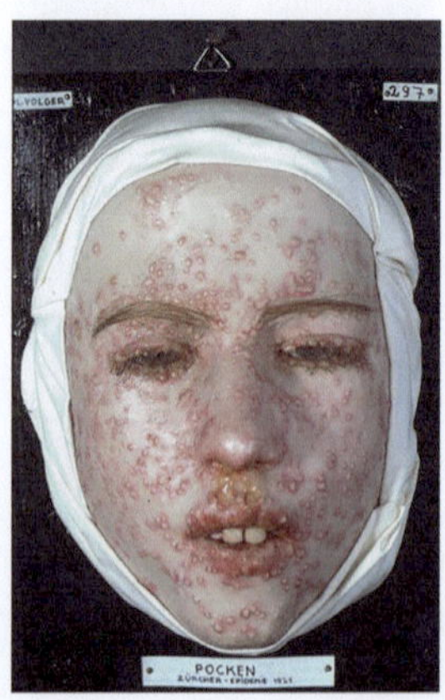

Fig. 6.27 Smallpox: wax moulage

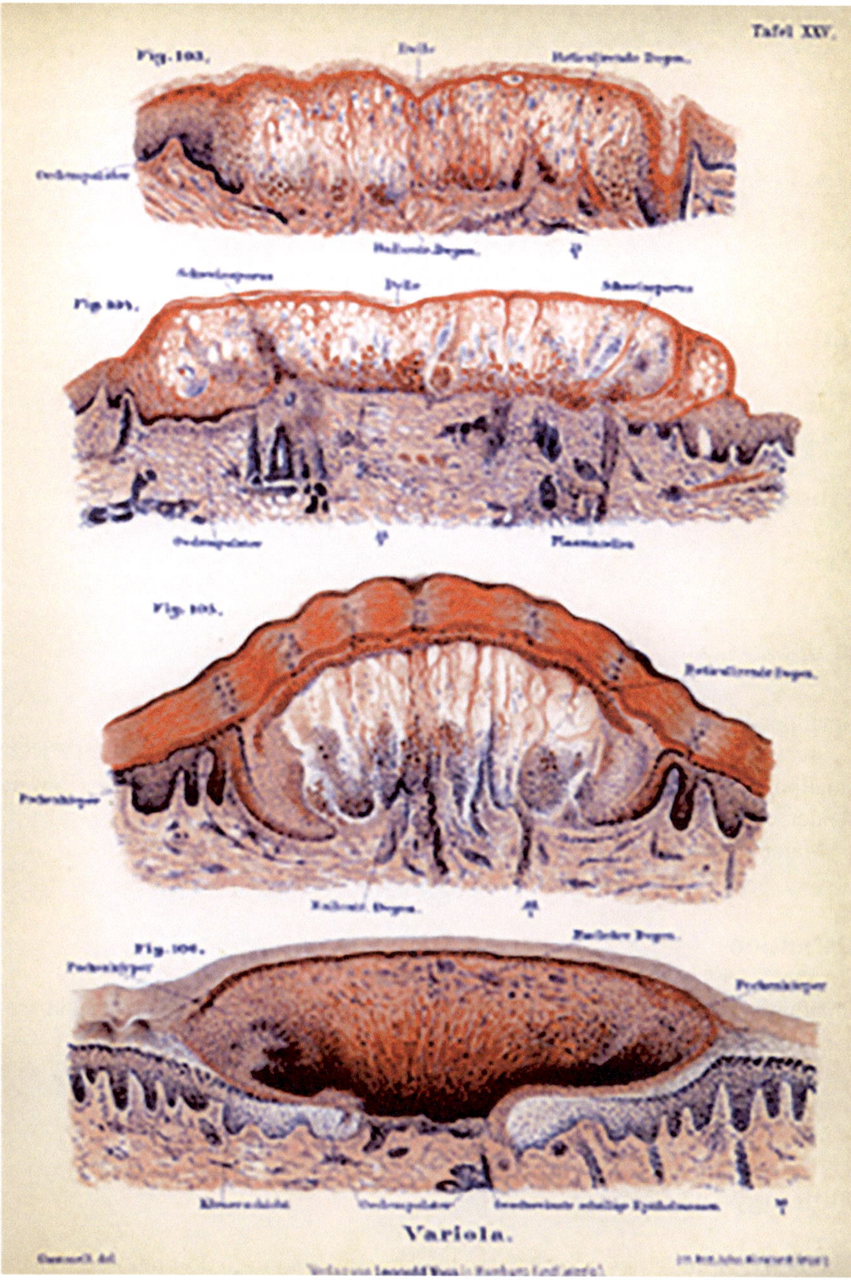

Fig. 6.28 Smallpox: schematic drawing of histology (Table XXV from PG Unna's Histologischer Atlas zur Pathologie der Haut, Leipzig 1910)

Grading of Importance

C

Level

Null

ICD-11

1E70

Synonyms

Variola.

Epidemiology

Smallpox is a human disease without animal reservoirs.

According to the 1980 declaration of the World Health Organization (WHO), smallpox has been eradicated, mainly due to effective immunisation (Edward Jenner, eighteenth century).

Major endemic areas were the Indian subcontinent and parts of Africa.

Definition

Smallpox is a member of the viral family poxvirus, genus *Orthopoxvirus* and species variola virus.

Highly contagious pustular disease caused by *Poxvirus variolae*. Overlap with *monkey* pox and cowpox/catpox.

Aetiology and Pathogenesis

The DNA-Virus *Poxvirus variolae* is the largest (300 nm to 350 nm long) of the human viral pathogens and has a brick-shaped appearance on electron microscopy. The virus is highly contagious and spreads through direct contact, by droplets, contaminated fomites, or airborne over long distances. The virus enters through the oro- or nasopharynx and replicates in the regional lymph nodes. On Day 3 to 4, viraemia with further dissemination to the bone marrow, spleen and additional lymph node chains occurs, followed by a secondary viraemia between Day 8 and 12 after infection and the start of fever and severe illness. At this stage the virus becomes localised in small blood vessels of the dermis, resulting in the appearance of rash.

Signs and Symptoms

The clinical course is severe. It begins with a non-specific febrile prodrome of general malaise, high fever, chills, vomiting, abdominal pain, headache. 1–3 days later, skin lesions appear, first at the forearms or face, scalp, palms and soles. Spread to the rest of the body with sparing of axillae and groins.

The lesions appear and mature simultaneously; in contrast to chicken pox, which present with lesions in different phases of development. Sequentially umbilicated papules, vesicles, pustules, crusts, finally leaving typical umbilicated "varioliform" scars with eschars, appear.

Localisation

Marked involvement of face, scalp, palms and soles with sparing of axillae and groins. In contrast in chickenpox palms and soles are not involved.

Classification

Poxviruses

- Orthopoxviruses
  - Smallpox
  - Vaccinia
  - Cowpox
  - Monkey pox (monkeypox virus (MPV, MPXV or hMPXV)
- Parapoxviruses
  - Ecthyma contagiosum (orf)
  - Milker's nodule
- Molluscum contagiosum

Laboratory and Other Workups

The relatively large virus can be identified by electron microscopy, by special culture or by PCR.

Dermatopathology

- Prominent reticular degeneration and necrosis of the epidermis
- Ballooning and necrosis of keratinocytes
- Intracytoplasmic globular deposits of virus capsid
- Blister formation may be minimal. Multinucleated giant cells usually are absent

Accompanying papillary oedema with erythrocyte extravasation and inflammatory infiltrate.

Course

Severe disease starting with general symptoms (fever, malaise). Skin lesions appear 3 days after infection, followed by generalised symptoms due to viraemia.

Complications

Bacterial superinfection.

Diagnosis

Typical clinical picture and course; electronmicroscopy, PCR.

Differential Diagnosis

Chickenpox, eczema herpeticum, disseminated zoster, hand-foot-mouth disease, drug eruptions, Stevens-Johnson syndrome, toxic epidermal necrolysis, generalised vaccinia, cowpox, monkeypox.

Prevention and Therapy

In the pre-eradication era, supportive care was the primary treatment available.

Tecovirimat was the first antiviral medicament for treatment of smallpox.

Finally, vaccination has been successful in the eradication of smallpox globally.

In 1798, Edward Jenner could demonstrate that cowpox protected against smallpox infection. By 1900 vaccinia virus, which is more closely related to horsepox, was globally used for vaccination. Today improved technology to develop tissue-culture-based live vaccines, live attenuated virus vaccines and viral subunit vaccine products may be used to protect personnel at increased special risk of exposure such as researchers and some healthcare workers.

Special

Vaccinia is a distinct poxvirus, probably evolved from the smallpox or the cowpox virus, that has been used for vaccination. Cowpox is more common in cats (catpox). Monkeypox are found in Zaire. They all may produce similar symptoms like smallpox.

Oral Hairy Leukoplakia [1]

Figure 6.29

Grading of Importance

C

Level

Advanced

Definition

Epstein-Barr virus associated hyperkeratotic changes on the tongue in HIV infection.

ICD-11

DA01.01

Signs and Symptoms

White, hyperkeratotic, often thread-like deposits on the sides and under surface of the tongue which cannot be wiped away (in contrast to oral candidiasis).

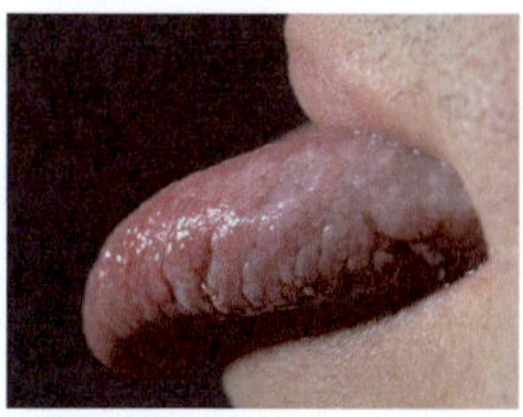

Fig. 6.29 Oral Hairy Leukoplakia

Differential Diagnosis

Leukoplakia, lichen planus, candidiasis.

References

1. Alramadhan S, Bhattacharyya I, Cohen D, Islam M (2021) Oral hairy leukoplakia in immunocompetent patients revisited with literature review. Head Neck Pathol 15:989–993
2. Bergqvist C, Kurban M, Abbas O (2017) Orf virus infection. Rev Med Virol 27(4):e1932
3. Cobb MW (1990) Human papillomavirus infection. J Am Acad Dermatol 22(4):547–566
4. Fatahzadeh M, Schwartz RA (2007) Human herpes simplex virus infections: epidemiology, pathogenesis, symptomatology, diagnosis, and management. J Am Acad Dermatol 57(5):737–763; quiz 764–736
5. Forbat E, Al-Niaimi F, Ali FR (2017) Molluscum contagiosum: review and update on management. Pediatr Dermatol 34(5):504–515
6. Kennedy PGE, Gershon AA (2018) Clinical features of varicella-zoster virus infection. Viruses 10(11):609
7. Park IU, Introcaso C, Dunne EF (2015) Human papillomavirus and genital warts: a review of the evidence for the 2015 Centers for Disease Control and Prevention Sexually Transmitted Diseases Treatment Guidelines. Clin Infect Dis 61(Suppl 8):S849–S855
8. Ren S, Gaykalova DA, Guo T, Favorov AV, Fertig EJ, Tamayo P, Callejas-Valera JL, Allevato M, Gilardi M, Santos J, Fukusumi T, Sakai A, Ando M, Sadat S, Liu C, Xu G, Fisch KM, Wang Z, Molinolo AA, Gutkind JS, Ideker T, Koch WM, Califano JA (2020) HPV E2, E4, E5 drive alternative carcinogenic pathways in HPV positive cancers. Oncogene 39(40):6327–6339
9. Simonsen K, Snowden J (2021) Smallpox. StatPearls – NCBI Bookshelf
10. Xiao A, Tsuchiya A (2020) Eczema Herpeticum. StatPearls, Treasure Island, FL

Bacterial Infections

7

Harald Gollnick, Martine Bagot, Adele De Masson, Veronique del Marmol, Gabor Dobos, and Evelyn Gaffal

Contents

H. Gollnick (✉)
Department of Dermatology & Venereology, Otto-von-Guericke University, Magdeburg, Germany
e-mail: Harald.Gollnick@med.ovgu.de

M. Bagot
Service de Dermatologie, Université Paris Cité, Hôpital Saint-Louis, Paris, France
e-mail: martine.bagot@gmail.com

A. De Masson · G. Dobos
Dermatology and Venereology, Université de Paris, Hopital Saint Louis, Paris, France
e-mail: adele.demasson@aphp.fr; gabor.dobos@charite.de

V. del Marmol
Département of Dermatology, Hôpital Erasme-HUB, Université Libre de Bruxelles, Brussels, Belgium
e-mail: veronique.delmarmol@hubruxelles.be

E. Gaffal
Department of Dermatology, University of Lübeck, Lübeck, Germany
e-mail: evelyn.gaffal@med.ovgu.de

H. Gollnick et al. (eds.), *Dermatology Cyberderm WebBook*,
https://doi.org/10.1007/978-3-031-78491-0_7

Test your learning and check your understanding of this book's contents: use the "Springer Nature Flashcards" app to access questions using ▶ https://sn.pub/1rhh6k.

To use the app, please follow the instructions in Chap. 1.

Erythrasma [7]

Figures 7.1, 7.2 and 7.3

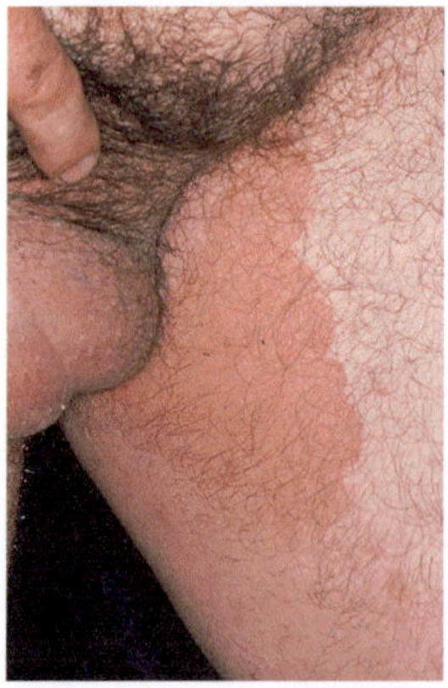

Fig. 7.1 Erythrasma: inguinal sharply demarcated brown-yellowish erythema

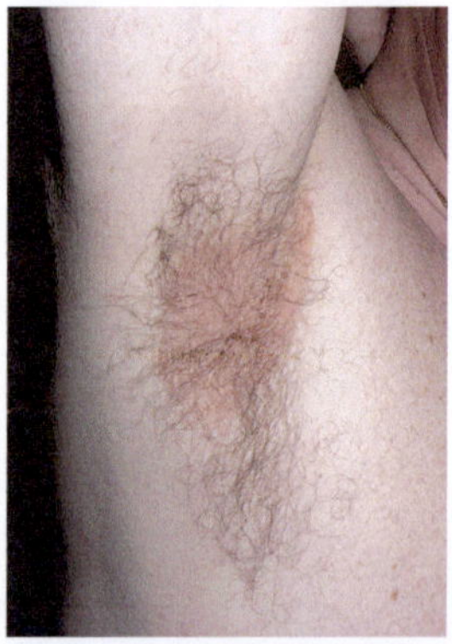

Fig. 7.2 Erythrasma: lesion in the axilla

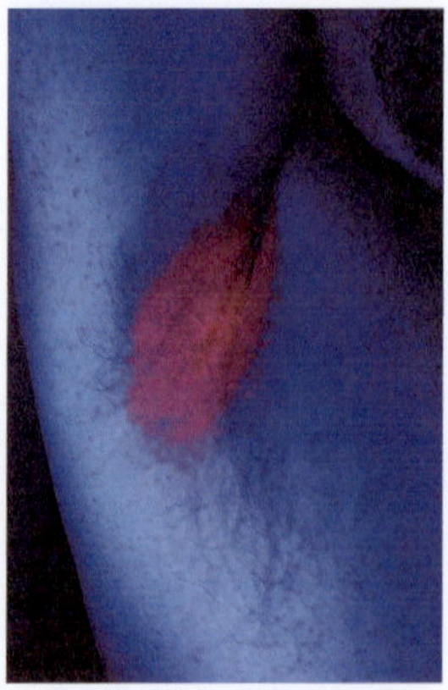

Fig. 7.3 Erythrasma: red fluorescence of axillar lesion under blue wood lamp

Grading of Importance

A

Level

Advanced

ICD-11

1C44

Synonyms

None

Definition

Superficial infection with diphtheroid bacteria mostly affecting intertriginous areas.

Etiology and Pathogenesis

Most infections are caused by *Corynebacterium minutissimum*.

Predisposing factors include obesity, diabetes, profuse sweating, occlusive clothing, and a warm humid climate.

Signs and Symptoms

Sharply demarcated, red-brown-yellowish, scaly patches, occasionally pruritic.

Localization

Axillary, inguinal, toe clefts. Occasionally sub-mammary areas.

Classification

Interdigital erythrasma, intertriginous erythrasma, generalized/disciform erythrasma.

Laboratory and Other Workups

None.

Dermatopathology

Usually not needed. Orthokeratosis with a minimal perivascular infiltrate in H&E staining. Gram staining shows positive rods and filaments in the stratum corneum.

Course

Chronic or frequent recurrences.

Complications

Scratching with secondary infection with other microbes.

Diagnosis

Wood's light: coral red fluorescence (porphyrins from bacterial metabolism), culture (difficult).

Differential Diagnosis

Tinea inguinalis and axillaris; contact dermatitis,psoriasis inversa, pityriasis versicolor, lichen planus.

Prevention and Therapy

Topical treatment including antiseptics. Erythromycin gel or solutions first choice in *Corynebacterium minutissimum* or fusidinic acid; ciclopirox or imidazoles (clotrimazole, econazole) in case of mycotic superinfection. Severe cases can be treated with oral antibiotics (erythromycin 4 × 250mg/d 2 weeks, tetracycline). Disappearance of red fluorescence indicates therapeutic success; hyperpigmentation may persist.

Impetigo Contagiosa [3, 20]

Figures 7.4 and 7.5

Grading of Importance

A

Level

Advanced

ICD-11

1B72

Synonyms

Superficial pyoderma. Superficial interfollicular and intrafollicular pyoderma

Epidemiology

Worldwide distribution, infants and small children mostly affected.

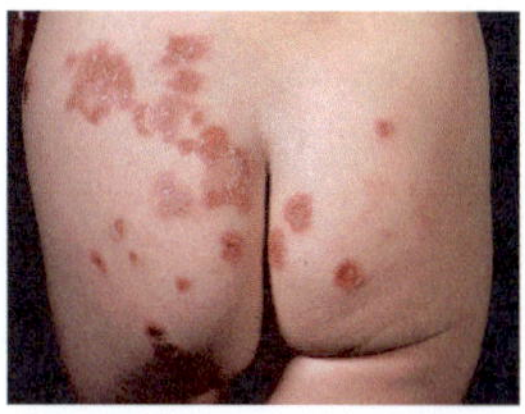

Fig. 7.4 Impetigo contagiosa: disseminated lesions on the buttocks

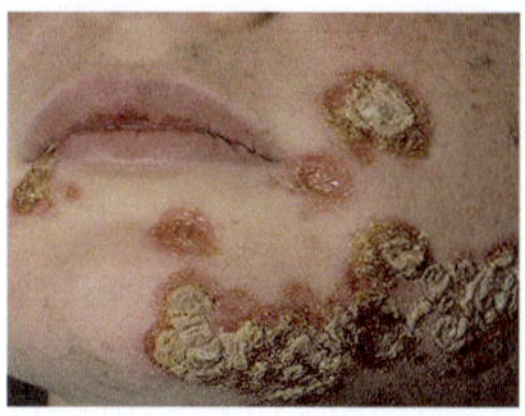

Fig. 7.5 Impetigo contagiosa: pustules with honey-yellow crusts in the face of a child

Definition

Superficial cutaneous bacterial infection of the interfollicular epidermis, more common in children, in those with atopic dermatitis, and in warm, humid environments.

Etiology and Pathogenesis

Staphylococcal and streptococcal bacterial infection spread by fomites or direct contact, usually to predisposed skin (disturbed epidermal barrier; under- or overwashing of children's skin; reduced local immune function in atopic dermatitis, angular stomatitis, rhinitis, herpes simplex, pruritus with scratching). Reservoir: nose. Causative agent usually 80% staphylococci, 10% ß-hemolytic streptococci, and 10% mixed infections.

Signs and Symptoms

Erythema, pustules, erosions and bullae, honey-yellow crusts.

Localization

Often face but can be anywhere.

Classification

Two types: a) small bullous and large bullous (10–20%), b) non-bullous (80–90%). Streptogenic are more crusted and red/inflammatory, staphylogenic more honey-like yellowish with small and large blisters. In addition, a *S. pyogenes*-related deep penetrating ecthyma type.

Laboratory and Other Workups

In widespread streptogenic type, differential blood count, CRP, urine for exclusion of glomerulonephritis and, in large bullous staphylogenic types, additionally exfoliatin toxin A/B.

Dermatopathology

Neutrophilic pustule within the follicles by staphylococci with small abscesses (intrafollicular pyoderma) or the stratum corneum in small bullous type, in large bullous type mid-epidermis by streptococci (interfollicular pyoderma).

Course

Usually self-limited, no scarring. Flat, then tiny vesicles followed by blisters, sero-crusts, and finally desquamation. Scratching leads to new lesions by autoinoculation.

Complications

Acute glomerulonephritis when infection is caused by certain strains of streptococci. Heavy producers of toxins can lead to staphylococcal scalded skin syndrome (2.2.6 SSSS) or staphylogenic/streptogenic toxic shock syndrome (2.2.7 STSS)

Diagnosis

Clinical features, Gram stain, culture.

Differential Diagnosis

Herpes simplex, eczema herpeticum, M.furfur folliculitis. Other skin diseases in particular eczemas with impetiginization.

Prevention and Therapy

- Topical: antiseptics such as polyvidone iodide or chlorhexidine; fusidic acid; wet-dry dressings if crusted
- Systemic: in widespread streptococcal and staphylococcal types, penicillinase-resistant antibiotics types, erythromycin, culture-directed secondary antibiotics
- MRSA carriers in the nostrils: mupirocin
- Contact tracing

Erysipelas [2, 4, 10, 16]

Figures 7.6, 7.7 and 7.8

Grading of Importance

A

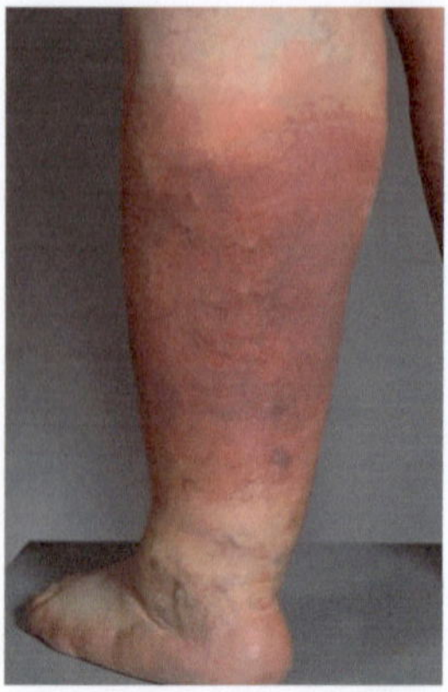

Fig. 7.6 Erysipelas: erythema and swelling of the lower leg

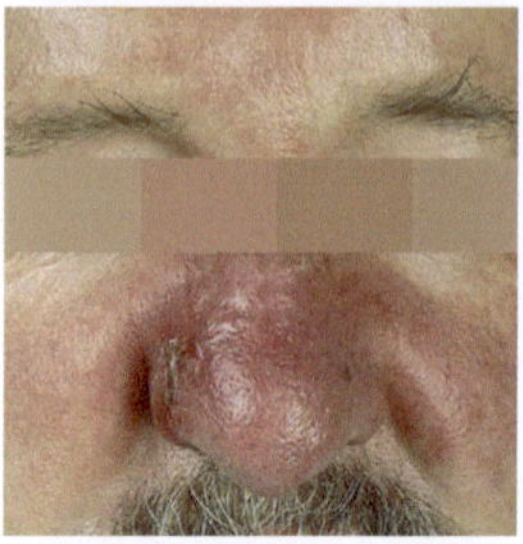

Fig. 7.7 Erysipelas: start of erythema from folliculitis of right nostril and swelling of the nose

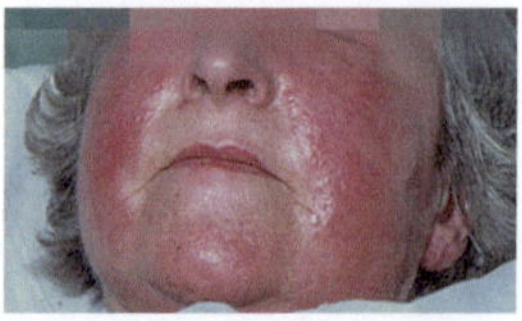

Fig. 7.8 Erysipelas: acute erythema and symmetrical swelling of the cheeks

Level

Advanced

ICD-11

1B70

Synonyms

Cellulitis (in Anglosphere).

Epidemiology

Prevalence around 1100 /100.000 per year.

Definition

Acute cutaneous bacterial infection involving the superficial lymphatics with fast spreading in the upper dermis. In rare cases it may penetrate into deeper layers including the adipose tissue, fascia, and muscle (necrotizing fasciitis).

Etiology and Pathogenesis

The site of entry often is in between toes, in skin folds, or in superficial erosions. Causative agents are about 90% beta-hemolytic group A streptococci or *Staphylococcus aureus* and sometimes other Gram-positive or Gram-negative bacteria. 90% are localized at the lower extremity and 2.5% in the face.

Signs and Symptoms

Acute illness with fever, chills (often missing in recurrent disease and in the elderly), sharply bordered, warm, tender, edematous, erythematous plaques with flame-like peripheral spread. Bullous, hemorrhagic, or necrotic presentations are more severe variants.

Localization

Erysipelas can affect any site, although it has a predilection for the face and legs. Chronic edema of the leg is predisposing. In the face often spreading to the opposite site. Visible symptoms (e.g., erythema) usually are proximal from bacterial site of entrance and leave a joint in between.

Classification

- Uncomplicated type
- Vesicular-bullous or hemorrhagic type
- Necrotic/gangrenous type

Laboratory and Other Workups

Erythrocyte sedimentation rate (ESR) and C-reactive protein (CRP) elevated, later ASL/AST titers, streptococcal DNA titer rises with a leukocytosis.

Dermatopathology

Dermal edema with dilation of upper and deep vessel plexus. Masses of polymorphous neutrophils between collagen bundles, later with necrotic areas.

Course

Flu-like presymptoms; then either short or high fever and fast response to anti-streptococcal antibiotics or complicated when deeper penetrating and host defense is low.

Complications

Lymphedema (especially with recurrent disease), myocarditis, pneumonia, glomerulonephritis. Sepsis <5%. Thrombosis (if occurring on the face this can result in venous sinus thrombosis). Necrotizing fasciitis is a severe complication, which may occur due to penetration of the infection into deeper layers including the adipose tissue, fascia, and muscle.

Diagnosis

Clinical features (fever, erythema), culture from possible entry point (tinea pedis between the toes or nasal swab), inflammatory markers.

Differential Diagnosis

Acute contact dermatitis, thrombophlebitis, erysipeloid, acrodermatitis chronica atrophicans (inflammatory stage), large phlegmon of the lower leg, be careful not to miss necrotizing fasciitis.

Prevention and Therapy

Bed rest, involved region elevated, cool moist compresses, systemic antibiotics (penicillin 4–five million IU daily i.v. or 4 x 500 mg oral or amoxicillin in uncomplicated cases, alternatively amoxicillin/clavulanate; severe erysipelas need hospitalization and thrice or four times daily 5 to 10 Mill. units penicillin, if resistant, cephalosporins) for around 7–10 days. Clindamycin is an alternative, especially in patients with penicillin allergy.

Special

In necrotizing deep penetrating type (necrotizing fasciitis), early and radical surgical intervention is mandatory.

In severe lymphedema with relapsing erysipelas: maintenance treatment (on/off). Inpatients can be treated with concomitant intermittent lymph-compression during antibiotic infusion.

Folliculitis [12]

Figures 7.9, 7.10 and 7.11

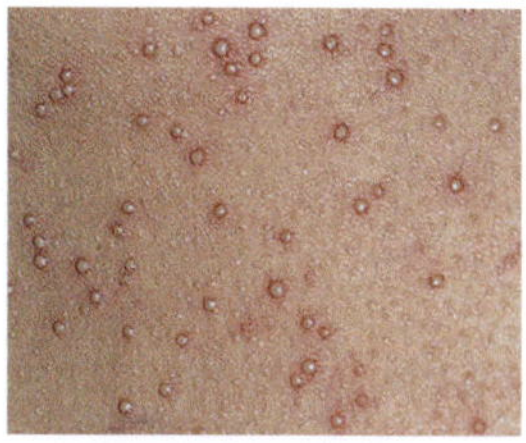

Fig. 7.9 Folliculitis: osteofolliculitis

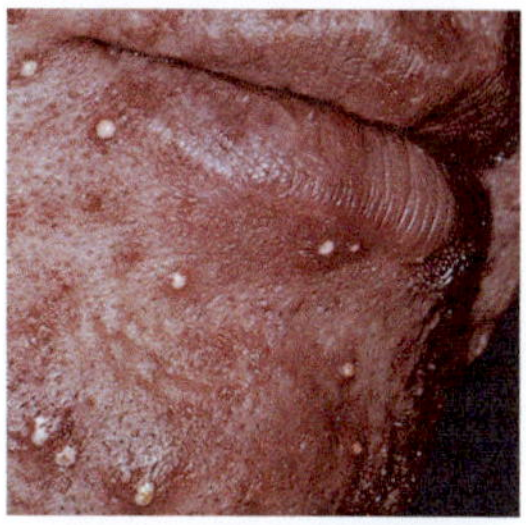

Fig. 7.10 Folliculitis: tiny pustules

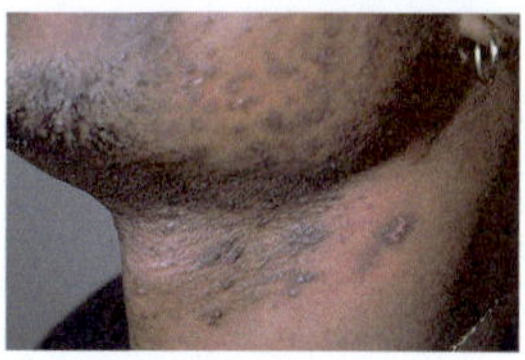

Fig. 7.11 Folliculitis: pseudofolliculitis barbae

Grading of Importance

A

Level

Advanced

ICD-11

1B74

Synonyms

Bacterial or mycotic folliculitis; infundibulo-folliculitis.

Definition

Intrafollicular pyoderma of microbial origin located at the hair follicles.

Etiology and Pathogenesis

Usually *Staphylococcus aureus* (coagulase positive), also Gram-negative bacteria or *Malassezia* spp. and other mycotic species. Predisposing factors: mechanical pressure (tight clothing, excoriations, increased humidity and sweating, occlusion by topical products or wound dressings, terminal hair shaving), immunosuppression (HIV, diabetes mellitus, corticosteroids), inadequate hygiene.

Signs and Symptoms

Papules and pustules involving the follicular canal at the acroinfundibulum and infrainfundibulum including surrounding tissue (perifolliculitis) of the hair follicles.

Localization

The skin with occlusion preferentially chest and back, intertriginous areas and buttocks, suprapubic area, belly folds, scalp, and neck.

Classification

- Ostiofolliculitis: pyoderma of the follicle ostia; often in intertriginous or occluded areas.
- Folliculitis et perifolliculitis: deeper penetration of infection into the infrainfundibulum with stronger inflammatory reaction and marked perifolliculitis. Final stage with deeper penetration leads to furuncle and involvement of several follicles to carbuncle.
- Folliculitis barbae: chronic ostiofolliculitis of terminal hair in beard area, often spread by shaving.

Laboratory and Other Workups

Culture. Blood glucose. In case of severe, widespread disease check immunodeficiency markers.

Dermatopathology

In superficial folliculitis, neutrophils invade the acroinfundibulum where Gram-positive and Gram-negative cocci or hyphae and spores colonize. The deeper the infectious agent penetrates into the follicle, the more perifollicular granulocytic neutrophils and mononuclear cells accumulate. Late stage of severe deep folliculitis leads to furuncle or carbuncle. Later granulomatous reaction and scarring repair.

Course

Acute and chronic depending on environment, type of microbe, and immune status of the patient.

Complications

Furuncle, carbuncle. Rarely sepsis. Scars.

Diagnosis

Clinical features and microbial culture (bacteria, fungi).

Differential Diagnosis

Other forms of folliculitis with sterile and non-sterile pustules: M. furfur folliculitis, eosinophilic folliculitis; pustular psoriasis; perforating folliculitis; acrosyringeal pustular eruption; pustular drug eruptions; pseudofolliculitis barbae; pili recurvati or incarnati with secondary foreign body reaction.

Prevention and Therapy

Depending on severity and location, first choice always antiseptics; avoid topical antibiotics. Systemic antibiotics in deep disseminated folliculitis and perifolliculitis or carbuncle. Topical or systemic (azoles) antimycotics when indicated.

Change and wash clothing regularly. Avoid humidity and occlusive dressing. Ph-neutral or acidic shower gels.

Furuncle/Carbuncle [6, 13, 21]

Figures 7.12 and 7.13

Grading of Importance

B

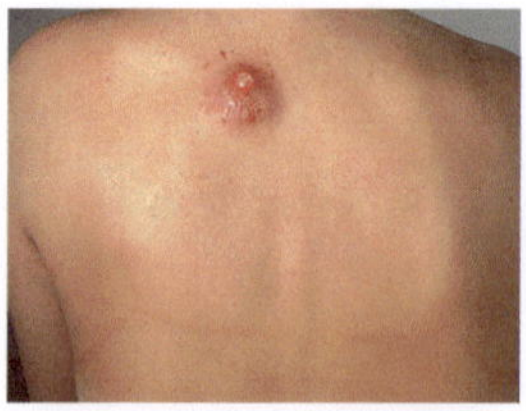

Fig. 7.12 Furuncle: purulen eruptive lesion on the back

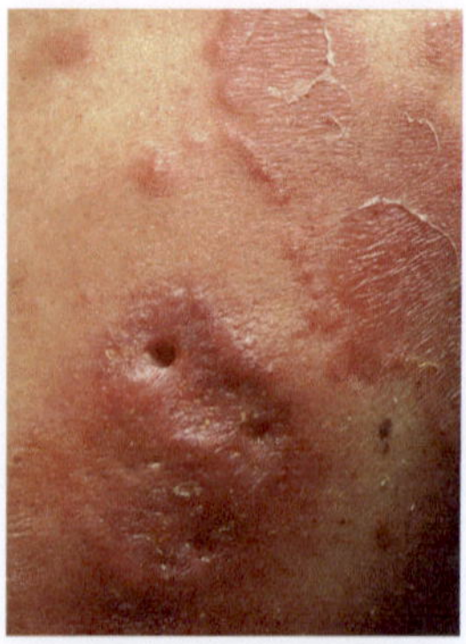

Fig. 7.13 Carbuncle: inflammatory infectious conglomerate with multiple fistular openings

Level

Advanced

ICD-11

1B75.0

Synonyms

Boil.

Epidemiology

10–20% of the population are carriers of staphylococci.

Definition

- Furuncle: deep follicular infection with abscess formation caused by *Staphylococcus aureus* or mixed infections.
- Carbuncle: conglomerate of multiple confluent deep follicular infections (furuncles), sometimes with multiple fistular openings.

Etiology and Pathogenesis

Infection either spreads via autoinoculation (from nose or throat) or exogenous. Site of entry is the follicular ostium; transfer from nostrils, armpits, groin, or natal cleft. It may be transferred to other sites from the nostrils via the finger nails.

Signs and Symptoms

Initially firm nodule, then fluctuant abscess with central necrotic plug, often edema, lymphangitis, lymphadenitis, spontaneous rupture and drainage, ulceration, later yellow-brown crusts, often painful.

Localization

All hair-bearing regions, often neck, face, axillae, or buttocks or upper shins.

Classification

None.

Laboratory and Other Workups

In case of carbuncle, check leucocytes, CRP, glucose.

Dermatopathology

Severe inflammation with accumulation of neutrophils and macrophages within and in the surrounding the follicular canal with destruction of follicle and dermal collagen and other adnexal structures. In carbuncle, fistular tunnels on serial sections.

Course

Painful and highly inflammatory course with spontaneous rupture of central follicular opening with masses of pus.

Complications

Septic course with hematogenous spread and bacterial involvement of heart valves, joints, or kidneys possible. In mid-face, risk of cavernous sinus thrombosis.

Diagnosis

Clinical feature and course.

Differential Diagnosis

Deep trichophyton infections (beard), hidradenitis suppurativa (axillae, groins, buttocks), necrotic herpes simplex, localized panniculitis, dracunculosis.

Prevention and Therapy

- Incision when fluctuation starts and continuous drainage with tamponade. Bed rest, elevation of involved area (face: talking, chewing forbidden).

- Systemic antibiotics for mid-face lesions and high-risk patients: penicillinase-resistant penicillins (oxacillin). Culture and sensitivity, since resistance is common and adjustments needed.
- Topical: no mechanical manipulation, wet antimicrobial dressings (chlorhexidine, povidone-iodine).

Staphylococcal Scalded Skin Syndrome (SSSS) [9, 14]

Figure 7.14

Grading of Importance

C

Level

Advanced

ICD-11

EA50.2

Synonyms

Staphylogenic Lyell's syndrome.

Epidemiology

The mean annual incidence of SSSS was about 8 per million US children, with prevalence in black females.

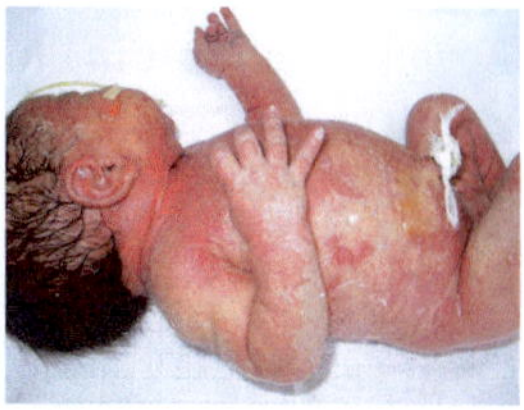

Fig. 7.14 Staphylococcal scalded skin syndrome (SSSS): widespread skin loss

Definition

SSSS: acute exfoliative dermatitis primarily in small children following staphylogenic infections with lysophage group II exfoliative toxins.

Etiology and Pathogenesis

Toxin-mediated epidermolytic dermatosis, characterized by erythema and widespread loss of the superficial epidermal layers, resembling burn. Causative agent is toxin-producing (exfoliative toxins A and B) *Staphylococcus aureus* toxins acting via serin proteases desmoglein 1 in the upper epidermal layers.

Signs and Symptoms

Following a staphylococcal infection, initially erythema resembling scarlet fever followed by small unstable blisters which quickly erode and lead to widespread skin loss similar to grade II burns. Acute course, systemically ill patients. Nikolsky sign positive.

Localization

All areas.

Classification

None.

Laboratory and Other Workups

Intensive care laboratory data regarding kidney, liver and blood, albumin.

Dermatopathology

Acantholytic cleft in the S. granulosum and blister roof only contains stratum corneum (in contrast to toxic epidermolytic necrolysis (1.1.3.5 TEN) with full-thickness epidermal damage), subcorneal blisters, and bullae.

Course

Rapid onset within hours to 2 days.

Complications

Sepsis, pneumonia.

Diagnosis

History, clinical feature, histology (frozen section of blister roof).

Differential Diagnosis

TEN (drug-induced), epidermolysis bullosa, chronic bullous disease of childhood (linear IgA disease). Streptogenic toxic syndrome; Kawasaki syndrome.

Prevention and Therapy

Children are to be admitted immediately to intensive care unit. Antibiotics covering resistant staphylococci according to resistogram; immunoglobulins are recommended. Fluid replacement as in burn patients, elimination of staphylococcal foci; antimicrobial disinfectant therapy (baths, compresses). Paracetamol, no NSAIDs.

Special

Immediate biopsy for cryosection to visualize the location of blister for differential diagnosis.

Staphylogenic/Streptogenic Toxic Shock Syndrome (STSS) [1, 8, 23]

Grading of Importance

C

Level

Advanced

ICD-11

EA50.2

Synonyms

Menstrual and non-menstrual STSS.

Epidemiology

Rare; about 50 cases per year in US.

Definition

STSS: acute *S. aureus* toxin TSST-1 and enterotoxin-related disease with fever, myalgia, nausea, headache, and vomiting and diffuse macular erythema followed by erythroderma and later exfoliation.

Etiology and Pathogenesis

Toxin-mediated epidermolytic dermatosis, characterized by erythema and widespread loss of the superficial epidermal layers, resembling burn.

- Menstrual type toxin TSST-1 and enterotoxins.
- Non-menstrual type toxin is related to *S. aureus* colonies from several infections.

Signs and Symptoms

Following a staphylococcal or streptococcal infection, initially erythema resembling scarlet fever followed by small unstable blisters which quickly erode and lead to widespread skin loss similar to grade II burns. Acute course, systemically ill patient. Nikolsky sign positive.

Localization

All areas.

Classification

Menstrual and non-menstrual STSS.

Laboratory and Other Workups

Intensive care laboratory data regarding kidney, liver and blood, albumin.

Dermatopathology

Acantholytic cleft in the S. granulosum and blister roof only contains stratum corneum (in contrast to toxic epidermolytic necrolysis (1.1.3.5 TEN)) with full-thickness epidermal damage), subcorneal blisters, and bullae.

Course

Rapid onset within hours to 2 days.

Complications

Sepsis, pneumonia. High mortality rate.

Diagnosis

History, clinical feature, histology (frozen section of blister roof).

Differential Diagnosis

TEN (drug-induced), epidermolysis bullosa, chronic bullous disease of childhood (linear IgA disease). Staphylococcal scalded syndrome (SSSS); Kawasaki syndrome.

Prevention and Therapy

Patients are to be admitted immediately to intensive care unit. Antibiotics covering resistant staphylococci or streptococci according to resistogram; immunoglobulins are recommended. Fluid replacement as in burn patients, elimination of bacterial foci; antimicrobial disinfectant therapy (baths, compresses). Paracetamol, no NSAIDs.

Special

Immediate biopsy for cryosection to visualize the location of blister for differential diagnosis.

Erythema (Chronicum) Migrans [5, 3, 14, 15, 19]

Figures 7.15, 7.16 and 7.17

Grading of Importance

A

Level

Advanced

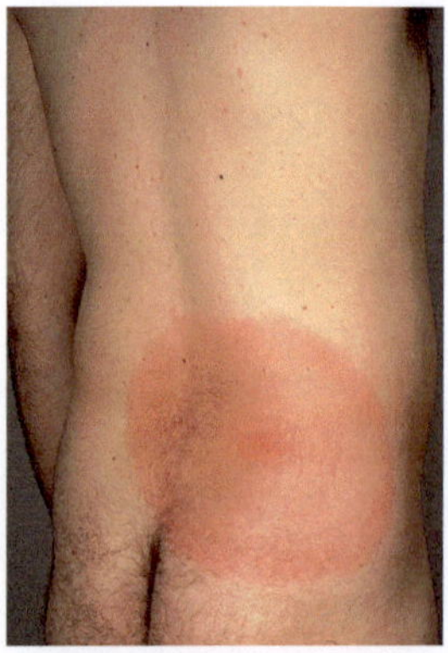

Fig. 7.15 Erythema (chronicum) migrans: centrifulal migating lesion on the hips

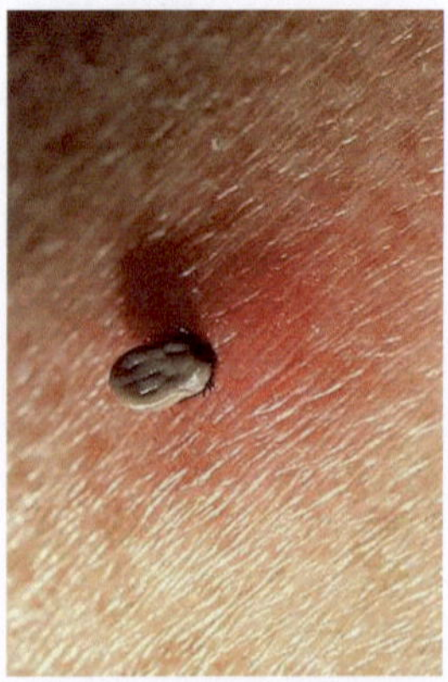

Fig. 7.16 Acute erythematous reaction to tick ixodes ricinus

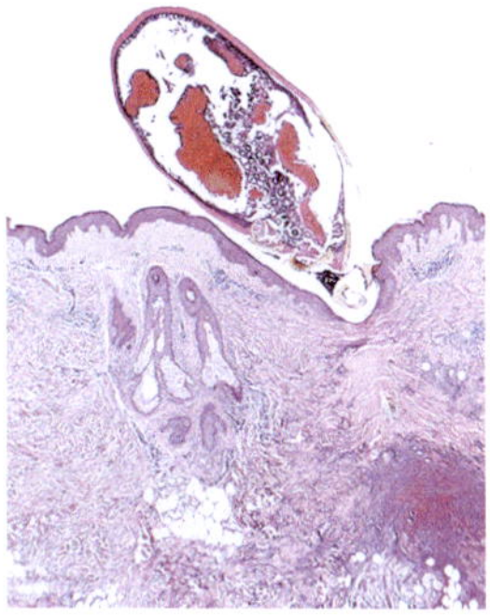

Fig. 7.17 Erythema (chronicum) migrans: histology ixodes ricinus filled with blood

ICD-11

1C1G.0

Synonyms

Stage 1 Lyme disease; early cutaneous lyme borreliosis; erythema migrans.

Epidemiology

In endemic areas in northern, middle, and eastern Europe up to 20% of *Ixodes ricinus* are infected by *B. afzelii*, *B. garinii*, *B. spielmanii*, and *Borrelia burgdorferi* sensu strictu. In the USA *B. burgdorferi* sensu *strictu* is most common. After a tick bite from an infected *Ixodes*, in 5% a local infection appears, and in up to 2%, if not treated, a manifestation of a borreliosis takes place. About 100–200 cases/100,000 people per year in Germany, Austria, or Slovenia even higher up to 400 cases. Individuals at special risk: farmers, joggers, hikers, dog owners, forest workers.

Definition

Vector (*Ixodes ricinus*)-mediated infection by various types of *Borrelia*, which belong to the family of *Spirochaetaceae*.

Etiology and Pathogenesis

Ixodes inserts (no bite!) hypostoma into the upper dermis. Factors help stabilizing its position and to open vessels and avoiding blood clotting when starting to suck.

Because of osmotic balance, saliva with *Borrelia* is deposited in the skin. *Borrelia* organisms are 20 μm long and 3 μm thick. The innate immune system reacts on the local site and the regional lymph node with a strong B-cell production of antibodies. Serological detection usually occurs by the third week after exposure.

Signs and Symptoms

- Incubation period: 1–4 weeks.
- Skin: sharply bordered erythematous ring with prominent border (sometimes with central hemorrhagic area) spreads peripherally and clears centrally, mostly 10–30 cm depending on body site.
- Center variable: pale, erythematous, hemorrhagic, vesicular. Multiple annular erythemas possible. Systemic symptoms can also occur: headache, neck pain, arthralgias, fever.

Localization

Preferentially: knee, lower leg, inguinal and buttocks, lumbar area, axilla, shoulder, chest, neck, auricle, mamilla.

Classification

- Early localized
- Early disseminated
- Late disseminated

Laboratory and Other Workups

Serology with IgM and IgG and additional early antigen markers in the immunoblot (p41, flagellin, OspE, Osp C) after about 3 weeks. Late stage Osp 17, A, B, p43.

Dermatopathology

Biopsy from the margin. Superficial dermal lymphocytic infiltrate with perivascular accumulation. Later more perineural and periglandular infiltrates and plasma cells appear. Initially some eosinophils.

Course

If not treated, dissemination may occur and manifestations in other organ systems take place: joints, muscles, peripheral and central nervous system, heart.

Complications

Meningoradiculitis, Guillain-Barré syndrome, arthritis, myocarditis (conduction disturbances), encephalopathy.

Diagnosis

History, clinical features, PCR from lesion: *Borrelia* DNA; *Borrelia* serology initially negative.

Differential Diagnosis

Other arthropodes (spider), urticaria, erythema, and granuloma annulare, other figurate erythemas like fixed drug eruption, tinea, erysipelas, and erysipeloid.

Prevention and Therapy

After exposure in fields, forest, or garden/parks inspection of total skin, children need help by parents. Doxycycline 100 mg b.i.d. for 14 days. Alternatively, amoxicillin 3 x 500 to 1000 mg/d 2 weeks. Azithomycin 2 x 250 mg / d for 10 days.

Lymphadenosis Cutis Benigna [17]

Figures 7.18, 7.19 and 7.20

Grading of Importance

B

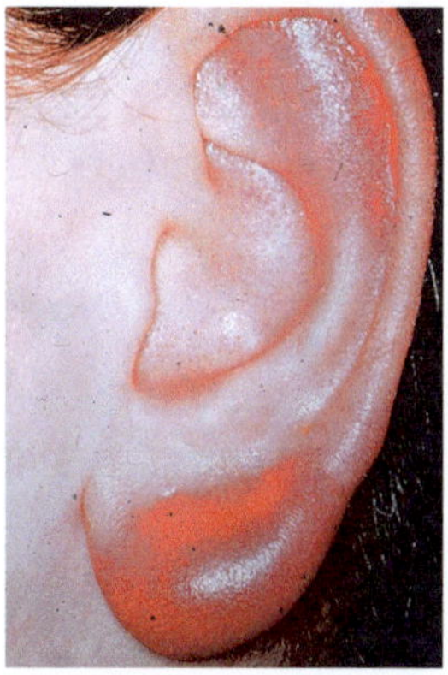

Fig. 7.18 Lymphadenosis cutis benigna: erythematous swelling of the earlobe

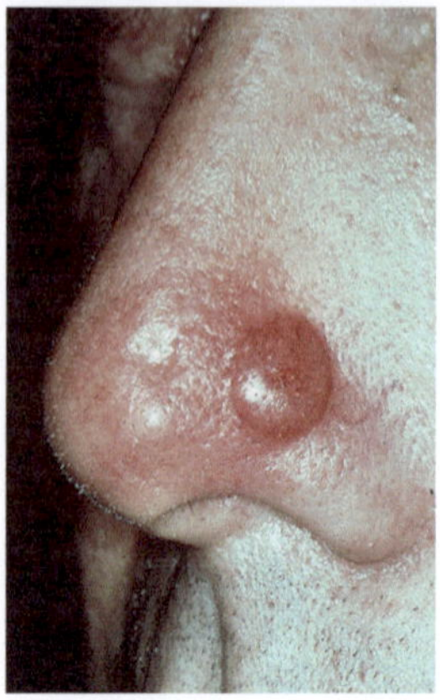

Fig. 7.19 Lymphadenosis cutis benigna: dome shaped lesion on the nose

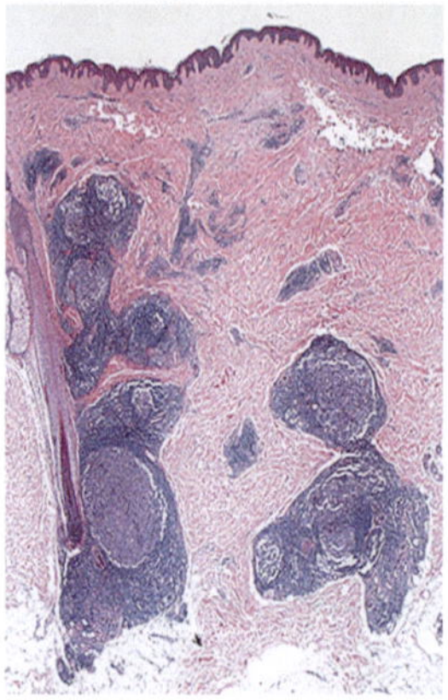

Fig. 7.20 Lymphadenosis cutis benigna: histology with follicular lesions in the dermis

Level

Advanced

ICD-11

EE91 / 1C1G.14

Synonyms

Pseudolymphoma, *Borrelia* lymphocytoma, Spiegler-Fendt-Sarcoid, lymphocytic infiltration, reactive lymphoid hyperplasia.

Epidemiology

Borrelial lymphocytoma occurs primarily in Europe, in areas in which *Ixodes ricinus* ticks are endemic (Scandinavia, parts of Austria and Eastern Europe). In Europe incidence >50 cases/100,000 inhabitants/year. Almost absent in the USA, where *Borrelia burgdorferi* sensu stricto is prevalent.

Definition

Harmless, reactive pseudolymphomatous infiltrate with follicular structures, which simulates cutaneous B-cell lymphoma (CBCL).

Etiology and Pathogenesis

Causative agents: *Borrelia garinii* and *Borrelia afzelii* living in the gut of *Ixodes ricinus* are transferred to the human host within 24 hours following the tick bite and induce a lymph follicle-like inflammatory reaction.

Rare forms include reactions following herpes zoster, scabies, *Hirudo medicinalis* (leeches).

Signs and Symptoms

Different forms: Soft, indolent, red-blue nodules (up to 5 cm) or infiltrated plaques; mostly solitary sometimes multiple. A lupoid infiltrate is seen with diascopy (under glass slide); occasionally lymphadenopathy.

Localization

Sites of predilection: loose skin (ear, nipple, scrotum, axillary folds).

Classification

None.

Laboratory and Other Workups

Borrelia IgG and IgM titers. Dermatopathology with immunochemistry. Blood cell count.

Dermatopathology

Typical B-cell pattern infiltrate, simulating an ectopic secondary (reactive antigen triggered) sharp demarcated nodular lymph follicle in the dermis, composed of small (centrocytes) and large (centroblasts) polyclonal B-lymphocytes (expression of B-cell-epitopes CD20, CD79a) and many macrophages with inclusions (tingible bodies) in the follicular center, accompanied by polyclonal (mixed kappa and lambda light chains) plasma cells and varying number of eosinophils. No monoclonal rearrangement of immunoglobulins heavy or light chains.

Course

Often heal spontaneously within weeks or some months or following adequate treatment; in contrast to malignant CBCL, which enlarges permanently.

Complications

None.

Diagnosis

Clinical features, serology, histology, PCR.

Differential Diagnosis

Malignant B–/T-cell lymphomas, cutaneous sarcoidosis, secondary syphilis.

Prevention and Therapy

Antibiotics (doxycycline 100 mg b.i.d. for 3 weeks). Topical glucocorticosteroids may be effective (apoptosis of lymphocytes).

Acrodermatitis Chronica Atrophicans [18]

Figures 7.21, 7.22 and 7.23

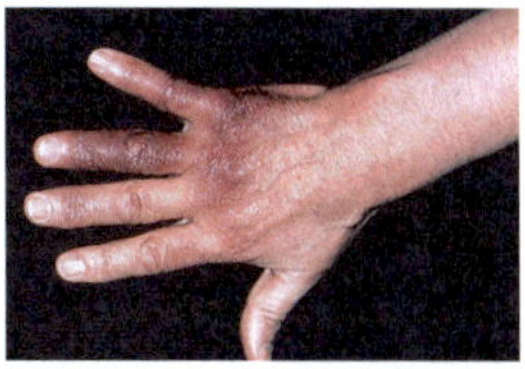

Fig. 7.21 Acrodermatitis chronica atrophicans: discoloration and atrophy of skin on the back of the hand

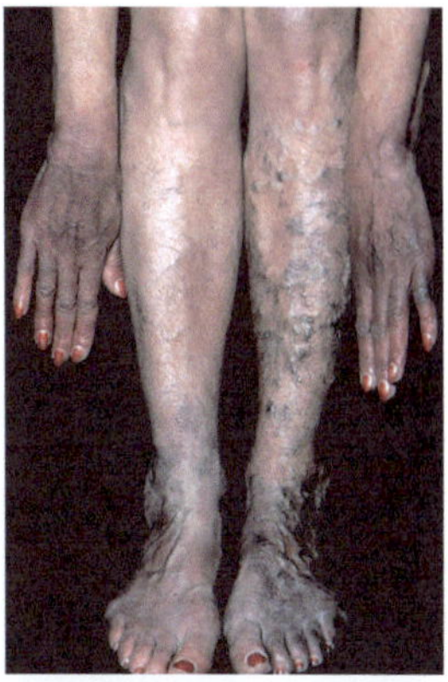

Fig. 7.22 Acrodermatitis chronica atrophicans: thinning of skin and discoloration on all extremities

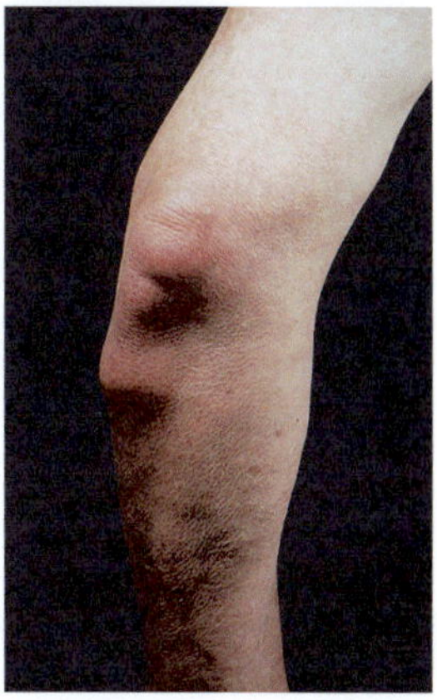

Fig. 7.23 Acrodermatitis chronica atrophicans: fibrinoid nodule on the elbow

Grading of Importance

B

Level

Advanced

ICD-11

1C1G.14

Synonyms

Lyme borreliosis; late cutaneous lyme borreliosis; Herxheimer's disease.

Epidemiology

In the European population < 10:100,000 per year. In the USA, rare; in northern Mexico, some infections. All ages can be involved, but adults are preferred. Individuals at special risk: farmers, joggers, hikers, dog owners, forest workers.

Definition

Cutaneous manifestation of chronic *Borrelia burgdorferi* sensu latu species and *B. afzelii* infection leading to a first step to inflammatory edematous changes and in a later step to irreversible atrophy. Concurrent neurological and /or cardiac involvement may occur.

Etiology and Pathogenesis

Late manifestation of chronic infection, mostly by spirochaete *Borrelia afzelii*. Transfer of *Borrelia* bacteria mostly via tick sting (*Ixodes ricinus*). History (mostly 2–6 months back) of insertion of hypostoma into the skin and sampling of blood and in parallel introduction of tick saliva and content of intestinal fluids with *Borrelia*.. Strong B-cell activation and accumulation of plasma cells in situ. Persistence of microbes over decades possible. Destruction of dermal tissue, nerves, and epidermal atrophy.

Signs and Symptoms

Stage I: inflammatory-edematous stage.

Stage II: atrophic stage (cigarette paper skin, telangiectases, pigmentary changes). Sclerosis (scleroderma-like collagen changes, ulnar and tibial bands) and hard fibrous nodules (up to several cm, cartilage-like nodules about joints). Associated allodynia and axonal peripheral neuropathy.

Localization

Hands and feet, elbows, knees, initially unilateral, later symmetrical. Unusual localization possible.

Classification

Early edematous inflammatory and late atrophic stage.

Laboratory and Other Workups

Sedimentation rate elevated, *Borrelia* IgG titer raised, sometimes IgM persisting. Typical outer surface proteins Osp 17 (p21), Osp A and B, p 30,43,45,58 83,100 persisting antigens.

Dermatopathology

Atrophy of epidermis. Infiltrate rich in plasma cells and additionally lymphomononuclear cells. No neutrophils or eosinophils. Collagen and elastic fiber destruction. Often adnexal structures with follicles and sweat glands are missing. Sometimes plasma cells around nerve bundles.

Course

Chronic over years.

Complications

Soft tissue and muscle atrophy. Polyneuropathy. Increased vulnerability of atrophic skin.

Diagnosis

Clinical features, histology, PCR, *Borrelia* serology positive with antigen subtype profiling necessary.

Differential Diagnosis

Thrombophlebitis, deep venous thrombosis, acrocyanosis, perniones, erysipelas, in stage I. Varicose veins in stage II. Sudeck's atrophy in both stages. Advanced aging of the skin with dermatoporosis.

Prevention and Therapy

Prevention of reinfection to tick stings. Treatment according to stage related guideline. First choice systemic antibiotic is doxycycline orally 3 weeks 200 mg/day. Infusions with ceftriaxone.

Leprosy (See Also Section "Leprosy" in Chap. 29) [11]

Figures 7.24, 7.25, 7.26, 7.27, 7.28 and 7.29

Grading of Importance

B

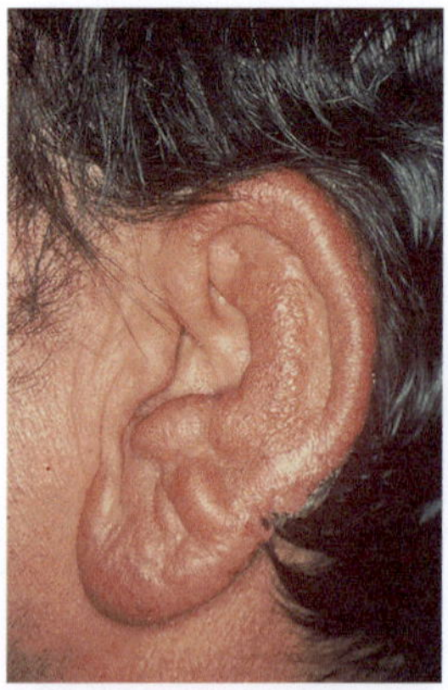

Fig. 7.24 Leprosy: swelling of the earlobe in paucibacillary leprosy

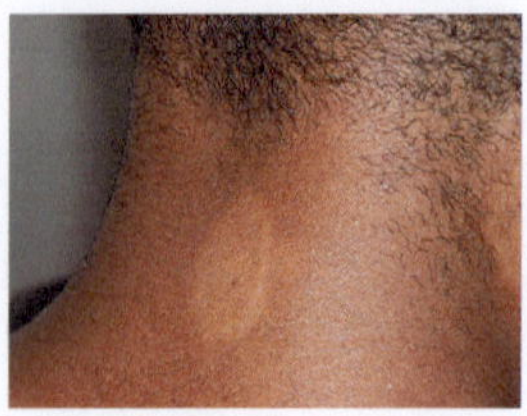

Fig. 7.25 Leprosy: circumscribed depigmented spot in the neck

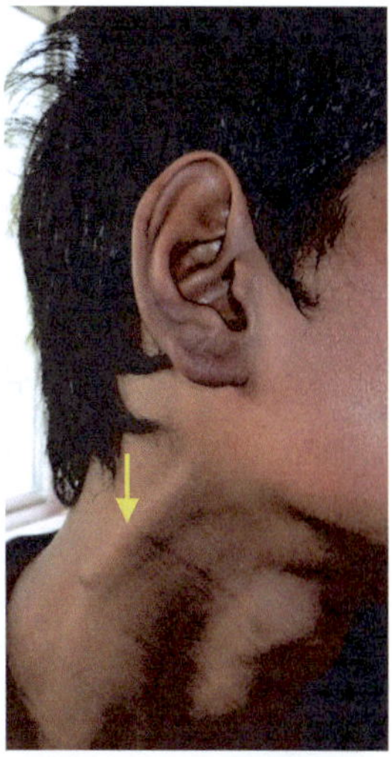

Fig. 7.26 Leprosy: swelling of nerve (arrow)

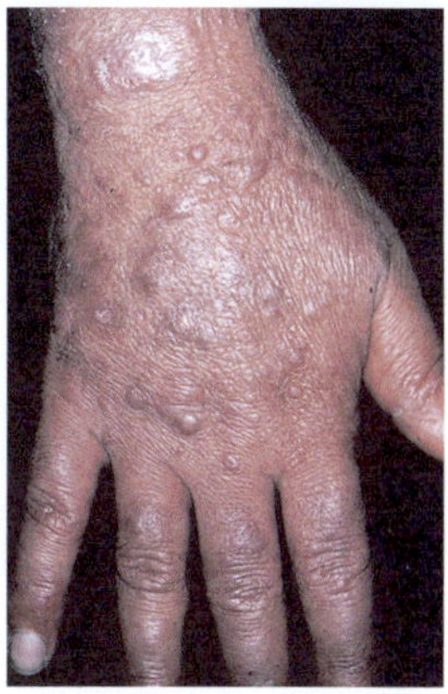

Fig. 7.27 Leprosy: popular lesions on the hand

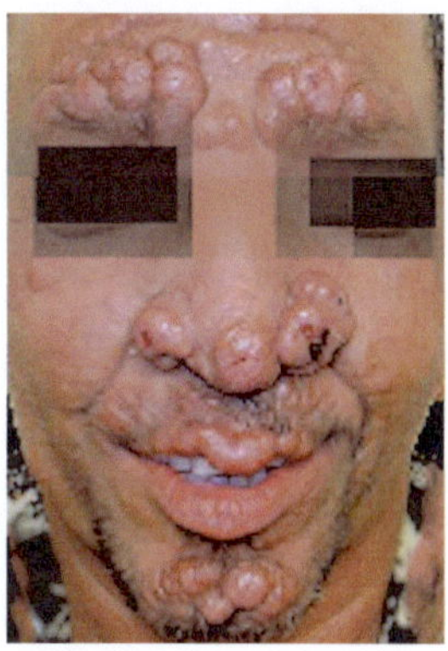

Fig. 7.28 Leprosy: facies leonina

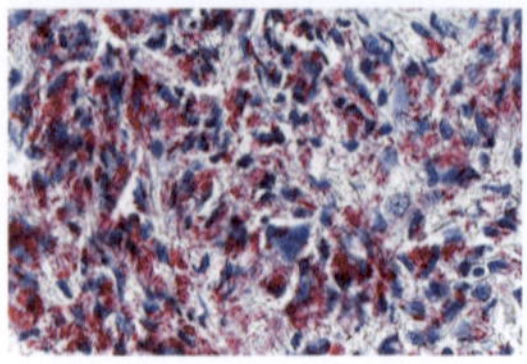

Fig. 7.29 Leprosy: acid fast positive rots in histology of lepromatous leprosy

Level

Advanced

ICD-11

1B20

Synonyms

Hansen's disease.

Epidemiology

Mainly a tropical disease, belonging to the group of neglected tropical diseases (section "Leprosy" NTD's) malnutrition; poverty is major risk factor. Worldwide around 200,000 new cases are registered every year (predominantly in India, Brazil, Indonesia, Nepal, Congo, Mozambique, Philippines). However as soon as therapy has started, patients drop out from the statistics.

Definition

Chronic, minimally contagious infection with *Mycobacterium leprae*, developing after an incubation period of 3 to 20 years, mainly affecting the skin and peripheral nerves.

Etiology and Pathogenesis

Leprosy is caused by *Mycobacterium leprae*, an intracellular Gram-positive acid-fast bacillus.

Signs and Symptoms

- **Skin involvement:** solitary or multiple hypopigmented, anhidrotic and hypoesthetic macules or plaques, nodules (leproma), red macules with peripheral papular spread, solitary or multiple hypopigmented areas with reduced sensation. Leonine face is a special feature.
- **Neurological features:** palpable thickening of nerves (e.g., ulnar), impaired sensation, motor and sensory problems (muscle atrophy), trophic ulcers.
- **Eye involvement** includes: lagophthalmia, uveitis, cataract, corneal involvement, optic neuropathy, diffuse involvement (panophthalmia leprosa), which can lead to loss of vision and blindness.

Localization

Hypopigmented macules with sensitivity loss can occur anywhere on the body. Leproma nodules are frequently located on the face, ears, or hands.

Classification

Leprosy can be classified by clinical manifestations, which span from indeterminate leprosy (IL, potential initial stage), tuberculoid leprosy (TT), lepromatous leprosy (LL), and borderline leprosy (spectrum of transient forms, BT, BL, BB). This disease also can be classified by the number of bacilli; paucibacillary leprosy (corresponding to tuberculoid leprosy) and multibacillary leprosy (corresponding to lepromatous leprosy).

Immune reactions associated with the presence of *M. leprae* are known as leprosy reactions:

- Type I: type IV immunologic reaction; flare-up of old skin lesions and neuritis. Occurs during therapy
- Type II: type III immunologic reaction in lepromatous or borderline leprosy. Skin changes known as erythema nodosum leprosum

Laboratory and Other Workups

Staining of swap from scarification (prevent bleeding) for acid-fast bacilli (Ziehl-Neelsen, Fite-Faraco, or immunohistochemistry). A polymerase chain reaction in the skin can be used to identify *Mycobacterium leprae* but can be negative in tuberculoid forms without ruling out the diagnosis.

Dermatopathology

Tuberculoid leprosy manifests as granuloma with epithelioid histiocytes surrounding small cutaneous nerves; giant cells may be seen. Bacilli are usually scarce but can be found by immunohistochemistry.

In lepromatous leprosy, macrophages (Virchow cells) can be found in poorly circumscribed nodules in the dermis; numerous bacilli are present especially in cutaneous nerves and in the vessels. Bacilli can be visualized by Ziehl-Neelsen and immunohistochemistry staining.

Course

The course can change in any direction between lepromatous, tuberculoid, and borderline forms.

Complications

Neurological deficiencies, amputation, mutilations, chronic ulcers, blindness.

Diagnosis

The diagnosis is suspected when clinically evocative skin lesions +/− palpable nerves or neurological defects are observed. The diagnosis is confirmed by the existence of a specific leproid granuloma histologically and/or by the identification of *M. leprae* (by Ziehl-Neelsen or Fite and immunohistochemistry staining and/or PCR) especially in lepromatous form.

Differential Diagnosis

Hypopigmented lesions: *eczema*, psoriasis, dermatophytes infection, seborrheic dermatitis, mycosis fungoides, vitiligo, pityriasis versicolor, pityriasis rosea.

Nodules: sarcoidosis, cutaneous lymphoma, leishmaniasis, syphilis.

Prevention and Therapy

The treatment is a combination of antibiotics (rifampicin, dapsone, and clofazimine), and the duration of the treatment depends on the form of disease. Paucibacillary leprosy is treated for 6 months. Multibacillary leprosy is treated for at least 12 months.

Skin Tuberculosis and Atypical Mycobacterioses (MOTT) [22, 24]

Figures 7.30, 7.31, 7.32, 7.33, 7.34, 7.35 and 7.36

Grading of Importance

B

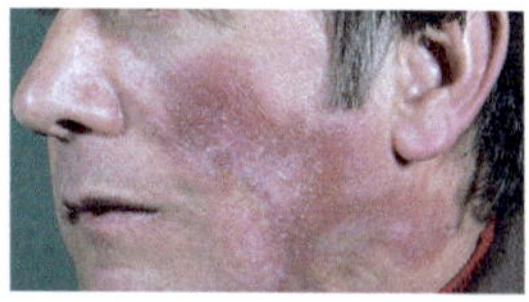

Fig. 7.30 Skin tuberculosis: red-brown discoloration of the face in lupus vulgaris

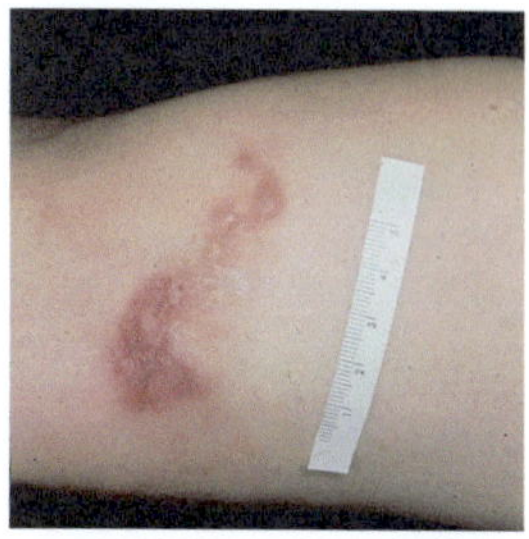

Fig. 7.31 Skin tuberculosis: red-brown lesion of the lower arm in lupus vulgaris

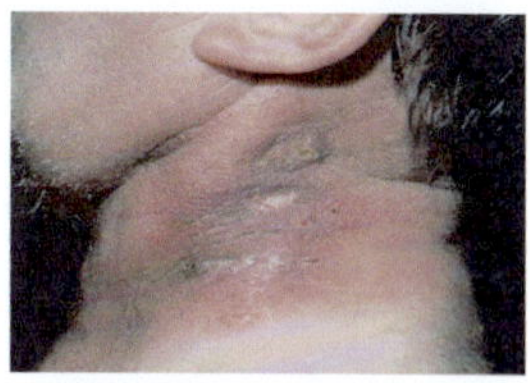

Fig. 7.32 Skin tuberculosis: tuberculosis colliquativa on the neck

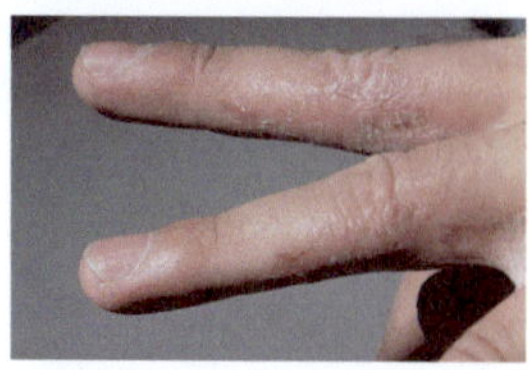

Fig. 7.33 Atypical mycobacterioses (MOTT): tuberculosis verrucosa

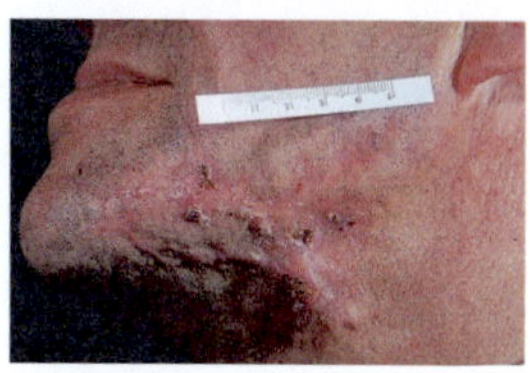

Fig. 7.34 Atypical mycobacterioses (MOTT): verrucous tuberculosis

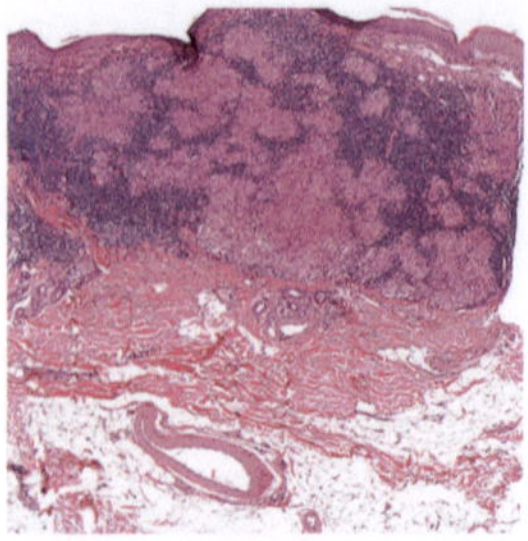

Fig. 7.35 Skin tuberculosis: granulomatous infiltrate (with caseating necrosis)

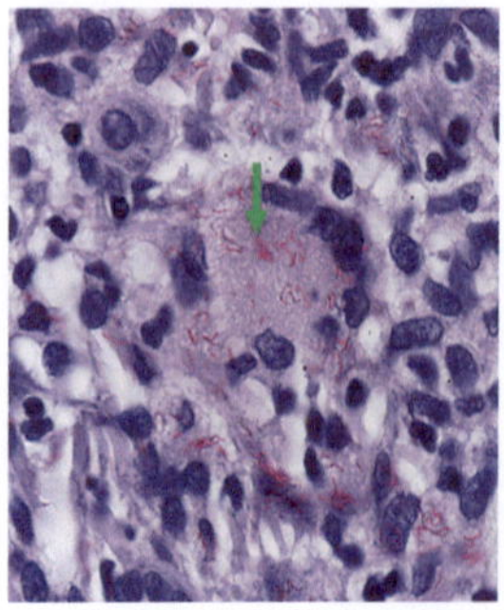

Fig. 7.36 Skin tuberculosis: acid fast resistant mycobacteriae (Ziehl-Neelsen)

Level

Advanced

ICD-11

1B12.8

Synonyms

Skin Koch disease, lupus vulgaris, tuberculosis cutis, MOTT (mycobacteria other than tuberculosis).

Epidemiology

Tuberculosis (TB) is a worldwide frequent infection with around ten million new cases each year. It affects frequently the lungs, the mediastinal or peripheral lymph nodes, urogenital tract, bone, nervous system, or the skin. Immune suppression is a risk factor of developing tuberculosis (malnutrition, AIDS). This disease occurs more frequently in developing countries.

Atypical mycobacterial skin infections include fish tank (or swimming pool) granuloma caused by *Mycobacterium marinum* (typically papulonodules or ulcers of the hands/limbs), Buruli ulcer caused by *Mycobacterium ulcerans* (cutaneous nodule or ulcer), present in tropical countries, and infections with *M. chelonae*, *M. abscessus*, or *M. fortuitum*, present worldwide, and most frequently found after skin injections, tattoos, skin trauma, or surgery.

Definition

Skin infection with *Mycobacterium tuberculosis* and MOTT complex.

Aetiology and Pathogenesis

Classical tuberculosis by *Mycobacterium tuberculosis* is transmitted by droplets. Infectious droplets are generated when persons with pulmonary or laryngeal TB disease cough, sneeze, shout, or sing. MOTT of the lungs may be transmitted via droplets (*M. avium* or *kansasii*) or on the skin by contact with defective skin barrier.

Signs and Symptoms

Cutaneous tuberculosis can appear in different forms depending on immune status. Lupus vulgaris: red-brown papules with apple-jelly color on glass diascopy. Tuberculosis cutis verrucosa or prosector's warts: verrucous plaque-like lesions.

Tuberculids: erythema induratum of Bazin, lichen scrofulosorum, and papulonecrotic tuberculids. Erythema induratum of Bazin presents typically as inflammatory nodules of the limbs in elderly women.

Localization

Lupus vulgaris and tuberculids can appear anywhere on the body. Tuberculosis cutis verrucosa is frequently found on the hands or face. Erythema induratum of Bazin presents on lower limbs; specific localization in *Mycobacterium marinum* at hands and lower arms.

Classification

Skin tuberculosis results from direct inoculation or systemic spread of *Mycobacterium tuberculosis* complex. Cutaneous atypical mycobacterial infections are non-tuberculous mycobacterial infections of the skin, excluding leprosy.

Laboratory and Other Workups

Mantoux-test: local inoculation with tuberculin toxin. After 2 or 3 days, the diameter of the induration is measured and is used to define positivity. A positive test indicates a previous contact with the *Mycobacterium tuberculosis* complex.

Quantiferon-TB-Gold-test (interferon-gamma release assay) is another indirect, highly sensitive and specific laboratory test that detects the presence of a cellular immune response against *M. tuberculosis.*

Bacterial culture (Lowenstein medium) has a slow growth. From biopsies PCR tests can be used to prove the presence of different types of mycobacteria.

Faster discrimination follows by PCR from biopsy.

Dermatopathology

Tuberculosis: granulomatous infiltrate with caseating necrosis. Bacilli are colored by Ziehl-Neelsen, Fite-Faraco, and immunohistochemistry staining.

Course

Tuberculosis is a chronic disease, and if untreated, the infection can spread to other organs.

Complications

Ulcerations, scaring, mutilations or systemic spread, squamous cell carcinoma on chronic skin ulcers.

Diagnosis

Detection of the different types of mycobacteria by Ziehl-Neelsen and immunohistochemistry staining, PCR, or mycobacterial direct examination and culture, associated with a consistent clinical context.

Differential Diagnosis

Early lupus vulgaris may mimic psoriasis vulgaris or discoid lupus erythematosus. MOTT can mimic different skin infections such as ulcers, deep impetigo, nodular vasculitis, and leprosy.

Prevention and Therapy

Treatment of TB is becoming more complicated today because of high worldwide distribution of resistance. It typically relies on isoniazid and rifampicin for 6 months, together with ethambutol and pyrazinamide in the first 2 months. Bacterial culture has to be initiated prior to treatment to evaluate resistance.

Treatment of MOTT is different to classical tuberculosis and is based on antibiotics such as tetracyclines, fluoroquinolones, macrolides (e.g., amikacin, clarithromycin), rifampicin, and sulfonamides (cotrimoxasole). Deep surgical debridement is often essential.

Special

Prior to the introduction of immunosuppressive or immunomodulatory therapies (e.g., TNF-alpha inhibitors), a latent underlying mycobacterial infection has to be excluded to avoid the risk of reactivation.

References

1. Angus DC, van der Poll T (2013) Severe sepsis and septic shock. N Engl J Med 369(9):840–851
2. Bläckberg A, Trell K, Rasmussen M (2015) Erysipelas, a large retrospective study of aetiology and clinical presentation. BMC Infect Dis. 15:402
3. Bowen AC, Mahé A, Hay RJ, Andrews RM, Steer AC, Tong SYC et al (2015) The Global Epidemiology of Impetigo: A Systematic Review of the Population Prevalence of Impetigo and Pyoderma. PLoS ONE 10(8):e0136789. https://doi.org/10.1371/journal.pone.0136789
4. Brindle RJ & Louise A. O'Neill LA & Williams OM (2020) Risk, Prevention, Diagnosis, and Management of Cellulitis and Erysipelas. Current Dermatology Reports 9:73–82
5. Cardenas-de la Garza JA, De la Cruz-Valadez E, Ocampo-Candiani J, Welsh O (2019) Clinical spectrum of Lyme disease. Eur J Clin Microbiol Infect Dis 38(2):201–208
6. Demos M, McLeod MP, Nouri K (2012) Recurrent furunculosis: a review of the literature. Br J Dermatol 167(4):725–732
7. Forouzan P, Cohen PR (2020) Erythrasma Revisited: Diagnosis, Differential Diagnoses, and Comprehensive Review of Treatment. Cureus. 12(9):e10733. https://doi.org/10.7759/cureus.10733. PMID: 33145138; PMCID: PMC7599055
8. Gottlieb M, Long B, Koyfman A (2018) The evaluation and management of toxic shock syndrome in the Emergency Department: a review of the literature. J Emerg Med. 54(6):807–814. https://doi.org/10.1016/j.jemermed.2017.12.048. Epub 2018 Jan 20. PMID: 29366615
9. Handler MZ, Schwartz RA (2014) Staphylococcal scalded skin syndrome: diagnosis and management in children and adults. J Eur Acad Dermatol Venereol 28(11):1418–1423
10. Kröger K, Schwarzkopf A, Eder S, Protz K, Münter C, Dissemond J (2021) Diagnostik und Therapie des Erysipels: Ein Positionspapier der Initiative Chronische Wunden (ICW) e. V [Diagnosis and therapy of erysipelas: A position paper of the Society Initiative Chronische Wunde (ICW) e. V.]. Dtsch Med Wochenschr 146(12):822–830. https://doi.org/10.1055/a-1392-8128. German. Epub 2021 Jun 15. PMID: 34130325
11. Kundakci N, Erdem C (2019) Leprosy: a great imitator. Clin Dermatol 37(3):200–212

12. Lin H-S, Lin P-T, Tsai Y-S, Wang S-H, Ching-Chi (2018) Interventions for bacterial folliculitis and boils (furuncles and carbuncles). Cochrane Database Syst Rev. 2018(8):CD013099. https://doi.org/10.1002/14651858.CD013099. PMCID: PMC6513076
13. Lin H-S, Lin PT, Tsai Y-S, Wang S-H, Chi C-C. Interventions for bacterial folliculitis and boils (furuncles and carbuncles). Cochrane Database Syst Rev 2021, Issue 2. Art. No.: CD013099. DOI: https://doi.org/10.1002/14651858.CD013099.pub2. Accessed 17 January 2025
14. Liy-Wong C, Pope E, Weinstein M, Lara-Corrales I (2021) Staphylococcal scalded skin syndrome: an epidemiological and clinical review of 84 cases. Pediatr Dermatol 38(1):149–153. https://doi.org/10.1111/pde.14470. Epub 2020 Dec 1. PMID: 33283348
15. Marques AR, Strle F, Wormser GP (2021) Comparison of Lyme Disease in the United States and Europe. Emerg Infect Dis. 27(8):2017–2024. https://doi.org/10.3201/eid2708.204763
16. Michael Y, Shaukat NM (2020) Erysipelas. StatPearls, Treasure Island, FL
17. Mitteldorf C, Kempf W (2020) Cutaneous pseudolymphoma-a review on the spectrum and a proposal for a new classification. J Cutan Pathol 47(1):76–97
18. Moniuszko-Malinowska A, Czupryna P, Dunaj J, Pancewicz S, Garkowski A, Kondrusik M, Grygorczuk S, Zajkowska J (2018) Acrodermatitis chronica atrophicans: various faces of the late form of Lyme borreliosis. Adv Dermatol Allergol XXXV(5):490–494. https://doi.org/10.5114/ada.2018.77240. Epub 2018 Jul 19. PMID: 30429707; PMCID: PMC6232541
19. Nadelman RB (2015) Erythema migrans. Infect Dis Clin N Am 29(2):211–239
20. Nardi NM, Schaefer TJ (2020) Impetigo. StatPearls, Treasure Island, FL
21. Ramakrishnan K, Salinas RC, Higuita N (2015) Skin and soft tissue infections. Am Fam Physician 92(6):474–483. PMID: 26371732k
22. Scollard DM, Dacso MM, Abad-Venida ML (2015) Tuberculosis and leprosy: classical granulomatous diseases in the twenty-first century. Dermatol Clin 33(3):541–562
23. Smith RJ, Schlievert PM, Himelright IM, Baddour LM (1994) Dual infections with Staphylococcus aureus and streptococcus pyogenes causing toxic shock syndrome. Possible synergistic effects of toxic shock syndrome toxin 1 and streptococcal pyrogenic exotoxin C. Diagn Microbiol Infect Dis 19(4):245–247
24. van Zyl L, du Plessis J, Viljoen J (2015) Cutaneous tuberculosis overview and current treatment regimens. Tuberculosis (Edinb) 95(6):629–638

Fungal Infections

8

Branka Marinović and Zrinka Bukvić Mokos

Contents

B. Marinović (✉) · Z. Bukvić Mokos
Department of Dermatology and Venereology, School of Medicine University of Zagreb, Zagreb, Croatia
e-mail: branka.marinovic@kbc-zagreb.hr

H. Gollnick et al. (eds.), *Dermatology Cyberderm WebBook*,
https://doi.org/10.1007/978-3-031-78491-0_8

Test your learning and check your understanding of this book's contents: use the "Springer Nature Flashcards" app to access questions using ▶ https://sn.pub/1rhh6k.

To use the app, please follow the instructions in Chap. 1.

Dermatophyte Infections [4, 7]

Figures 8.1, 8.2, 8.3, 8.4, 8.5, 8.6, 8.7, 8.8 and 8.9

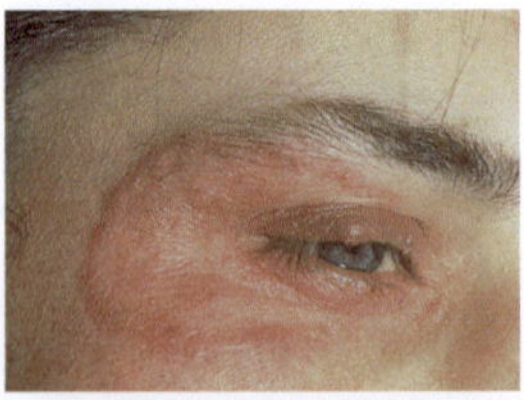

Fig. 8.1 Dermatophyte infections: erythema with elevated border

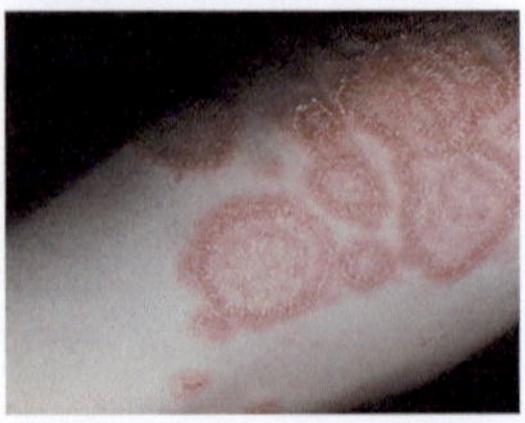

Fig. 8.2 Dermatophyte infections: target lesions on the lower arm

Fig. 8.3 Dermatophyte infections: sharply demarcated inguinal lesion

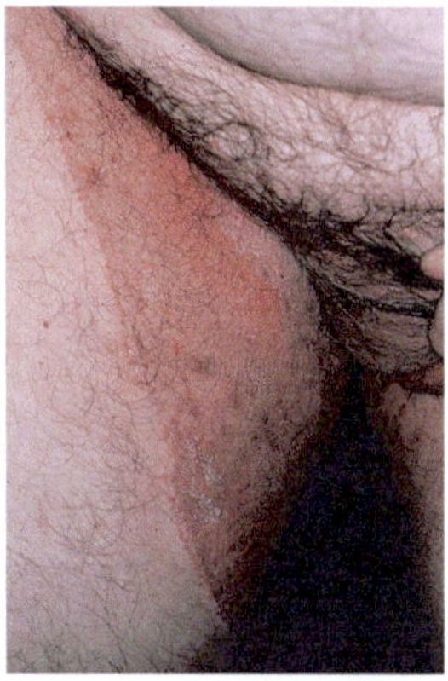

Fig. 8.4 Dermatophyte infections: centrifugal spreading lesions on the buttocks with central regession

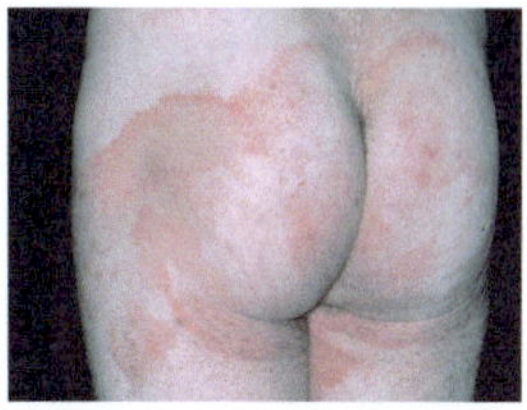

Fig. 8.5 Dermatophyte infections: sycosis barbae

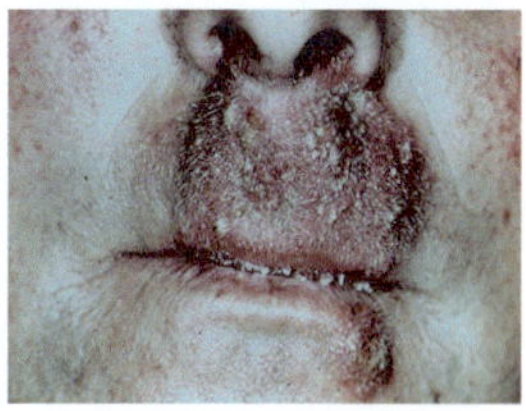

Fig. 8.6 Dermatophyte infections: alopecia due to fungal infection

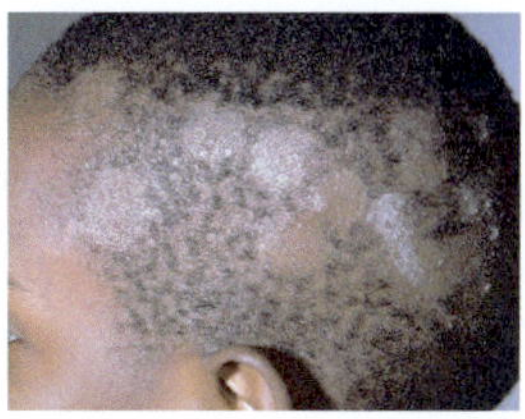

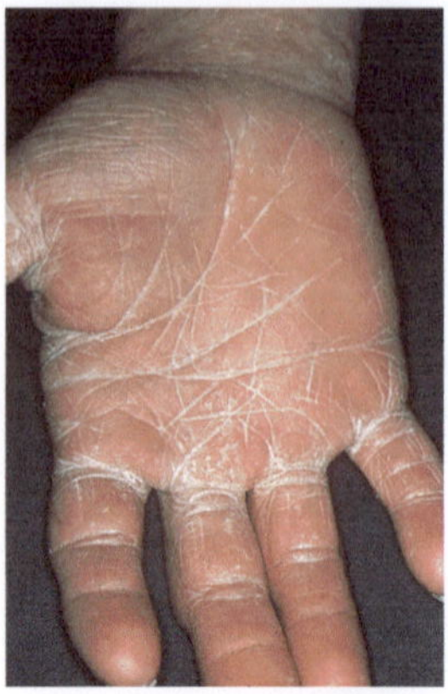

Fig. 8.7 Dermatophyte infections: pityriasiforme scaling in the palms

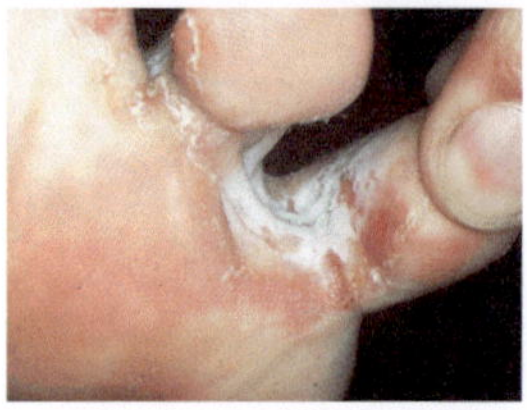

Fig. 8.8 Dermatophyte infections: erosio interdigitalis blastomycetica

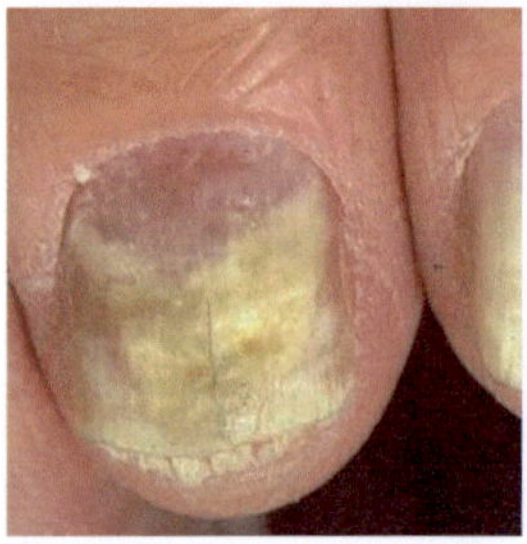

Fig. 8.9 Dermatophyte infections: dystrophy and discoloration in fungal nail infection

Grading of Importance

A

Level

Advanced

ICD-11

1F28; 1F28.Y

Synonyms

Tinea, the term is usually followed by the Latin name for the involved anatomic site such as tinea corporis (body), tinea capitis (scalp), tinea faciei (face), and others.

Epidemiology

- Tinea corporis and tinea capitis: more common in children
- Favus: rarely found
- Tinea barbae: exclusively in males
- Tinea pedis and onychomycosis: 20% prevalence among adults
- Tinea manuum: almost always following tinea pedis

Definition

Infections caused by dermatophytes (keratinophilic fungi which infect hair, nails, and scales) of the species *Microsporum*, *Trichophyton*, and *Epidermophyton*. Transmission: human to human and animal to human (more inflammatory).

Mycoses are often divided into three classes: dermatophytes, yeasts, moulds.

Aetiology and Pathogenesis

- Anthropophilic dermatophytes (*T. rubrum*): little inflammatory chronic infection
- Zoophilic types (*Microsporum canis*, *Trichophyton verrucosum*): intense inflammation
- Geophilic species: rarely cause mycoses in humans

Signs and Symptoms

- Tinea in the skin usually presents with annular, erythematous, circumscribed plaques with peripheral scale (caused by the spread of the fungus within the stratum corneum); centrifugal growth with tendency towards central clearing. Itching is variable. Occasionally dyshidrosiform or pustular when caused by zoophilic agents.
- Trichomycoses: dermatophytes of terminal hairs; clinically one should distinguish between *Trichophyton* infections (classic tinea capitis or scalp ringworm), *Microsporum* infection, and favus. Trichomycoses are caused by spread of the agent from the stratum corneum into hair follicles and shafts; only anagen hairs are affected.

- Classic tinea capitis is the most common dermatophyte infection in childhood. In anthropophilic endothrix infection, the hair is filled with spores, visible as small black dots in the follicle opening ("black dot ringworm").
- Zoophilic dermatophytes extend deep into the follicles and induce an intense inflammation, pustules, and massive purulent secretion ("kerion").
- Microsporum infections often lead to bland deep folliculitis without abscess formation caused by anthropophilic *M. audouinii* or *by M. canis* (zoophilic; particularly in cats). Hairs break off shortly after emerging above the scalp surface. These hairs fluoresce yellow-green on Wood's light examination.
- Favus: features exuberant masses of fungal elements, scales, and secretions producing scutula (Latin for small shield). They heal with scaring (cicatricial alopecia or pseudopelade). Tinea barbae: deep abscess-forming folliculitis of the beard hair caused in particular by *T. verrucosum* (common dermatophyte in cows) or the zoophilic form of *T. interdigitale.*

Ringworm of the palms and soles: Tinea pedis is one of the most common dermatological diseases. There are three clinical forms:

- Interdigital: maceration and coarse scaling, most commonly between closely approximated third and fourth toes. Shedding of the macerated skin produces erosions and fissures.
- Hyperkeratotic: non-inflammatory diffuse scaling of the entire plantar surface of soles; often mistaken for dry skin
- Vesicular/dyshidrotic: most often on the arch of the foot, as well as the tips of the small and great toes. Presents with scattered, intensely pruritic vesicles which may be cloudy.

Tinea manuum: usually only affects one hand, but may be bilateral in chronic cases; clinically there may be fine collarette scaling on the cup of the palm, especially along the palmar creases.

Dyshidrosiform type: itchy vesicles on palm and sides of fingers. Special type: one-hand/two-feet mycosis which always affects both soles as well as one palm. Onychomycosis (tinea unguium): more than 80% of all nail infections are caused by dermatophytes (usually *T. rubrum*). Impaired nail growth is a predisposing factor. More frequently affects the feet (starting from tinea pedis) rather than the hands.

Several forms of **fungal nail infection** can be clinically distinguished:

- Unilateral subungual onychomycosis is the most common form.
- White superficial onychomycosis (white macules).
- Proximal subungual onychomycosis.
- Complete dystrophic onychomycosis with marked destruction of the nail plate as final state of the first three forms.

Laboratory and Other Workups

Identification of fungi (KOH examination –> immediate result; culture –> takes 3–4 weeks), PCR

Diagnosis

Clinical features, mycology laboratory. (KOH examination detects fungal elements but does not identify species; culture: takes 1–4 weeks; PCR: just 24 hours).

Differential Diagnosis

Pyodermas, dermatitis, psoriasis, pityriasis rosea, discoid or subacute cutaneous lupus erythematosus. “If a lesion is scaly, a fungal infection should be excluded”.

Prevention and Therapy

- General measures include correction of predisposing factors (sweating, improper shoes), treatment of (asymptomatic) carriers.
- Antimycotics: azoles, amorolfine, ciclopirox olamine, terbinafine. Polyenes (amphotericin B, nystatin) are ineffective against dermatophytes.
- Keratolytics: salicylic acid, urea (nails, hair). Fabry’s tincture (salicylic acid, phenol).
- Formalin to disinfect shoes.
- For **systemic** therapies, terbinafine is the gold standard; alternatively, triazoles such as itraconazole and fluconazole can be used. Griseofulvin is restricted to *Microsporum* infections in childhood.

Candidiasis [1, 3]

Figures 8.10, 8.11, 8.12, 8.13, 8.14 and 8.15

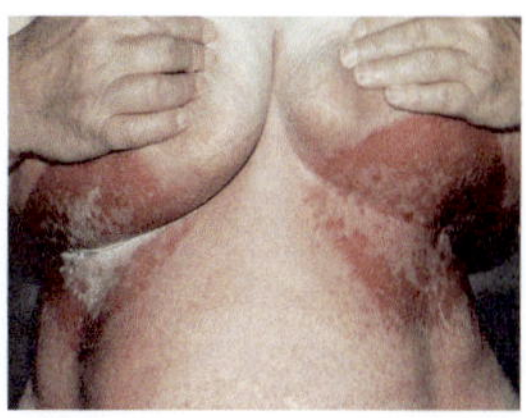

Fig. 8.10 Candidiasis: intertriginous infection in a patient with diabetes

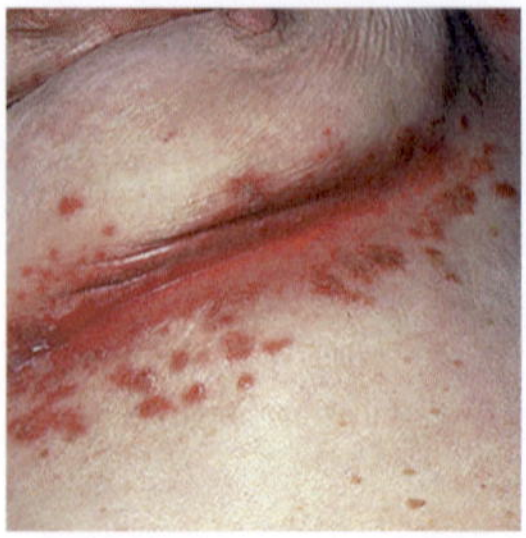

Fig. 8.11 Candidiasis: sub-mammary erythema and papules

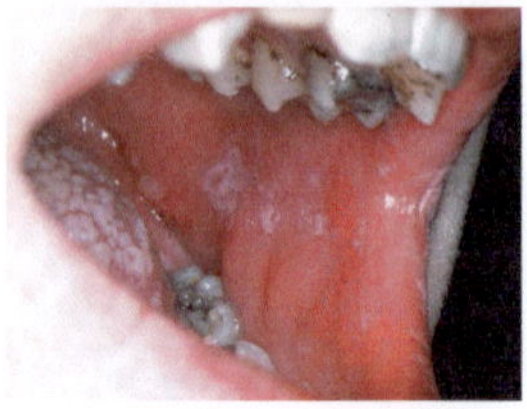

Fig. 8.12 Candidiasis: involvement of tongue and oral mucosa

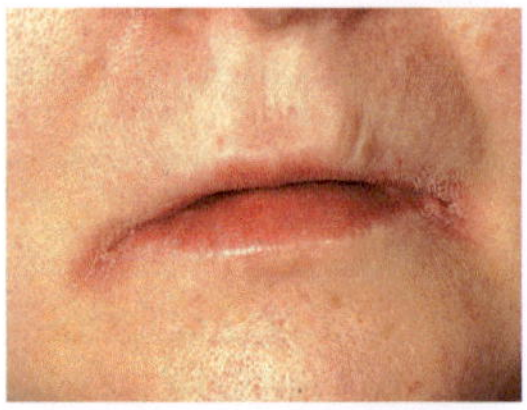

Fig. 8.13 Candidiasis: perlèche in the corners of the mouth

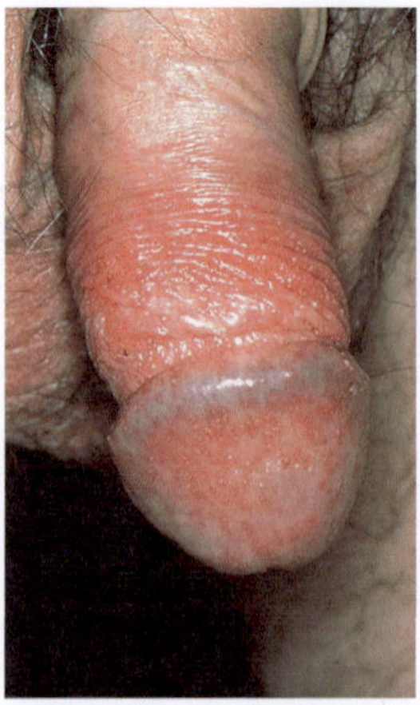

Fig. 8.14 Candidiasis: erythema of the penis

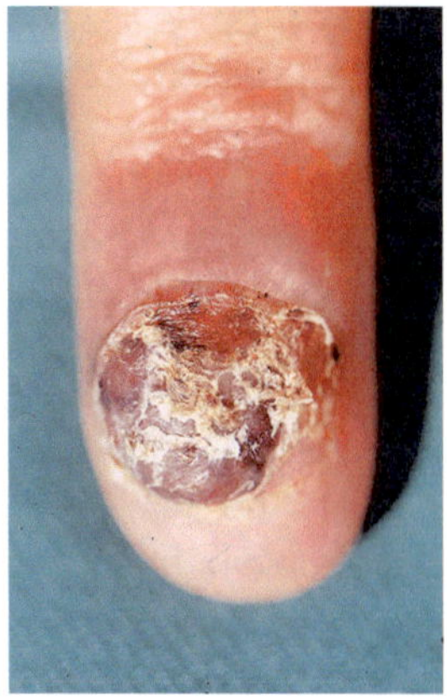

Fig. 8.15 Candidiasis: paronychia and nail dystrophy

Grading of Importance

B

Level

Advanced

ICD-11

1F23.Z

Synonyms

Moniliasis; candidiasis; yeast infection; thrush.

Epidemiology

Frequent finding; it occurs at least once during the lifetime of every individual.

Definition

Candidiasis is a harmless commensal colonisation with yeast of the genus *Candida* (normal flora of the gastrointestinal tract, upper respiratory tract, female genitalia) which in the presence of predisposing factors can develop into an infection. Main species is *Candida albicans*; other less common *Candida* (C.) species are *C. tropicalis*, *C. stellatoidea*, *C. parapsilosis*, and *C. glabrata*.

Aetiology and Pathogenesis

Predisposing factors in generating infection are: very old, very young, very ill. Pre-existing diseases of skin and mucous membranes, use of topical corticosteroids, chronic maceration, intertrigo, increased sweating, in-dwelling plastic lines or implants that can serve as entry sites; diabetes mellitus, obesity, pregnancy, severe illness, malnutrition, antibiotic therapy, and immunosuppression (autoimmune disease, transplant patients, HIV). The disease is caused by the growth of sporophytic yeasts (skin, GI tract) or by infection (birth canal, sexual contact).

Signs and Symptoms

Candida infections can involve skin and mucous membranes, but in immunocompromised patients can be also systemic.

- Intertriginous and anogenital candidasis, onychomycosis, paronychia, oral candidiasis, intestinal candidiasis, systemic candidiasis, mucocutaneous candidasis. Candidal intertrigo is the most common complication of intertrigo with macerations and fissures and scattered outbreaks (satellite lesions) in the surrounding area.
- In candidal paronychia and candidal nail infection, there may be a red, swollen nail wall with suppuration.
- Candida folliculitis can lead to small follicular pustules, particularly in the beard area of adult males.
- In chronic mucocutaneous and vulvovaginal candidiasis, pregnancy, oral contraceptives, and mechanical stress are predisposing factors. Vaginal involvement: whitish discharge forming a removable coat on the vaginal wall. *Candida* balanitis: circumscribed redness, grey-whitish coating or erosions with overlying exudate on the foreskin (balanoposthitis), predisposing factors are as follows: wet-warm environments in the preputial space, bad hygiene, specifically insufficient drying after washing or sexual intercourse with a partner that has *Candida* vulvovaginitis. There is a risk of phimosis when the inflammation is chronic.

Localisation

Mainly in moist areas (intertriginous regions, mucosa).

Classification

See Symptoms.

Laboratory and Other Workups

KOH examination of mycology scrapings. Culture over the course of 1 to 4 days; white or cream colonies with a dull surface and without air mycelium; differentiation by means of micromorphology on rice agar (chlamydospores in *C. albicans*) or biochemical/PCR.

Dermatopathology

PAS stain shows hyphae and spores and neutrophilic inflammatory infiltrate sometimes with pustular accumulation in the stratum corneum.

Course

Generally good. Outlook poor in candidal sepsis, depending on underlying disease.

Complications

Predisposition to bacterial superinfection.

Diagnosis

Clinical features, laboratory findings.

Differential Diagnosis

Depends on location: lichen planus, leukoplakia, food remnants, secondary syphilis, flexural psoriasis, bacterial infections, other fungi.

Prevention and Therapy

Stop predisposing factors (often opportunistic infections). Topical and, where appropriate, systemic antifungal therapy. Polyenes (nystatin, amphotericin B) and azoles are effective in treating these fungal infections. Griseofulvin is not effective for some yeasts, depending on localisation: creams and ointments (trunk and extremities), pastes (intertrigines), lacquer paint (nails), suppositories/vaginal tablets (vaginal), lozenges, and suspensions (oral mucosa). Systemic therapy of a severe local candidiasis (fluconazole, itraconazole, posaconazole). For invasive candidiasis: amphotericin, echinocandin, and intravenous flucytosine.

Pityriasis Versicolor [2, 5, 6]

Figures 8.16 and 8.17

Grading of Importance

B

Level

Advanced

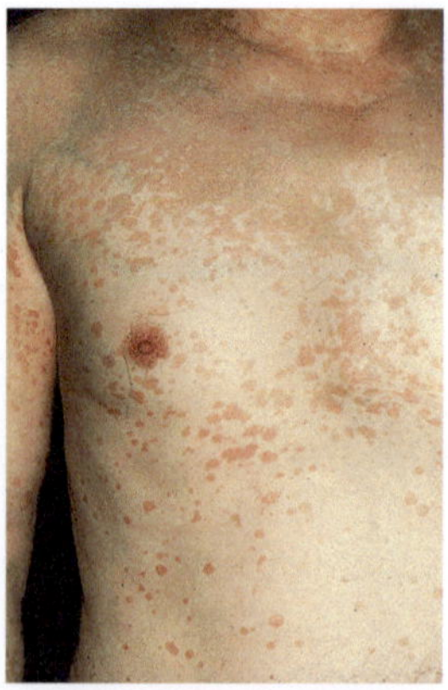

Fig. 8.16 Pityriasis versicolor: pigmented macular lesions in winter

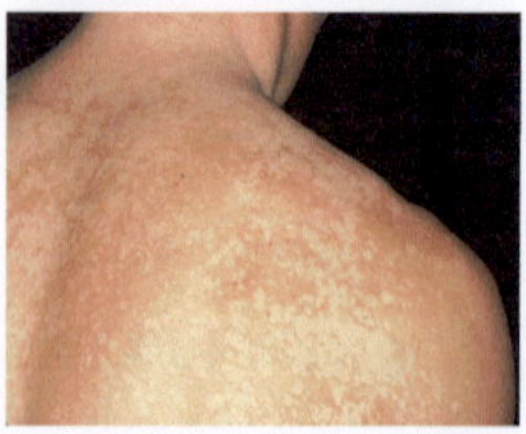

Fig. 8.17 Pityriasis versicolor: depigmented macules in summer

ICD-11

1F2D.0

Synonyms

Tinea versicolor.

Epidemiology

Most common in young adults during spring and summer seasons.

Definition

Superficial cutaneous mycosis caused by lipophilic *Malassezia* yeasts (primarily *M. globosa*) with hypo- and hyperpigmented macules.

Aetiology and Pathogenesis

Causative lipophilic *Malassezia* yeasts belong to the resident flora of human skin. Various predisposing factors trigger hyphal growth stage.

Predisposing factors: sweating, humid climate, immunosuppression.

Signs and Symptoms

Variable picture; several clinical types:

- Hyperpigmented type: small, yellow-brown macules, disseminated, fine scale, sometimes modest pruritus.
- Depigmented type (pityriasis versicolor alba): small white macules in dark-skinned or tanned individuals.
- Erythematous type: erythematous macules with infiltrate and only minimal scale.
- Follicular type: acneiform, often at the back.
- Atypical forms: solitary or few lesions, often in atypical sites.

Localisation

Upper trunk, less often lower trunk and proximal extremities.

Classification

Non applicable.

Laboratory and Other Workups

KOH examination or stripping with cellophane tape; methylene stain for grouped spores and hyphae on scales under microscope (spaghetti and meatballs pattern).

Dermatopathology

Hyphae and spores in the stratum corneum and in the acroinfundibula.

Course

Usually persistent or recurrent, sometimes clears spontaneously.

Complications

Cosmetic irritation.

Diagnosis

Clinical features, microscopic examination of scales, yellow-orange fluorescence under Wood's light (365 nm).

Differential Diagnosis

Guttate hypomelanosis, vitiligo, pityriasis alba, pityriasis rosea, tinea corporis, seborrheic dermatitis, erythrasma.

Prevention and Therapy

Prevention: careful drying of skin after shower, wearing breathable fabrics to decrease sweating, avoidance of tight clothing, avoidance of highly moisturising skin products. Treatment of scalp reservoir.

Topical treatment of the entire body (shampoos containing imidazoles, selenium sulphide, ciclopirox, or zinc pyrithione); in cases with frequent recurrences or widespread involvement: systemic antifungals such as itraconazole.

References

1. Arya NR, Rafiq N (2020) Candidiasis. StatPearls – NCBI Bookshelf
2. Karray M, McKinney WP (2020) Tinea Versicolor. StatPearls, Treasure Island (FL)
3. Meunier F (1989) Candidiasis. Eur J Clin Microbiol Infect Dis 8(5):438–447
4. Odom R (1993) Pathophysiology of dermatophyte infections. J Am Acad Dermatol 28(5 Pt 1):S2–S7
5. Prohic A, Jovovic Sadikovic T, Krupalija-Fazlic M, Kuskunovic-Vlahovljak S (2016) Malassezia species in healthy skin and in dermatological conditions. Int J Dermatol 55(5):494–504
6. Thoma W, Kramer HJ, Mayser P (2005) Pityriasis versicolor alba. J Eur Acad Dermatol Venereol 19(2):147–152
7. Yee G, Al Aboud AM (2020) Tinea Corporis. StatPearls, Treasure Island, FL

Parasitic Infections

9

Zrinka Bukvić Mokos, Günter Burg, Harald Gollnick, Branka Marinović, and John A. McGrath

Contents

Z. Bukvić Mokos (✉) · B. Marinović
Department of Dermatology and Venereology, School of Medicine University of Zagreb, Zagreb, Croatia
e-mail: branka.marinovic@kbc-zagreb.hr

G. Burg
Dermatology, Zurich, Switzerland
e-mail: g.burg@access.uzh.ch

H. Gollnick
Department of Dermatology & Venereology, Otto-von-Guericke University, Magdeburg, Germany
e-mail: Harald.Gollnick@med.ovgu.de

J. A. McGrath
St John's Institute of Dermatology, King's College London, London, UK
e-mail: john.mcgrath@kcl.ac.uk

H. Gollnick et al. (eds.), *Dermatology Cyberderm WebBook*,
https://doi.org/10.1007/978-3-031-78491-0_9

Test your learning and check your understanding of this book's contents: use the "Springer Nature Flashcards" app to access questions using ▶ https://sn.pub/1rhh6k.

To use the app, please follow the instructions in Chap. 1.

Leishmaniasis [3, 7, 10, 16]

Figures 9.1 and 9.2

Grading of Importance

B

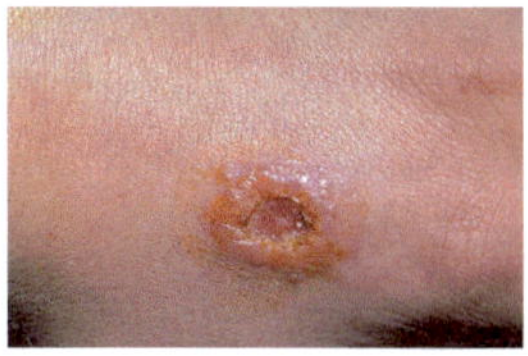

Fig. 9.1 Leishmaniasis: ulceration with elevated border in the face

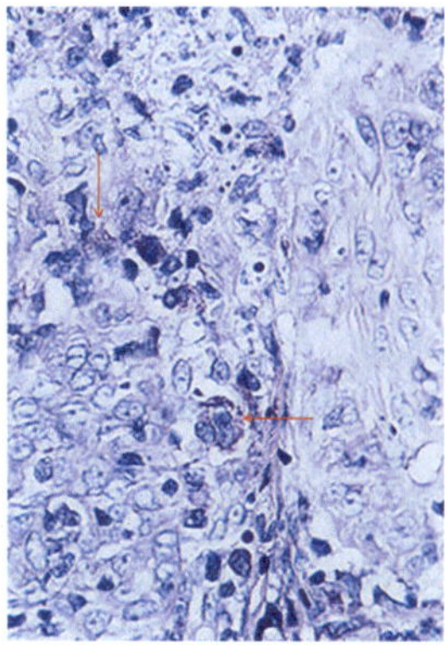

Fig. 9.2 Leishmaniasis: macrophages filled with amastigotes (arrow)

Level

Advanced

ICD-11

1F54.1

Synonyms

Old World cutaneous leishmaniasis: oriental sore, Aleppo/Baghdad boil, Delhi boil.

New World cutaneous leishmaniasis: chiclero ulcer; uta; jungle yaws.

Mucocutaneous leishmaniasis: espundia.

Epidemiology

Approximately one million new cases of cutaneous leishmaniasis worldwide per year. Geographical distribution: cutaneous leishmaniasis (CL): Middle East and South America; mucocutaneous leishmaniasis (MCL): Central and South America.

Definition

Infection with *Leishmania*, a protozoan. Three typical clinical forms (see Classification).

Aetiology and Pathogenesis

Transmission by the female *Phlebotomus* sandflies only. Depending on species and different animal reservoirs (e.g. wild rabbits and dogs for *L. infantum*), different clinical patterns occur (see Classification).

Cutaneous leishmaniasis (CL):

- The Old World: *L. major*, *L. tropica*, *L. aethiopica*, *L. infantum*
- The New World: *L. mexicana* and *L. brasiliensis*
- MCL species: *L. braziliensis*

Signs and Symptoms

CL: an erythematous papule at the site of the sting progresses within weeks to months to an ulcerated hyperkeratotic plaque. Occasional satellite papules are present. Usually the lesion heals spontaneously over a period of months with scarring.

MCL: mutilating mucosal lesions (the nose or mouth mainly in New World infections).

Localisation

Usually on exposed sites (face, forearms, legs).

Classification

Different forms of cutaneous leishmaniasis include:

- Self-healing localised cutaneous leishmaniasis
- Leishmaniasis recidivans
- Mucocutaneous leishmaniasis
- Anergic diffuse cutaneous leishmaniasis
- Disseminated leishmaniasis
- Post-kala-azar dermal leishmaniasis (PKDL): cutaneous manifestation observed in some visceral leishmaniasis patients after successful treatment

Laboratory and Other Workups

Giemsa-stained smears (tissue impression smears, dermal scrapping or needle aspiration) or biopsy specimens: the presence of amastigote parasites; culture (Novy-MacNeal-Nicolle (NNN)medium); serology (ELISA and immunofluorescence studies), PCR assay.

Dermatopathology

Early lesions: amastigote parasites in dermal macrophages. Chronic form: granulomatous inflammation (tuberculoid-like granulomas).

Course

CL may resolve spontaneously.

MCL: progressive course; potentially lethal due to secondary infections and aspiration pneumonia.

Visceral leishmaniasis: serious and progressive disease; if untreated, lethal in 75–95% of patients.

Complications

Diffuse cutaneous leishmaniasis, persistence of the infection, relapses, involvement of mucous membranes (*L. braziliensis*) and systemic spread (*L. donovani*, *L. infantum*), particularly in immunosuppressed patients.

Diagnosis

Travel history and clinical features. Identification of a parasite in a smear preparation or skin biopsy, PCR assay or with culture.

Differential Diagnosis

Tropical ulcers: infiltrates due to other causes; ecthyma in travellers.

Prevention and Therapy

Prevention: vector control, use of insect repellents, protective clothing, fine-mesh screens.

Therapy includes cryosurgery, local heat therapy, excision, topical paromomycin, intralesional or systemic antimony compounds, oral miltefosine and oral itraconazole. Cutaneous leishmaniasis of Old-World subtypes is often self-limited.

Scabies [4, 5, 8, 19]

Figures 9.3, 9.4, 9.5, 9.6 and 9.7

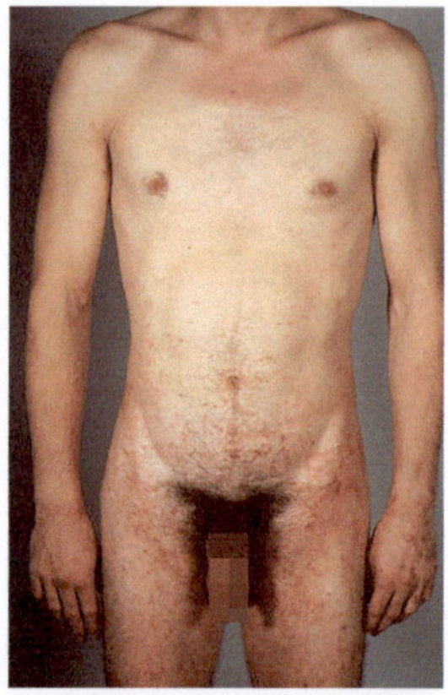

Fig. 9.3 Scabies: exanthematic lesions in an adult

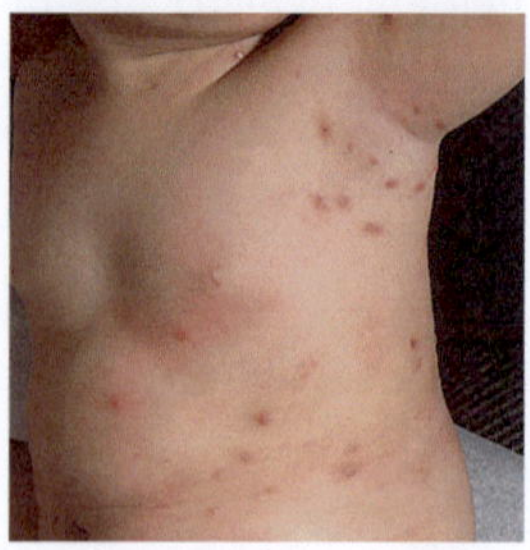

Fig. 9.4 Scabies: papular lesions in a child

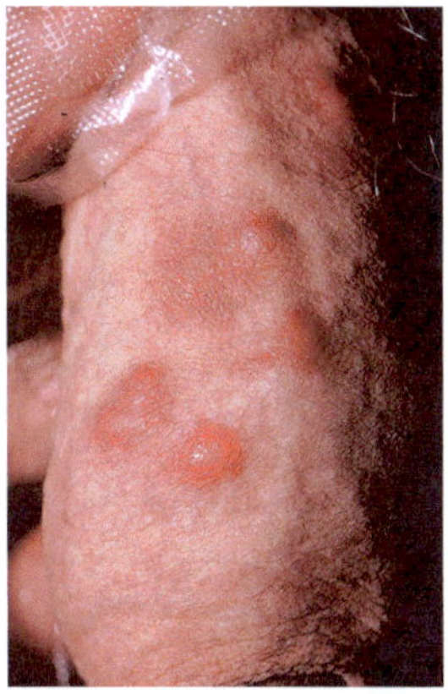

Fig. 9.5 Scabies: penile nodules

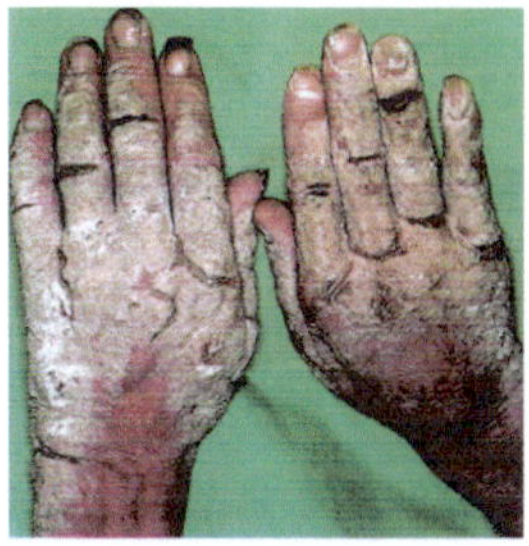

Fig. 9.6 Scabies: scabies custosa

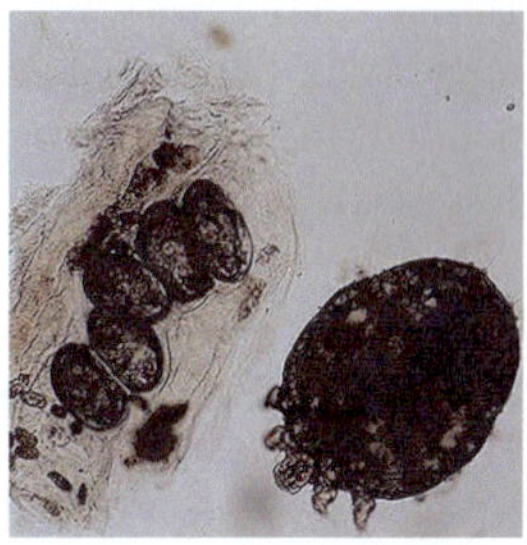

Fig. 9.7 Scabies: mite and scybalae

Grading of Importance

A

Level

Advanced

ICD-11

1G04

Synonyms

Sarcoptic itch; 7-year itch.

Epidemiology

Approximately 300 million individuals are affected worldwide each year. Overcrowding promotes the spread of the disease. Refugee camps are hotspots. Residential homes.

Definition

Intensely pruritic infestation caused by the mite *Sarcoptes scabiei* var. *hominis*.

Aetiology and Pathogenesis

Sarcoptes scabiei var. *hominis* is a human ectoparasite with marked host specificity. Human-to-human transmission occurs with close personal contact, sometimes via clothing or bedding. Female mites (0.3–0.5 mm) dig a burrow in the stratum corneum of the epidermis to lay their eggs; sexually mature mites develop in 3 weeks. Immunologic reaction to mite antigens causes inflammation and pruritus.

Signs and Symptoms

Marked pruritus, especially at night. Initially the mites burrow and develop elongated inflamed papules; in infants there can be evidence of vesicles. An exanthema with tiny papules and fine crusts and tiny tunnels may be found symmetrically over the flanks and proximal extremities, indicating a cellular immunologic reaction against scabies antigens. Face and interscapular regions are spared.

Localisation

The predilection sites for burrows: interdigital, anterior axillary folds, nipples, umbilicus, groin, penis, scrotum, wrists and dorsal aspects of the feet. In children the face, scalp, palms and soles can be affected.

Classification

Special form: Crusted ("Norwegian") scabies—massive infestation in immunosuppressed individuals, clinically presents as hyperkeratotic papules/plaques with thick scales.

Laboratory and Other Workups

Identification of the mite, its eggs or scybala (feces) under the dermatoscope or microscope.

Dermatopathology

Usually not necessary, however, consider a biopsy in cases of persisting lesions causing pseudolymphomatous papules or small nodules.

Course

Can be chronic. Recurrences may occur.

Complications

Complications include impetiginisation, post scabetic papules (nodular scabies) and persistent inflammatory reaction without presence of mites. Itching often persists after successful eradication of the mites (post scabies dermatitis).

Diagnosis

Characteristic clinical features, including severe pruritus, worsening at night; a history of contact with a person with pruritus. Microscopic identification of mites, their eggs or scybala (feces) from specimen obtained by skin scraping or de-roofing burrow with scalpel blade.

Differential Diagnosis

Pruritic dermatoses, prurigo, dermatitis herpetiformis, urticaria, psoriasis (in crusted scabies).

Prevention and Therapy

Check of environment and in particular sexual partner.

The treatment of choice is topical permethrin cream (5%) applied from top to toe once for 8–12 hours. Repeat the second course after 7 days. If there are still signs of active scabies after 14 days, repeat treatment with an alternative drug. Second-line treatments include benzyl benzoate used on 3 consecutive days or crotamiton.

Ivermectin orally for crusted scabies or if topical treatment is difficult. Increasing amount of resistancies to topical permethrin

Prevention of reinfection: Change clothing and bedding, and wash everything. All non-washable items should be aired for 4 days (mites can live for 2–3 days at room temperature). Identify and treat in parallel contact persons (family, kindergarten, sexual partner).

Trombidiosis [2]

Figures 9.8 and 9.9

Grading of Importance

B

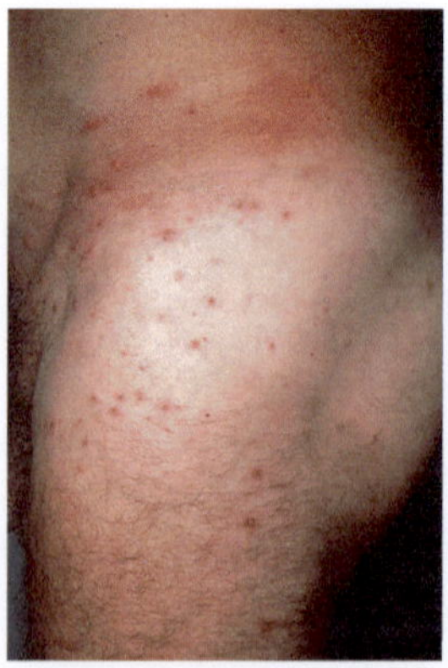

Fig. 9.8 Trombidiosis: tiny papular lesions

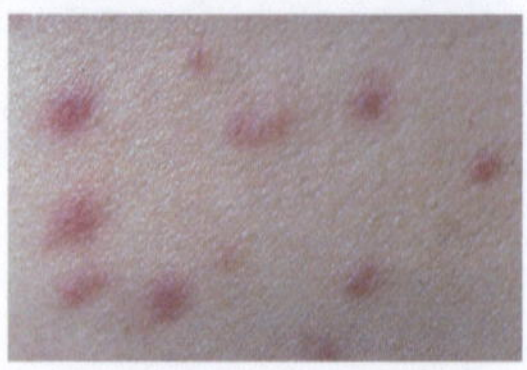

Fig. 9.9 Trombidiosis: pruritic papules

Level

Advanced

ICD-11

NE61

Synonyms

Harvest itch, chigger itch.

Epidemiology

Larvae are most prevalent in forests and long and overgrown grass in fields and gardens in late summer and fall. In tropical areas, the infection may occur at any time of the year. The natural hosts are small rodents.

Definition

Pruritic skin lesions caused by mite larvae (chiggers) of the Trombiculidae family.

Aetiology and Pathogenesis

Larval mites (*Trombicula autumnalis*): 0.3 mm, transfer from vegetation to skin, usually late summer, bite human as accidental host, inject proteolytic agent then suck up debris and drop off.

Signs and Symptoms

Intensely pruritic papules and macules with haemorrhagic central punctae (site of bite), sometimes vesicles.

Localisation

Sites where clothing is tight (belt line, tight cuffs), proximal thighs, popliteal fossae, ankles. Often several lesions in a linear pattern.

Classification

None.

Laboratory and Other Workups

Not required.

Dermatopathology

Lymphomononuclear cell infiltrate with eosinophiles in the dermis. Focal parakeratosis and spongiosis in the epidermis, sometimes vesicles around sting.

Course

Usually resolves spontaneously.

Complications

Bacterial superinfection; "summer penile syndrome".

Diagnosis

Clinical features and history (exposure in known endemic areas). Almost impossible to find larva on human. Sometimes larva found outdoors.

Differential Diagnosis

Prurigo, other arthropod bites.

Prevention and Therapy

Topical antipruritic agents (zinc or corticosteroid lotion). Systemic antihistamines. Prophylaxis: avoidance of risk areas (gardens, parks, compost piles), insect repellents for garden work.

Pediculosis Capitis [4, 14, 19]

Figures 9.10, 9.11 and 9.12

Grading of Importance

A

Level

Advanced

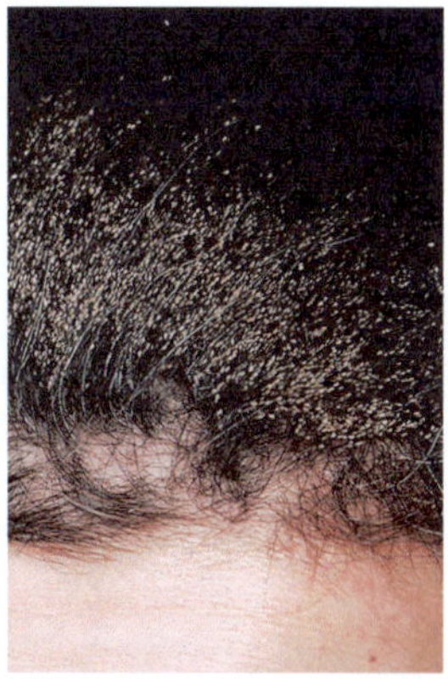

Fig. 9.10 Pediculosis capitis: nits in the hair

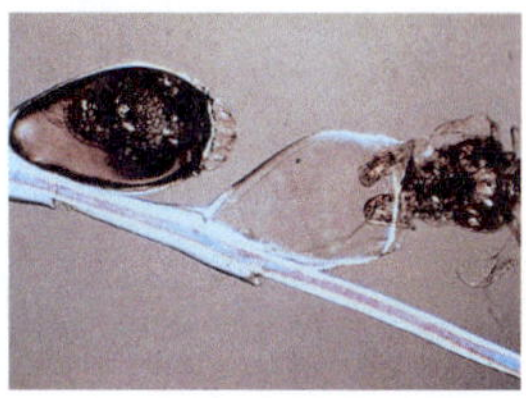

Fig. 9.11 Pediculosis capitis: nits attached to a hair

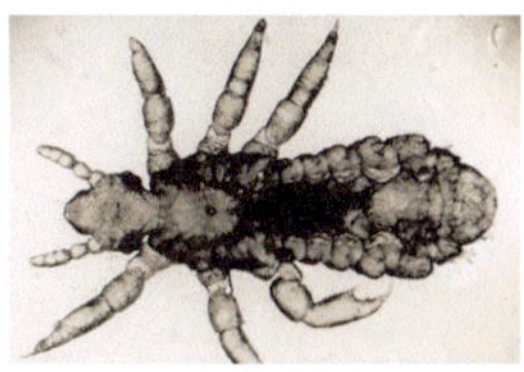

Fig. 9.12 Pediculosis capitis: head louse

ICD-11

1G00.0

Synonyms

Head lice infestation; head lice; nits.

Definition

Pruritic scalp lesions usually in children caused by bites of the head lice, followed by strong itching.

Aetiology and Pathogenesis

Head lice (*Pediculus capitis*, 2.25–4 mm) are strictly human-specific ectoparasites. The larvae hatch from eggs after 7 days, and after a total of 2–3 weeks, the adult lice are sexually mature. Transmission is from human-to-human, especially under cramped living conditions.

Signs and Symptoms

Sometimes markedly pruritic erythematous papules, especially found on the retroauricular and occipital areas and the nape of the neck. Nits (eggs) are firmly attached to hair shafts, whereas adult lice move freely.

Localisation

Usually scalp, especially retroauricular and occipital.

Classification

Not applicable.

Laboratory and Other Workups

Dermatoscopic examination of the hair shaft may show the lice and the nits attached to the hair.

Dermatopathology

Not necessary.

Course

Recurrences are common if improperly treated or re-contamination.

Complications

Impetiginisation with associated occipital and/or cervical lymphadenopathy; hairs can become matted with pus and crust.

Diagnosis

Clinical features. Identification of nits or lice.

Differential Diagnosis

Seborrheic dermatitis, folliculitis, impetigo.

Prevention and Therapy

Prevention measures: Combs, brushes and hats should not be shared.

Prevention of reinfection: Contact persons should be examined and treated as required in parallel. It is important to wash clothing, bedding and towels at 60 °C minimum and dry well. Place items which cannot be washed in airtight plastic bags for 14 days and clean combs and hair brushes in hot soapy water. Vacuum carpets, rugs, furniture and mattresses.

Therapy: Wet combing (nit comb, fine-toothed comb), first-line dimethicone, 5% topical permethrin, pyrethrins, malathion, ivermectin.

Pediculosis Pubis [15]

Figures 9.13, 9.14 and 9.15

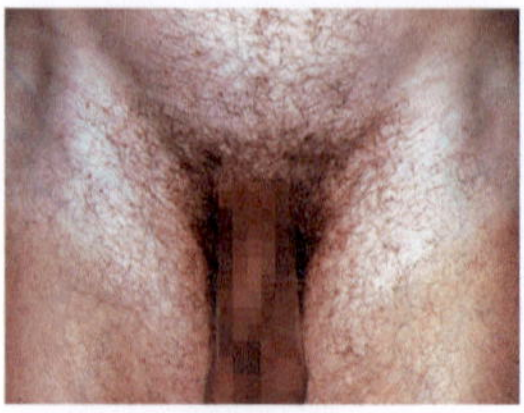

Fig. 9.13 Pediculosis pubis: eczematous lesion in the inguinal region

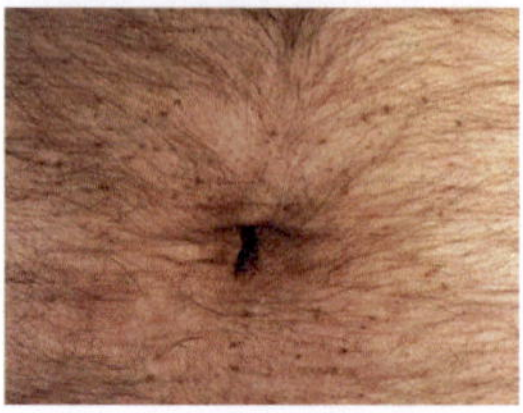

Fig. 9.14 Pediculosis pubis: involvement of periumbilical hairs

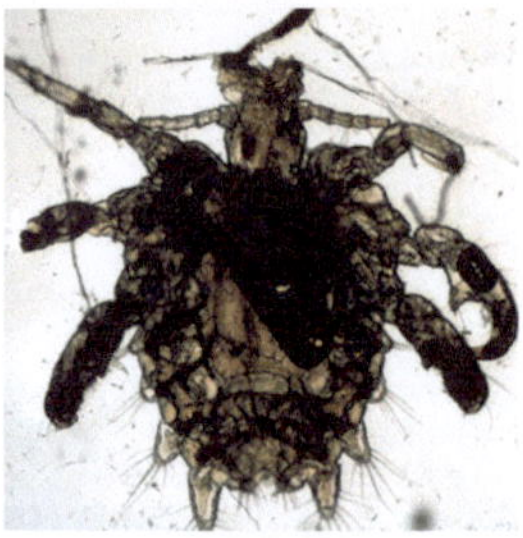

Fig. 9.15 Pediculosis pubis: pubic louse (phthiri)

Grading of Importance

B

Level

Advanced

ICD-11

1G03

Synonyms

Phthiriasis; infestation by crab lice; crabs.

Definition

Pruritic skin lesions in the pubic, perianal and axillary regions caused by bites from the pubic louse.

Aetiology and Pathogenesis

Pubic louse (*Pthirus pubis*): 1.3–1.6 mm. Pubic lice live for only 2 days at room temperature without a host. Transmission by close personal contact, particularly sexual contact.

Signs and Symptoms

Pruritus in pubic or other hairy regions. Distinctive (but not common finding): slate grey to blue-grey macules as a result of haemosiderin degradation products at the bite site. Nits attached to hair shafts and adult lice are tightly attached to the hairs near the skin surface.

Localisation

Hair bearing regions, especially pubic and perianal regions; can also affect the axillae, chest, abdomen, thighs and beard region. In children, eyelashes, eyebrows and rarely scalp can also be involved.

Classification

Not applicable.

Laboratory and Other Workups

The lice and nits can be identified by dermatoscopic examination.

Dermatopathology

Not necessary.

Course

Persistence with inappropriate treatment. Re-infection with recurrences may occur.

Complications

Impetiginisation. Spreading to other people.

Diagnosis

Clinical features. Identification of nits and lice.

Differential Diagnosis

Scabies, arthropod bites.

Prevention and Therapy

Prevention: Sexual contact should be avoided until both sexual partners have been successfully treated.

Therapy: General measures; similar management to pediculosis capitis. It is also important to treat sexual contacts. Topical treatment: malathion shampoo; permethrin cream rinse; synergised pyrethrin shampoo. Consider repeating treatment after 10 days. Oral ivermectin in resistant cases.

Special

Examine the patient for other sexually transmitted diseases.

Demodicosis [9]

Figure 9.16

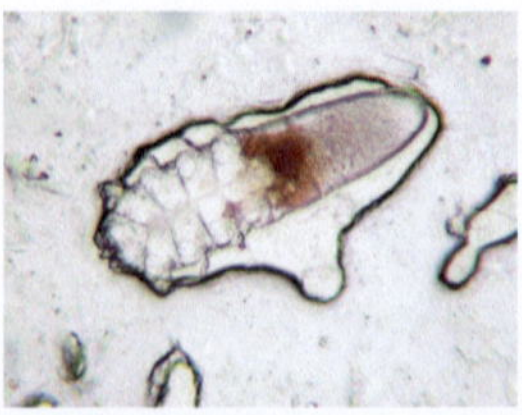

Fig. 9.16 Demodicosis: follicle mite

Grading of Importance

B

Level

Null

ICD-11

1G07.0

Synonyms

Pityriasis folliculorum.

Epidemiology

Around 90% of the world population have some demodex mites on the body surface, but around 5 to 10% only suffer from demodicosis.

Definition

Demodex mites are living in the follicular canal of the skin. In case of an infectious course with inflammation and a high density of demodex mites (> 5/cm^2), it is called demodicosis.

Aetiology and Pathogenesis

Most infections are caused when demodex mites are overpopulating, penetrating the follicular wall, colonising the follicular opening and interfollicular epidermal surface. Two types have to be differentiated:

- *Demodex folliculorum* (0.2–0.4 mm), mostly in sebaceous follicles
- *Demodex brevis* (0.15–0.2 mm), mostly found in the follicles of the eye lashes

Predisposing factors: aged skin (wider follicular openings), actinic elastosis, immunodeficiency (HIV) or chemotherapy, alcoholism and diabetes, rosacea

Signs and Symptoms

Demodex mites move in the night 8–16 mm /h over the skin, deposit eggs and can produce itching. Light makes them move back to the follicle to hide. The skin feels sensitive and sometimes more scaly, may produce tiny rough feeling by moving over the surface (spinula-like pattern) and shows some redness. The appearance of papules and pustules mimic an acneiform feature. Sometimes small abscesses and granulomatous reactions may develop. In particular the eye lashes are prone to involvement.

Localisation

Demodex mites are preferentially found on the facial skin; not symmetrical. The forehead with high density of sebaceous gland follicles are predisposed followed by the nose cheeks, chin, eye lashes and outer ear canal. In males with long-standing alopecia, demodex mites are also found on the naked scalp.

Classification

Primary demodicosis (*sui generis*): due to abnormal increase in mite colonisation.

- Demodex folliculorum (spinulate demodicosis or pityriasis folliculorum)
- Papulopustular/nodulocystic or conglobate demodicosis
- Ocular demodicosis

Secondary demodicosis: due to immunosuppression or presence of pre-existing or concurrent inflammatory dermatoses (acne, rosacea perioral dermatitis).

Laboratory and Other Workups

Dermatoscope can make the spinula visible. A cyanoacrylate tape stripe can help to visualise the mites under the microscope.

Dermatopathology

Not necessary. The mites are in masses populating the follicular canal with folliculitis and perifolliculitis, sometimes granulomatous reactions.

Course

Chronic; frequent recurrences.

Complications

Scratching with secondary infection with other microbes. Furuncle. Severe conjunctivitis and loss of eye lashes can occur. Increased scaling and itching at the external ear canal.

Diagnosis

Clinical picture, dermatoscopy, KOH preparation, cyanoacrylate stripe.

Differential Diagnosis

Seborrhoeic dermatitis, periorificial dermatitis, acne, folliculitis.

Others: follicular T-cell lymphoma, spinula follicular pattern in plasmacytoma (Nazzaro sign), atopic dermatitis, tinea follicularis and *Candida*.

Prevention and Therapy

Prevention: regular use of facial cleansers; avoiding UV light (promoter of actinic elastosis).

Topical: weekly application of 5% permethrin ointment including antiseptics in case of papulopustular pattern over 4 weeks. Other options are 1.0% ivermectin cream daily long term.

In granulomatous and absceding courses: oral ivermectin treatment is necessary.

Arthropod Reactions [1, 11]

Figures 9.17, 9.18 and 9.19

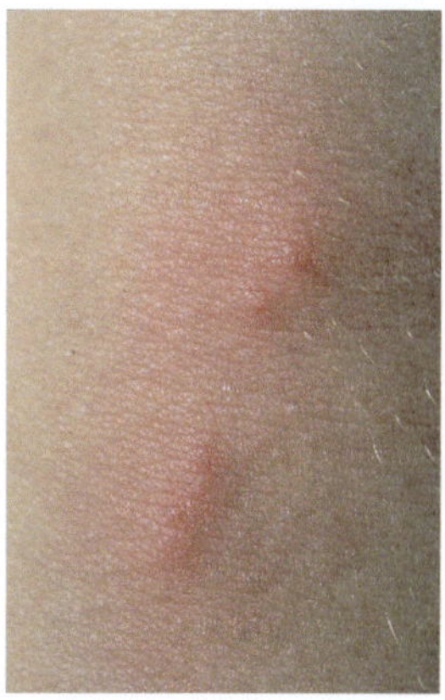

Fig. 9.17 Arthropod reactions: light reaction; itching urticarial papules

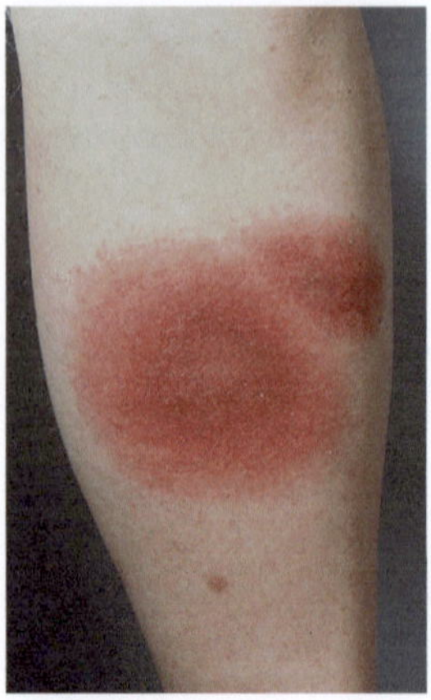

Fig. 9.18 Arthropod reactions: stronger reaction

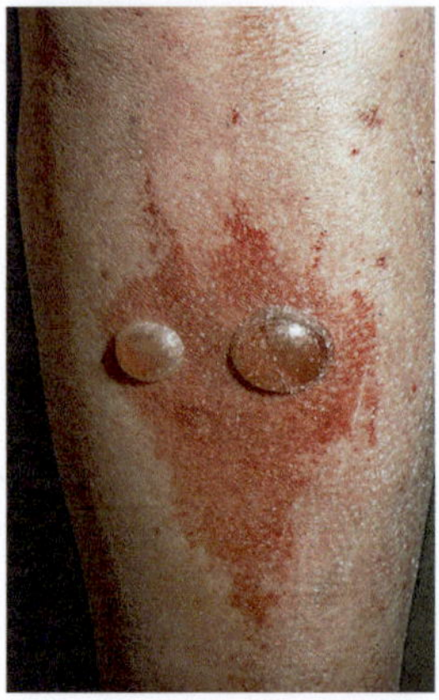

Fig. 9.19 Arthropod reactions: bullous reaction

Grading of Importance

B

Level

Advanced

ICD-11

EK50.0

Synonyms

Ticks, stings, arthropod reaction.

Epidemiology

Prevalence: hard to estimate because of different types of arthropods and environmental considerations. Most cases do not require medical intervention; more often in tropical climates.

Definition

Types of reaction

- Reactions to toxins from insect, spider, mites and tick bites
- Reactions to bites of parasitic insects, spider, mites and ticks
  Types of ectoparasites
- Permanent ectoparasites: parasitic insects (or arachnids = mites, ticks) live and/or feed on humans are highly adapted and may be found on human hosts.
- Temporary-accidental ectoparasites: bite humans by chance, the bite reaction varies greatly, and the parasite is rarely found on patients.

Aetiology and Pathogenesis

Human ectoparasites.

Permanent ectoparasites insects: head louse, clothing louse, pubic louse. Arachnids: Demodex and Sarcoptes scabiei. Spiders of different types.

Accidental parasitic insects: bed bugs, fleas, mosquitoes, sandflies, gnats, flies and horse flies.

Accidental parasitic arachnids: ticks, *Neotrombicula* (see Trombiculosis), bites mites (*Dermanyssus*), non-burrowing animal mites (Cheyletiellidae = walking mange), animal forms of scabies (Sarcoptidae and others).

Sometimes symptoms may be due to neurotoxins.

Signs and Symptoms

Immediate and delayed reactions at site of sting: erythema, macules, papules, wheals and blisters.

The nature of the reaction depends more on the sensitivity of the victim, rather than the nature of the stinging insect.

Localisation

Exposed skin areas: head, neck, extremities.

Classification

See Aetiology and Pathogenesis.

Laboratory and Other Workups

None specific.

Dermatopathology

Not necessary.

Course

Varies from self-limited mild local reaction to life threatening anaphylactic reactions.

Complications

Persistent arthropod reaction with other complications: pseudolymphomatous reactions, persistent prurigo nodularis-like lesions, secondary bacterial infection. Arthropod borne systemic infections.

Diagnosis

Clinical features (grouped or linearly arranged pruritic papules, sometimes with haemorrhagic centre (purpura pulicans).

Differential Diagnosis

For insect bites reactions: folliculitis, impetigo, furuncle, carbuncle, prurigo, dermatitis herpetiformis, erysipelas, blistering diseases.

Prevention and Therapy

Prevention: protective clothing, sleep under fine-mesh nets, repellents.

Insect bite reaction from parasitic insects: topical antipruritic agents (zinc oxide lotion, anti-pruritic cream, corticosteroid lotions). Antihistamines in special situations of IgE-mediated reactions (e.g. mosquitoes).

Bee and Wasp [12, 13, 17]

Grading of Importance

B

Level

Basic

ICD-11

XM7930

Synonyms

Hymenoptera stings.

Epidemiology

According to the European network of severe allergic reactions (NORA), 20% of all cases of anaphylaxis in children and 48% of documented anaphylaxis in adults were due to insect venom. Patients with increased number of mast cells and mastocytosis with increased blood tryptase levels (about 8% of population) have a higher risk of local and systemic reactions. Serious systemic reactions are 2–3 times higher in beekeeping.

Definition

Allergic and pseudoallergic reactions to stings of bees and wasps.

Aetiology and Pathogenesis

Honeybee stings are generally not more severe than wasp stings, but they inject more venom. Both liberate different pain inducer peptide 401, prostaglandins, serotonin, kinins and acetylcholine. Bees can sting once but wasps multiple times. Insect sting allergy may cause local, large local (>10 cm) or even systemic reactions (SR) and potentially life-threatening anaphylactic reactions. Anaphylaxis is IgE mediated. In individuals who have previously been sensitised to bee venom, IgE antibodies attach to tissue mast cells and basophils. Once these cells are activated, the progression of the cascade reaction increases vasoactive substances, which stimulate release of leukotrienes, histamine and eosinophil chemotactic factor-A. The number of mast cells in the skin and mucosa influences the release of histamine, bradykinin and platelet activating factor (PAF). IgG4 antibodies block spIgE.

Signs and Symptoms

In addition to local reaction, systemic reactions are classified in stages. First sign is usually pruritus. Complete picture includes flushing, urticaria, angioedema, hypotension, bronchospasm, nausea, abdominal colic, cramping, incontinence of urine and stool. 50% of symptoms appear within 5 minutes, another 40% within 30 minutes (see classification of allergic reactions/Mueller grading system 1–4).

Localisation

Exposed skin areas: head, neck, extremities. Mucosal area mouth, tongue and by swallowing larynx, trachea and oesophagus.

Classification

Symptoms and grading of allergic reaction against hymenoptera according to Mueller:

- Grade 0: increased local reaction (>10 cm, >24 h).
- Grade 1 (mild generalised reaction): widespread urticaria, pruritus, malaise, anxiety.
- Grade 2 (moderate generalised reaction): the above symptoms and two or more of the following: angioedema (Grade 2 even if solitary), tightening of chest, nausea, vomiting, diarrhoea.
- Grade 3 (severe generalised reaction): any of the above and two or more of the following: dyspnoea (Grade 3 even if solitary), stridor, dysphagia, dysarthria, excitement, confusion, fear of death.

- Grade 4 (shock reaction): any of the above and two or more of the following—cyanosis, hypotension, collapse, incontinence of urine or stool, loss of consciousness.

Laboratory and Other Workups

Identification of total and specific IgE in serum (ImmunoCAP, RAST). Tryptase. IgG4 subclassification as sign for autoantibodies against specific IgE (and for hyposensitisation follow-up).

Dermatopathology

Not necessary.

Course

Varies from self-limited mild local reaction to life-threatening anaphylactic reaction.

Diagnosis

Clinical features (local reaction, general features). After thorough case history specific IgE titre in serum, scratch, prick and intracutaneous testing can be performed to identify threshold of reactivity (titration with aqueous solutions of wasp and bee toxins).

Differential Diagnosis

Bites from other insects, particularly order Hymenoptera (hornets and bumblebees), hives, angioedema (see chapter Arthropod reactions and Angioedema).

Prevention and Therapy

Prevention: protective clothing, sleep under fine-mesh nets, repellents. Local reaction: topical steroids or antipruritic agents, short-term ice packs, oral antihistamines.

Hymenoptera allergy: mild generalised reaction—antihistamines i.v., perhaps corticosteroids p.o. or i.v. (at least 100 mg prednisolone or equivalent).

Severe generalised reaction: treat as anaphylactic reaction. Counselling for future exposure, emergency set (soluble prednisolone liquid 100 mg to swallow, two tablets of a rapid-acting antihistamine, epinephrine self-injector—e.g. EpiPen—or metered aerosol inhaler).

Venom Immunotherapy (always with Grade 3–4 reactions), initial hyposensitisation under in patient condition (rush/ultrarush hyposensitisation). Peripheral tolerance to allergens can be achieved by specific immunotherapy or by regular exposure to them, which may induce allergen-specific IgG4 that can contribute to reducing hypersensitivity reactions by competing with IgE for binding to allergen and by other mechanisms.

Flea Bites [6, 18]

Figures 9.20 and 9.21

Grading of Importance

B

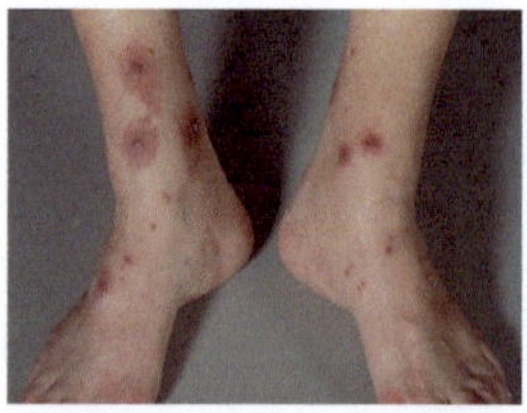

Fig. 9.20 Flea bites: on the legs

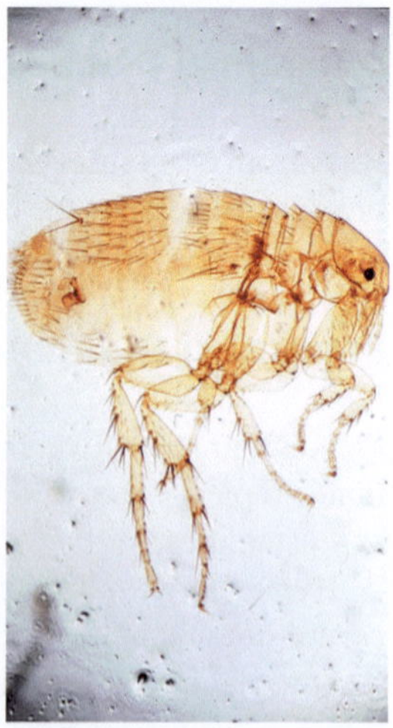

Fig. 9.21 Flea bites: the malefactor

Level

Advanced

Synonyms

Pulicosis.

ICD-11

NE61

Definition

Pruritic lesions caused by bites of from human or animal fleas.

Aetiology and Pathogenesis

Human flea (pulex irritans), various animal fleas (such as dog fleas, cat fleas, pigeon fleas, European rat fleas): flightless insects, 1–6 mm.

Signs and Symptoms

Multiple, very pruritic urticarial papules with central haemorrhagic centre. Typically present in an asymmetry.

Localisation

Exposed body areas, preferentially around the ankles and lower legs.

Classification

Can occur with more erythema in infants.

Complications

Impetiginisation. Fleas can also transmit concurrent infectious diseases (e.g. *Xenopsylla cheopis* and plague).

Diagnosis

Clinical features. History of exposure and look for fleas in the affected individuals; immediate environment; to confirm diagnosis and allow for treatment of primary host.

Differential Diagnosis

Urticaria, other arthropod bites such as bed bugs.

Prevention and Therapy

Keep the affected area dry and use topical antipruritic measures (zinc oxide lotion, corticosteroid lotion). Systemic antihistamines. Insecticides and repellents. Treat potential primary hosts in the immediate environment such as pets and pigeons. Prophylactic measures include flea bands for dogs and cats.

References

1. Adib-Tezer H, Bayerl C (2018) Honeybee and wasp venom allergy: sensitization and immunotherapy. J Dtsch Dermatol Ges 16(10):1228–1247
2. Alexander L, Buckley CJ (2020) Chigger bites. StatPearls, Treasure Island, FL
3. Aronson NE, Joya CA (2019) Cutaneous leishmaniasis: updates in diagnosis and management. Infect Dis Clin N Am 33(1):101–117
4. Arora P, Rudnicka L, Sar-Pomian M, Wollina U, Jafferany M, Lotti T, Sadoughifar R, Sitkowska Z, Goldust M (2020) Scabies: a comprehensive review and current perspectives. Dermatol Ther 33(4):e13746
5. Balestri R, Magnano M, Infusino SD, Rizzoli L, Girardelli CR, Rech G (2021) Scabies is becoming less sensitive to permethrin therapy. J Eur Acad Dermatol Venereol 35(12):e889–e891
6. Bolivar-Mejia A, Alarcon-Olave C, Rodriguez-Morales AJ (2014) Skin manifestations of arthropod-borne infection in Latin America. Curr Opin Infect Dis 27(3):288–294
7. Burza S, Croft SL, Boelaert M (2018) Leishmaniasis. Lancet 392(10151):951–970
8. Chandler DJ, Fuller LC (2019) A review of scabies: an infestation more than skin deep. Dermatology 235(2):79–90
9. Chen W, Plewig G (2014) Human demodicosis: revisit and a proposed classification. Br J Dermatol 170:1219–1225
10. de Vries HJ, Reedijk SH, Schallig HD (2015) Cutaneous leishmaniasis: recent developments in diagnosis and management. Am J Clin Dermatol 16(2):99–109

11. Fitzgerald KT, Flood AA (2006) Hymenoptera stings. Clin Tech Small Anim Pract 21(4):194–204
12. Guillet C, Martin OY, Meincke C, Joerg L, Schmid-Grendelmeier P (2022) Part I: insect stings and bites—beyond the realm of bee and wasp allergies. Allergo J Int 31(6):183–193
13. Hemmer W, Wantke F (2020) Insect hypersensitivity beyond bee and wasp venom allergy. Allergologie Select **4**:97–104
14. Ko CJ, Elston DM (2004) Pediculosis. J Am Acad Dermatol 50(1):1–12; quiz 13–14
15. Powers J, Badri T (2020) Pediculosis corporis. StatPearls, Treasure Island, FL
16. Reithinger R, Dujardin JC, Louzir H, Pirmez C, Alexander B, Brooker S (2007) Cutaneous leishmaniasis. Lancet Infect Dis 7(9):581–596
17. Sahiner UM, Durham SR (2019) Hymenoptera venom allergy: how does venom immunotherapy prevent anaphylaxis from bee and wasp stings? Front Immunol 10:1959
18. Singh S, Mann BK (2013) Insect bite reactions. Indian J Dermatol Venereol Leprol 79(2):151–164
19. Thomas C, Coates SJ, Engelman D, Chosidow O, Chang AY (2020) Ectoparasites: Scabies. J Am Acad Dermatol 82(3):533–548

Sexually Transmitted Infections

10

Annamari Ranki, Eija Hiltunen-Back, and Alexander Salava

Contents

Annamari Ranki has died before the publication of this book.

A. Ranki · E. Hiltunen-Back · A. Salava (✉)
Department of Dermatology and Allergology, Helsinki University Hospital, Helsinki, Finland
e-mail: eija.hiltunen-back@hus.fi; alexander.salava@hus.fi

H. Gollnick et al. (eds.), *Dermatology Cyberderm WebBook*,
https://doi.org/10.1007/978-3-031-78491-0_10

Test your learning and check your understanding of this book's contents: use the "Springer Nature Flashcards" app to access questions using ▶ https://sn.pub/1rhh6k.

To use the app, please follow the instructions in Chap. 1.

Gonorrhoea [16]

Figures 10.1, 10.2 and 10.3

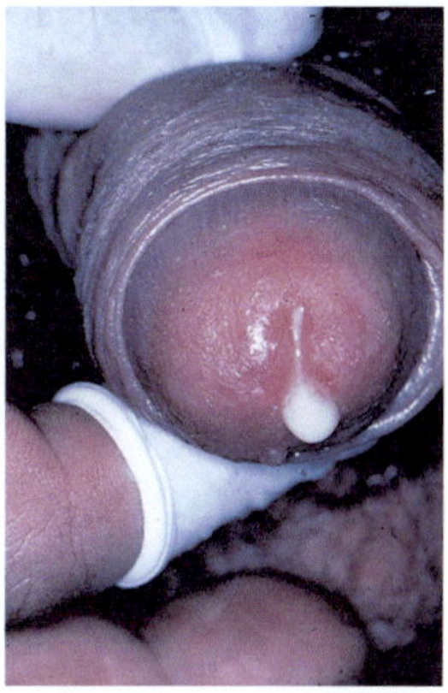

Fig. 10.1 Gonorrhoea: urethral discharge of pus

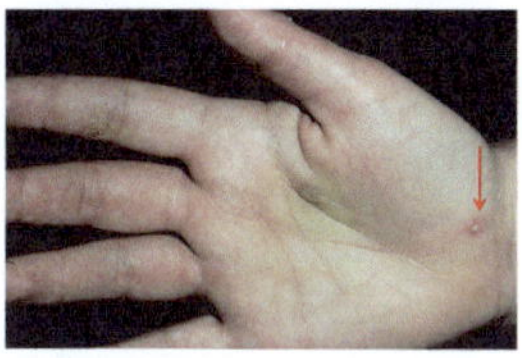

Fig. 10.2 Gonorrhoea: pustule (arrow) in benign gonococcal sepsis

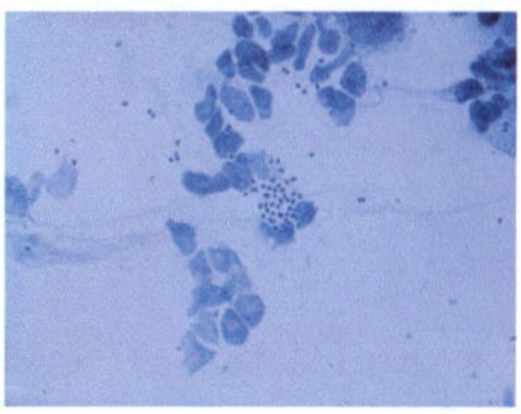

Fig. 10.3 Gonorrhoea: discharge with intracellular diplococci

Grading of Importance

A

Level

Advanced

ICD-11

1A7Z

Synonyms

Blennorrhoea; tripper.

Epidemiology

After chlamydial urethritis, the second most common bacterial sexually transmitted infection. In many European countries, incidence is increasing especially among young adults and homosexual men.

Definition

Urogenital, anorectal, or oral infection by *Neisseria gonorrhoeae*; rarely systemic infection (disseminated gonorrhea).

Aetiology and Pathogenesis

Gram-negative bacterium *Neisseria gonorrhoeae*. Incubation period 4–7 days, may be as short as 24 hours. Transmission by infected secretions during genital, anorectal, or oral sex. Co-infection with *Chlamydia trachomatis* is detected in 10–40% of the cases. Perinatal gonococcal infection can cause neonatal conjunctivitis (ophthalmia neonatorum).

Signs and Symptoms

Infection of columnar epithelium of urethra, endocervix, rectum, pharynx, and conjunctivae. Typical manifestation in men: acute urethritis with urethral discharge, pain on urination, and dysuria. Generally asymptomatic in women; sometimes abnormal vaginal discharge, dysuria, and lower abdominal pain. Rectal infections often asymptomatic, but can cause rectal and anal pain or discharge. Pharyngeal gonorrhea is mainly asymptomatic, but sore throat and pharyngitis can occur.

Localisation

See symptoms

Classification

Acute and chronic course; localised and disseminated infection.

Laboratory and Other Workups

Direct microscopy of smear (intracellular diplococci). Further investigation by nucleic acid amplification tests (NAATs) and culture. NAATs are highly sensitive and specific tests that can detect *N. gonorrhoeae* in first void urine and urethral, cervical, pharyngeal, and rectal swab. Appropriate tests should be directed by the locations of sexual activity. NAATs cannot provide information on antimicrobial susceptibility. Thus, specimens should be collected also for culture and antimicrobial susceptibility testing.

Dermatopathology

Not necessary.

Course

Acute or chronic course; beware of resistant strains.

Complications

Untreated infection in women can cause pelvic inflammatory disease. In men epididymo-orchitis and prostatitis. Rarely bacteraemia with fever, arthritis, perihepatitis (Fitz-Hugh-Curtis syndrome) and skin lesions (disseminated gonococcal infection).

Diagnosis

Diagnosis is based on clinical features and microbiological confirmation: intracellular diplococci.

Differential Diagnosis

Chlamydial and other microbial urethritis/vaginitis causes. Herpes simplex meatitis.

Prevention and Therapy

Empirical first-line dual therapy with ceftriaxone 500 mg intramuscularly (i.m.) together with azithromycin 2 g as a single oral dose. Fluoroquinolones (ciprofloxacin 500 mg as a single oral dose) can be used only if resistance is excluded by susceptibility testing. Test of cure (TOC) to identify persisting infection and emerging resistance >2 weeks after the treatment.

Special

Tests for other STIs, like chlamydial urethritis, syphilis, and HIV is strongly recommended. Evaluation and tracing of sex partners within the preceding 2 months and offer them testing and treatment. Infection report according to the national communicable disease legislation.

Chlamydial Urethritis [5] [11]

Figure 10.4

Grading of Importance

B

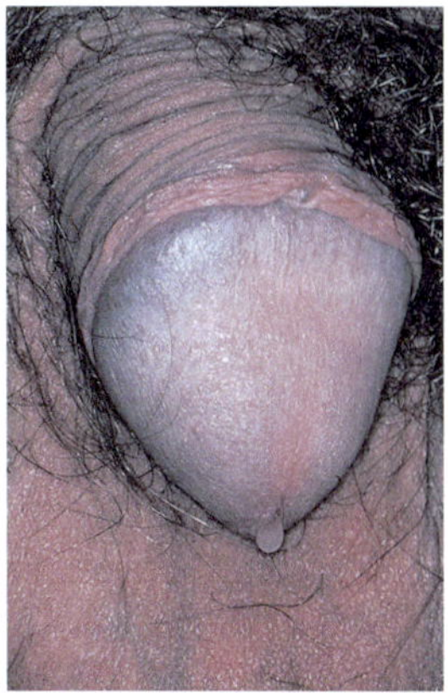

Fig. 10.4 Chlamydial urethritis: Mild mucoid urethral discharge

Level

Advanced

ICD-11

1A81.0

Epidemiology

Most common sexually transmitted infection (STI) in Europe. Worldwide 127 million adults aged 15–49 years had chlamydia infection in 2016. For 2017, 26 EU member states reported almost 410′000 cases of chlamydia infection, with the crude notification rate of 146 cases per 100,000 population.

Definition

Chlamydia trachomatis caused urogenital infection.

Aetiology and Pathogenesis

Caused by strains D-K of the intracellular Gram-negative bacterium *Chlamydia trachomatis*. Can also cause acute eye infections, trachoma, anorectal infections, and lymphogranuloma venereum. Sexually active young people are at the greatest risk.

Signs and Symptoms

Incubation period usually 1–3 weeks. Often asymptomatic. 70% of genital *C. trachomatis* infections in women and 50% in men are asymptomatic at the time of diagnosis. Mild mucoid or mucopurulent urethral discharge in the morning is less profuse than in gonorrhea. Males may complain testicular pain and epididymitis. In women, chlamydia urethritis can similarly cause dysuria and pollakisuria. Cervicitis can cause vaginal discharge, postcoital bleeding, and abdominal pain. Proctitis and pharyngitis are often asymptomatic. Anorectal infection can cause discharge and discomfort and pharyngeal chlamydia mild sore throat. Conjunctivitis can be the result of contact with contaminated hands or direct exposure to semen and vaginal fluids.

Localisation

See Symptoms.

Classification

Based on localisation.

Laboratory and Other Workups

Nucleic acid amplification tests (NAAT) are the most sensitive and the most widely used tests for the detection of genital chlamydia. Positive NAAT result can be observed within a few days of exposure but at the latest 2 weeks later. Point-of-care tests can be used for self-collected swabs and allows for self-testing outside the clinic.

Complications

Complications in men include epididymitis, epididymo-orchitis, and sexually acquired reactive arthritis. In women chronic pelvic pain and infertility can be sequelae.

Diagnosis

Based on clinical features and confirmatory microbiological tests.

Differential Diagnosis

Gonorrhoea and other causes of urethritis (*Mycoplasma genitalium*, *Ureaplasma urealyticum*, *Trichomonas vaginalis*); urethral Herpes simplex infection.

Prevention and Therapy

Prevention: barrier contraception.

First-line treatment: doxycycline 100 mg twice a day for 7 days (contraindicated in pregnancy) or azithromycin 1 g as a single dose. The second-line treatment includes erythromycin 500 mg twice a day for 7 days or levofloxacin 500 mg once a day for 7 days. Tests for other STIs, like gonorrhea, syphilis, and HIV are strongly recommended.

Special

Test-of-cure 4 weeks not recommended routinely but should be offered to pregnant women, in patients with complicated or persisting clinical findings, with second-line treatment, and suspicion of non-compliance or re-exposure. Evaluation and testing of the patient's sex partners from a period of the preceding 6 months.

Lymphogranuloma Venereum (LGV) [11]

Figure 10.5

Grading of Importance

C

Level

Advanced

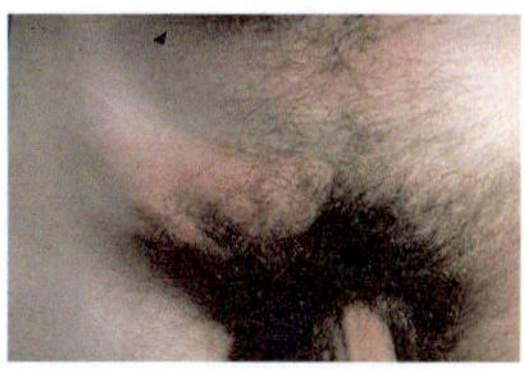

Fig. 10.5 Lymphogranuloma venereum: swelling of inguinal lymph node

ICD-11

1A80

Synonyms

Chlamydial lymphogranuloma; Frey disease; Durand-Nicolas-Favre disease; climatic bubo.

Epidemiology

In Europe the current LGV epidemic has been detected among homosexual men, causing mainly proctitis. Some cases of heterosexual LGV have been seen in Europe; most of them were imported from endemic countries (Africa, India).

Definition

Uro- and anogenital infection by *C. trachomatis*, serovars L1–3

Aetiology and Pathogenesis

LGV is caused by the invasive L1–3 strains (serovars) of *C. trachomatis* that disseminate via underlying connective tissue and spread to regional lymph nodes. Most cases in Europe have been detected among homosexual men.

Signs and Symptoms

Three stages of the infection:

Stage 1 develops after an incubation period of 1–4 weeks. In the current LGV epidemic among homosexual men, proctitis is the primary manifestation of infection. Patients complain severe anorectal pain, purulent discharge and bleeding from the rectum, tenesmus, and constipation. In classical LGV the primary lesion is often an unnoticed, small, painless papule or pustule that erodes to an ulcer and heals within 1 week.

Stage 2 (inguinal) begins 2 to 6 weeks after the onset of primary lesion. There is painful inflammation of the inguinal and/or femoral lymph nodes causing unilateral enlargement, inflammation, and abscesses (buboes) that may rupture. Constitutional symptoms like low-grade fever, chills, malaise, myalgias, and arthralgias may occur.

Stage 3 (anogenitorectal syndrome) is more often present in women and homosexual men. Patients develop proctocolitis followed by perirectal abscesses, fistulas, strictures, and stenosis of the rectum.

Classification

See above

Laboratory and Other Workups

C. trachomatis NAAT test is used for screening, and if positive, the diagnosis is confirmed by the detection of LGV biovar-specific *C. trachomatis* DNA from the same specimen. Many LGV-positive men are also HIV-positive, so screening for other STIs including HIV, hepatitis B, and hepatitis C should be offered.

Complications

Systemic spread of *C. trachomatis* occasionally results in arthritis or (peri-) hepatitis. Rare systemic complications include cardiac involvement, aseptic meningitis, and ocular inflammatory disease. Anogenitorectal syndrome with chronic progressive lymphangitis can lead to chronic oedema and sclerosing fibrosis, resulting in strictures and fistulas of the involved region, which can ultimately lead to elephantiasis.

Diagnosis

Based on clinical features and confirmed by microbiological tests.

Differential Diagnosis

LGV proctitis mimics chronic inflammatory bowel diseases like Crohn's disease both clinically and histopathologically. Inguinal lymph node enlargements and ulceration can mimic boils, hidradenitis suppurativa, and lymphomas.

Prevention and Therapy

First-line treatment is doxycycline 100 mg twice a day orally for 21 days and second-line erythromycin 500 mg four times a day orally for 21 days. Fluctuant buboes should be aspirated promptly through healthy adjacent skin. A test of cure for LGV is not considered necessary if the recommended 21-day course of doxycycline is completed.

Special

Sexual partners within the last 3 months are strongly recommended testing for chlamydia/LGV and epidemiological treatment with antibiotic therapy commenced until chlamydia/LGV has been excluded in the partner. All LGV cases should be reported according to the national legislation of communicable diseases.

Nonspecific Urethritis [10, 13]

Grading of Importance

C

Level

Advanced

ICD-11

GC02.1

Synonyms

Non-venereal urethritis; non-gonococcal-non-chlamydial urethritis (NGNCU).

Epidemiology

Probably underreported or not correctly diagnosed.

Definition

The term nonspecific urethritis (NSU) applies to non-gonococcal, non-chlamydial urethritis (NGNCU).

Aetiology and Pathogenesis

In many men with acute urethritis, a known pathogen is not detected. The most common organism detected is *Mycoplasma genitalium*, which accounts for approximately 15–40% of cases, and there is a high concordance of infection in sexual partners. Other causes: *Trichomonas vaginalis*, adenoviruses, or herpes simplex virus types 1 and 2 (HSV1–2).

Signs and Symptoms

Patients complain of clear urethral discharge, dysuria, penile tip irritation, urethral discomfort, or itch but can be asymptomatic, too. Clinical signs are often modest or missing; the presence of a mucopurulent or purulent urethral discharge or penile tip erythema can be detected on examination.

Localisation

Lower and upper urethral duct.

Classification

Usually based on causative agent.

Laboratory and Other Workups

The diagnosis of urethritis can be confirmed by demonstrating ≥5 polymorphonuclear leukocytes (PMNLs) per high power microscopic field from the urethral smear.

Dermatopathology

Not necessary.

Course

Spontaneous resolution may occur; some cases are persistent or recurrent.

Complications

Epididymo-orchitis; sexually acquired reactive arthritis.

Diagnosis

Based on clinical feature and exclusion of gonococcal and chlamydial urethritis.

Differential Diagnosis

Chlamydia, gonorrhoea, genital herpes simplex, chronic pelvic pain syndrome.

Prevention and Therapy

Prevention: barrier contraception.

Infection should be treated according to the etiological findings.

Azithromycin for 5 days (500 mg stat then 250 mg od for 4 days) in eradicating macrolide-susceptible *M. genitalium* infection. If macrolide-resistant *M. genitalium* is detected, moxifloxacin 400 mg orally once daily for 7–14 days is recommended. Test of cure >3 weeks after treatment.

Trichomoniasis [6, 15]

Figure 10.6

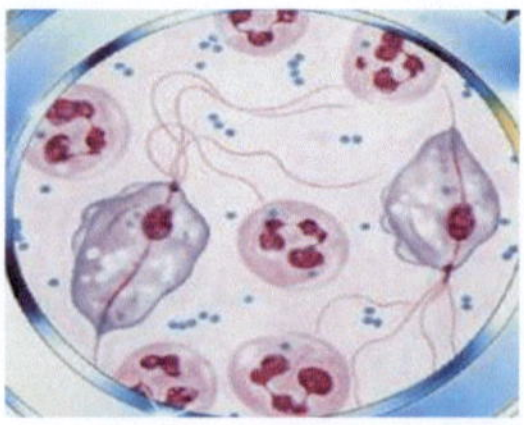

Fig. 10.6 Non-specific urethritis: *Mycoplasma genitalium*

Grading of Importance

B

Level

Advanced

ICD-11

1A92

Synonyms

None.

Epidemiology

3% of women of reproductive age in the USA infected; estimated rate of asymptomatic cases is 50%. 180 million new infections worldwide annually, according to WHO.

Definition

A sexually transmitted infection caused by the protozoan parasite *Trichomonas vaginalis*.

Aetiology and Pathogenesis

The causative agent *T. vaginalis* is a flagellated protozoan parasite transmitted during sexual intercourse. Transmission usually occurs via direct, skin, or mucosal contact with an infected individual, most often through vaginal intercourse. Females can acquire the disease from infected males or females, but males usually acquire it only from infected females.

Signs and Symptoms

The incubation time is usually 1–2 weeks, but up to half of infected females have no symptoms and can be asymptomatic carriers for years. Most symptomatic females have vaginal discharge with an offensive odour. The classic symptom is a yellow-green, frothy discharge, which is present in less than 10% of symptomatic females. Other symptoms include pruritus vulvae and vaginal burning sensation. There can also be dysuria and pain or bleeding during sexual intercourse. The cervix may have a punctate or strawberry-like appearance.

T. vaginalis is present in 30–70% of the male partners of infected females, but most infected males have no symptoms. If there are symptoms, they are usually a result of urethritis (urethral discharge, meatal irritation, and dysuria).

Localisation

See Symptoms.

Classification

No classification applicable.

Laboratory and Other Workups

In women, a vaginal or cervical smear with direct microscopy. In men a urethral swab (women: a high vaginal or cervical swab) for culture. Nucleic acid amplification test and tests detecting Trichomonas antigens in urethral or cervical smears are also available.

Dermatopathology

Not necessary.

Course

The infection may cause acute symptoms, but the majority of patients have no symptoms and can be asymptomatic carriers for years.

Complications

None.

Diagnosis

Based on typical clinical features and microbiological confirmation. Mixed STI infections to be excluded.

Differential Diagnosis

Vulvovaginitis due to other causes (candida, bacterial vaginosis, aerobic vaginitis); chlamydial urethritis, gonorrhoea, and mycoplasma urethritis. Genital herpes simplex can also cause similar symptoms.

Prevention and Therapy

Transmission can be prevented by barrier contraception.

First-line treatment consists of metronidazole p.o. 400–500 mg × 2–3 for 5–7 days or as a single dose of 2 g and is usually effective. The alternative is tinidazole as a 2 g single dose p.o. It is important also to treat the sexual partner of the patient. Sexual activity should not take place until symptoms have cleared.

Bacterial Vaginosis [1, 9, 14]

Grading of Importance

B

Level

Advanced

ICD-11

MF3A

Synonyms

Nonspecific vaginitis, *Gardnerella vaginitis*, bacterial vaginitis.

Epidemiology

A very common cause of vaginal symptoms in women of reproductive age; lifelong prevalence in Europe 15–20%.

Definition

A disturbance of the normal bacterial flora of the vulva and/or vagina causing a malodorous discharge.

Aetiology and Pathogenesis

Pathogenesis not completely understood; disturbances of normal vaginal microbiota (*Lactobacillus* spp.) suspected. Detectable overgrowth of anaerobic bacteria with an elevation of the vaginal pH. Predisposing factors: recent use of broad-spectrum antibiotics, use of an intrauterine device, high number of sexual partners.

Signs and Symptoms

Main symptom is a malodorous, milky or grey-white homogeneous vaginal discharge. The discharge can cause irritation of the vulvar skin. The odour of the discharge has a fishy smell and is a common complaint.

Localisation

Usually localised to vulvar skin and vaginal mucosa.

Classification

Not applicable.

Laboratory and Other Workups

Microscopy of a vaginal smear shows epithelial cells with many adherent cocci (clue-cells) with almost no leucocytes. Vaginal pH strip test (pH > 4.5). If drops of potassium hydroxide solution are applied on the speculum, a fishy smell can be provoked (KOH-test). Some patients with positive test results do not have symptoms. Findings of bacterial vaginosis can be normal in asymptomatic postmenopausal women.

Dermatopathology

Not necessary.

Course

Symptoms usually wax and wane; may last some days to weeks.

Complications

During pregnancy, there have been reports associating bacterial vaginosis with premature labour and perinatal infections (chorioamnionitis).

Diagnosis

Based on typical clinical features and complementary tests suggestive for bacterial vaginosis.

Differential Diagnosis

Vaginal discharge caused by other causes of vulvovaginitis (candida, aerobic, and trichomonas vaginitis). If there is discharge from the cervix, genital chlamydia and gonorrhoea should be excluded; in recurrent cases and elderly women, a colposcopy to exclude malignancies.

Prevention and Therapy

Usually not preventable. Recurrences after treatment are common due to the biofilm produced by *G. vaginalis*. Oral combined contraceptives can reduce recurrence.

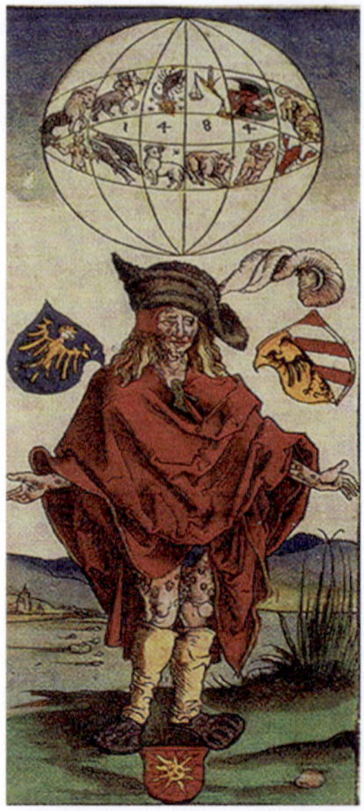

Fig. 10.7 Syphilis: Depiction of a syphilis patient by Albrecht Dürer (1496)

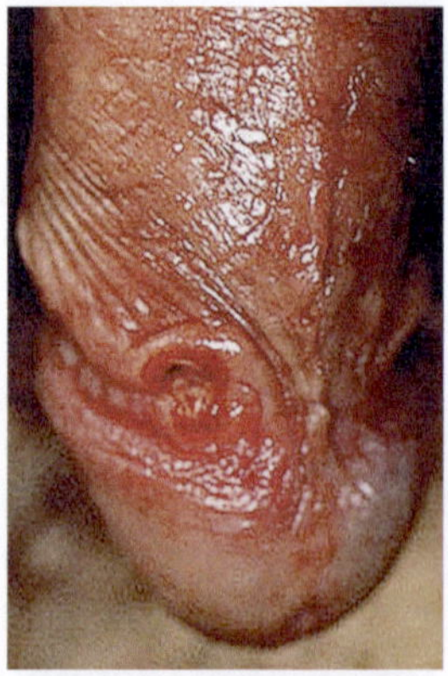

Fig. 10.8 Syphilis: stage I; ulcus durum on the penis

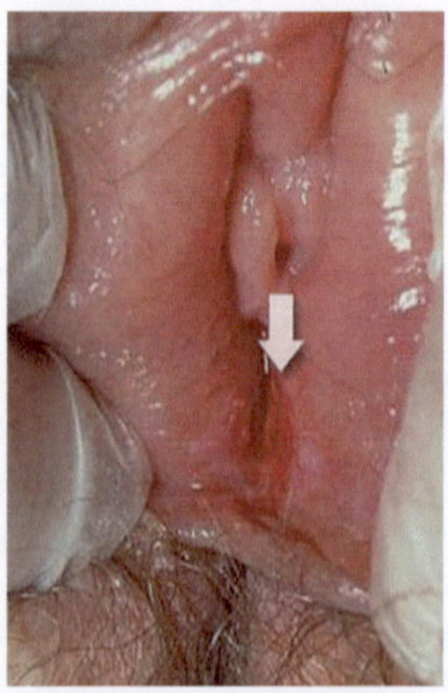

Fig. 10.9 Syphilis: stage I; vulva ulcus durum

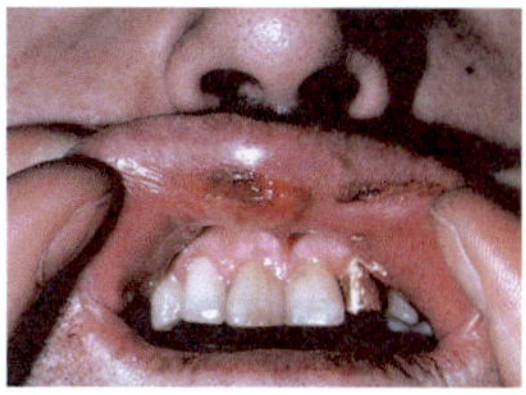

Fig. 10.10 Syphilis: stage I; lip ulcus durum

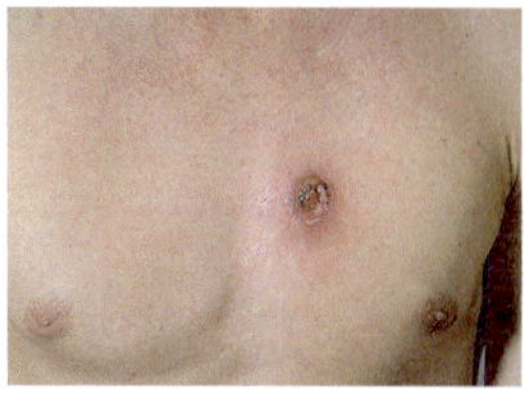

Fig. 10.11 Syphilis: stage I; ulcus durum on the breast

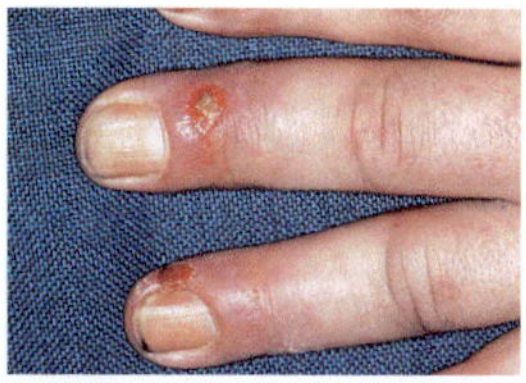

Fig. 10.12 Syphilis: stage I; ulcus durum on the finger

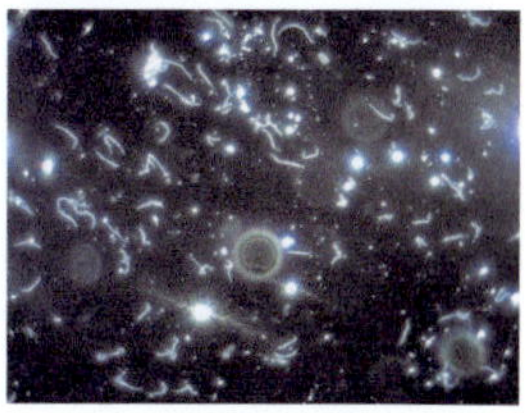

Fig. 10.13 Syphilis: stage I; *Treponema pallidum* spirochete in microscopic darkfield examination

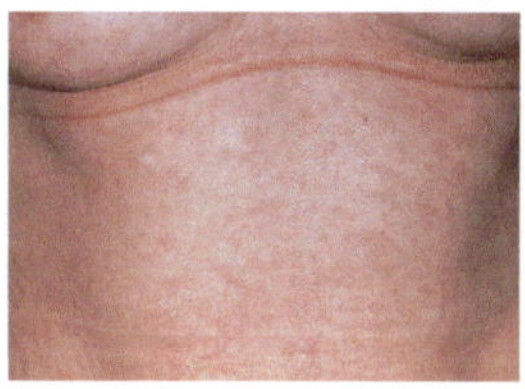

Fig. 10.14 Syphilis: stage II; non-itching skin rash

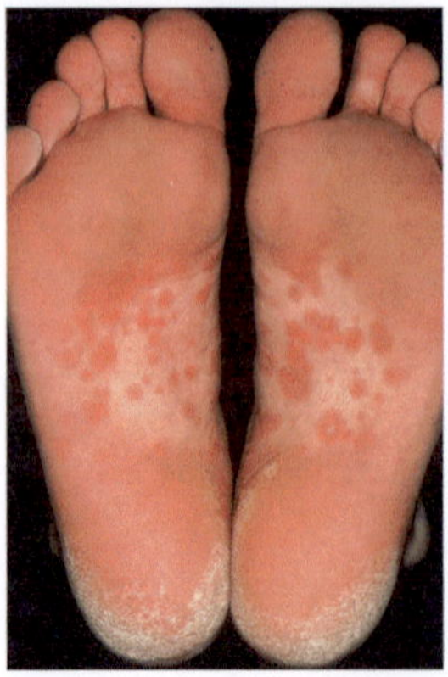

Fig. 10.15 Syphilis: stage II; lesions on the plantae

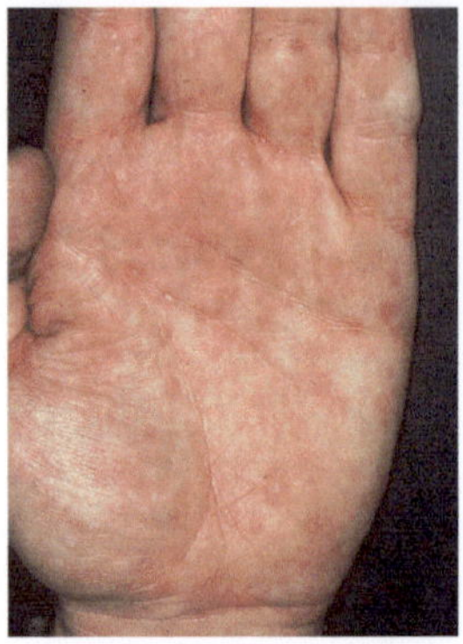

Fig. 10.16 Syphilis: stage II; lesions on the palm

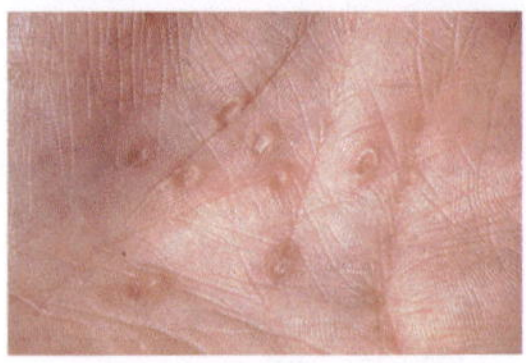

Fig. 10.17 Syphilis: stage II; small keratotic lesions on the palm

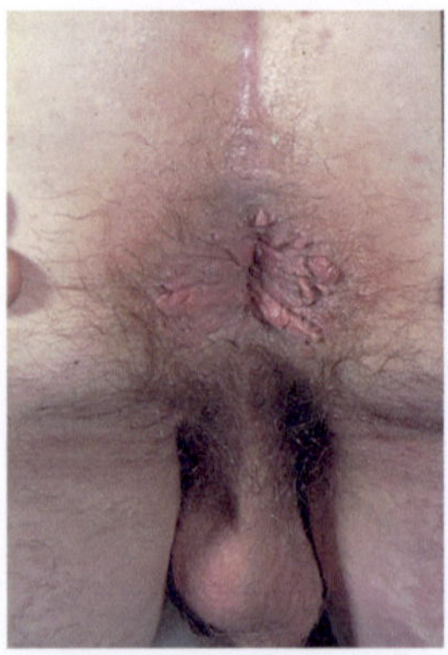

Fig. 10.18 Syphilis: stage II; anal condylomata lata

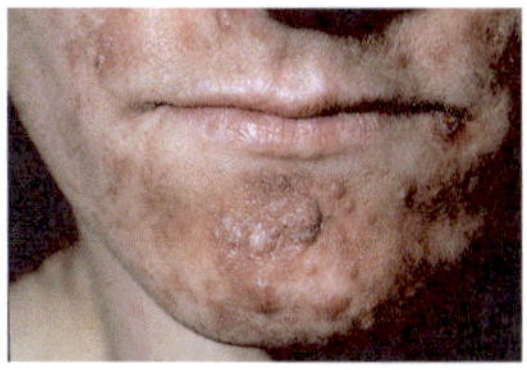

Fig. 10.19 Syphilis: stage II; condylomata lata in the face

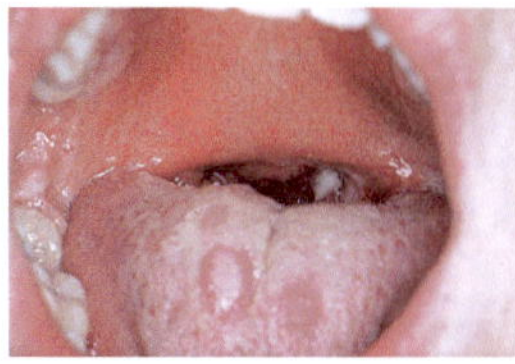

Fig. 10.20 Syphilis: stage II; plaque muceuse of the tongue

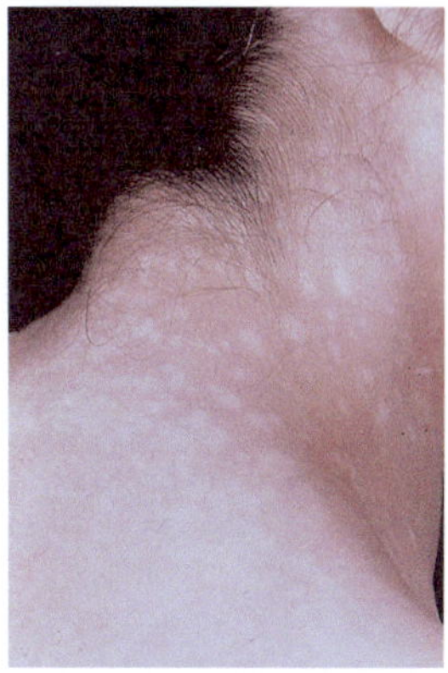

Fig. 10.21 Syphilis: stage II; leukoderma specificum of the neck

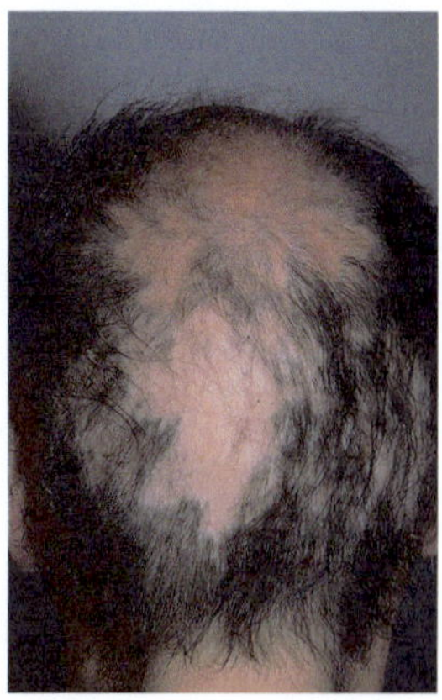

Fig. 10.22 Syphilis: stage II; alopecia areolaris

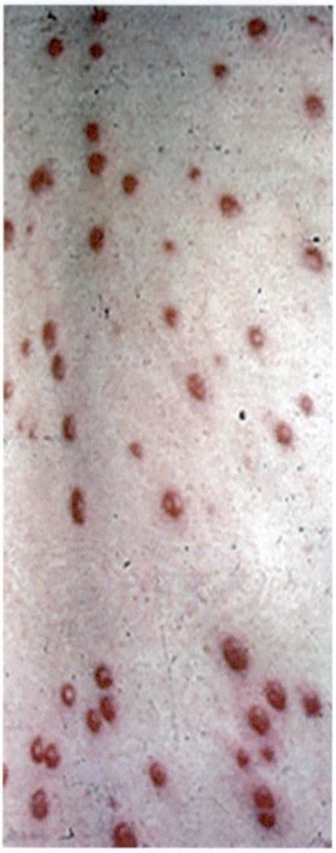

Fig. 10.23 Syphilis: stage II; papular eruptions

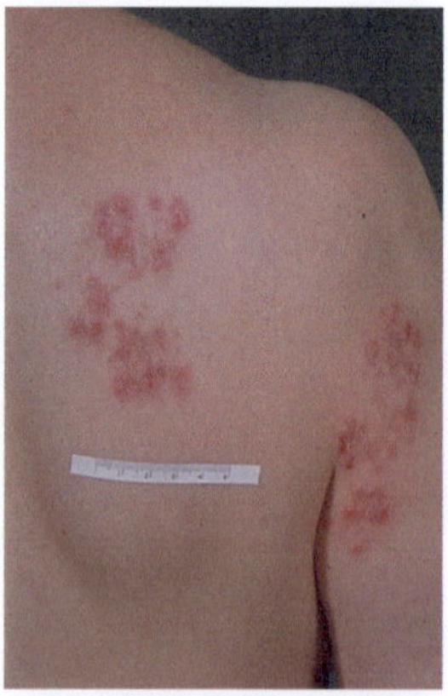

Fig. 10.24 Syphilis: stage II; late stage lesions (corymbiform syphilid)

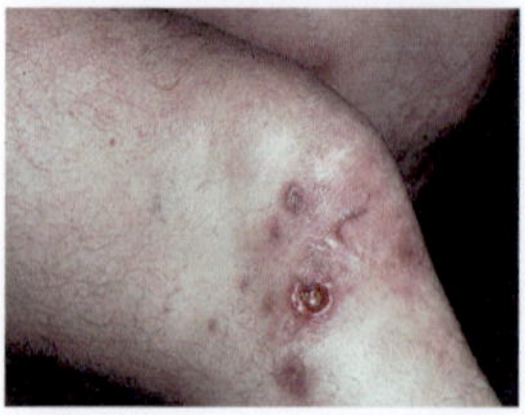

Fig. 10.25 Syphilis: stage III; gumma with ulceration

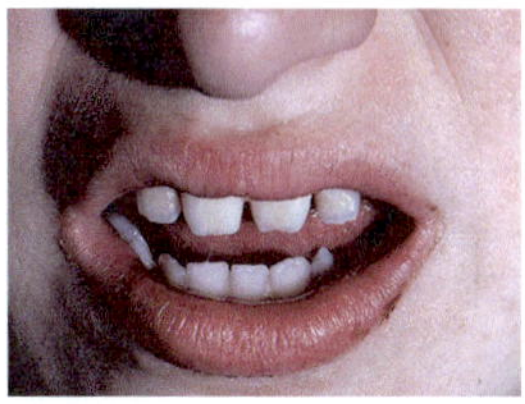

Fig. 10.26 Syphilis: lues connata, Hutchinson's teeth

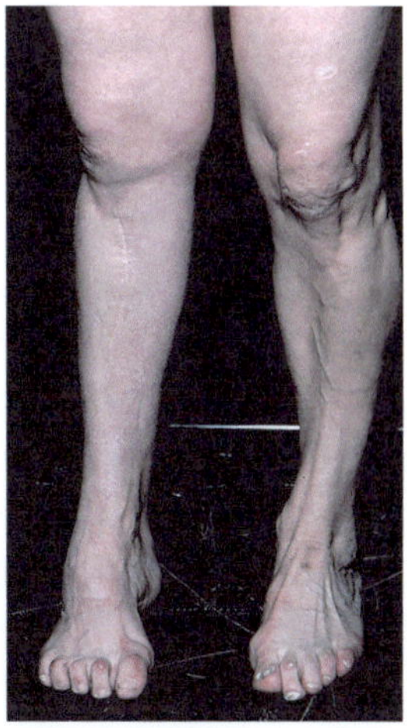

Fig. 10.27 Syphilis: lues connata, late sign; saber tibia

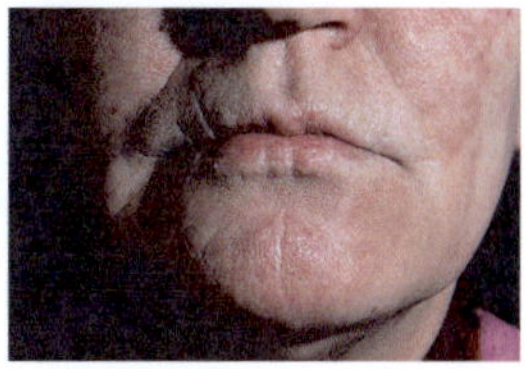

Fig. 10.28 Syphilis: lues connata, late sign; Parrot's lip furrows

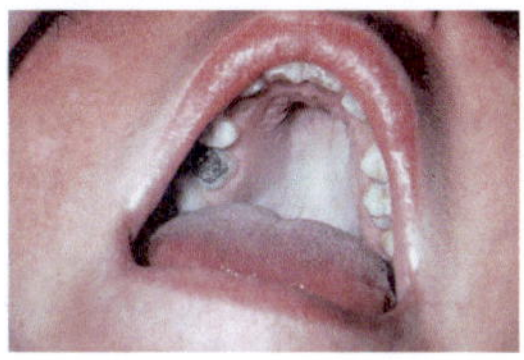

Fig. 10.29 Syphilis: lues connata, late sign; high palate

Bacterial vaginosis has a tendency to spontaneously subside, and treatments are not always necessary. Should be treated during pregnancy because of possible association with perinatal complications.

Effective treatments are a single dose of p.o. metronidazole 2 g or a course of p.o. metronidazole 400–500 mg t.i.d. for 5–7 days.

Syphilis [3, 12]

Figures 10.7, 10.8, 10.9, 10.10, 10.11, 10.12, 10.13, 10.14, 10.15, 10.16, 10.17, 10.18, 10.19, 10.20, 10.21, 10.22, 10.23, 10.24, 10.25, 10.26, 10.27, 10.28 and 10.29

Grading of Importance

B

Level

Advanced

ICD-11

1A6Z

Synonyms

Lues.

Epidemiology

World Health Organization (WHO) estimates that in 2017 six million new cases occurred among adolescents and adults aged 15–49 years worldwide. In Europe, almost 30,000 syphilis cases (6.1 /100000) and still congenital syphilis cases were reported. The reported syphilis rates were eight times higher in men than in women and peaked among 25–34-year-old men. Two-thirds of the syphilis cases with information on transmission were among men who have sex with men (MSM).

Definition

Mainly sexually transmitted systemic infection by *Treponema pallidum.*

Aetiology and Pathogenesis

Syphilis is a systemic infection caused by *Treponema pallidum* spirochete and has four stages; primary, secondary, latent, and tertiary syphilis.

- The incubation period from infection to the primary stage is 10–90 days.
- Secondary syphilis develops in 30% of untreated patients 2–3 months after the onset of chancre.
- Tertiary syphilis is rare and develops in 10% of untreated patients. Syphilis is mostly considered as a sexually transmitted infection (STI), but a foetus of the untreated mother can get...
- Congenital syphilis.

The European Centre for Disease Prevention and Control (ECDC) defines early or infectious syphilis as an infection acquired ≤1 year earlier, and it includes primary, secondary, and early latent syphilis stages. Late syphilis, which is divided to late latent and tertiary stages, has been acquired more than a year earlier. Patients are considered infectious during the first year (primary and secondary syphilis). Later transmission vertically.

Signs and Symptoms

- The typical symptom of primary syphilis is a single, painless, indurated ulcer (chancre) at the inoculation site, mainly in the anogenital area but can also be detected extragenitally, such as in the oral area. Regional lymphadenopathy is usually observed. The primary stage may be asymptomatic or chancres, which are difficult to detect if located in the vagina or rectum.
- The typical feature of secondary syphilis is a non-itching skin rash (roseola) on the trunk and later, papular syphilids on the palms and soles and mucocutaneous lesions. Constitutional symptoms like fever, chills, malaise, generalised lymphadenopathy, myalgias, and arthritis occur due to bacteremia. During the secondary stage of syphilis, symptoms of early neurosyphilis, like uveitis, retinitis, otitis, meningitis, and cranial nerve dysfunction, may occur
- Latent syphilis is clinically asymptomatic
- The symptoms of tertiary syphilis are like erosive cutaneous or mucosal lesions (gumma), neurological (late neurosyphilis), and cardiovascular (aortic aneurysm) disorders.

Localisation

Stage I: anogenital, oral or elsewhere, draining lymph node enlarged.

Stage II: all over the body, localised and generalised, general lymphadenopathy.

Stage III: all over the body, localised and generalised, central and peripheral nerve system, cardiovascular.

Classification

Syphilis stages are clinically defined, and they may overlap each other.

Primary stage: ulcer (ulcus durum) at the inoculation site; regional lymphadenopathy.

Secondary stage: eruptive skin rash (roseola exanthem); papular syphilids on palms and soles; mucocutaneous lesions; fever with generalised lymphadenopathy.

Tertiary: plaque-like lesions (gumma), neurological (late neurosyphilis), and cardiovascular (aortic aneurysm) disorders.

Laboratory and Other Workups

The direct verification of the spirochete is done with darkfield examination by microscopy in the early chancre. Serological tests for syphilis (STS) are obligatory; additionally they are used for screening and follow-up. Both treponemal tests (TT) and non- treponemal tests (NTT) are available. NTTs like the Venereal Diseases Research Laboratory (VDRL) test and the rapid plasma reagin (RPR) test become positive 10–15 days after the onset of the primary chancre (i.e. around 6 weeks after infection). After a previously adequately treated syphilis, the STS often stay positive. A person with a positive STS should be asked about earlier treatments of syphilis and treated as for syphilis if not known.

Titres of NTT correlate with the disease activity and are used to monitor disease activity and efficacy of treatment.

Dermatopathology

Usually not necessary. In cutaneous secondary and tertiary stages, a biopsy may become essential to exclude differential diagnoses such as viral exanthemas, hand eczema, psoriasis, cutaneous pseudolymphoma, and malignant lymphomas.

Course

Untreated cases run according to classification and symptoms (see above).

Complications

Comorbidity with HIV and other sexually transmitted infections is frequent. The clinical picture and disease course can be severe (disseminated ulcerative skin lesions, severe constitutional symptoms, neurosyphilis, aortic aneurysm) in immunocompromised patients (lues maligna). HIV infection increases the propensity of syphilis to progress into neurosyphilis and ocular syphilis.

Diagnosis

The diagnosis of syphilis is done by a thorough case history, clinical picture, and laboratory test (see above) for correct staging. A biopsy should be done in several differential diagnoses (see below).

Differential Diagnosis

Primary chancres may be atypical, multiple, painful, deep, and indistinguishable from genital and oral herpes. In female, the chancre may be misdiagnosed as Bartholinitis. Roseola can mimic other dermatological exanthemas (drug reactions,

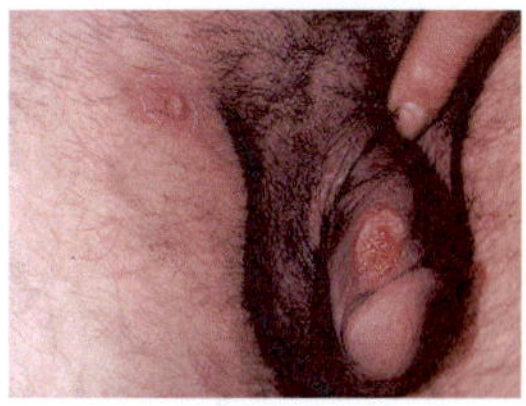

Fig. 10.30 Chancroid: ulcus molle on the penis

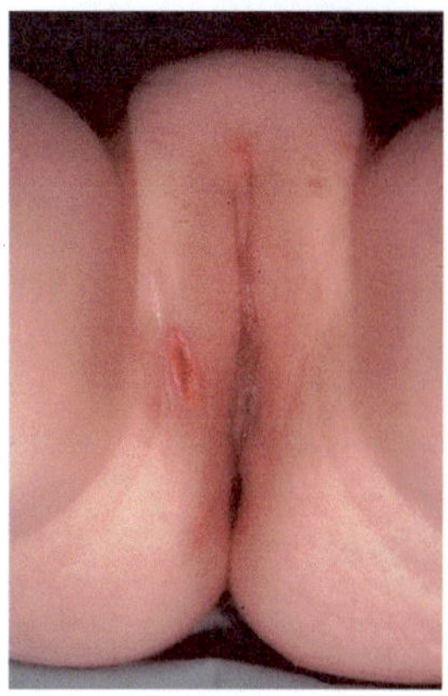

Fig. 10.31 Chancroid: ulcus molle on the female labia

viral infections) and eruptive papulosquamous dermatoses (e.g. guttate psoriasis,

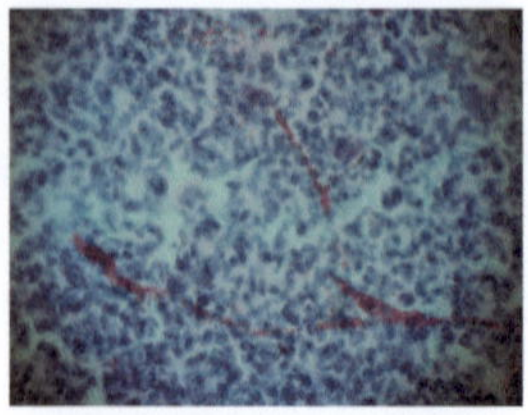

Fig. 10.32 Chancroid: the rod shaped gram negative bacteria *Haemophilus ducreyi*

pityriasis rosea, pityriasis lichenoides). Pseudolymphomas and malignant lymphomas have to be ruled out in nodular and infiltrated plaque lesions (gumma).

Prevention and Therapy

The first-line therapy for the early syphilis is single dose of benzathine penicillin G (BPG) 2.4 million units intramuscularly (i.m.). The treatment of late latent syphilis is benzathine penicillin G (BPG) 2.4 million units i.m. weekly on Days 1, 8, and 15. In case the patient is allergic to penicillin or refuses the parenteral treatment, oral doxycycline 200 mg daily (2x100) can be used for 14 days (early syphilis) and for 21–28 days (late latent). Benzyl penicillin 18–24 million units intravenously daily and (3–four million units every 4 h) during 10–14 days is the first choice of treatment for neurosyphilis and ocular and auricular syphilis. Consider Jarisch-Herxheimer reaction.

NTTs are used for monitoring the effectiveness of treatment at 1, 3, and every 6 months thereafter, until it becomes negative or attains a low plateau (1:1–1:4).

All syphilis cases should be reported and contact tracing performed according to the local communicable disease legislation.

Chancroid [3, 8]

Figures 10.30, 10.31 and 10.32

Grading of Importance

C

Level

Advanced

ICD-11

1A90

Synonyms

Bubo; soft chancre; ulcus molle.

Epidemiology

Very rare in Europe except endemic hotspots and most commonly found in tropical and subtropical regions of Africa, the Caribbean, South America, and southwest Asia; in Europe, mainly seen in travellers and patients originating from endemic areas.

Definition

Sexually transmitted infection caused by *Haemophilus ducreyi* with characteristic painful ulcers in the genital area; often unilateral swollen inguinal lymph nodes.

Aetiology and Pathogenesis

The causative agent *Haemophilus ducreyi* is a rod-shaped Gram-negative bacterium, which is transmitted during sexual intercourse by direct inoculation from affected skin and mucosal sites.

Signs and Symptoms

Appear during the first week after transmission. Typically, there are one or more painful ulcers in the genital area. The site of most infections in men is the foreskin and other parts of the penis. In women ulcers may be located on the labia, perineum, or intravaginal. Women may demonstrate less specific symptoms such as dysuria, vaginal discharge, or rectal bleeding. Some women may have less or no symptoms at all.

Localisation

See Symptoms.

Classification

No classification applicable.

Laboratory and Other Workups

Bacterial culture of *Haemophilus ducreyi* requires special culture media which are not widely available. Other swab tests using nucleic acid amplification are available only in specialised laboratories.

Dermatopathology

Usually not necessary.

Course

Ulcers usually last for some weeks; if not treated many patients develop chronic inguinal lymphadenopathy.

Complications

If not treated, many patients develop painful inflammation of the inguinal lymph nodes (i.e. buboes), typically on one side. Chancroid increases the risk of HIV-transmission, so HIV testing and screening for other STI should be undertaken.

Diagnosis

Usually the diagnosis is based on typical clinical features (related to foreign travel to endemic areas) and ruling out syphilis and genital herpes simplex.

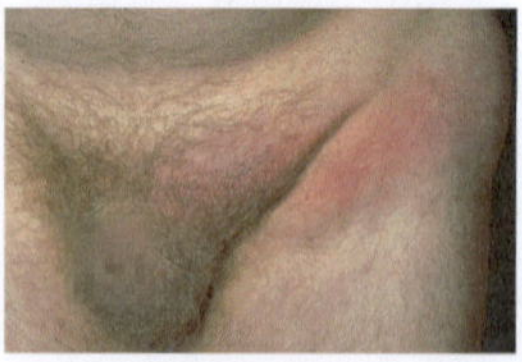

Fig. 10.33 Granuloma inguinale: swelling of the inguinal lymph node

Differential Diagnosis

Genital herpes simplex and syphilis (primary chancre) and in travel related cases to endemic regions granuloma inguinale. Lymphogranuloma venereum, if inguinal lymphadenopathy is present.

Prevention and Therapy

Prevention: barrier contraception.

A single dose of p.o. azithromycin 1 g or i.m. Ceftriaxone 250 mg is usually effective. Alternatives are p.o. Ciprofloxacin 500 mg b.i.d. (3 days) or p.o. Erythromycin 500 mg t.i.d. (7 days). Rarely, surgical treatments are required to drain infected lymph nodes.

Sexual activity should not take place until all lesions have healed. Sexual partners should be requested for clinical examination and treatment.

Granuloma Inguinale [2]

Figure 10.33

Grading of Importance

C

Level

Advanced

ICD-11

1A91

Synonyms

Donovanosis.

Epidemiology

Very rare in Europe. Most cases are travel-related; quite frequent and endemic in the tropical and subtropical regions of Africa, India, and the Caribbean.

Definition

Sexually transmitted infection caused by *Klebsiella granulomatis* with characteristic ulcerated nodules in the genital and perianal area.

Aetiology and Pathogenesis

The causative bacterium *Klebsiella granulomatis* is a Gram-negative rod-shaped bacterium. Transmission usually occurs via direct, skin, or mucosal contact with an infected individual.

Signs and Symptoms

The symptoms appear weeks after transmission, and there is great individual variation of the incubation time, which may be from 1 week up to 3 months (most frequently 4–6 weeks). Characteristic lesions: ulcerated nodules or plaques appearing on genital and perianal skin and mucous membranes. Some patients develop hypertrophic nodules (verrucous, resembling warts) or necrotic ulcers. Lesions are typically painless and symptoms are mild. Local lymph nodes (mostly inguinal) may be enlarged and drain abscesses into the overlying skin.

Localisation

See Symptoms.

Classification

Not applicable.

Laboratory and Other Workups

Tests such as bacterial culture, nucleic acid amplification tests, or serology are usually available only in specialised laboratories.

Course

Primary infection usually lasts 2–3 weeks, but recurrences are shorter, usually 7–10 days; prolonged course is possible in immunocompromised patients (HIV).

Complications

Permanent scarring of the genitals and secondary genital lymphedema.

Diagnosis

Based on typical clinical features and the detection of microscopically visible Donovan bodies. Screening tests for other STI should be carried out.

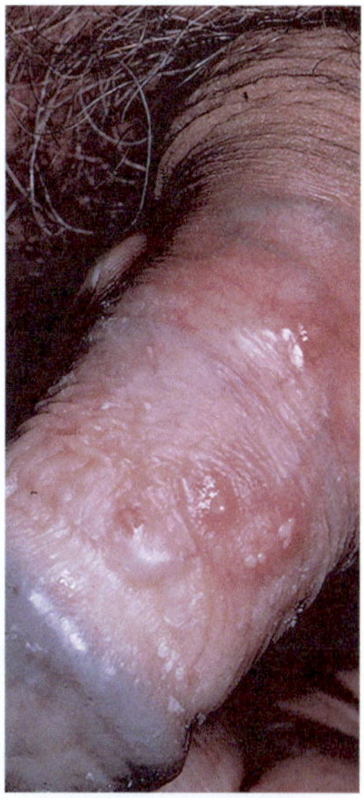

Fig. 10.34 Genital herpes simplex: vesicles on the penis

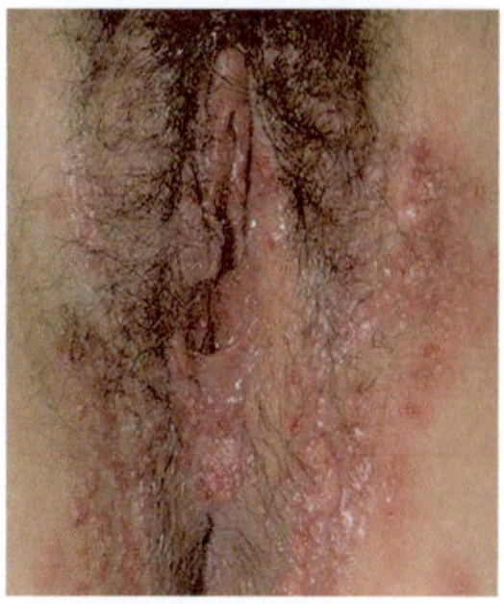

Fig. 10.35 Genital herpes simplex: vesicles on vulva labia

Differential Diagnosis

Genital herpes simplex and syphilis (primary chancre) and in travel-related cases chancroid. If inguinal lymphadenopathy is present, also lymphogranuloma venereum. In chronic genital ulcers, one must also rule out penile or vulvar cancer (squamous cell carcinoma).

Prevention and Therapy

Transmission can be prevented by barrier contraception.

Antibiotic treatment is recommended for at least 3–4 weeks or longer until visible lesions have completely healed. Oral azithromycin 1 g (once a week) is considered the first-line treatment. Alternatives are p.o. doxycycline 100 b.i.d. and p.o. Erythromycin 500 mg q.i.d.

Sexual activity should not take place until all lesions have healed. Sexual partners should be requested for clinical examination and treatment. A follow-up examination may be necessary to ensure complete recovery.

Genital Herpes Simplex [7]

Figures 10.34 and 10.35

ICD-10

A60.0

Grading of Importance

A

Level

Advanced

Synonyms

None.

Epidemiology

One of the most frequent sexually transmitted infections in Europe. Seroprevalence 15–20% but varies substantially between countries. Incidence in Europe ranges from 5 to 24 per 100 persons per year. 1 in 5 adults have evidence of HSV-2 infection.

Definition

Primary infection or recurrence of the genital mucosa or adjacent skin by human herpes simplex virus (HSV) type 2 (or less commonly type 1).

Aetiology and Pathogenesis

Causative pathogens are both HSV types, mostly type 2, which both belong to the most common human viral infections worldwide. Clinical symptoms can be caused by primary infection or recurrences. After the primary infection, HSV remains latent in regional neuronal ganglia from where the virus spreads to the mucous membrane or skin epithelial cells via sensory neurons. HSV infection can recur spontaneously on different stimuli.

Signs and Symptoms

Primary Infection

In males the most common clinical features are grouped vesicles and erosions on the glans and corona glandis penis and the shaft. The erosions are painful and, if untreated, can last 2–3 weeks. The inguinal lymph nodes can be tender and patients can have flu-like symptoms with fever and myalgia.

In females, the lesions tend to be more erosive and ulcerative. Typical sites are the vulvar area and the mucosae of the vagina and cervix. Many patients have dysuria and pelvic pain. Although infection may be asymptomatic in some cases, fever may occur and the disease course may be more severe in females.

Recurrence

Symptoms are usually milder and of shorter duration than in the primary infection. They can occur spontaneously or be triggered by individual provoking factors: minor trauma (e.g. after sexual intercourse), genital infections (e.g. *Candida* vaginitis), menstrual cycle (especially before menstrual bleeding), immunocompromised patients, and emotional stress.

Localisation

See symptoms. Anal intercourse can also lead to perianal and rectal HSV infection.

Classification

Based on causative agent HSV2 or less commonly HSV1 or on suspected clinical course as primary infection or a recurrence.

Laboratory and Other Workups

HSV can be detected from the skin and mucosal lesions of the skin by viral culture, HSV antigen test (direct immunofluorescence), or nucleic acid amplification tests. Serological tests are not helpful.

Dermatopathology

Usually not necessary.

Course

See symptoms.

Complications

In rare cases, chronic neurogenic pain in the pelvic and genital areas. In pregnancy, genital herpes simplex can lead to infection of the foetus and should be managed by doctors of the maternity care or the obstetrician. Genital herpes increases the risk of HIV transmission. Severe ulcerative and disseminated herpes infection possible in immunocompromised patients.

Diagnosis

Based on typical clinical features and optional confirmatory microbiological tests. Additional HIV testing and screening for other STI should be undertaken.

Differential Diagnosis

Trauma-induced ulcers (e.g. during sexual intercourse), genital aphthae, herpes

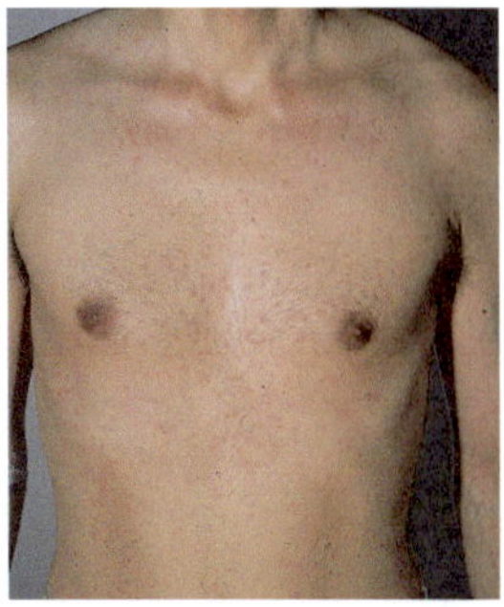

Fig. 10.36 Skin manifestations of HIV infection: faint exanthematous reaction in early stage of infection

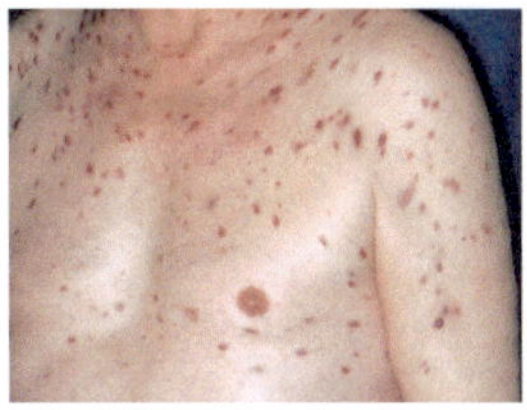

Fig. 10.37 Skin manifestations of HIV infection: disseminated AIDS associated Kaposi disease

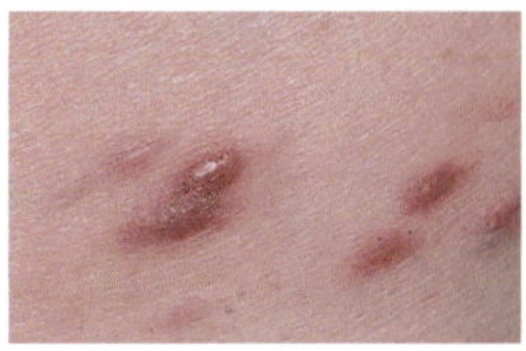

Fig. 10.38 Skin manifestations of HIV infection: smal papules and nodules in AIDS associated Kaposi disease

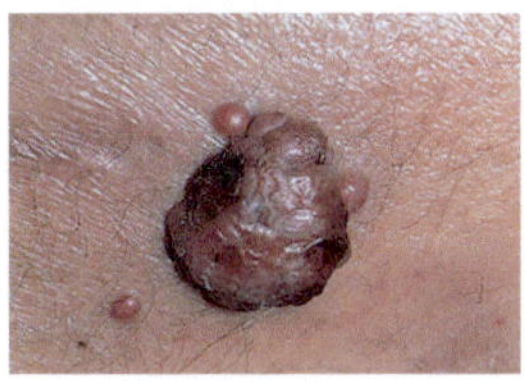

Fig. 10.39 Skin manifestations of HIV infection: Bacillary angiomatosis in AIDS

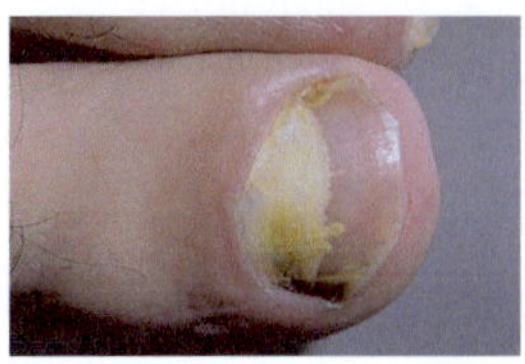

Fig. 10.40 Skin manifestations of HIV infection: fungal infection of the nail

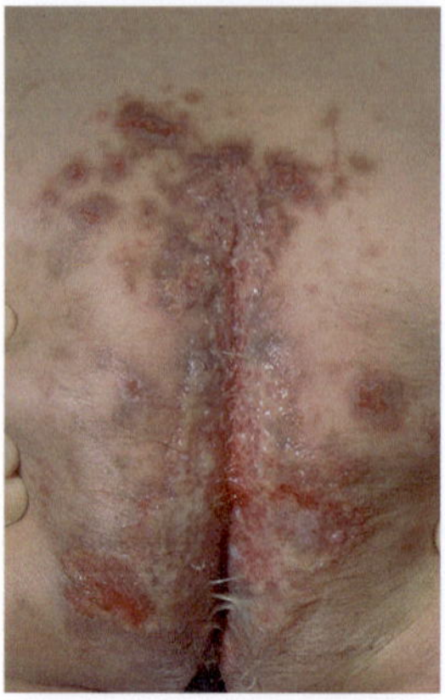

Fig. 10.41 Skin manifestations of HIV infection: cytomegalovirus infection with perianal lesions

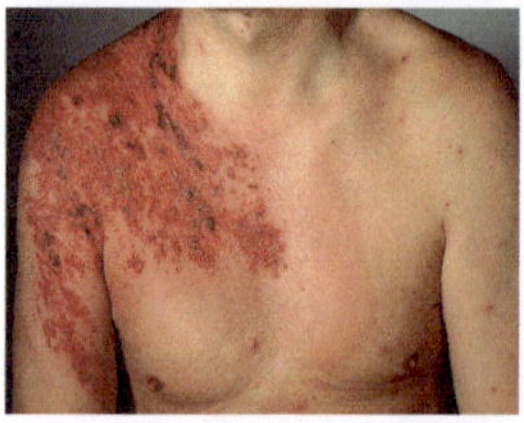

Fig. 10.42 Skin manifestations of HIV infection: herpes zoster

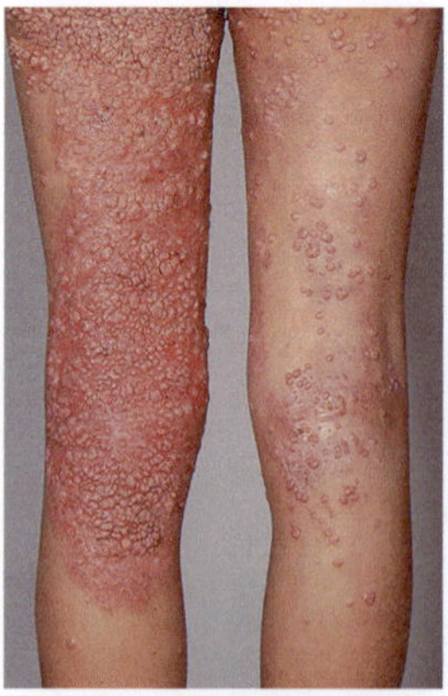

Fig. 10.43 Skin manifestations of HIV infection: widespread warts

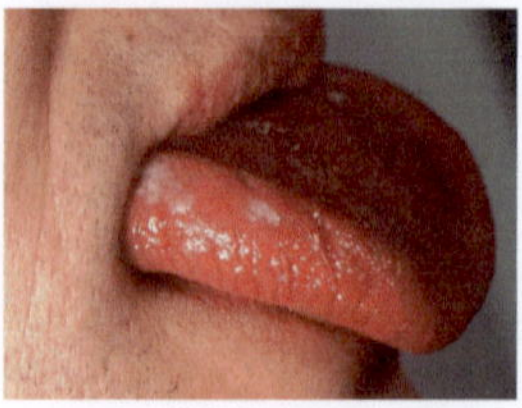

Fig. 10.44 Skin manifestations of HIV infection: hairy leukoplakia

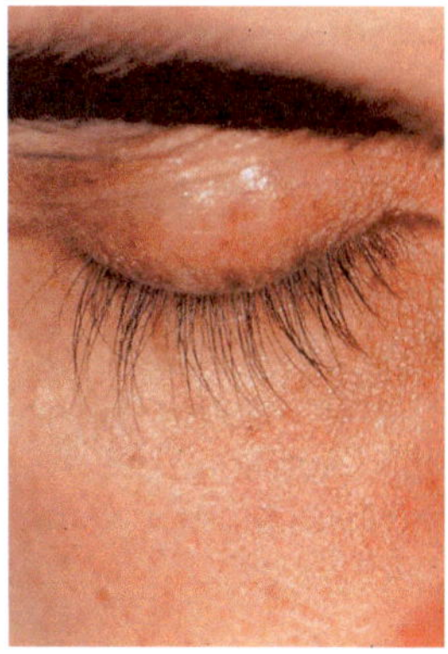

Fig. 10.45 Skin manifestations of HIV infection: elongation of eyelashes

zoster (shingles), syphilis (primary chancre), ulcerative candida-infections, streptococci, and weeping irritant and allergic contact dermatitis. In travel-related cases, chancroid (ulcus molle) and granuloma inguinale.

Prevention and Therapy

Barrier contraception may prevent the transmission of the infection.

Systemic anti-viral medicaments shorten symptomatic period and may decrease pain and itching caused by the infection. Antivirals should be started early when symptoms occur. Patients with frequent recurrences and high disease burden may profit from repeated courses or continuous antiviral medication.

Primary infection (course duration 3–10 days): acyclovir 400 mg t.i.d. or 200 mg q5h; valaciclovir 500 mg b.i.d.; famciclovir 250 mg t.i.d.

Recurrences (course duration 5 days): aciclovir 400 mg t.i.d. or 200 mg q5h; valaciclovir 500 mg b.i.d.; famciclovir 125 mg b.i.d.

Immunosuppressed patients may require initial administration of aciclovir intravenously 10 mg/kg body weight t.i.d.

Sexual activity should not take place until all lesions have healed.

Skin Manifestations of HIV Infection [4]

Figures 10.36, 10.37, 10.38, 10.39, 10.40, 10.41, 10.42, 10.43, 10.44 and 10.45

Grading of Importance

C

Level

Advanced

Definition

Human immune deficiency virus (HIV)—infected patients have significantly more skin problems than the general population. Some of the skin manifestations may have an indicator character and should awake the need for prompt HIV-testing.

ICD-11

EL3Y

Aetiology and Pathogenesis

HIV infection is transmitted by sex, contaminated needles or blood products, and across the placenta from infected mothers to the infants. HIV causes a lifelong infection, slowly destroying the body's immune defences and ending in the acquired immune deficiency syndrome (AIDS). Along the decrease of CD4 cells and immune response deterioration, numerous skin and mucous membrane symptoms develop, such as infections, dermatoses, malignancies, and drug eruptions.

Signs and Symptoms

Primary infection of the HIV virus can cause acute flu-like symptoms with a generalised transient maculopapular exanthematous skin eruption affecting face, throat, trunk, and proximal limbs. The other symptoms include fever, fatigue, sore throat with occasional apthae, and sometimes also diarrhoea but no respiratory infection symptoms. The primary infection can also be asymptomatic; usually the acute infection ends with clinical recovery in 2–4 weeks. Chronic HIV infection is a period of clinical latency. This stage can last for years or even decades. During this time, a multitude of skin problems (e.g. infections, dermatoses, skin cancer/Kaposi sarcoma) often develop. There is not any specific skin symptom. Skin manifestations have a tendency to recur and may show an atypical or more severe course.

Secondary symptoms in HIV may be viral, bacterial, and parasitic infections and may have a clinical different pattern to the usual course (herpes zoster, molluscum contagiosum, HPV condyloma, hairy leukoplakia, chronic pruritus, seborrhoeic dermatitis).

Most important is to consider a possible HIV infection in patients with skin problems that follow uncommon or severe disease courses or are recurrent and refractory to standard therapy.

Localisation

Anywhere on the skin, localised or disseminated, oral cavity, anogenital region.

Classification

Acute and chronic phase of HIV infections (see above "Symptoms").

Laboratory and Other Workups

Diagnosis of the HIV-infection with HIV antigen/antibody test and confirmation with Western blot. The HIV AgAb test becomes positive earliest at 2 weeks and latest at 3 months after infection. A positive screening test always requires a second confirmatory test. In new-borns detection of the HIV-virus with nucleic acid quantitation (viral copies/ml). Pregnant women should be routinely offered HIV testing and counselling, since infection of the foetus can be prevented with ART during pregnancy.

Dermatopathology

Depends on the stage of the disease and the type of associated disease. Lymphomas or Cerebrovascular accident (CVA).

Course

Unlike the sporadic forms of the listed skin problems, in HIV-infected patients they may be refractory to standard therapy and may follow an untypical and more severe course. HIV-associated psoriasis and Kaposi's sarcoma usually respond rapidly to antiretroviral therapy.

Course of the HIV Infection

Acute retroviral syndrome (primary HIV infection)/WHO stage 1

During the acute symptoms, HIV viral load (viremia) is very high in the body and the infected person is highly infectious. HIV-antibody test usually turns positive

2–4 weeks after the onset of symptoms while a combined antibody-antigen test (HIVAgAb) becomes positive already 2–4 weeks after the transmission of HIV infection; in rare cases it may take up to 3 months for the antibodies to turn positive. In newborns, HIV-infection can be confirmed by PCR-based quantitation of HIV RNA.

Chronic HIV-infection (clinical latency))/WHO stages 2–3

The severity of the skin problems often progresses corresponding to the immunosuppression. The total amount CD4-positive T-lymphocytes in the blood is used as a marker of the severity of the immunosuppression (normally over 0,4 E9/l).

AIDS stage (WHO stage 4)

In this advanced stage, the CD4 cell count has dropped below 0.2 E9/l, HIV viral load is high, and the person is highly infectious. Typically Kaposi's sarcoma, caused by HHV-8, occurs in this stage.

AIDS-defining skin conditions include Kaposi's sarcoma, caused by HHV-8.

Complications

Complications of an early infectious stage: none.

In the latency stage depends on the type of infectious agents or dermatoses; causative agents may become resistant to standard therapy regimens. Severe drug reactions due to HIV drugs may occur.

Diagnosis

Primary infection of HIV exanthema. Latency stage with different associated skin diseases (see above).

HIV-specific skin manifestations are usually suspected based on clinical features; laboratory, microbiological (skin infections), and histopathological tests (dermatoses, malignancies) are necessary for confirmation. The viral load (virus copies/ml) and degree of immunosuppression (CD4-cell count) should be determined; screening tests for other STIs should be carried out.

Differential Diagnosis

In particular the early HIV exanthema is difficult to differentiate. The amount of differential diagnoses in the latency stage of HIV infection depends on the type of skin symptom.

Prevention and Therapy

Avoidance of skin associated symptoms is depending on prevention programs of HIV infection.

Early initiation of antiretroviral therapy (ART) enables people living with HIV to stay alive and reduces the risk of transmitting the virus to partners. WHO guidelines recommend ART is to be started for all patients diagnosed with HIV, irrespective of their CD4 cell count. Today, about 30 different anti-retroviral drugs are available. The treatment is lifelong. Management of antiretroviral medication is usually carried out by an HIV specialist.

Skin infections might require more effective (e.g. intravenous) and longer antibiotic, antiviral, and antifungal therapies; (e.g. infections due to *Candida albicans*, herpes simplex). Similarly, dermatoses in HIV-infected patients often require a longer and more efficient therapy to achieve remission.

Special

It is important that the patients with unclear skin lesions are referred to dermatologists and specialist centres.

References

1. Bagnall P, Rizzolo D (2017) Bacterial vaginosis: a practical review. JAAPA 30(12):15–21
2. Basta-Juzbasic A, Ceovic R (2014) Chancroid, lymphogranuloma venereum, granuloma inguinale, genital herpes simplex infection, and molluscum contagiosum. Clin Dermatol 32(2):290–298
3. Çakmak S, Tamer E, Karadağ A, Waugh M (2019) Syphilis: a great imitator. Clin Dermatol 37:182–191
4. Chelidze K, Thomas C, Chang AY, Freeman EE (2019) HIV-related skin disease in the era of antiretroviral therapy: recognition and management. Am J Clin Dermatol 20(3):423–442
5. Crofts M, Horner P (2015) Chlamydia (uncomplicated, genital). BMJ Clin Evid 2015:1607
6. Galadari I, Galadari H (2004) Nonspecific urethritis and reactive arthritis. Clin Dermatol 22(6):469–475
7. Gnann JW Jr, Whitley RJ (2016) CLINICAL PRACTICE. Genital Herpes. N Engl J Med 375(7):666–674
8. Irizarry L, Velasquez J, Wray AA (2020) Chancroid. StatPearls, Treasure Island, FL
9. Kairys N, Garg M (2020) Bacterial vaginosis. StatPearls, Treasure Island, FL
10. Kaufman RE, Wiesner PJ (1974) Nonspecific urethritis. N Engl J Med 291(22):1175–1177
11. Mohseni M, Sung S, Takov V (2020) Chlamydia. StatPearls, Treasure Island, FL
12. Peeling RW, Mabey D, Kamb ML, Chen XS, Radolf JD, Benzaken AS (2017) Syphilis. Nat Rev Dis Primers 3:17073
13. Rawla P, Thandra KC, Limaiem F (2020) Lymphogranuloma Venereum. StatPearls, Treasure Island, FL
14. Schumann JA, Plasner S (2020) Trichomoniasis. StatPearls, Treasure Island, FL
15. Schwebke JR, Burgess D (2004) Trichomoniasis. Clin Microbiol Rev 17(4):794–803. table of contents
16. Unemo M, Seifert HS, Hook EW 3rd, Hawkes S, Ndowa F, Dillon JR (2019) Gonorrhoea. Nat Rev Dis Primers 5(1):79

Part III

Nevi, Tumours and Cysts

This part includes various types of skin changes, exhibiting an increase of tissue either due to permanent "structural flaws" of the nature (nevi) or due to benign or malignant proliferations of tissues.

Naevi

11

Martine Bagot, Zrinka Bukvić Mokos,
Veronique del Marmol, Adele De Masson, Gabor Dobos,
Giampiero Girolomoni, Paolo Gisondi, Branka Marinović,
Martina Maurelli, and Jonathan M. White

Contents

M. Bagot (✉)
Service de Dermatologie, Université Paris Cité, Hôpital Saint-Louis, Paris, France
e-mail: martine.bagot@gmail.com

Z. Bukvić Mokos · B. Marinović
Department of Dermatology and Venereology, School of Medicine University of Zagreb, Zagreb, Croatia
e-mail: branka.marinovic@kbc-zagreb.hr

V. del Marmol
Département of Dermatology, Hôpital Erasme-HUB, Université Libre de Bruxelles, Brussels, Belgium
e-mail: veronique.delmarmol@hubruxelles.be

A. De Masson · G. Dobos
Dermatology and Venereology, Université de Paris, Hopital Saint Louis, Paris, France
e-mail: adele.demasson@aphp.fr; gabor.dobos@charite.de

G. Girolomoni · P. Gisondi · M. Maurelli
Department of Medicine, Università degli Studi di Verona, Verona, Italy
e-mail: giampiero.girolomoni@univr.it; paolo.gisondi@univr.it

J. M. White
Ecole de Santé Publique, Université libre de Bruxelles, Brussels, Belgium
e-mail: Jonathan.White@ulb.be

H. Gollnick et al. (eds.), *Dermatology Cyberderm WebBook*,
https://doi.org/10.1007/978-3-031-78491-0_11

Test your learning and check your understanding of this book's contents: use the "Springer Nature Flashcards" app to access questions using ▶ https://sn.pub/1rhh6k.
To use the app, please follow the instructions in Chap. 1.

Melanocytic Nevus [1]

Figures 11.1, 11.2, 11.3, 11.4, 11.5 and 11.6

Grading of Importance

B

Level

Advanced

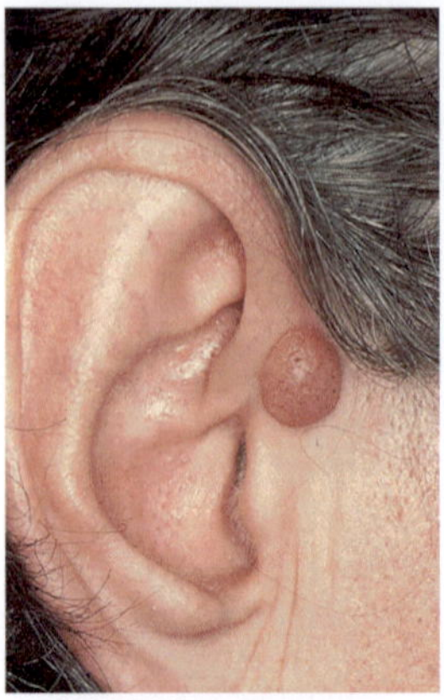

Fig. 11.1 Melanocytic nevus: non pigmented dome shaped dermal nevus at the ear

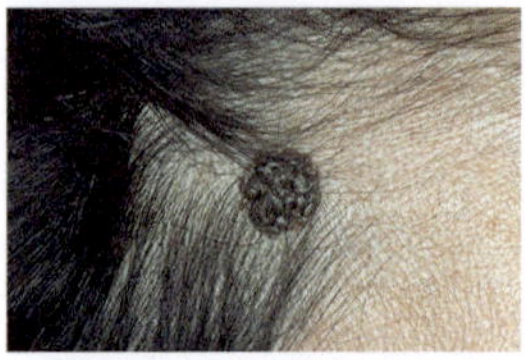

Fig. 11.2 Melanocytic nevus: pigmented morula-like dermal nevus

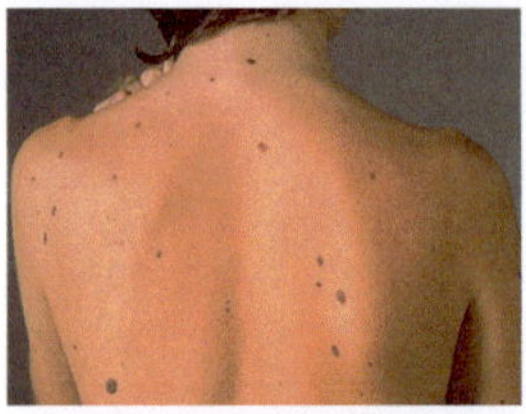

Fig. 11.3 Melanocytic nevus: multiple nevi on the back

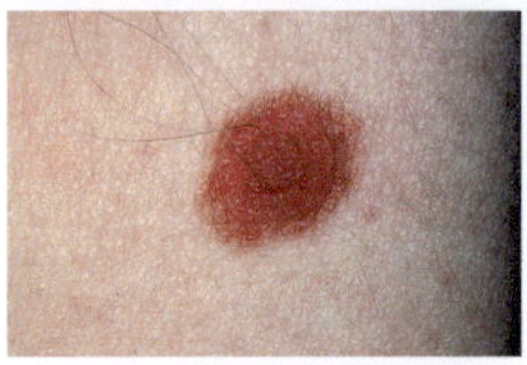

Fig. 11.4 Melanocytic nevus: junctional nevus

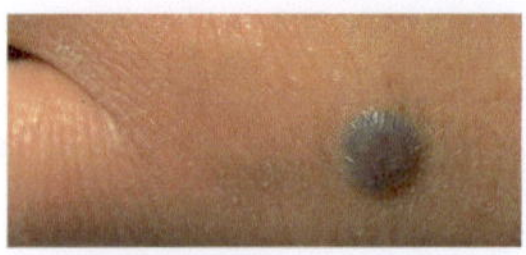

Fig. 11.5 Melanocytic nevus: blue nevus

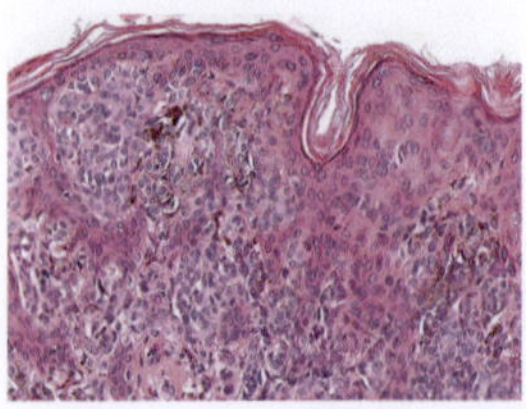

Fig. 11.6 Melanocytic nevus: histology of blue nevus

ICD-11

2F20.Z

Synonyms

Mole, sometimes just called "nevus".

Epidemiology

Melanocytic naevi are very common (even ubiquitous, even in African populations) and may be present at birth. The number of melanocytic naevi increases with age until the age of around 30 years, but there may be involution over time as well. A new melanocytic lesion appearing after the age of 30 years should raise clinical suspicion for malignant melanoma.

Definition

Acquired benign neoplasms of melanocytic lineage are termed melanocytic nevi (the plural of nevus). They are collections of melanocytes (naevus cells) in the epidermis, dermis or both.

Aetiology and Pathogenesis

Acquired melanocytic nevi express a high diversity of clinical appearance and histomorphology, age of onset mostly during first two decades of life, anatomic site and genetic alterations. Melanocytes arise from the neural crest and migrate to the skin during embryogenesis. Most melanocytic naevi appear during the first two decades of life. Increased exposure to UV light in childhood seems to be a promoting factor, particularly episodes of sunburn. Melanocytic nevi tend to disappear with aging.

Signs and Symptoms

These skin-coloured or mostly pigmented macular, papular or nodular lesions are usually asymptomatic, but can occasionally be itchy or uncomfortable if irritated. They should be symmetrical, with a smooth outline, homogeneous, with a regular border, of small diameter (<6 mm) and stable over time (see ABCDE rules/"ugly duck" concept in section "Malignant Melanoma" in Chap. 13; for atypical melanocytic nevus, see section "Atypical Melanocytic Naevus and Syndrome").

Localisation

Melanocytic nevi may occur anywhere on the body, sometimes on the oral and genital mucosa or in the sclera or retina of the eye.

Classification

Variants of common acquired nevus cell nevus:
- Junctional nevus
- Dermal nevus
- Compound nevus (combination of both)

  More structural and clinical variants:
- Blue nevus
- Combined nevus (acquired plus blue nevus)
- Mongolian spot
- Congenital (hairy) nevus
- Halo naevus
- Spindle and epithelioid cell nevus

Laboratory and Other Workups

No laboratory tests are needed. Dermatoscopy (see section "Dermscopy").

Dermatopathology

Proliferation of melanocytes, single or in nests, epidermal (junctional nevus), dermal (dermal nevus) or at both levels (compound nevus). Melanocytic naevi with histological signs of atypia are referred to as dysplastic naevi (see separate section "Atypical Melanocytic Naevus and Syndrome").

Course

Progression towards atypical melanocytic nevi possible, for melanoma, is exceptional (except in cases of giant congenital nevus, see section "Congenital Melanocytic Nevus"), but patients with more than 100 nevi are at higher risk of developing a melanoma. Multiple enlarged acquired nevi have increased melanoma risk.

Complications

The number of melanocytic naevi (>50), along with skin type and history (severe sunburns in childhood), is the most important risk factors for melanoma. Irritated or excoriated naevi are sometimes mistaken for cancer.

Diagnosis

ABCDE rules/"ugly duck"/ "mole out of context" concept may help distinguish benign from malignant lesions (see section "Malignant Melanoma" in Chap. 13). Clinical features, dermatoscopy (see section "Dermscopy", where images are magnified x10), histology.

Differential Diagnosis

Other pigmented, usually acquired skin lesions including seborrheic keratosis, pigmented basal cell carcinoma; less often dermatofibroma, haemangioma. Different subtypes of early melanomas.

Prevention and Therapy

Excision if there is aesthetic discomfort, irritated nevi by trauma or localization or in case of atypical nevi or suspicious melanoma.

Excision if there is an irritated nevus by trauma or localization with constant irritation. Usually observation/abstention (using the ABCDE rules to guide decision; see section "Malignant Melanoma" in Chap. 13) if there is diagnostic doubt or functional problems. Digital images in the clinical record may be helpful to facilitate accurate long-term follow-up. Visible change in the digital record within 3 months of follow-up is an absolute indication for excision.

Congenital Melanocytic Nevus [1, 4]

Figures 11.7, 11.8 and 11.9

Grading of Importance

B

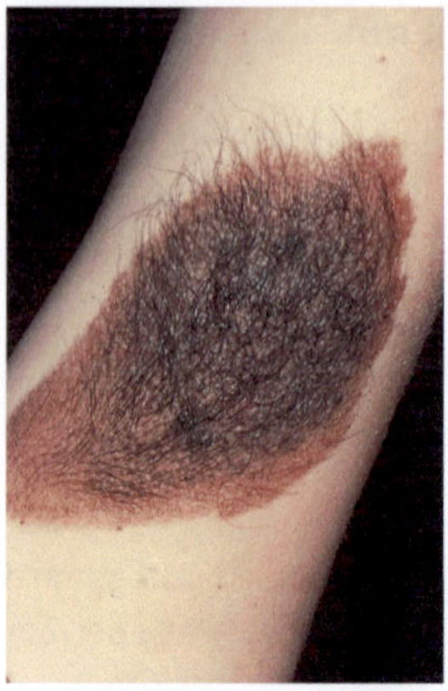

Fig. 11.7 Congenital melanocytic nevus: medium sized nevus pigmentosus et pilosus

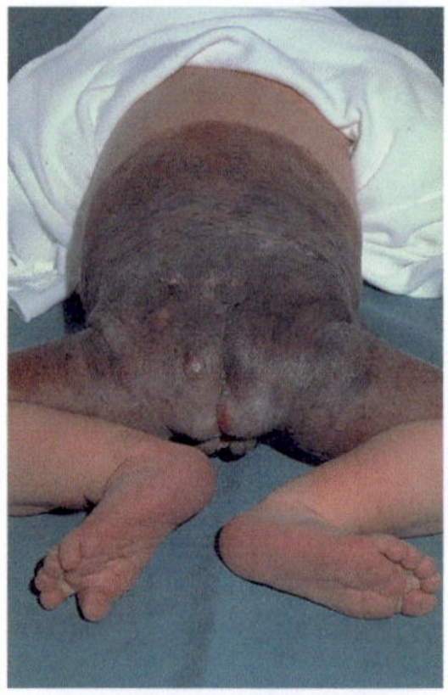

Fig. 11.8 Congenital melanocytic nevus: large giant (bathing trunk) naevus

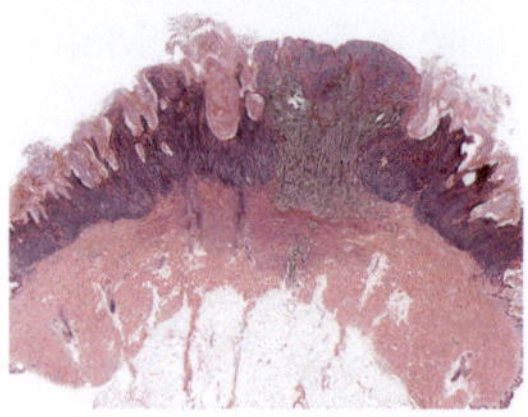

Fig. 11.9 Congenital melanocytic nevus: histology of congenital nevus

Level

Advanced

ICD-11

2F20.2

Synonyms

Pigmented birth mark.

Epidemiology

The incidence is 0.2–2.1% in newborns. The incidence in large/giant congenital nevi is 0.005%. M:F = 1:1.17–1:1.4.

Definition

Collection of pigmented melanocytes in epidermis and dermis, usually present at birth, often associated with increased numbers of hair follicles.

Aetiology and Pathogenesis

Embryonal acquired mutation in the tyrosine kinase NRAS (neuroblastoma RAS) in cells of the neural crest. Rarely, lesions may appear up to 2 years after birth. They are not different from congenital nevi, but sometimes are called tardive congenital nevi.

Signs and Symptoms

Circumscribed brown to black nodules or plaques, often with hypertrichosis. At the very early beginning after birth, it may be even a macular lesion which then increase in volume and size.

Localisation

Trunk, head, as well as extremities.

Classification

Estimated size of nevus at birth expected to reach in adulthood:

Type I. Size 1–3 cm: common and harmless, 1:100

Type II. Size 3–20 cm: uncommon, 1:1000–1:20000, rarely malignant change

Type III. Size >20 cm: usually on the trunk (giant or bathing trunk naevus) 1:500000, risk of melanoma 3–5%

Laboratory and Other Workups

Measurement of thickness by ultrasound could be useful.

Dermatopathology

Accumulation of melanocytes at the epidermal-dermal junction and in the dermis, often extending deeply, into the lower reticular dermis, subcutaneous fat and fascia and even deeper.

Course

Permanent, life-long. No tendency to regression.

Complications

In giant naevi, risk of leptomeningeal melanosis. Lumbosacral: spina bifida, myelomeningocele. Increased risk of neurological disorders expected in giant nevi (> 40 cm) or those reaching this size in adulthood. In patients with congenital nevi Type III, the mean age at diagnosis of developing melanoma is around 15 to 16 years.

Diagnosis

Clinical features, histology.

Differential Diagnosis

Haemangioma, dermatofibroma, melanoma, melanocytic nevi, *plexiform neurofibromas*; see also section "Nevus Sebaceus".

Prevention and Therapy

Type II and Type III congenital nevi should have an annual follow-up or whenever parents see significant changes.

Small lesions: excision if desired for cosmetical reasons.

Medium-sized lesions: consider excision after puberty.

Large lesions: dermabrasion shortly after birth (does not influence leptomeningeal melanosis), close clinical follow-up and excision of suspicious areas.

Atypical Melanocytic Naevus and Syndrome [6]

Grading of Importance

B

Level

Basic

ICD-11

2F20.1

Synonyms

Atypical navus; atypical mole syndrome; dysplastic naevus syndrome; familial atypical multiple mole melanoma (FAMMM) syndrome.

Epidemiology

Approximately 5–10% of Caucasian populations show atypical melanocytic naevi, with likely lower rates in populations with darker skin types. Increasing numbers of atypical melanocytic naevi increase the risk of developing malignant melanoma.

Atypical melanocytic naevus syndrome is much rarer: only around 5–12% of melanomas are considered to have an inherited component. In the familial atypical nevus type, one or more first-degree or second-degree relatives diagnosed with malignant melanoma are at a young age (< 40 years). They show a large number of naevi (often more than 50), some of which are atypical.

Definition

Atypical melanocytic naevi are pigmented lesions similar to ordinary melanocytic naevi but they:

- Usually measure more than 0.6 cm
- Have irregular or poorly defined borders
- Irregular pigmentation within the lesion
- Possibly irregular texture

There are sporadic and family associated subtypes. They can also arise over the second to third decade of life. On examination this is referred to as a clinically atypical naevus; however, when the abnormalities are microscopically confirmed, the term dysplastic is used (see ABCDE rules in the melanoma, section "Malignant Melanoma" in Chap. 13).

Atypical melanocytic naevus syndrome is where there are more than 50 pigmented lesions on the same individual. The lesion is confirmed to be dysplastic on histological analysis and there is a family history of confirmed melanoma in one or more first- or second-degree relative under the age of 40.

Aetiology and Pathogenesis

Various genetic mutations have been described reducing the efficacy of tumour-suppressor genes. These mutations may be magnified by repeated sunburn. The most important are primary oncogenic mutations such as BRAF and germline mutations *CDKN2A* (600160).

Signs and Symptoms

Apart from the appearance and potential changes in the appearance, atypical naevi are asymptomatic but occasionally may be itchy or bleed.

Localisation

Sun-exposed sites are the most commonly affected; however any body site may be affected.

Classification

- Sporadic
- Familial

Histological classification is by the subjective degree of change of dysplasis of melanocytes and amount of atypical cells: mild, moderate and severe.

Laboratory and Other Workups

Additional laboratory tests are not usually required unless a melanoma is diagnosed.

Dermatopathology

When the clinical abnormalities of an atypical nevus are microscopically confirmed, the term dysplastic is used.

Melanocytic cells may have a different appearance to typical melanocytes (unusually spindle-shaped, or broad) and they may be of an unusual size (small or large) or the cytoplasm shows dot-like pigment distribution. The cells may be arranged in an unusual pattern, such as with bridging between nests of melanocytes. An inflammatory infiltrate, fibrosis in the papillary dermis and increased vascularization may also be present.

Course

The course of atypical naevi is controversial, since the most unusual ones are almost always excised once noticed. Some clinically atypical naevi probably never become malignant, but some may also develop into melanoma. However, there are lesions which represent a genomic profile intermediate between a benign naevus and a melanoma, and their malignant potential is uncertain.

Complications

Malignant transformation to a melanoma may occur. As excision is essential for the diagnosis, scarring complications may occur after the procedure including hypertrophic or keloid scars, as well as functional impairment in large procedures.

Diagnosis

The diagnosis is clinical for an atypical melanocytic naevus. It follows the ABCD(E) rule (section "Malignant Melanoma" in Chap. 13). It is mandatory to obtain a complete excision with a 0.5 cm margin for histological analysis if a melanoma is clinically possible. Histological confirmation is necessary to be able to diagnose the atypical melanocytic naevus syndrome. See also section "Melanocytic Nevus".

Differential Diagnosis

The differential diagnosis includes seborrhoeic keratoses, benign melanocytic naevi, blue and combined nevi, pigmented basal cell carcinomas and melanomas.

Prevention and Therapy

Avoidance of sun burn is important; however with strict sun avoidance, vitamin D replacement therapy is advisable. Regular dermatological follow-up (including digital photography to track changes in individual lesions) is required for those with the atypical melanocytic naevus syndrome or numerous atypical naevi. The acute eruption of an atypical nevus is also an option for excision. Screening of relatives should be offered. Histological excision of doubtful clinical lesions and those with changes during follow-up to exclude development of a melanoma is essential. Consider genetic testing in appropriate individuals.

Special

Familial screening

Nevus Flammeus [5]

Figures 11.10, 11.11, 11.12 and 11.13

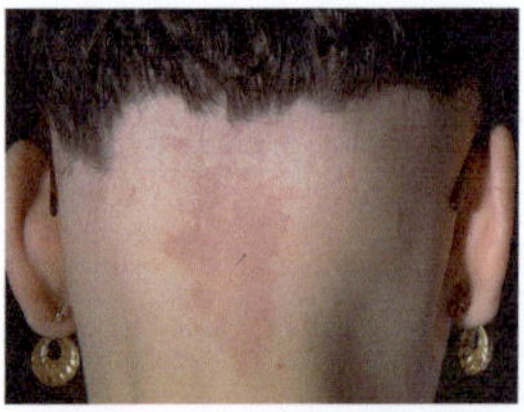

Fig. 11.10 Nevus flammeus: axial nevus flammeus of the neck (Unna's nevus)

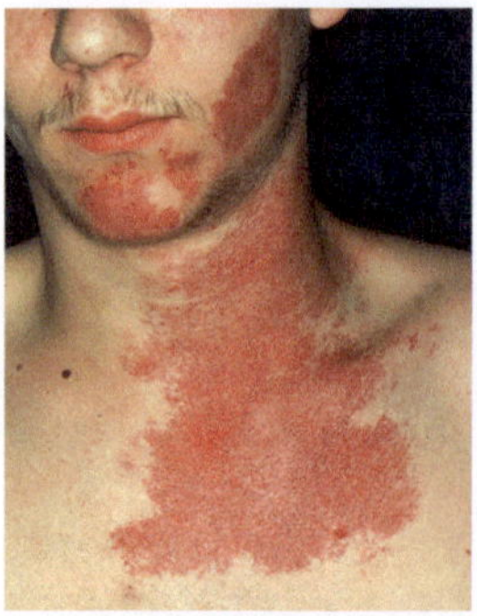

Fig. 11.11 Nevus flammeus: lateral nevus of cheek, chin and neck

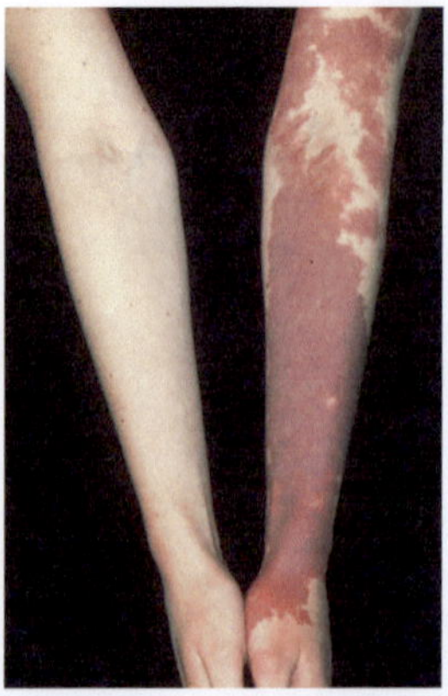

Fig. 11.12 Nevus flammeus: lateral nevus in Klippel-Trénaunay syndrome

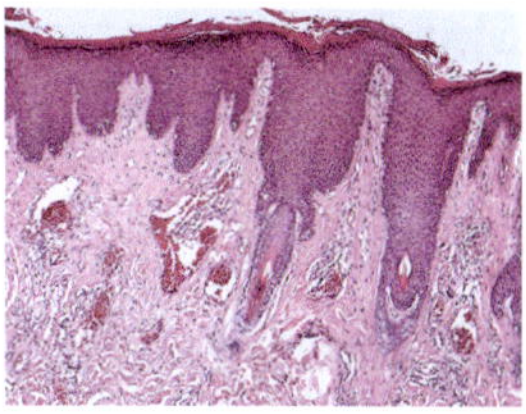

Fig. 11.13 Nevus flammeus: histology showing dilated vessels in the upper dermis

Grading of Importance

B

Level

Advanced

ICD-11

LC50.1

Synonyms

Nevus vinosus, portwine nevus, naevus teleangiectaticus.

Epidemiology

0.3–1% of the Population; F 2xM.

Definition

Benign vascular malformation since birth. Sharply demarcated red spots, due to dilatation and augmentation of small superficial vessels in the affected area.

Aetiology and Pathogenesis

Inherited. May be in the nosologic context of angiodysplasia syndromes (Sturge-Weber syndrome, von Hippel-Lindau syndrome, Klippel-Trénaunay/Parkes-Weber syndrome).

Signs and Symptoms

Sharply demarcated red spots and patches without augmentation of tissue.

Localisation

- Axial nevi flammei: (Unna-nevus; angel's kiss of the forehead; salmon patch); never associated with syndromatic angiodystrophy.
- Lateral nevi flammei, syndrome-associated quadrant nevus:
  - Trigeminus area: unilateral portwine nevus; potential association with meningeal or central nervous angiomas of eyes, meninges and brain (Sturge-Weber syndrome)
  - Extremities: possible association with venous malformation and increased growth of soft tissue and bones of the respective limb (Klippel-Trénaunay syndrome)

Classification

- True nevoid not self-regressing capillary malformations
- Temporary and regressing capillary malformation "salmon patches" (neck, forehead)

Laboratory and Other Workups

None. Ultrasound for the determination of depth.

Dermatopathology

Not needed. Dilated vessels in the dermis.

Course

In contrast to axial nevi, the lateral nevi do not regress spontaneously, but enlarge with body growth, change colour to deep red and can show tuberous transformation (i.e. macrocheilia) and pyogenic granuloma.

Complications

Exclude involvement of eye (glaucoma) in periorbital nevus flammeus. Additional complications may be found in conjunction with angiodysplastic syndromes (CNS-involvement; haemorrhage; thromboses; limb deformities).

Diagnosis

Typical clinical features.

Differential Diagnosis

Infantile haemangioma: red-blue vascular tumour (not nevus!), developing in the first week of life, grows proportionally and regresses spontaneously after months.

Prevention and Therapy

Laser, intense pulse light, cosmetic camouflage.

Ophthalmologic control for nevi covered by trigeminus I and II.

Nevus Sebaceus [2, 3]

Figure 11.14

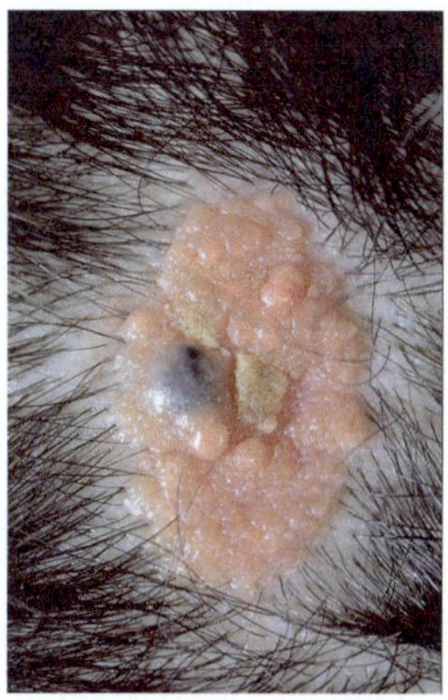

Fig. 11.14 Nevus sebaceus: yellowish bumpy plaque on the scalp, partly pigmented

Grading of Importance

C

Level

Basic

ICD-11

LC02

Synonyms

Naevus sebaceous of Jadassohn.

Epidemiology

Affects 0.3% of newborns. The prevalence is equal in males and females. Most frequent scalp lesion in newborns and childhood.

Definition

A congenital epidermal hamartoma that comprises sebaceous, follicular and apocrine elements.

Aetiology and Pathogenesis

Postzygotic somatic mutations of the Ras gene family, most commonly HRAS, less common KRAS.

Signs and Symptoms

At birth: a slightly raised, solitary plaque with a smooth, yellowish surface. Most commonly present on the scalp, hairloss at the site. At puberty, the lesion becomes thicker, and the surface is more verrucous. In adulthood, neoplasms (most commonly benign) may develop within the lesion.

Localisation

Most commonly scalp area (90%), but it may also appear on the face and neck and rarely on the trunk.

Classification

None. Association with syndromal constellation: Schimmelpenning-Feuerstein-Mims syndrome, didymosis aplasticosebacea.

Laboratory and Other Workups

Not necessary. Genetic counselling may be necessary in some cases.

Dermatopathology

In **infancy**: epidermal changes include acanthosis and papillomatosis; pilosebaceous units are immature.

At **puberty**: the epidermis becomes more hyperplastic, papillomatous and verrucous. Numerous sebaceous glands with an increased number of sebaceous lobules are found in the superficial dermis.

Course

See Symptoms.

Complications

In adulthood, secondary neoplasms may develop. The most common tumour within the naevus sebaceous is trichoblastoma, followed by syringocystadenoma papilliferum. Basal cell carcinoma develops in less than 1% of lesions.

Diagnosis

History; clinical features.

Differential Diagnosis

In early infancy: aplasia cutis congenita, mastocytoma. In later stages: epidermal nevus, congenital nevus, sebaceoma, seborrheic keratosis, verruca vulgaris, juvenile xanthogranuloma.

Prevention and Therapy

Observation, surgical excision (depending on the size and location of the tumour).

References

1. Burian EA, Jemec GBE (2019) Eruptive melanocytic nevi: a review. Am J Clin Dermatol 20(5):669–682
2. Eisen DB, Michael DJ (2009a) Sebaceous lesions and their associated syndromes: part I. J Am Acad Dermatol 61(4):549–560; quiz 561–542
3. Eisen DB, Michael DJ (2009b) Sebaceous lesions and their associated syndromes: part II. J Am Acad Dermatol 61(4):563–578; quiz 579–580
4. Schaffer JV (2015) Update on melanocytic nevi in children. Clin Dermatol 33(3):368–386
5. Slaughter K, Chen T, Williams E III (2016) Vascular lesions. Facial Plast Surg Clin N Am 24:559–571
6. Wiedemeyer K, Hartschuh W, Brenn T (2021) Dysplastic Nevi: morphology and molecular and the controversies in-between. Surg Pathol Clin. 14:341–357

Benign Tumors and Cysts

12

Günter Burg, Martine Bagot, Adele De Masson,
Gabor Dobos, Harald Gollnick, and Christos C. Zouboulis

Contents

G. Burg (✉)
Dermatology, Zurich, Switzerland
e-mail: g.burg@access.uzh.ch

M. Bagot
Service de Dermatologie, Université Paris Cité, Hôpital Saint-Louis, Paris, France
e-mail: martine.bagot@gmail.com

A. De Masson · G. Dobos
Dermatology and Venereology, Université de Paris, Hopital Saint Louis, Paris, France
e-mail: adele.demasson@aphp.fr; gabor.dobos@charite.de

H. Gollnick
Department of Dermatology & Venereology, Otto-von-Guericke University, Magdeburg, Germany
e-mail: Harald.Gollnick@med.ovgu.de

C. C. Zouboulis
Departments of Dermatology, Venereology, Allergology and Immunology, Staedtisches Klinikum Dessau, Brandenburg Medical School Theodor Fontane and Faculty of Health Sciences Brandenburg, Dessau, Germany
e-mail: christos.zouboulis@mhb-fontane.de

H. Gollnick et al. (eds.), *Dermatology Cyberderm WebBook*,
https://doi.org/10.1007/978-3-031-78491-0_12

Test your learning and check your understanding of this book's contents: use the "Springer Nature Flashcards" app to access questions using ▶ https://sn.pub/1rhh6k.
To use the app, please follow the instructions in Chap. 1.

Seborrheic Keratosis [3, 4]

Figures 12.1, 12.2, 12.3 and 12.4

Grading of Importance

B

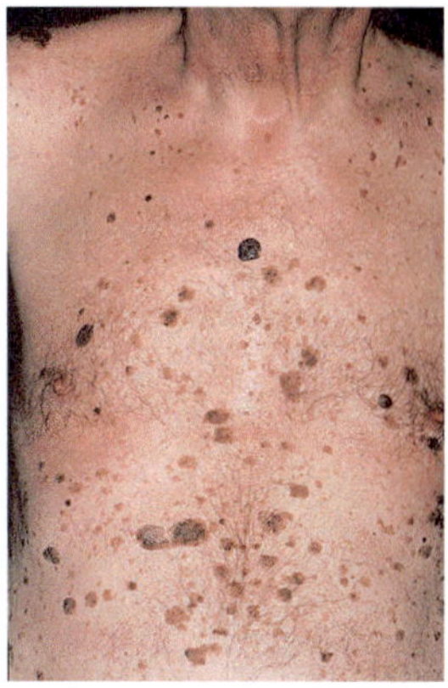

Fig. 12.1 Seborrheic keratosis: multiple seborrheic keratoses on the trunk

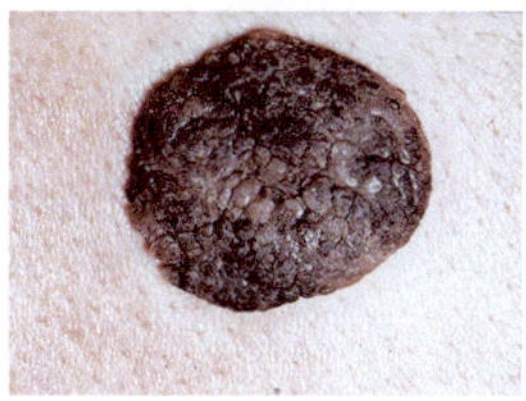

Fig. 12.2 Seborrheic keratosis: exophytic solitary seborrheic keratosis

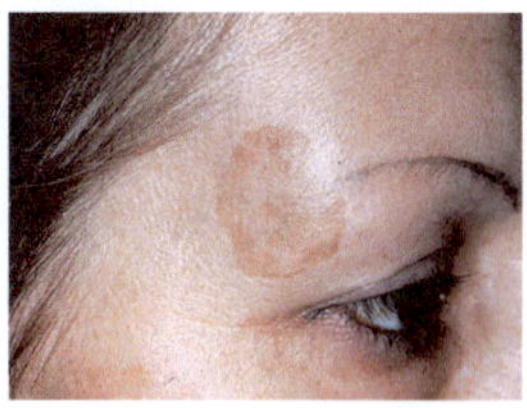

Fig. 12.3 Seborrheic keratosis: flat growing variant on the forehead

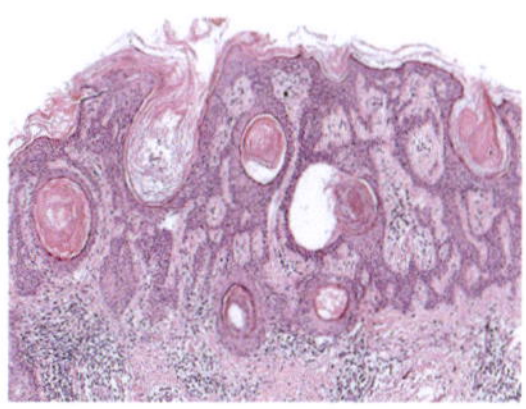

Fig. 12.4 Seborrheic keratosis: histology showing verruciform acanthosis and hyperkeratosis with horny pseudocysts filled with keratin

Level

Advanced

ICD-11

2F21.0

Synonyms

Seborrheic wart, basal cell papilloma.

Epidemiology

90% of older people >60 years. The seborrheic keratosis is the most frequent benign skin tumor.

Definition

The seborrheic keratosis is a benign verrucous epithelial tumor, commonly seen in patients over 50 years.

Etiology and Pathogenesis

The cause of seborrheic keratosis is not completely known. Stable and clonal mutations or activation of FRFR3, PIK3CA, RAS, AKT1 and EGFR genes are found in seborrheic keratoses.

Signs and Symptoms

It is a soft, wart-like (verrucous), keratotic yellowish to brown or black papule or plaque of the skin. The lesions can vary in size from a few millimeters to several centimeters. They are sometimes itchy.

Localization

Seborrheic keratoses can be localized on all areas of the body, most often on trunk and face. Dermatome-like pattern may occur.

Classification

Exophytic or flat subtypes. Stucco keratosis and black papular dermatitis (dermatosis papulosa nigra) are variants of seborrheic keratosis.

Laboratory and Other Workups

Laboratory tests are not needed for the diagnosis

Dermatopathology

Major criteria are acanthosis, hyperkeratosis, and horn pseudo-cysts, usually accompanied by epidermal hyperpigmentation.

Course

Seborrheic keratoses show slow growth and may reach several centimeters in size and become numerous. Leser-Trélat sign is the extremely rare explosive onset of multiple seborrheic keratoses in a segmental like pattern and may indicate an underlying internal solid tumor (paraneoplasia; see section "Paraneoplastic Disorders" in Chap. 13).

Complications

Seborrheic keratoses may sometimes become irritated, infected, or bleeding (trauma). Malignant transformation is extremely rare.

Diagnosis

Seborrheic keratoses can be identified by clinical features. Dermoscopy is helpful in visualizing the horn pearls. Histology is generally not necessary except melanoacanthoma type. Easily removable by curettage.

Differential Diagnosis

It is important to distinguish seborrheic keratoses from other new pigmented lesions (melanoma, pigmented basal cell carcinoma, melanocytic nevus, long-standing angioma).

Prevention and Therapy

Treatment of seborrheic keratosis is generally not needed except in severely symptomatic lesions or in specific localizations or disfiguring patterns. Treatment options include curettage, cryosurgery, laser ablation, and shave excision.

Keratoacanthoma [10]

Figures 12.5, 12.6, 12.7 and 12.8

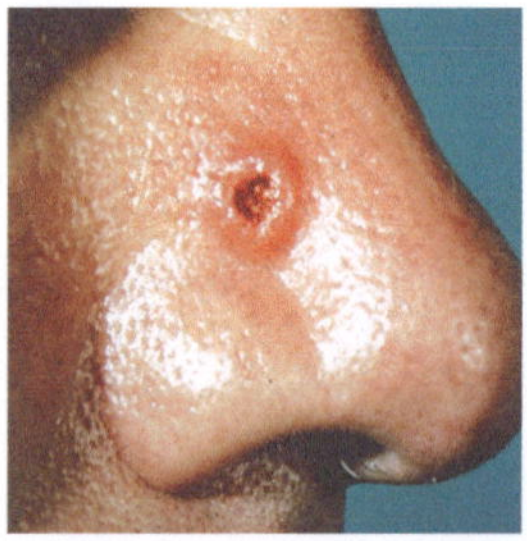

Fig. 12.5 Keratoacanthoma: nodule with central crater arising on normal skin

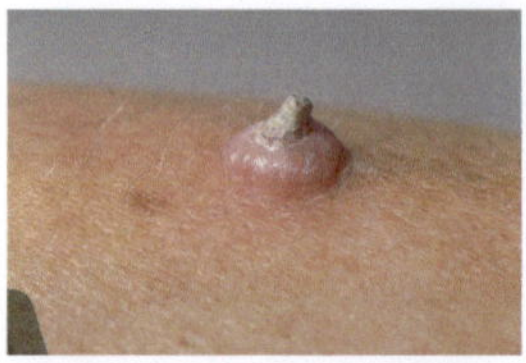

Fig. 12.6 Keratoacanthoma: cutaneous horn on keratoacanthoma

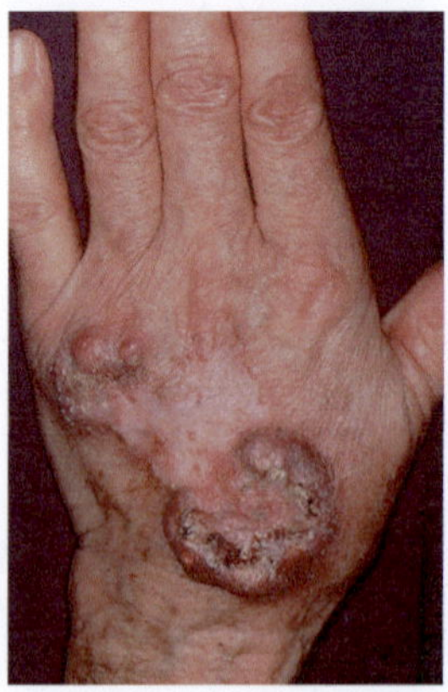

Fig. 12.7 Keratoacanthoma: variant KA centrifugum marginatum

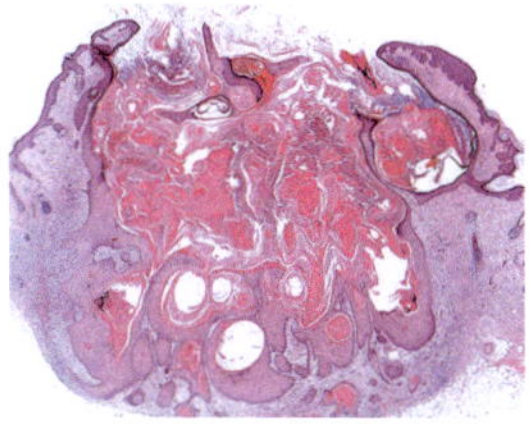

Fig. 12.8 Keratoacanthoma: histology showing crater filled with horn

Grading of Importance

B

Level

Basic

ICD-11

2C31.1

Synonyms

Pseudocarcinoma; verrucous carcinoma.

Epidemiology

Quite common tumor mostly affecting males with fair skin over 60 years. Smoking and solar damage are risk factors.

Definition

Keratoacanthoma (KA) is a clinically benign (no metastases) proliferation of highly differentiated squamous cells arising on normal skin. It belongs to the group of so-called pseudocarcinomas: papillomatosis carcinoides (carcinoma verrucosum), florid oral papillomatosis, genital condylomata gigantea (Buschke-Löwenstein), epithelioma (carcinoma) cuniculatum (L. Ackerman) of the foot, and papillomatosis cutis carcinoides (Gottron).

Etiology and Pathogenesis

Human papilloma virus (HPV types 16, 21, others) infection in 25% of cases. UV light may play a pathogenetic role. Transforming growth factor beta receptor 1 (TGFBR1) can cause multiple self-healing squamous cell carcinomas. In multiple familial and syndromatic cases, an autosomal-dominant inheritance is discussed. Proliferation of epithelial cells with strong keratinization.

Signs and Symptoms

Rapidly growing (weeks) dome-shaped solitary nodule, with a central crater filled with keratotic and necrotic material. Even though sun-exposed skin is preferentially involved, the underlying skin is normal (no scarring). Rare variants include flat and migratory lesions with elevated margins, aggregated or generalized forms. Association with other symptoms is seen in Muir-Torre syndrome.

Localization

Developing on normal skin, in contrast to malignant squamous cell carcinoma, which always develops on predamaged skin (scars). Head and neck most common sites, followed by extremities. Rarely the oral cavity is affected.

Classification

This includes other pseudocarcinomas

- Solitary keratoacanthoma (most frequent type)
- KA centrifugum marginatum
- Multiple generalized or aggregated keratoacanthomas (Ferguson-Smith; Grzybowski)
- Syndromic keratoacanthomas (Muir-Torre syndrome)
- Papillomatosis cutis carcinoides (Gottron)
- Giant keratoacanthomas (Buschke-Löwenstein)
- Intraoral and mucosal keratoacanthoma

Laboratory and Other Workups

Biopsy.

Dermatopathology

Revealing of the typical features only in full size biopsies or excisions: symmetrical cup-shaped tumor, filled with cornified debris and with smooth outer margins; central keratotic plug with massive acanthosis and papillomatosis; bilateral epithelial lip formation of adjacent rete ridges; proliferation of atypical keratinocytes and mitoses; intraepidermal formation of microabscesses, filled with mixed inflammatory cells and debris; mixed cellular infiltrate in the dermis. Necrotic masses in regressing lesions.

Course

Developing within a few weeks, in contrast to malignant squamous cell carcinoma, which develops over months. Clinically benign with tendency for spontaneous regression; no metastasis.

Complications

Scarring. Misdiagnosis of fast growing malignant squamous cell carcinoma.

Diagnosis

Diagnosis relies on clinical features and histology.

Differential Diagnosis

Squamous cell carcinoma, nodular basal cell carcinoma, verruca vulgaris, prurigo nodularis, and hypertrophic lichen planus in disseminated types of KA, tumors of skin appendages.

Prevention and Therapy

Wait and see. Biopsy often leads to spontaneous regression. Intralesional injection of glucocorticosteroids (leads to apoptosis of cells) or methotrexate. If still growing removal by surgical excision.

Special

Radiotherapy is ineffective because of the high cellular differentiation and even may induce malignant transformation.

Dermatofibroma [13, 14]

Figures 12.9 and 12.10

Grading of Importance

B

Level

Advanced

ICD-11

2F23.0

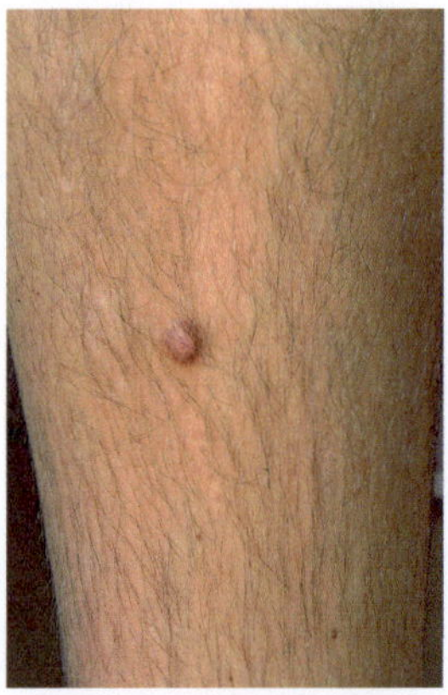

Fig. 12.9 Dermatofibroma: firm nodule on the leg

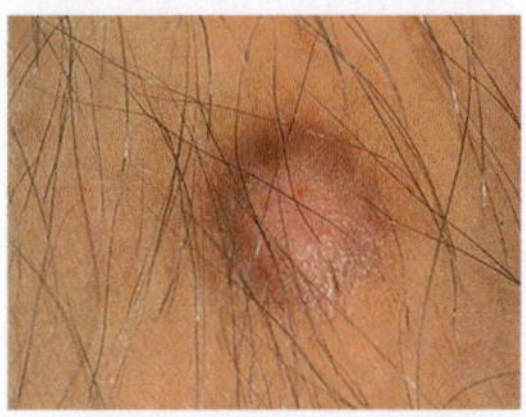

Fig. 12.10 Dermatofibroma: closeup view, showing hyperpigmented ring

Synonyms

Fibrous histiocytoma; histiocytoma, histiocytofibroma. Benign fibrous histiocytoma.

Epidemiology

Dermatofibroma is one of the most common skin tumor-like lesions.

Definition

Frequent, benign fibrohistiocytic dermal tumor.

Etiology and Pathogenesis

The etiology of dermatofibromas is not known; they sometimes occur after cutaneous trauma including persisting stings.

Signs and Symptoms

Solitary or multiple brownish, lentil-shaped, firm sometimes itchy papules or small nodules.

Localization

Dermatofibromas can occur on the whole body except palms and soles.

Classification

The histopathological types include cell-rich fibrous histiocytoma (80%) and other types: hemosiderotic, epithelioid, cellular, lipidized, atrophic and clear cell variants.

Laboratory and Other Workups

None.

Dermatopathology

Fibrous histiocytomas are benign dermal fibrohistiocytic tumors, made up of a mixture of fibroblastic and histiocytic cells, collagen, and blood vessels. Variable hemosiderin, chronic inflammatory cells may be found at the margin of the lesion.

Course

Dermatofibromas have a chronic course and may remain unchanged or flatten with time.

Complications

Usually none.

Diagnosis

Clinical feature; histology is rarely needed.

Differential Diagnosis

Basal cell carcinoma, melanocytic nevus, old regressing congenital nevi, melanoma, scars, and hemangioma. Large dermatofibromas must be differentiated from dermatofibrosarcoma protuberans, a rare infiltrating soft tissue sarcoma.

Prevention and Therapy

Abstention, surgical excision, cryosurgery, or laser ablation.

Keloid [12]

Figures 12.11, 12.12, 12.13, 12.14, and 12.15

Grading of Importance

C

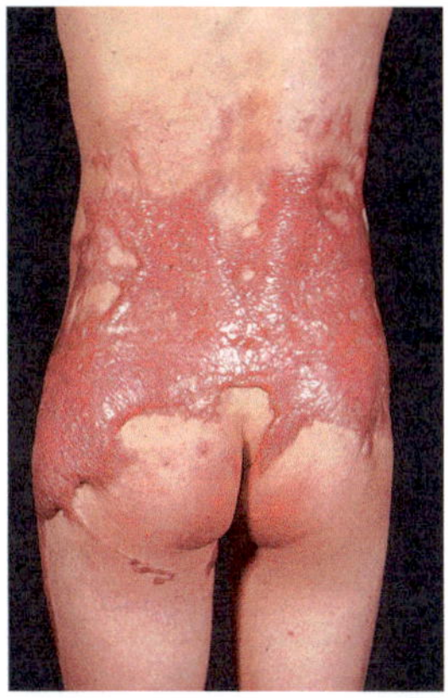

Fig. 12.11 Keloid: extensive keloid following scald-injury in childhood

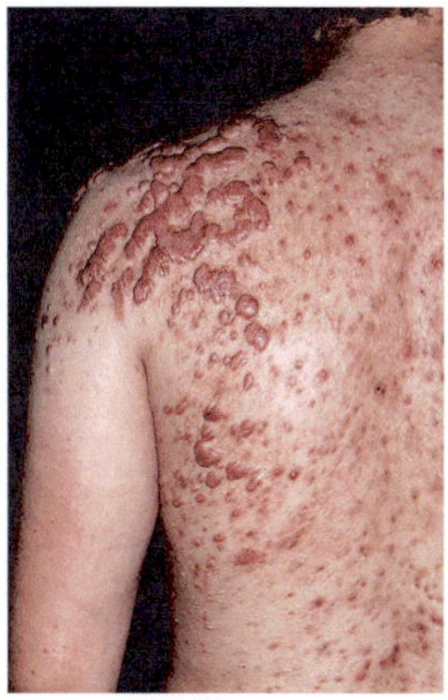

Fig. 12.12 Keloid: following acne conglobata

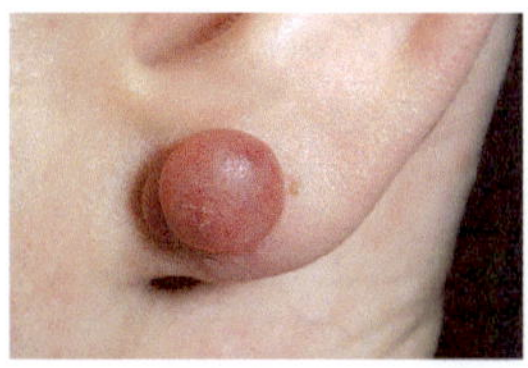

Fig. 12.13 Keloid: after ear piercing

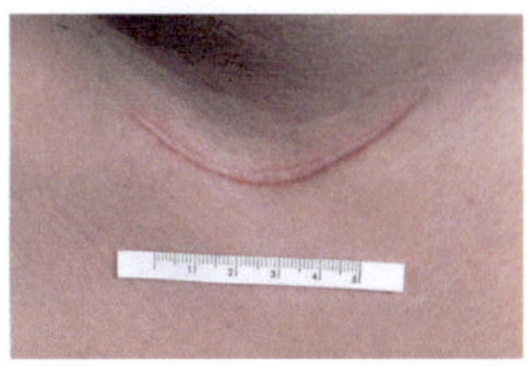

Fig. 12.14 Keloid: after operation of thyroid

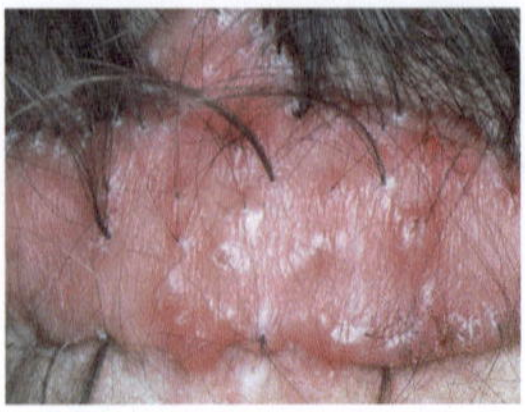

Fig. 12.15 Keloid: acne keloidalis nuchae

Level

Advanced

ICD-11

EE60

Synonyms

Cheloid, cicatrix keloidalis.

Epidemiology

Higher incidence in dark-pigmented populations, during puberty and pregnancy and in positive family history.

Definition

Benign scar tissue which grows beyond the borders of the original injury or surgical defect.

Etiology and Pathogenesis

Aberrant wound healing of surgical wounds, injuries (piercings, tattooing, scarification, insect bites, vaccinations), burns, skin-damaging infections, acne, increased skin tension, spontaneous (no trigger found). Overproduction of collagen I and III (20x greater than that of healthy skin and 3x greater than a hypertrophic scar).

Signs and Symptoms

Bizarre sharply bordered nodular proliferation of connective tissue with erythema, pruritus, and sometimes pain. Keloid extends beyond original defect.

Localization

Predilection sites: presternal, neck, shoulders, tense wounds, and joints.

Classification

No international classification exists, clinically: suppurative keloid, presternal keloid, juxta-articular keloid, folliculitis keloidalis nuchae.

Dermatopathology

Increased whorls of thickened, hyalinized collagen bundles of the dermis.

Course

Keloids may develop 1 to 12 months after injury. Do not improve with time and do not heal spontaneously.

Complications

Contractures over joints hamper motion, chronic itching/pain.

Diagnosis

History, clinical features.

Differential Diagnosis

Hypertrophic scar (remains confined to area of surgery or damage), sarcoidosis, dermatofibroma, and dermatofibrosarcoma.

Prevention and Therapy

Prevention is essential, cosmetic and elective surgical procedures should be performed considering the development of keloids. Rapid primary closure, adequate hemostasis, reduction of wound tension, and compression therapy may reduce keloid development.

Intralesional corticosteroids mostly in combination with contact cryosurgery, intralesional cryosurgery, surgical excision with post-surgical radiation or intralesional steroids, radiotherapy, and LASER treatment can be considered. Topical imiquimod, intralesional botulinum toxin, intralesional bleomycin or 5-fluorouracil, and silicone gel tapes.

Lipoma [9]

Figures 12.16 and 12.17

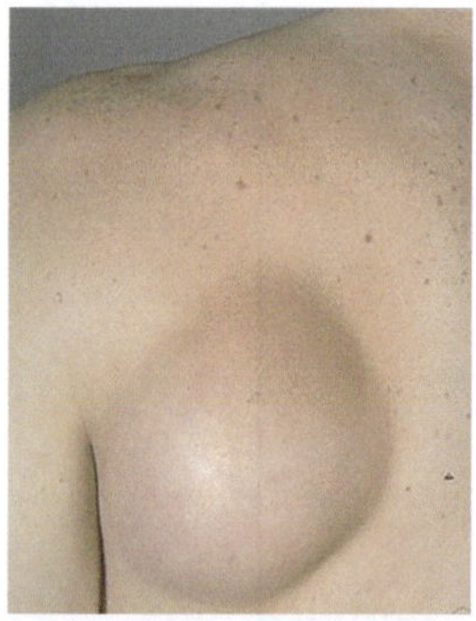

Fig. 12.16 Lipoma: solitary lesion

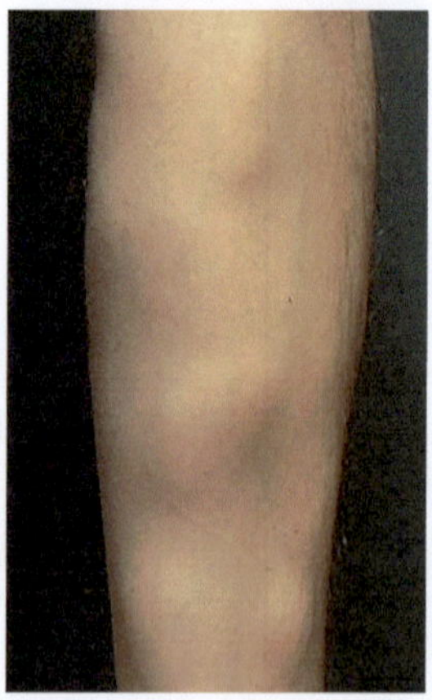

Fig. 12.17 Lipoma: lipomatosis (arm)

Grading of Importance

B

Level

Advanced

ICD-11

2E80.0

Synonyms

Fatty tumor or steatoma.

Epidemiology

Relatively frequent tumor. Lipomas occur in 1–2% of the adult population. Males > females.

Definition

Adipocytic tumors are benign soft tumors of the skin, arising from the subcutaneous fat tissue.

Etiology and Pathogenesis

Most frequently spontaneous but there may be a genetic predisposition (see subtypes).

Signs and Symptoms

Rubbery feeling, indolent (slowly growing), soft, mobile, circumscribed, round, and subcutaneous mass.

Localization

Lipoma may be solitary, multiple, or disseminated, and may occur anywhere.

Classification

- Single or multiple (lipomatosis) non-pain-associated lipomas
- Subtypes:
  - Familial multiple lipomatosis, adiposis dolorosa (Dercum disease), a condition marked painful lipomas
  - Familial multiple lipomatosis, a hereditary condition that causes multiple lipomas
  - Benign symmetric lipomatosis (Madelung disease), a rare condition marked by lipomas forming around the upper body

Laboratory and Other Workups

No laboratory tests are needed. Ultrasound.

Dermatopathology

Well-limited fatty tissue lobules, frequently with a connective tissue capsule. Lipomas with vessel proliferation: angiolipomas; lipomas with connective tissue proliferation: fibrolipomas and mixed types: angiofibrolipomas.

Course

The typical course is a slow growth followed by stabilization.

Complications

Pressure on adjacent tissues and vessel thrombosis within the lipoma may rarely lead to pain, esthetic discomfort.

Diagnosis

Clinical characteristic features, ultrasonography, and histological confirmation if needed.

Differential Diagnosis

Malignant liposarcoma well-differentiated liposarcoma (WDL)/atypical lipomatous tumor (ALT) must be suspected if the tumor is rapidly growing or painful, and in this case the lesion must be removed surgically for histopathological examination. Other differential diagnoses: cysts, connective tissue tumors, and benign symmetrical lipomatosis.

Prevention and Therapy

Excision is performed in case of discomfort or to rule out a malignant tumor if the clinical presentation is atypical (e.g. rapid growth, pain).

Hemangioma [7, 11]

Figures 12.18, 12.19, 12.20, and 12.21

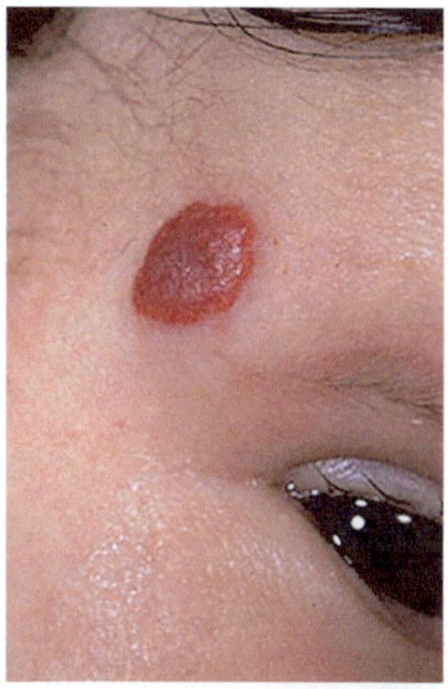

Fig. 12.18 Hemangioma: flat lesion on the temple

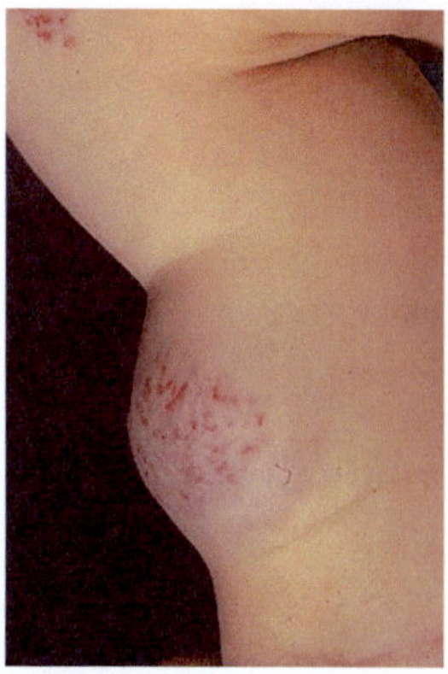

Fig. 12.19 Hemangioma: subcutaneous variant

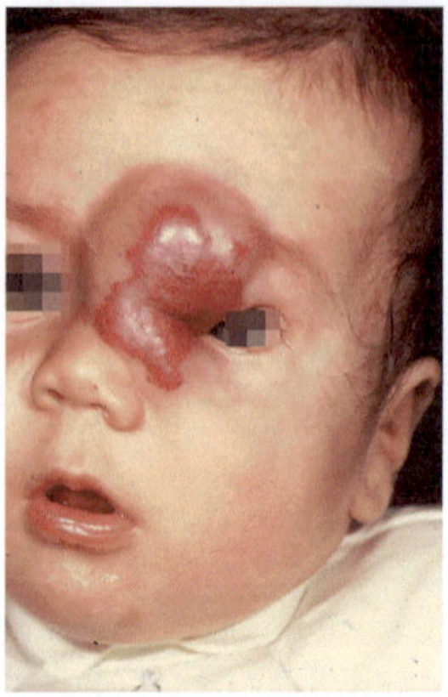

Fig. 12.20 Hemangioma: threatening visus

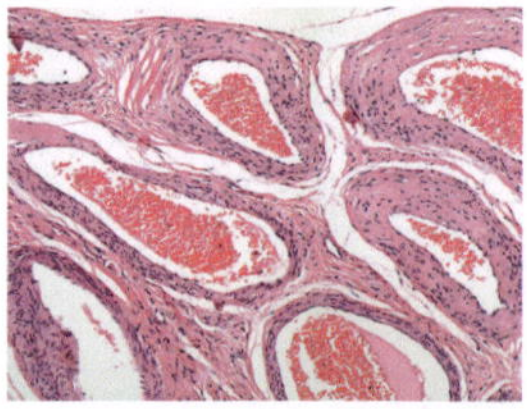

Fig. 12.21 Hemangioma: histology showing dilated blood vessels

Grading of Importance

B

Level

Advanced

ICD-11

XH5AW4

Synonyms

Infantile hemangioma, strawberry nevus, hemangioma of infancy (HI).

Epidemiology

Relatively frequent (4–5% of infants).

Definition

Benign vascular tumors that appear in the first weeks after birth.

Etiology and Pathogenesis

Unknown.

Signs and Symptoms

Dome-shaped circumscribed bright red nodules (cutaneous hemangioma) or pink to blue soft swelling (subcutaneous hemangioma), or both (mixed type) or superficial.

Localization

They can be located in any area of the body.

Classification

Superficial (cutaneous), deep (subcutaneous), or mixed (superficial and deep).

Laboratory and Other Workups

Laboratory tests are not needed.

Dermatopathology

Histology is not needed for the diagnosis. A proliferation of dermal mature vessels without inflammatory infiltrate is observed if a biopsy is performed. However, growing hemangioma of infancy express more GLU-1 receptor by immunohistochemistry. This should prompt the clinician to consider intervention.

Course

Childhood hemangiomas are not present at birth, appear in the first weeks of life, grow during a few months and then spontaneously regress in the first or first years of life. Those which are rapidly and continuously growing need intervention.

Complications

Ulceration (infection, pain), scar with esthetic consequences, bleeding (uncommon). Depending on hemangioma location:

- Eye: amblyopia
- Nose: cartilage deformation
- Lips: feeding difficulties
- Lower jaw: associated subglottic hemangioma with possible stridor and respiratory obstruction

Segmentary facial hemangiomas and perineal/lombo-sacral hemangiomas may be associated with underlying malformations (rare); miliary hemangiomatosis may be associated with visceral hemangiomas and high output cardiac insufficiency (rare).

Diagnosis

Most cases: clinical. Diagnostic uncertainty: ultrasonography. Suspicious subglottic hemangioma: referral to ENT (ear-nose-throat) specialist. Suspicious PHACES or PELVIS syndrome: brain or medullary MRI, respectively. Glut-1 staining.

Differential Diagnosis

Differential diagnoses include vascular malformations (such as nevus flammeus), granuloma pyogenicum, angiosarcoma, other malignant tumors (rhabdomyosarcoma, infantile fibrosarcoma). Kasabach-Merritt syndrome is characterized by profound thrombocytopenia, consumptive coagulopathy with a hemorrhagic risk, in association with vascular tumors (rare).

Prevention and Therapy

In most cases: no treatment. In case of complications related to localization or rapid growth: beta-blockers (propranolol).

Special

Aggressive early treatment (laser) may be needed in fast growing lesions in anatomical risky localizations (i.e. eyes); however, in this situation, systemic ß-blocker administration for inpatients may be required.

Pyogenic Granuloma [6]

Figure 12.22

Grading of Importance

C

Level

Basic

ICD-11

2F26

Synonyms

Granuloma pediculatum, granuloma teleangiectaticum, lobular capillary hemangioma, pseudobotryomycoma, eruptive angioma, proliferating angioma; epulis granulomatosa (gingiva).

Epidemiology

Frequent; all ages; M = F; more common in white than in black people.

Definition

Misnomer, since this exophytic benign reactive proliferation of small vessels has nothing to do with bacterial "pyogenic" (pus producing) infection, like "botryomycosis," which again is a misnomer (mostly due to staphylococcal, not fungal infection).

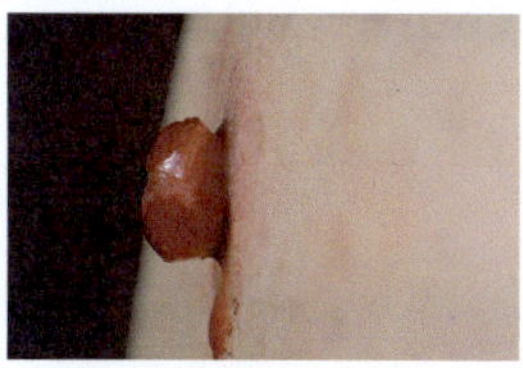

Fig. 12.22 Pyogenic granuloma: eruptive nodule on a small base

Aeiology and Pathogenesis

Injuries, wounds, and hormones (pregnancy) are initiating factors. Nitrogen monoxide synthase (NOS), fibroblast growth factor (FGF), and connective tissue growth factor (CTGF) are important pathogenetic factors.

Signs and Symptoms

Friable, bleeding exophytic proliferation with collarette by the surrounding epidermis. Occasionally small angiomatous satellites in the vicinity.

Localization

Wounds; areas exposed to injuries; extremities, face, tips of the fingers and toes; lips, tongue, gingiva (epulis).

Classification

- Eruptive pyogenic granuloma
- Subcutaneous intravascular pyogenic granuloma
- Pyogenic granuloma with satellites
- Pyogenic granuloma on lips, gingiva (epulis)

Laboratory and Other Workups

Not needed; micobiologic swab (see differential diagnoses).

Dermatopathology

Erosion on the surface with hemorrhagic crust formation; proliferation of newly formed capillaries with many mitoses around a central vessel. Mixed cellular inflammatory infiltrate in the dermis. Collarette of the epidermis.

Course

Spontaneous involution possible; prognosis good following complete removal.

Complications

Bleeding; superinfection; recurrence if not completely removed.

Diagnosis

Typical clinical feature and history (trauma, pregnancy).

Differential Diagnosis

Granulation tissue, amelanotic melanoma, hemangiosarcoma, botryomycosis (bacterial infection), bacillary angiomatosis (*Bartonella henselae* infection, i.e. in HIV).

Prevention and Therapy

Avoid injuries. Removal by excision or laser.

Special

Cave: Confusion with malignant melanoma.

Cutaneous Mastocytosis [1, 2, 5]

Figures 12.23, 12.24, 12.25 and 12.26

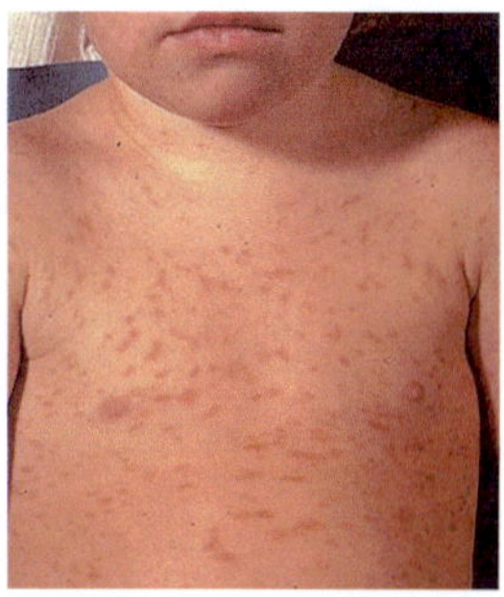

Fig. 12.23 Cutaneous mastocytosis: juvenile form

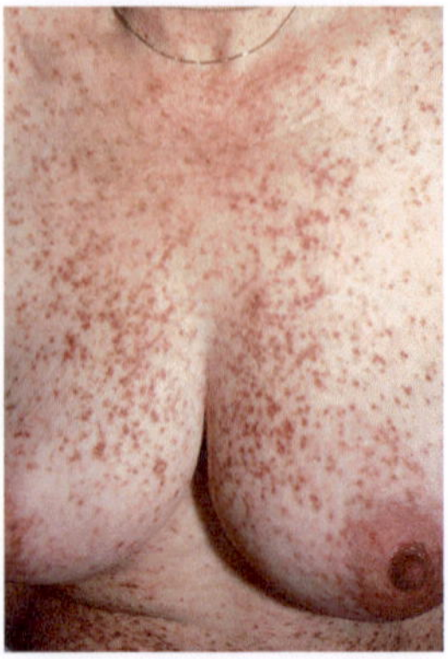

Fig. 12.24 Cutaneous mastocytosis: adult form

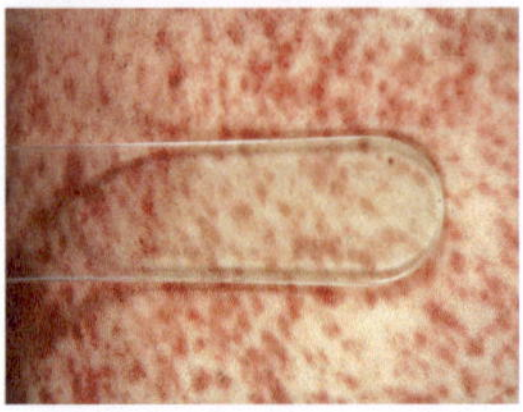

Fig. 12.25 Cutaneous mastocytosis: apple jelly like pigmentation under pressure

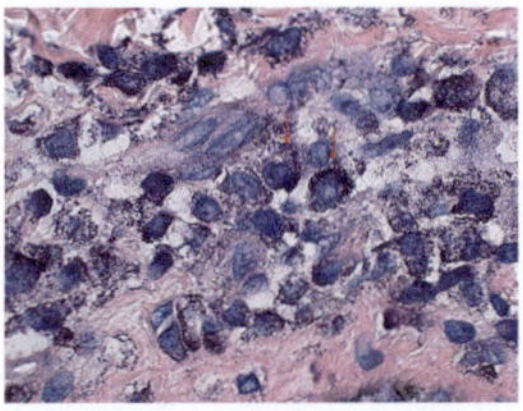

Fig. 12.26 Cutaneous mastocytosis: granular mast cells

Grading of Importance

B

Level

Advanced

ICD-11

2A21.1

Synonyms

Mastocytosis, mast cell disease.

Epidemiology

Rare disease, most common in children. Prevalence 0.1 to 0.8% of dermatology consultations.

65% are observed in children below 15 years. Two peaks of incidence, one between 6 months and 2 years (55%) and one between 20 and 40 years (35%).

Definition

Proliferation of mast cells in the skin.

Aeiology and Pathogenesis

It is most often sporadic but may be caused by mutations in the KIT gene (KIT D816V). MRGPRX2 activates mast cells, which in turn release tryptase and histamine with local or systemic symptoms.

Signs and Symptoms

- Urticaria pigmentosa (maculopapular mastocytosis): many red-brown, maculopapular lesions, with variable flushes and pruritus (most common form).
- Diffuse cutaneous mastocytosis: diffuse erythema, skin infiltration, blistering (rare, in the first month of life).
- Localized mastocytosis (mastocytoma) is a single lesion (or sometimes 1–3 lesions), most often found in children.
- Furthermore, a so-called idiopathic mast cell activation syndrome (MACS) was recently introduced as an entity within the mast cell disorders.

Mastocytosis skin lesions respond with an urticarial reaction spontaneously or after irritation (Darier's sign: wheal, erythema, itch).

Localization

Cutaneous mastocytosis (urticaria pigmentosa and diffuse cutaneous mastocytosis) shows a disseminated appearance on the entire body. Mastocytoma is a unique lesion or multiple (generally one to three) lesions localized anywhere on the skin.

MACS is a disorder, in which products are released from mast cells without specific localization and without diffuse increase of mast cells, as in the diffuse type.

Classification

The 2016 updated current WHO classification of mastocytosis identifies three forms of cutaneous mastocytosis:

- Urticaria pigmentosa
- Diffuse cutaneous mastocytosis
- Mastocytoma

Laboratory and Other Workups

Serum tryptase levels are correlated with the mast cell tumor burden. A complete blood count is useful to screen for hematologic (medullary) involvement.

Dermatopathology

Dense perivascular infiltrates of mast cells, which stain positively with Giemsa, toluidine blue (heterochromasia), or chloroacetate esterase (Leder-stain). Immunohistochemistry to stain mast cells (anti-CD117 = KIT, anti-tryptase, and anti-CD25 antibodies).

Course

If the disease appears in childhood, spontaneous remission is frequent. The adult version is generally clinically stable, but mast cells may proliferate and lead to systemic symptoms.

Complications

In adults, flushes, hives, diarrhea, vomiting, headache, depression, breathing problems, osteoporosis, visceral involvement, and anaphylaxis (rare). Worsening of symptoms may be provoked by alcohol and certain food or drugs. Malignant transformation very rare.

Diagnosis

Diagnosis is based on typical clinical features and confirmed by histopathology. At baseline, no additional workup is required in children. Serum tryptase levels, complete blood count, abdominal ultrasonography, and osteodensitometry are performed in adults. In diffuse type of mastocytosis and KIT anomaly, a bone marrow aspiration is indicated.

Differential Diagnosis

Lichen planus, disseminated granuloma annulare or sarcoidosis, secondary syphilis (not permanent, no swelling), plane warts, multiple leiomyomas, various adnexal tumors, and pseudolymphoma.

Prevention and Therapy

None is required if no functional disturbance. Non-sedating antihistamines; H2 blockers or cromoglycate for gastrointestinal symptoms; PUVA; short-term high-potency topical glucocorticoids.

Cutaneous Cysts [8]

Figures 12.27, 12.28 and 12.29

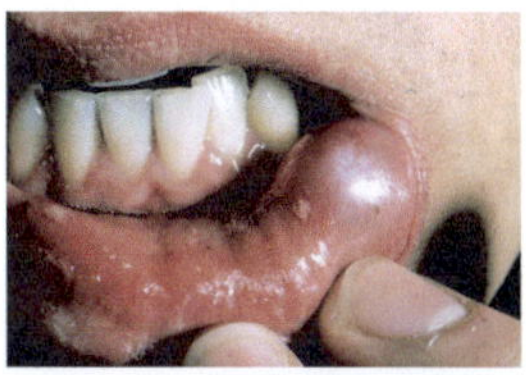

Fig. 12.27 Cutaneous cysts: mucoid pseudocyst of the lip

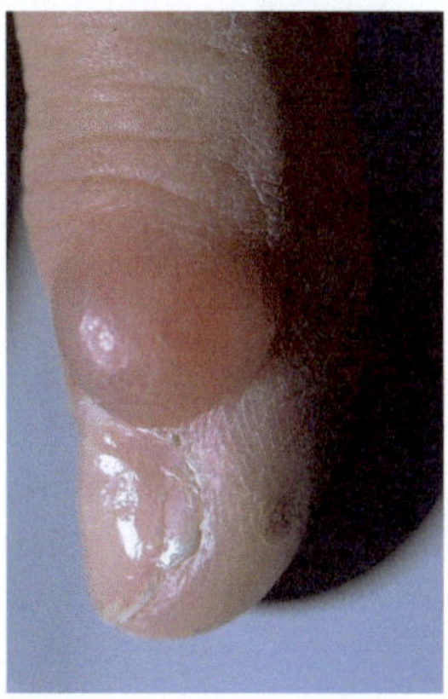

Fig. 12.28 Cutaneous cysts: digital pseudocyst

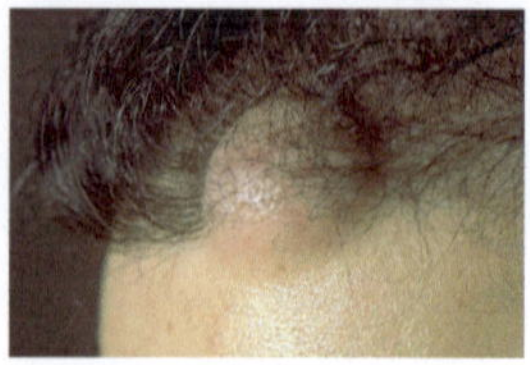

Fig. 12.29 Cutaneous cysts: sebaceous cyst on the scalp

Grading of Importance

B

Level

Basic

ICD-11

EK70

Synonyms

Cysts of skin, lips, mucous membrane.

Epidemiology

Frequent. M > F.

Definition

- Cysts with epithelial lining (CEL): benign encapsulated firm or fluctuant lesions, containing material of various types (squamous material, sebum, sweat, hair, oily fluid).
- Cysts without epithelial lining (pseudocysts) (PC): clinically are similar to CEL, but do not have a capsule.

Etiology and Pathogenesis

Often superficial trauma, small injuries or subepidermal blistering diseases (milia due to blisters in porphyria cutanea tarda or epidermolysis).

Dispersion of epidermal or follicular germs or ductal structures into the dermis.

Signs and Symptoms

CEL: Round, slowly growing nodule, showing a central pore in some cases. Fixed or slightly movable beyond the overlying erythematous smooth skin surface.

PC: Translucent submucosal node developing on lip, tongue, or buccal mucosa in the vicinity of salivary glands, following minor injury.

Milia (sing. milium) are tiny epidermal cysts arising from the infundibular portion of vellus hairs or dermal sweat ducts, without connection to the overlying epidermis. They present as yellowish tiny papules and usually disappear within a few weeks.

Ganglion: synovial pseudocyst with wall formed by fibrous tissue, surrounding amorphous myxoid material and with connection with the joint capsule.

Localization

CEL: Preferred localizations are face, neck, capillitium, and back.

PC: Lips or mucous membranes, site of injury.

Classification

- Epithelial cysts
  - Sebaceous cysts
  - Epidermal cysts
  - Trichilemmal cysts
  - Milia
  - Hybrid cysts
- Mucous (pseudo-) cysts (mucocele)
  - Oral mucous cyst
  - Lip cyst
  - Digital myxoid cyst
  - Synovial cyst (ganglion)

Laboratory and Other Workups

None or biopsy; diaphanoscopy (translucency), ultrasound.

Dermatopathology

Cysts with epithelial lining (CEL): epithelial wall surrounding squamous debris with or without follicular structures. Reactive inflammatory infiltrate of the dermis, sometimes after rupture of wall with granulomatous features and multinucleated foreign body giant cells.

Cysts without epithelial lining (pseudocysts) (PC): fibrous wall including oily liquid or amorphous myxoid material.

Course

Sometimes self-healing by spontaneous regression, especially in mucous cysts.

Complications

CEL: frequent rupture of the epithelial cyst wall with subsequent inflammatory reaction with or without bacterial superinfection leading to granulomatous foreign body reaction, abscess formation, bursting, and draining.

PC: none.

Diagnosis

Clinical and histologic features.

Differential Diagnosis

Acneiform reactions, fibroma, lipoma, and adnexal tumor.

Prevention and Therapy

Prevention not possible. Superinfected epidermal cysts developing an abscess need an incision and tamponade. Antibiotics if severely superinfected and additional surrounding tissue inflamed. Surgical removal including capsule in the native non-inflamed status. PC of mucous membranes may regress spontaneously.

References

1. Abid A, Malone MA, Curci K (2016) Mastocytosis. Prim Care 43(3):505–518
2. Di Raimondo C, Del Duca E, Silvaggio D, Di Prete M, Lombardo P, Mazzeo M, Spallone G, Campione E, Botti E, Bianchi L (2021) Cutaneous mastocytosis: a dermatological perspective. Australas J Dermatol 62(1):e1–e7
3. Greco MJ, Bhutta BS (2020) Seborrheic keratosis. StatPearls, Treasure Island, FL
4. Hafner C, Vogt T (2008) Seborrheic keratosis. J Dtsch Dermatol Ges 6(8):664–677
5. Hartmann K, Escribano L, Grattan C, Brockow K, Carter MC, Alvarez-Twose I, Matito A, Broesby-Olsen S, Siebenhaar F, Lange M, Niedoszytko M, Castells M, Oude Elberink JNG, Bonadonna P, Zanotti R, Hornick JL, Torrelo A, Grabbe J, Rabenhorst A, Nedoszytko B, Butterfield JH, Gotlib J, Reiter A, Radia D, Hermine O, Sotlar K, George TI, Kristensen TK, Kluin-Nelemans HC, Yavuz S, Hagglund H, Sperr WR, Schwartz LB, Triggiani M, Maurer M, Nilsson G, Horny HP, Arock M, Orfao A, Metcalfe DD, Akin C, Valent P (2016) Cutaneous manifestations in patients with mastocytosis: consensus report of the European Competence Network on mastocytosis; the American Academy of Allergy, Asthma & Immunology; and the European Academy of Allergology and Clinical Immunology. J Allergy Clin Immunol 137(1):35–45
6. Jafarzadeh H, Sanatkhani M, Mohtasham N (2006) Oral pyogenic granuloma: a review. J Oral Sci 48(4):167–175
7. Johnson EF, Davis DM, Tollefson MM, Fritchie K, Gibson LE (2018) Vascular tumors in infants: case report and review of clinical, histopathologic, and immunohistochemical characteristics of infantile hemangioma, pyogenic granuloma, noninvoluting congenital hemangioma, tufted angioma, and kaposiform hemangioendothelioma. Am J Dermatopathol 40(4):231–239
8. Kaya G, Saurat JH (2018) Cutaneous adnexal cysts revisited: what we know and what we think we know. Dermatopathol (Basel) 5(2):79–85
9. Kolb L, Yarrarapu SNS, Ameer MA, Rosario-Collazo JA (2020) Lipoma. StatPearls, Treasure Island, FL
10. Kwiek B, Schwartz RA (2016) Keratoacanthoma (KA): an update and review. J Am Acad Dermatol 74(6):1220–1233
11. Leaute-Labreze C, Harper JI, Hoeger PH (2017) Infantile haemangioma. Lancet 390(10089):85–94
12. McGinty S, Siddiqui WJ (2020) Keloid. StatPearls, Treasure Island, FL
13. Myers DJ, Fillman EP (2020) Dermatofibroma. StatPearls, Treasure Island, FL
14. Zelger B, Zelger BG, Burgdorf WH (2004) Dermatofibroma-a critical evaluation. Int J Surg Pathol 12(4):333–344

Premalignant and Malignant Tumours

13

Martine Bagot, Günter Burg, Adele De Masson, Gabor Dobos, Evelyn Gaffal, and Harald Gollnick

Contents

M. Bagot (✉)
Service de Dermatologie, Université Paris Cité, Hôpital Saint-Louis, Paris, France
e-mail: martine.bagot@gmail.com

G. Burg
Dermatology, Zurich, Switzerland
e-mail: g.burg@access.uzh.ch

A. De Masson · G. Dobos
Dermatology and Venereology, Université de Paris, Hopital Saint Louis, Paris, France
e-mail: adele.demasson@aphp.fr; gabor.dobos@charite.de

E. Gaffal
Department of Dermatology, University of Lübeck, Lübeck, Germany
e-mail: evelyn.gaffal@med.ovgu.de

H. Gollnick
Department of Dermatology & Venereology, Otto-von-Guericke University, Magdeburg, Germany
e-mail: Harald.Gollnick@med.ovgu.de

H. Gollnick et al. (eds.), *Dermatology Cyberderm WebBook*,
https://doi.org/10.1007/978-3-031-78491-0_13

Test your learning and check your understanding of this book's contents: use the "Springer Nature Flashcards" app to access questions using ▶ https://sn.pub/1rhh6k.
To use the app, please follow the instructions in Chap. 1.

Actinic Keratosis [7, 28]

Figures 13.1, 13.2 and 13.3

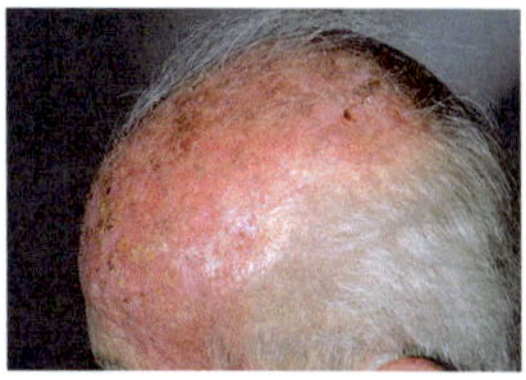

Fig. 13.1 Actinic keratosis: sun exposed bald had

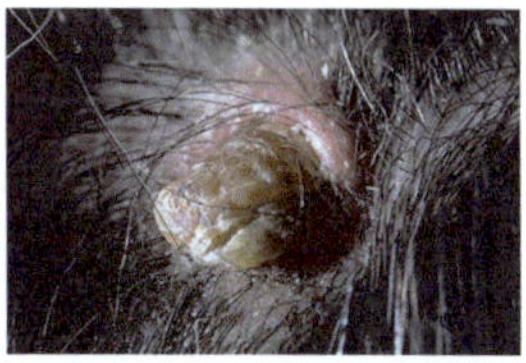

Fig. 13.2 Actinic keratosis: cutaneous horn on actinic keratosis

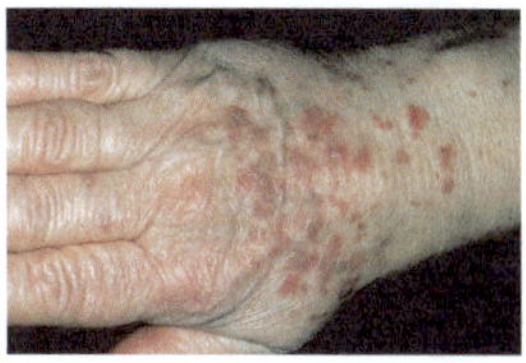

Fig. 13.3 Actinic keratosis: hand of a farmer woman

Grading of Importance

B

Level

Advanced

ICD-11

EK90

Synonyms

Solar keratosis.

Epidemiology

Dependent on skin type and life conditions. Prevalence in the UK, 6% in female and 15% in male.

Definition

Carcinoma in situ caused by chronic UV light exposure.

Aetiology and Pathogenesis

Chronic UV exposure followed by mutations of keratinocyte-DNA. In addition human papilloma virus (HPV), chemicals, genetic predisposition, immunosuppression.

Signs and Symptoms

Circumscribed hyperkeratotic yellow-brownish papules or plaques, sometimes flat or atrophic

Localisation

Sun-exposed areas (scalp, face, back of hands, shins, forearms).

Classification

Grades 1 to 3.

Laboratory and Other Workups

None.

Dermatopathology

Hyperkeratosis, epidermal disarray, atypical keratinocytes, inflammatory infiltrate, actinic elastosis.

Course

Chronic over years.

Complications

Transition to squamous cell carcinoma possible.

Diagnosis

Clinical features, histology.

Differential Diagnosis

Bowen's disease, seborrhoeic keratoses.

Prevention and Therapy

Prevention: sun protection.

Treatment: physical methods (cryosurgery, curettage, photodynamic therapy), topical methods (5-fluorouracil or immune modifiers: imiquimod cream, diclofenac, ingenol mebutate).

Carcinoma in Situ [2]

Figures 13.4, 13.5 and 13.6

Grading of Importance

B

Level

Advanced

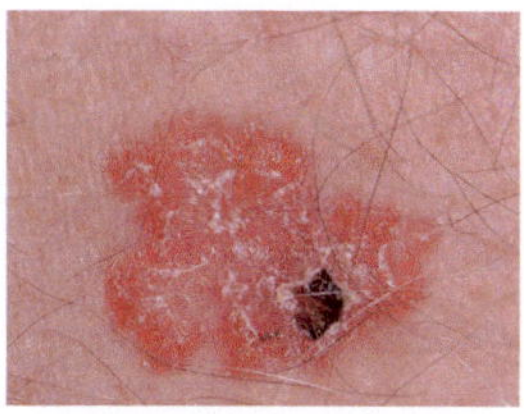

Fig. 13.4 Carcinoma in situ: plaque-lie flat tumor on the breast

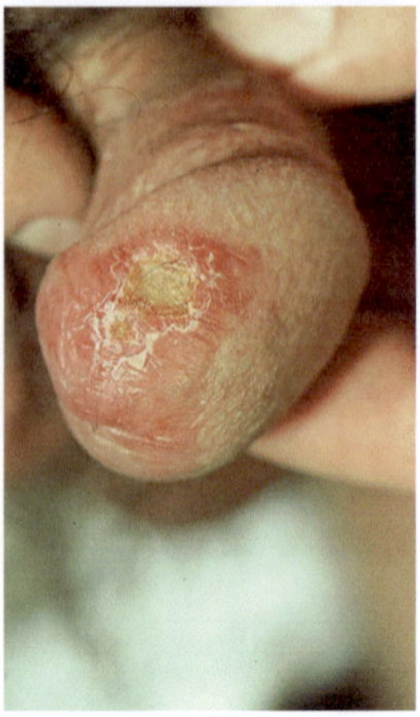

Fig. 13.5 Carcinoma in situ: flat lesion on the glans penis (erythroplasia)

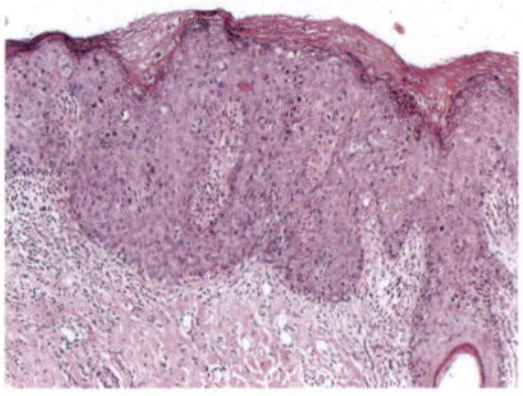

Fig. 13.6 Carcinoma in situ: histology showing acanthosis with large, atypical cells in all levels of the epidermis

ICD-11

2E64

Synonyms

Bowen's disease (skin), erythroplasia of Queyrat (glans penis), leukoplakia (mucous epithelia).

Epidemiology

Incidence 15/100,000/year in persons with white skin.

Definition

Carcinoma in situ (intraepidermal and intraepithelial carcinoma).

Aetiology and Pathogenesis

UV exposure, immunosuppression, HPV, tobacco, betel nut.

Signs and Symptoms

Circumscribed erythematous (sometimes scaly) patch or plaque, persistent whitish mucosal lesions.

Localisation

Sun-exposed skin, genitalia, buccal mucosa.

Classification

Grades 1 to 3 according to progression and involvement by histology.

Laboratory and Other Workups

None

Dermatopathology

Orthohyperkeratosis (pink) alternating with parakeratosis (blue). Abnormal keratinocytes. Pseudopod-like proliferation of the epidermis. Solar elastosis in the upper dermis.

Complications

Transition to invasive cutaneous or mucosal squamous cell carcinoma.

Diagnosis

Diagnosis relies on clinical picture and histology.

Differential Diagnosis

Depending on localisation (lips, buccal or genital mucosa): superficial basal cell carcinoma, bowenoid papulosis, extramammary Paget's disease. Confirmation by histology.

Prevention and Therapy

Depends on localisation and histological type. For example: excision, cryosurgery, photodynamic therapy, radiotherapy, 5-fluorouracil or imiquimod cream.

Paget's Disease [18]

Figures 13.7, 13.8 and 13.9

Grading of Importance

B

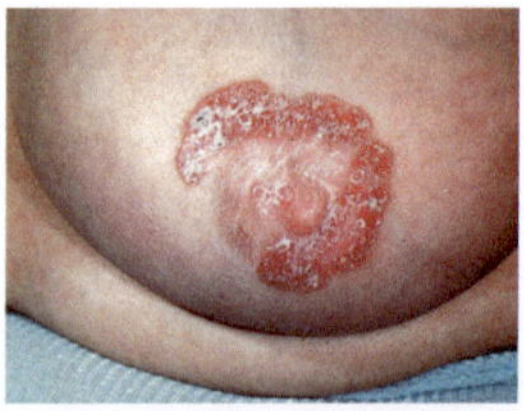

Fig. 13.7 Paget's disease: of the nipple

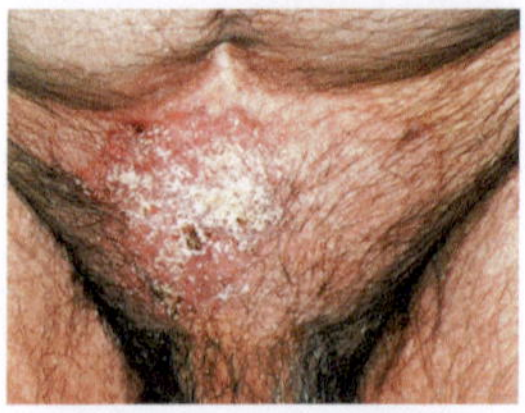

Fig. 13.8 Paget's disease: extramammary

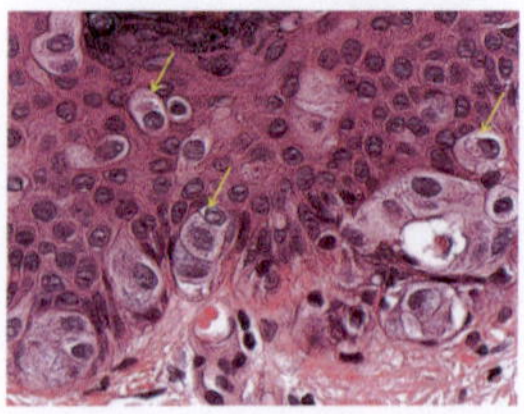

Fig. 13.9 Paget's disease: histology showing large, clear intraepithelial tumor cells

Level

Advanced

ICD-11

Breast: XH3E21

Extramammary: XH70F8

Epidemiology

Rare disease. 3% of all breast cancers.

Definition

Uncommon intraepidermal adenocarcinoma, arising from intraductal carcinoma in the breast (mammary Paget's disease). Can also arise from apocrine sweat glands or underlying carcinomas, e.g. rectum, prostate (extramammary Paget's disease).

Aetiology and Pathogenesis

Associated breast cancer is of the intraduct variety.

Signs and Symptoms

Circumscribed, erythematous, sometimes scaly, increasingly infiltrated plaque. Nipple (unilateral), axilla, groin or perianal.

Cave: for chronic dermatitis involving one nipple – > rule out Paget's disease.

Localisation

Nipple, axilla, genitalia, lower abdomen, perianal.

Dermatopathology

Large clear intraepithelial tumour cells, PAS positive.

Course

Slowly and gradually spreads.

Complications

Association with intraductal carcinoma (Paget's disease) or adenocarcinoma (extra-mammary Paget's disease).

Diagnosis

Clinical features and histology.

Differential Diagnosis

Nipple dermatitis, perianal dermatitis, psoriasis.

Prevention and Therapy

Surgical excision adjusted to tumour size and underlying disease, multidisciplinary approach.

Squamous Cell Carcinoma [23, 30]

Figures 13.10, 13.11 and 13.12

Grading of Importance

B

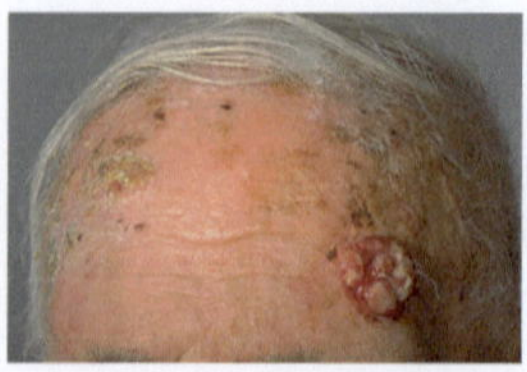

Fig. 13.10 Squamous cell carcinoma: tumor on sun damaged skin of an elderly patient

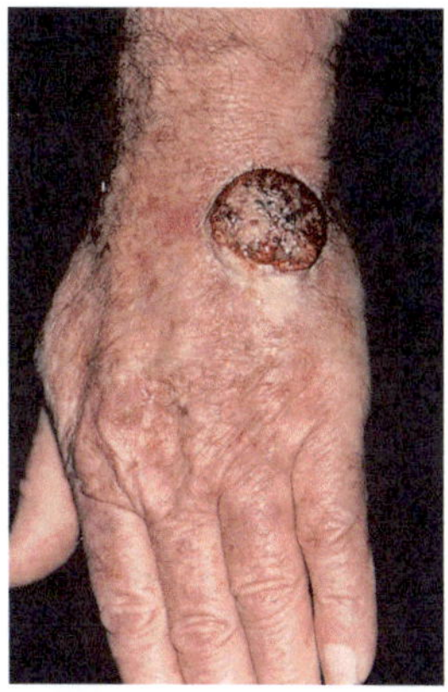

Fig. 13.11 Squamous cell carcinoma: exophytic tumor

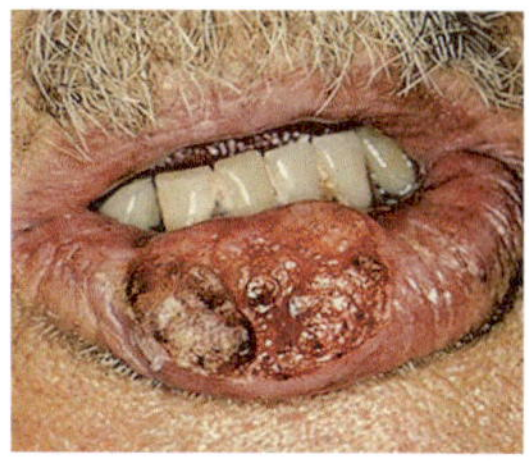

Fig. 13.12 Squamous cell carcinoma: lower lip in a pipe smoker

Level

Advanced

ICD-11

2C31

Synonyms

Epidermoid carcinoma.

Epidemiology

Incidence 30–50 /100,000 per year.

Definition

Malignant keratinocytic tumour with tendency to progressively invade and metastasise.

Aetiology and Pathogenesis

Arises on previously damaged skin: UV, ionising radiation, arsenic, tar, soot, abnormal scars, HPV. Precursors: actinic keratoses, in situ carcinoma, scars, chronic ulcers. Predisposing factors: skin types I and II, occupations with marked UV exposure (farmers, mountaineers, sailors, roofers and construction workers), transplanted patients and those with chronic immunosuppression.

Signs and Symptoms

Usually in sun-exposed areas, irregular, often hyperkeratotic papules or nodules, easily ulcerate.

Localisation

May appear all over the skin, in particular sun-exposed sites (head, ear, neck, lower lip, back of hands, forearms, shins).

Classification

According to keratinocyte differentiation (Broder's grades 1 to 3) by histology.

Laboratory and Other Workups

Not necessary.

Dermatopathology

Hyperkeratosis, strands of epithelium extending into dermis, atypia, mitoses, inflammatory infiltrate, dyskeratosis, single cell necrosis (apoptosis with eosinophilic cytoplasm), keratin pearls. Degree of differentiation: grade 1 (well-differentiated, risk of metastasis 1–2%), grade 3 (poorly differentiated with high risk).

Course

Patients with immunosuppression and transplantation have higher risk of metastasis.

Complications

Depending on the localisation: local invasion of deeper structures and metastasis.

Diagnosis

Clinical features and histology. Continuously growing, hyperkeratotic, sometimes ulcerated nodular usually non-pigmented lesions.

Differential Diagnosis

Keratoacanthoma, actinic keratoses, Bowen's disease, basal cell carcinoma, verrucae vulgaris, hypertrophic lichen planus.

Prevention and Therapy

Depends on size and localisation. Excision should be done with histologically proven margins, radiotherapy, radiofrequency therapy with bleomycin, immune modulators (check point inhibitors).

Basal Cell Carcinoma [16, 20, 25]

Figures 13.13, 13.14, 13.15, 13.16, 13.17, 13.18 and 13.19

Grading of Importance

B

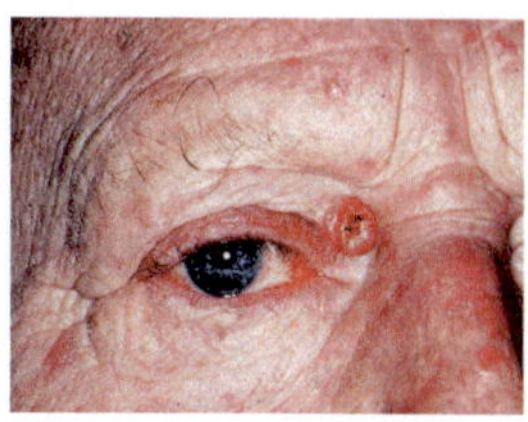

Fig. 13.13 Basal cell carcinoma: nodular crateriform lesion in a typical localization

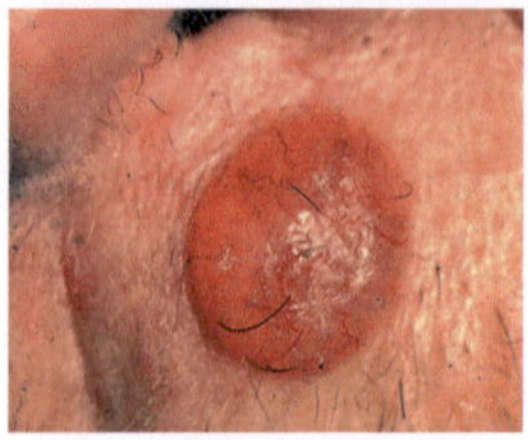

Fig. 13.14 Basal cell carcinoma: nodular tumor with telangiectasias

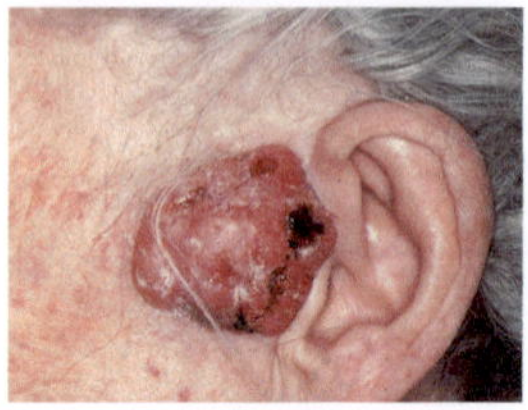

Fig. 13.15 Basal cell carcinoma: preauricular nodular tumor

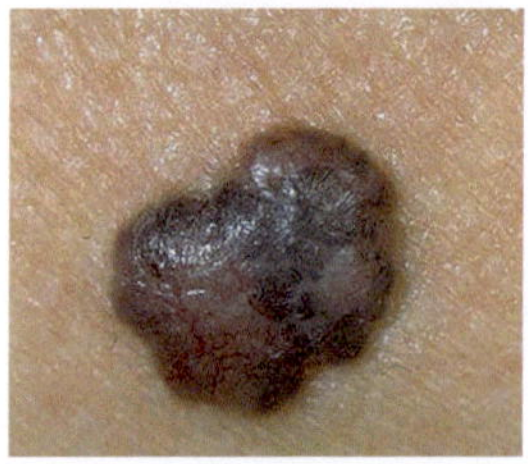

Fig. 13.16 Basal cell carcinoma: pigmented BCC

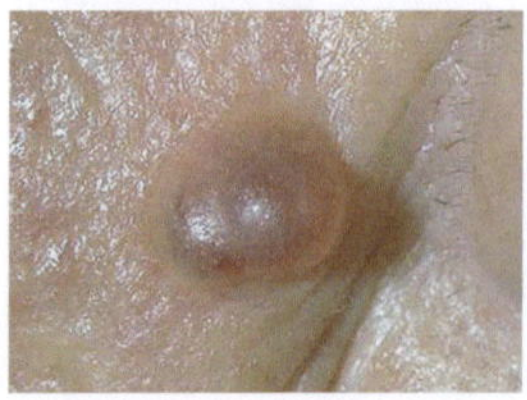

Fig. 13.17 Basal cell carcinoma: cystic BCC

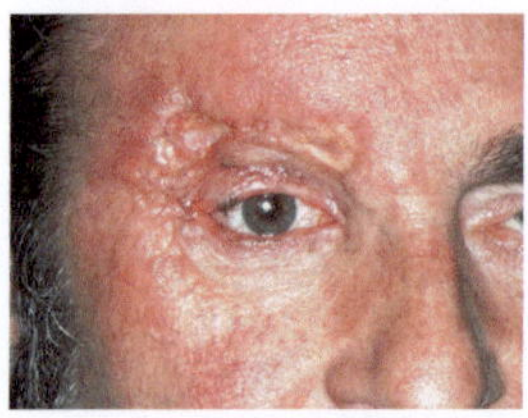

Fig. 13.18 Basal cell carcinoma: sclerodermiform (morphea-like) BCC

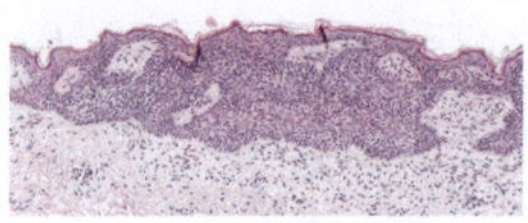

Fig. 13.19 Basal cell carcinoma: proliferation of epidermal cells

Level

Advanced

ICD-11

2C32

Synonyms

Basal cell epithelioma, basalioma.

Epidemiology

Incidence in Europe: 450 to 500/100000/year, most common skin malignancy.

Definition

Locally destructive malignant tumour derived from pluripotential epidermal stem cells, almost never metastasises.

Aetiology and Pathogenesis

Risk factors: Skin types I and II (pale white and fair skin), UV exposure, immunosuppression, radiation, arsenic exposure/ingestion, specific genetic predisposition. Naevoid basal cell carcinoma syndrome (Gorlin-Goltz syndrome) is a genetic disease with predisposition for multiple basal cell carcinomas.

Signs and Symptoms

Pearly nodule with telangiectases, often raised border and central ulceration in superficial type (most common). Solid or nodular type. Sclerodermiform type infiltrating without sharp borders. Other types: cystic, rodent ulcer, metatypic (aggressive), pigmented.

Localisation

Face, trunk, extremities. In contrast to squamous cell carcinoma, not restricted to sun exposed area.

Classification

No precursor lesions. Typing by histology.

Laboratory and Other Workups

Not necessary.

Dermatopathology

Proliferation of progenitor cells in the basal layer of the epidermis and acroinfundibulum. Tumour cells invade different layers of the dermis. Peripheral palisading (darker row of cells at periphery), mitoses, single cell necrosis (apoptosis).

Types:

- Solid or nodular type
- Sclerodermiform type infiltrating without sharp borders
- Other types: cystic, rodent ulcer, metatypic (aggressive), pigmented

Course

Slowly progressing. May be locally destructive of deeper tissues.

Complications

Recurrence rate after surgery or radiotherapy up to 5% within 5 years.

Diagnosis

Depending on clinical and histological type.

Differential Diagnosis

Sebaceous hyperplasia, dermal naevi, dermatofibroma, pseudolymphoma, melanoma, carcinoma in situ (Bowen disease or Paget disease), actinic keratosis, tumours of skin appendages.

Prevention and Therapy

Depends on the type, size and location. Excision of nodular and sclerodermic type because of recurrences in particular sclerosing tumours with micrographic control of margins (Mohs surgery, see section "Basics of Dermatosurgery Techniques" in Chap. 28); radiation therapy in nodular types, cryosurgery. For superficial variants, also consider cryosurgery, photodynamic therapy, topical 5-fluorouracil, immunomodulators (imiquimod), ablative laser with monitoring follow-up. Advanced lesions: hedgehog inhibitors.

Lentigo Maligna [13, 14, 27, 29]

Figures 13.20 and 13.21

Grading of Importance

B

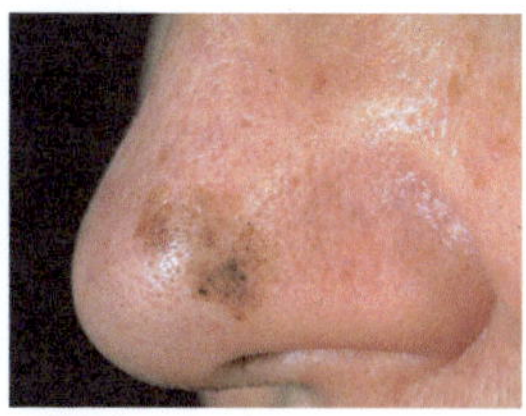

Fig. 13.20 Lentigo maligna: flat lesion on the nose

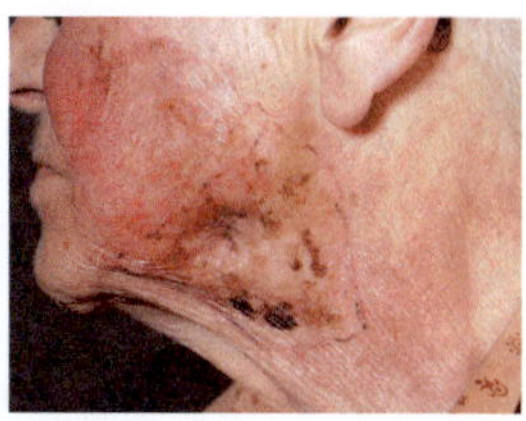

Fig. 13.21 Lentigo maligna: remnants of a lesion on the jaw following superficial soft x-rax therapy

Level

Advanced

ICD-11

2E63.00

Synonyms

Hutchinson melanotic freckle; lentigo maligna melanoma in situ.

Epidemiology

10–15% of all melanoma. Slight female predominance.

Definition

Intraepithelial proliferation of atypical melanocytes mostly in sun-damaged skin and in elderly patients.

Aetiology and Pathogenesis

Chronic natural and artificial UV exposure.

Signs and Symptoms

Irregularly pigmented macule or patch with irregular borders, not palpable, slow growing.

Localisation

Sun-exposed areas (face and neck area, forearms, shins).

Classification

In situ melanocytic proliferation.

Laboratory and Other Workups

Not necessary.

Dermatopathology

Epidermal atrophy, increased number of atypical melanocytes in basal layer, also extending into hair follicle, dermal lymphocytic infiltrate, melanophages, solar elastosis.

Course

Lesions slowly extending and finally developing into a lentigo maligna melanoma.

Complications

Lentigo maligna melanoma and metastasis.

Diagnosis

Clinical features and histology.

Differential Diagnosis

Lentigo simplex, solar lentigo, flat seborrhoeic keratoses, melanoma (lentigo maligna melanoma, superficial spreading melanoma Level 1), naevoid lentigo, atypical naevi.

Prevention and Therapy

Depends on the size and location. Excision is preferred. If excision is not possible or otherwise contraindicated, soft X-ray treatment.

Malignant Melanoma [1, 11, 24]

Figures 13.22, 13.23, 13.24, 13.25, 13.26, 13.27, 13.28, 13.29, 13.30, 13.31 and 13.32

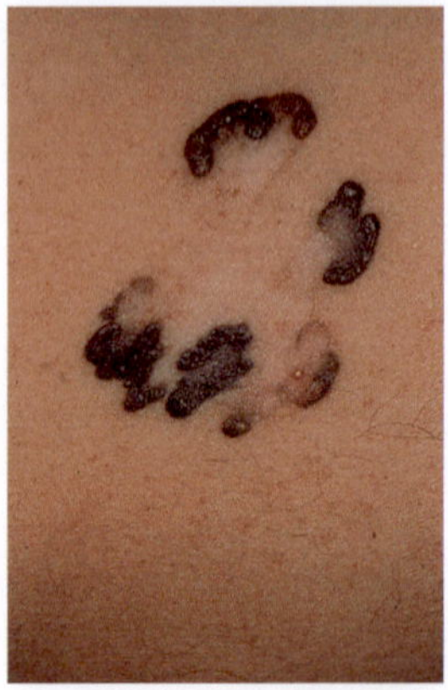

Fig. 13.22 Malignant melanoma: regressing lesion

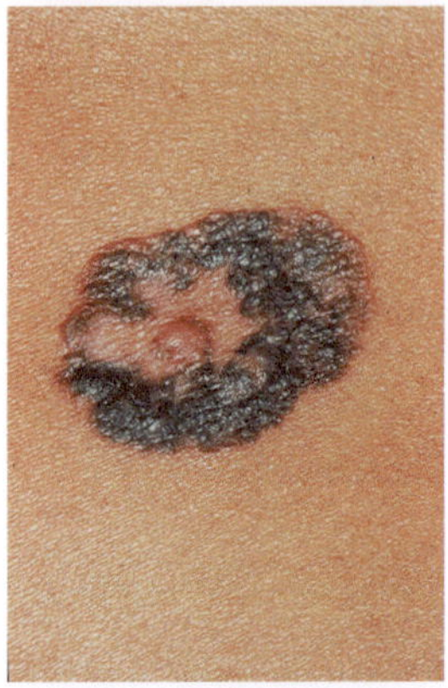

Fig. 13.23 Malignant melanoma: regressing lesion with amelanotic tumor in the center

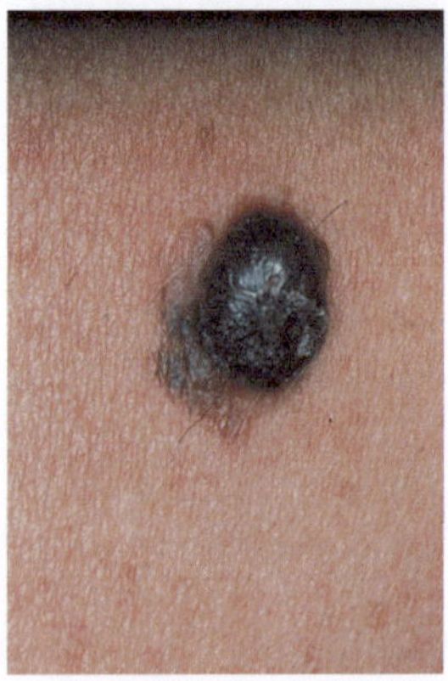

Fig. 13.24 Malignant melanoma: on nevus

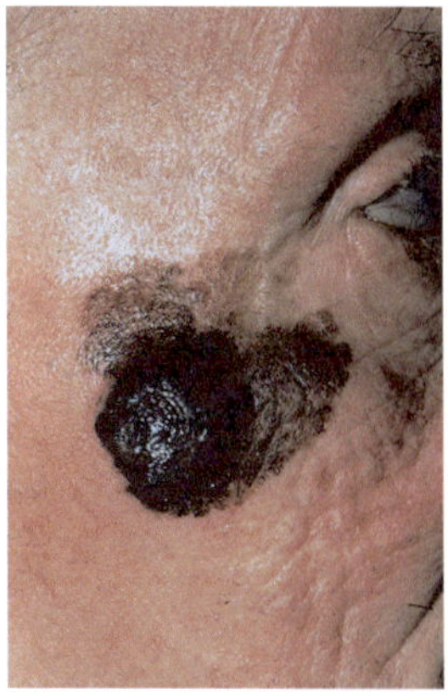

Fig. 13.25 Malignant melanoma: on lentigo maligna

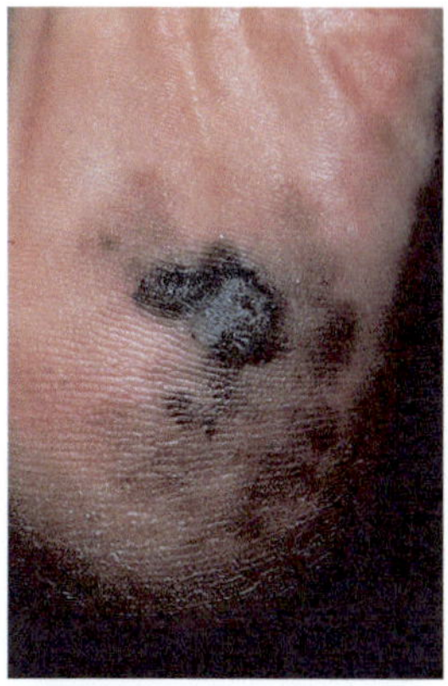

Fig. 13.26 Malignant melanoma: acrolentiginous melanoma of the heel

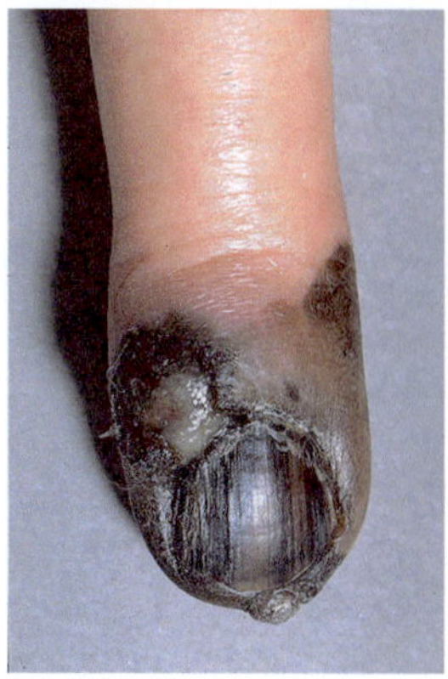

Fig. 13.27 Malignant melanoma: acrolentiginous melanoma of the finger

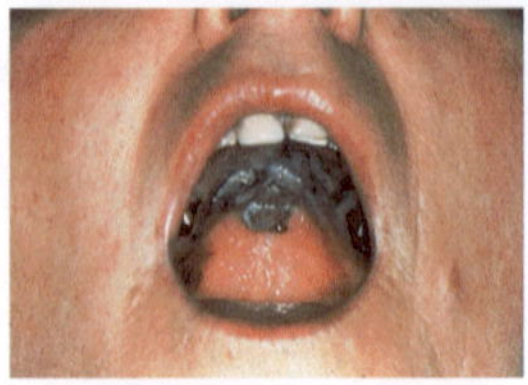

Fig. 13.28 Malignant melanoma: of the oral cavity

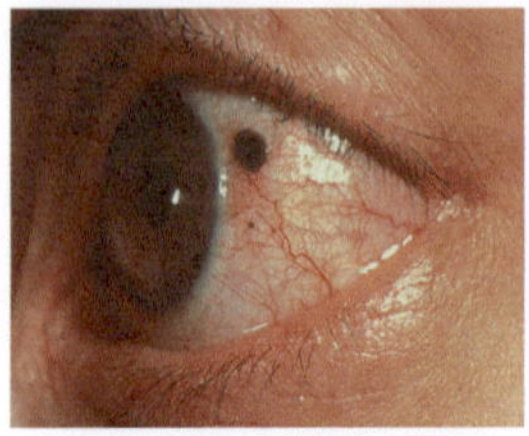

Fig. 13.29 Malignant melanoma: of the conjunctiva

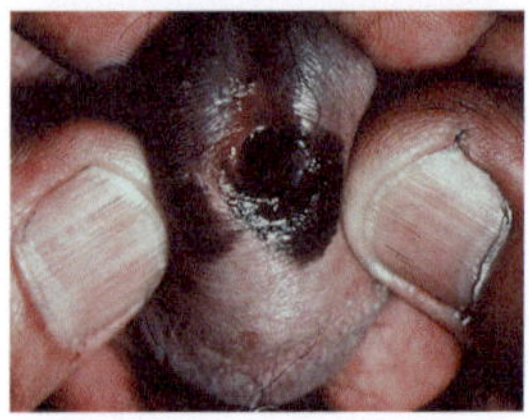

Fig. 13.30 Malignant melanoma: of the penile orificium urethrae

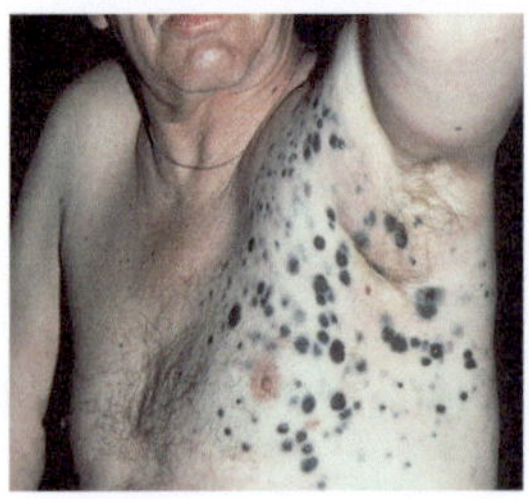

Fig. 13.31 Malignant melanoma: superficial metastases

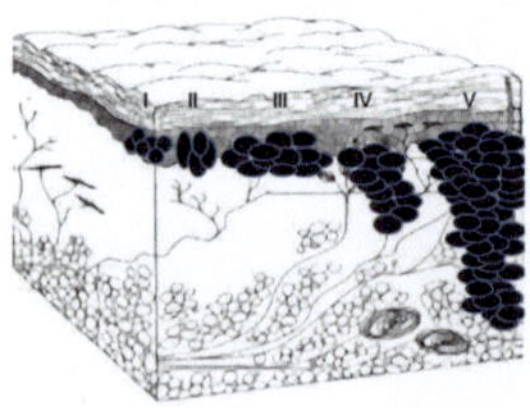

Fig. 13.32 Malignant melanoma: drawing showing depth of infiltration levels I-V

Grading of Importance

B

Level

Advanced

ICD-11

2C30.Z

Synonyms

Often referred to just as melanoma.

Epidemiology

In Europe, the incidence rate is <10–25 new melanoma cases per 100,000 inhabitants and is increasing by 5% yearly; in the USA 20–30 per 100,000; and in Australia, where very high incidence is observed, 50–60 per 100,000.

Melanoma occurs mainly in adults and is exceptional in children.

In order of decreasing frequency: Superficial spreading melanoma (SSM) 41%, nodular melanoma (NMM) 14%, lentigo maligna melanoma (LMM) 2.7–14%, acral lentiginous melanoma (ALM) 1–5% with lower in white colour population, higher in black colour.

Definition

Malignant tumour arising from neuroectodermal cells (melanocytes, naevus cells) with a high risk of metastasis.

Aetiology and Pathogenesis

Risk factors: fair skin, red-blond hair, freckles, blue eyes, history of sunburns as a child, UV exposure, large number (>100) of melanocytic naevi, and personal or family history of melanoma.

Signs and Symptoms

Lesions should be classified as suspicious according to **ABCDE rule**:

- A for asymmetry
- B for irregular border
- C for inhomogeneous colour
- D for diameter over 6 mm
- E for rapid evolution

Types of Melanoma

- Superficial spreading melanoma (SSM): heterogeneous, irregular, pigmented skin lesion with first a radial, later vertical growth, moderate time of evolution.
- Lentigo maligna melanoma arising from a longstanding lentigo maligna (Dubreuilh) is an irregular pigmented lesion of sun-exposed areas.
- Nodular melanoma: predominant aggressive rapid vertical growth phase. Pigmented (or not) nodule of the skin.
- Acrolentiginous melanoma is found on the extremities, sometimes appearing like a long-standing wart on the sole or a pigmented stripe in the nail plate.

Localisation

Melanoma can arise anywhere on the skin and occasionally also on mucosa (anus/rectum, vagina, mouth, sinuses, choroids, retina). Rarely, the diagnosis may be performed at the metastatic stage and the primary tumour is not found.

Classification

- Superficial spreading melanoma (SSM): heterogeneous, irregular, pigmented skin lesion with a variable evolution (low cumulative sun damage melanoma).
- Nodular melanoma: pigmented (or not) often eroded or bleeding nodule of the skin. No UV exposure preference.
- Acrolentiginous melanoma is found on the extremities (plantar, nails). Low to no UVR exposure (or variable/incidental).
- Lentigo maligna melanoma is an irregular pigmented lesion of sun-exposed areas arising from an intraepidermal lentigo maligna (Dubreuilh) high cumulative sun damage melanoma.
- Other subtypes are melanoma arising in a congenital naevus, desmoplastic melanoma, mucosal melanoma and uveal melanoma.

Laboratory and Other Workups

Dermatoscopy (see section "Dermscopy") essential for differentiation of precursor lesions (atypical naevi). Other methods confocal laser scan, electric impedance measures.

Genetic profiling.

According to type and histopathological grading, imaging procedures are essential: ultrasound, MRI, CT or PET-CT.

Metastatic melanoma can be associated with elevated serum LDH (lactate dehydrogenases).

Dermatopathology

Varying types of histopathologic patterns in all MMs. Highlight is an asymmetrical tumour growth with atypical melanocytes (clear cytoplasm, pleomorphic nuclei) growing in nests or singly, extending from the epidermal-dermal junction involving the upper layers of the epidermis, then invading the dermis or subcutaneous fat (thickness (Breslow depth) in mm). Early invasion of lymph vessels or capillaries possible. Mitosis rate, immunohistochemistry and molecular diagnostic of mutation type status are for further examination necessary. TNM classification.

Course

The clinical course is strongly associated with the tumour type and the presence of ulceration on histological examination. The 10-year survival is around 95% for thin melanomas (<1 mm) compared to 40% for thick melanomas (>4 mm). The main other prognostic factors are the presence of nodal and visceral involvement and are summarised in the AJCC TNM (tumour, node, metastasis) stage (I–IV).

Complications

About 90% of melanomas are diagnosed as primary tumours without any evidence of metastasis. The tumour-specific 10-year-survival for such tumours is 75 to 95%. The 10-year survival is 30 to 50% for patients with satellite and in-transit metastases, 69–75% for patients with lymph node micrometastases, and 40 to 60% for those with clinically apparent regional lymph node metastases.

Diagnosis

The diagnosis is suspected clinically, supported by dermatoscopy and confirmed by the histopathological examination.

The clinical diagnosis by the dermatologist is based on a combination of three analyses of any pigmented lesion: (1) visual analysis including ABCDE rule; (2) intra-individual comparative analysis with other pigmented lesions on patients skin; and (3) chronologic analysis of changes (evolution).

Prognosis is evaluated by AJCC pathological (pTNM) prognostic stage grouping.

Differential Diagnosis

Differential diagnoses include melanocytic naevi of different types, pigmented basal cell carcinoma, seborrhoeic keratoses, dermatofibroma.

Prevention and Therapy

The treatment of a suspected lesion is by immediate excision under local anaesthesia. Usually in atypical neavi (intraepidermal dysplasia), 0.5 cm safety margin is sufficient. If lesions are clinically highly suspicious for a melanoma, the primary safety margin is 1–2 cm. A sentinel lymph node biopsy may be performed (if the Breslow is >1 mm). Therapeutic decisions in stage III/IV patients should be primarily made by an interdisciplinary oncology team.

Adjuvant therapy is discussed in patients with a high risk of metastasis (micrometastases in sentinel lymph node) and may include targeted therapy (in cases with a V600 mutation of the oncogene BRAF) or immunotherapy.

Therapy of systemic metastases include immunotherapy with checkpoint inhibitors (anti-PD1 +/− anti-CTLA-4), targeted therapy (BRAF and MEK inhibitors) if BRAF V600 mutation is present (around half of the cases).

Follow-up: 5 years in intervals of 3–6 months with clinical examination and imaging, depending on risk group; looking for signs of recurrence and second primary melanomas, then life-long surveillance is recommended.

Prevention is based on the education of the population starting already in childhood including the parents, kindergarten and school. Important factors: sun protection factor cream, shadow, sunglasses, umbrella and UV-protecting clothes. Self-skin screening (ABCDE criteria), and skin screening of at-risk patients via themselves and partner/parents, and digital photo assessment. Governmental skin cancer screening campaigns. Telemedicine can be helpful for screening.

Kaposi's Sarcoma [12, 26]

Figures 13.33, 13.34, 13.35, 13.36 and 13.37

Grading of Importance

C

Level

Advanced

ICD-11

2B57.1

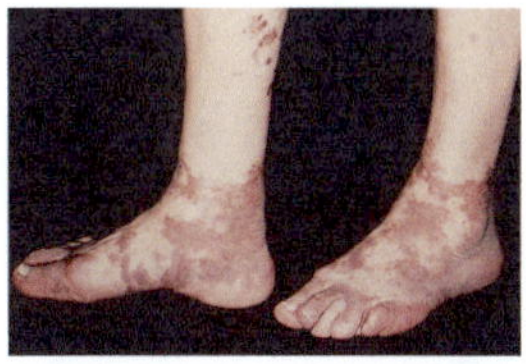

Fig. 13.33 Kaposi's sarcoma: plaque stage

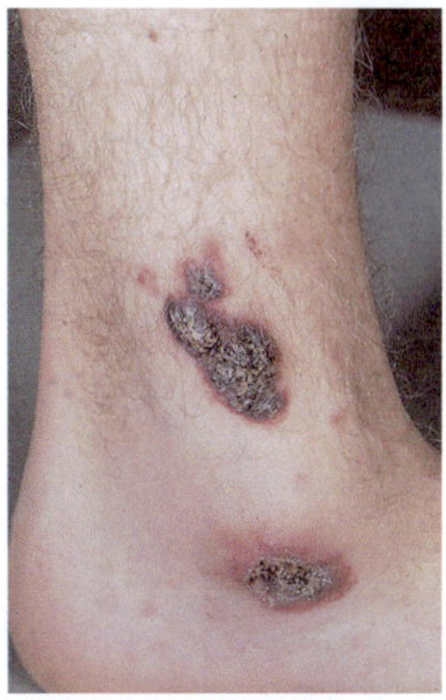

Fig. 13.34 Kaposi's sarcoma: hyperkeratotic lesions on the leg

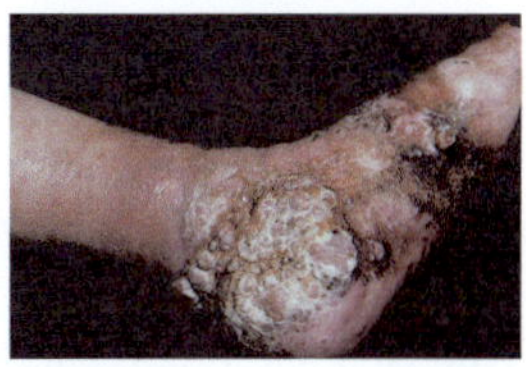

Fig. 13.35 Kaposi's sarcoma: tumorous stage

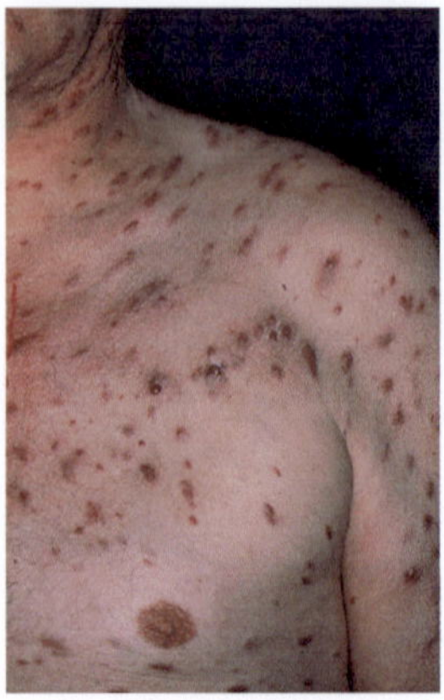

Fig. 13.36 Kaposi's sarcoma: small papules in AIDS-associated Kaposi

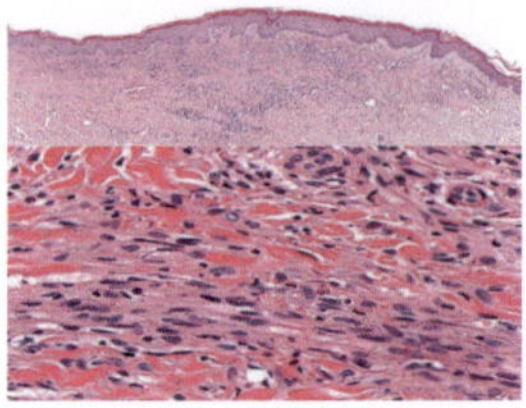

Fig. 13.37 Kaposi's sarcoma: histology showing proliferation of spindle cells

Synonyms

Sarcoma idiopathicum multiplex haemorrhagicum (old terminology).

Epidemiology

Rare disease, more common in HHV-8 endemic areas (Mediterranean, African) and in immunocompromised subjects.

Definition

Multifocal neoplasm of spindle-shaped lymphatic-endothelium-derived cells infected with HHV-8 (human herpes virus 8).

Aetiology and Pathogenesis

Kaposi's sarcoma is associated with HHV-8 infection. Immunosuppression is a well-known risk factor (HIV and transplantation).

Signs and Symptoms

Blue-red (purple) macules, plaques or tumours on the skin and mucosae, with or without lymphoedema.

Localisation

Classic Kaposi's sarcoma typically begins as nodules of the legs and has a slow progression. In immunosuppressed patients disseminated macules are frequently found on the skin and mucous membranes, along with involvement of lymph nodes, gastrointestinal or respiratory tract (lungs).

Classification

Kaposi's sarcoma is classified into four types:

- Classic Kaposi's sarcoma (older men in southeastern Europe and the Mediterranean basin).
- Endemic (African) Kaposi's sarcoma.
- HIV-associated (epidemic) Kaposi's sarcoma.
- Kaposi's sarcoma in immunosuppressed patients (iatrogenic) may occur, for example, in solid organ transplant recipients.

Laboratory and Other Workups

HIV serology and standard blood tests in all cases. HHV-8 viraemia and CD4 T cell count in epidemic (HIV) and iatrogenic forms.

Dermatopathology

Biopsy is mandatory: proliferation of spindle-cells that stain for endothelial cell markers such as CD34 and CD31. Immunohistochemistry against HHV-8 antigen.

Course

Classic, endemic: rare systemic involvement. Epidemic, iatrogenic: more frequent systemic involvement.

Complications

Untreated Kaposi sarcoma can show a local, slow progression. Lymphedema may occur. Visceral involvement (lung, oesophagus, colon) may lead to bleeding or breathing difficulties.

Diagnosis

Clinical features, histology and detection of HHV-8. A total body CT scan, with lung and digestive endoscopies can be performed depending on the clinical form.

Differential Diagnosis

Benign and malignant vascular tumours (angiosarcomas/lymphangiosarcomas), bacillary angiomatosis, T- and B-cell lymphomas, pseudo-Kaposi's sarcoma (acroangiodermatitis), described in more detail in section "Infantile Skin" in Chap. 25.

Pseudo-Kaposi sarcoma (acroangiodermatitis Mali) is a reactive process. It presents as red-brown (haemosiderin deposits) plaques on the back of the toes or on the ankle in patients with chronic venous insufficiency. Histology reveals the feature of stasis dermatitis with fibrosis and grouped capillary vessels.

Prevention and Therapy

Reduction of the immunosuppression in epidemic (antiretroviral therapy) and iatrogenic (reduction of immunosuppressants, switch to mTOR inhibitors) forms. In classic Kaposi sarcoma, no treatment is needed in many cases. Surgery or laser may be used to destroy lesions. Radiotherapy, intralesional chemotherapies and electrochemotherapy. Topical treatments such as imiquimod. Systemic treatments are reserved for locally aggressive extensive and disseminated Kaposi sarcoma: pegylated liposomal doxorubicin, paclitaxel, pegylated interferon.

Special

Interdisciplinary approach in epidemic forms of disseminated Kaposi sarcoma.

Dermatofibrosarcoma Protuberans [10]

Figure 13.38

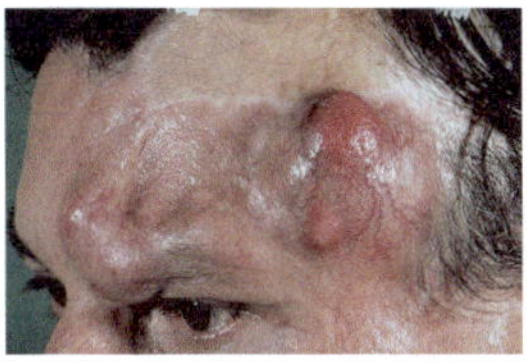

Fig. 13.38 Dermatofibrosarcoma protuberans: cutaneous subcutaneous nodules on the forehead

Grading of Importance

C

Level

Null

ICD-11

2B53.Y

Synonyms

DFSP

Epidemiology

Rare tumour, but on the skin the most frequent sarcoma type, panethnic, 1:100.000/year, male/female ratio 1:1,5, mean age around 40 years. Children mostly not affected.

Definition

Dermatofibrosarcoma protuberans (DFSP) is a rare usually non-metastising mesenchymal malignant tumour with an undermining-infiltrative, aggressive growth pattern and high local recurrence rate.

Aetiology and Pathogenesis

The cause of DFSP is unknown, but a traumatic initiation is discussed. A trauma has been reported in about 10–20% of cases. In 90% of cases a translocation of genetic material 17q22; 22q13 with fusion of genes COL1A1 and PDGFß has been detected. The gen product, a COL1A1-PDGFß- fusion protein, binds to a constitutive expressed PDGF-receptor acting thereafter as an autocrine growth stimulus for DFSP-cells. It usually does not metastasise (< 1%); however, it is highly aggressively growing horizontally in the surrounding, therefore classified as G2.

Signs and Symptoms

DFSP arises from deeper layers of the dermis. Typically, at the beginning, no subjective symptoms are reported. DFSP appears solitary and starts as a small, firm skin-coloured patch and may turn into purplish, reddish or flesh-coloured and is usually without clear margins. A rare variant is pigmented. The tumour grows slowly and infiltrative horizontally and polycyclic but becomes later a plaque and/or classical derma a big node. At late stage it can exulcerate.

Localisation

It is commonly found on the trunk, usually in the shoulder and chest area.

Classification

- Dermatofibrosarcoma protuberans, classical type
- Bednar tumour, pigmented type
- Myxoid type
- Pleomorphic—storiform type

Laboratory and Other Workups

None specific.

Dermatopathology

The biopsy is essential to diagnose the tumour. For the diagnosis, one needs a representative tart piece like biopsy; a punch biopsy is usually less helpful. By low power magnification, one can see the whole dermis infiltrating mesenchymal tumour composed of bundles of spindle cells. A fascicular and radiary growth produces the typical cartwheel pattern. Infiltrating the subcutis produces a honey comb pattern with large bundles of tumour cells surrounding the adipose cells. By immunohistochemistry, the tumour cells express the CD 34 antigen.

Course

A regular follow-up is essential after tumour removal to monitor for recurrence. Local relapses appear in 10–20% of DFSP's, usually within 3 years of the initial surgery. Despite being locally aggressive, the tumour spreads to other parts of the body (metastasises) in only 5% of cases.

Complications

Infiltration with joint involvement, exulceration. Scarring.

Diagnosis

Diagnosis relies on clinical features and dermatopathology.

Differential Diagnosis

- Nodular basal cell carcinoma
- Dermatofibroma including giant type
- Keloid
- Pleomorphic sarcomas, nodular B-cell lymphoma, pigmented or non-pigmented malignant melanoma (spindle cell type)

Prevention and Therapy

Treatment depends on size and localisation. Typically, it is treated with complete wide surgical excision of >3 cm (lowest recurrence rate of 7%); Mohs surgery (see section "Dermscopy") is performed dependent on localisation.

The chemotherapeutic agent imatinib mesylate is approved for adults with unresectable, recurrent or metastatic dermatofibrosarcoma protuberans.

Cutaneous Metastases [9]

Figures 13.39, 13.40, 13.41 and 13.42

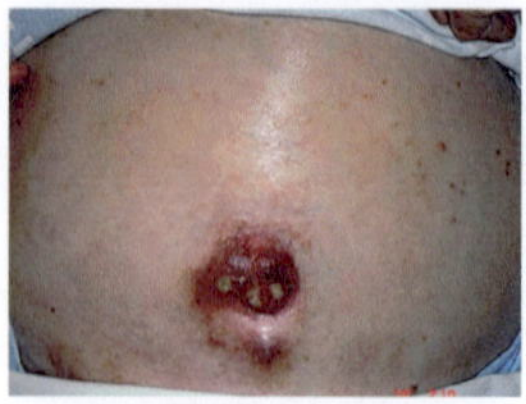

Fig. 13.39 Cutaneous metastases: sister Mary nodule in a patient with abdominal cancer

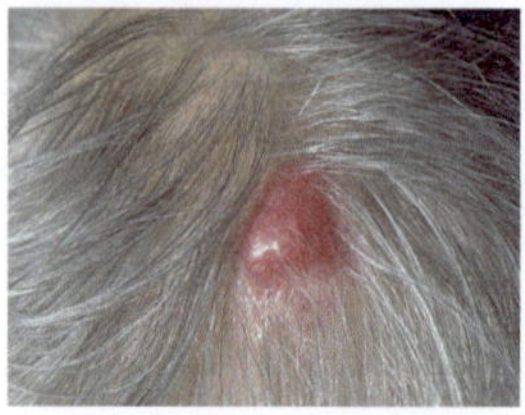

Fig. 13.40 Cutaneous metastases: metastasis on the scalp

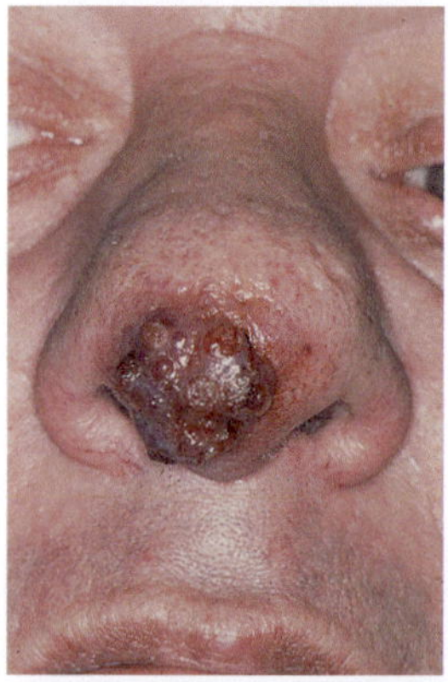

Fig. 13.41 Cutaneous metastases: hypernephroma metastasis in the nose

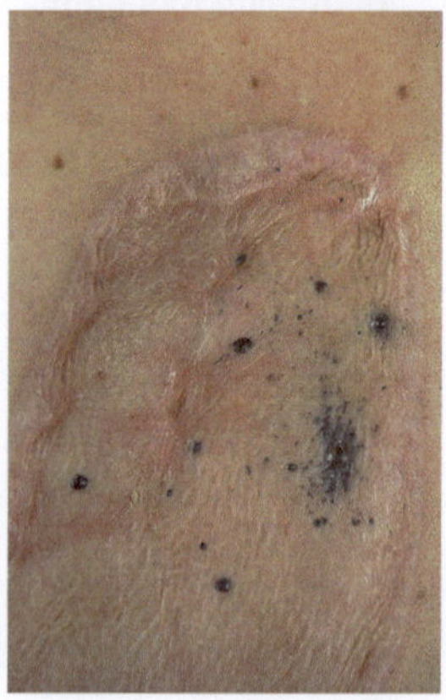

Fig. 13.42 Cutaneous metastases: satellite metastases after excision of a melanoma

Grading of Importance

C

Level

Advanced

ICD-11

2E08

Synonyms

Skin metastases.

Epidemiology

Prevalence is around 2%, incidence varying from 8 to 10%. In up to 10% of visceral tumours, skin metastases are the first sign, most commonly in carcinomas of the breast, colon and lung carcinomas as well as in leukaemias.

Definition

Cutaneous spread of malignant tumours of internal organs or haematological system, direct penetrating or via blood vessels, perineural sheet or lymphatics.

Aetiology and Pathogenesis

There is no clear pathological explanation why metastases spread to the skin except by direct penetrating. Some homing factors can play a role in leukaemia dissemination. Sometimes skin metastases home into herpes zoster scars.

Signs and Symptoms

Solitary or multiple, aggregated, zosteriform or disseminated firm blue-red to yellow papules and nodules in various levels of the skin with rapid growth with a short history. Sometimes erysipelas or lymphangiosis-like pattern (cancer en cuirasse) in breast cancer.

Localisation

If the skin metastasis is contiguous with the underlying primary, the precise type of cancer may be deduced.

Special localisations of metastasis

- Breast cancer metastases are often thoracic
- Prostate: suprapubic
- Sister Mary Joseph nodules located at the umbilicus derive from ovarian and gastro-intestinal origin

Oesophageal, gastric and colonic cancers, biliary tract, pulmonary and renal carcinomas prefer hairy scalp, neck and face.

Classification

No clear classification of cutaneous metastases.

Laboratory and Other Workups

Histological, immunohistochemical or molecular in conjunction with tumour screening.

Dermatopathology

Immunohistochemical profiling of tumour cells.

Course

Often metastases appear in tumour-free interval. Survival after detection of metastases in most cases less than 1 year.

Complications

Depending on the type of primary tumour, stage and pretreatment. Some metastases melt away, become necrotic, bleed or become superinfected.

Diagnosis

Metastasis has to be considered in case of a rapidly growing non-classifiable lesions in the skin.

Differential Diagnosis

Primary skin tumours and primary skin lymphomas, granulomatous infiltrates.

Prevention and Therapy

There is no prevention. Histological evaluation is a first step to decision algorithms for therapy of the primary tumour.

Special

Interdisciplinary approach and tumour boards must be involved.

Parapsoriasis Group [3, 4]

Figures 13.43, 13.44 and 13.45

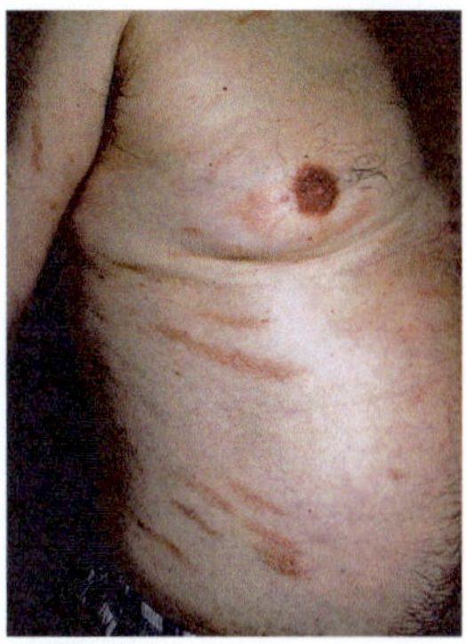

Fig. 13.43 Parapsoriasis: small plaques (patches) following the tension lines

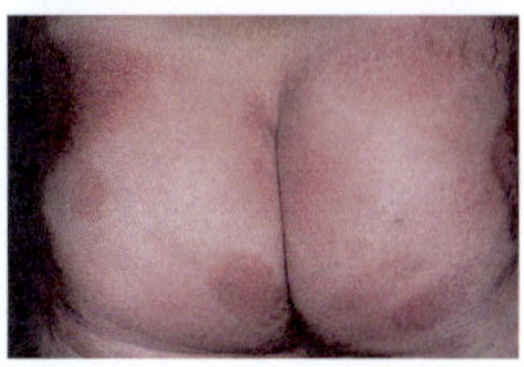

Fig. 13.44 Parapsoriasis: large plaques (mycosis fungoides)

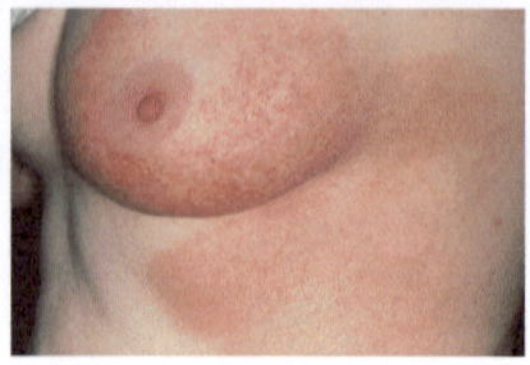

Fig. 13.45 Parapsoriasis: poikiloderma vasculare atrophicans

Grading of Importance

C

Level

Basic

ICD-11

Small Plaque Parapsoriasis (SPP) EA95
Large Plaque Parapsoriasis (LPP) EK91.0
Poikiloderma vasculare atrophicans (PVA) EK91.1

Synonyms

None

Epidemiology

Rare. Second half of life (>50 years).

Definition

The clinical picture and the terminology in some cases remain that of psoriasis, without any aetiopathogenetic relationship. However, there is a nosologic relationship to mycosis fungoides or other cutaneous T-cell lymphomas (CTCL).

Aetiology and Pathogenesis

Unknown.

Signs and Symptoms

SPP: Small red-brown, indolent (no itch), slightly scaling macules (1–2 cm), following the split skin lines.

LPP: large geographic irregular but sharply demarcated, slightly scaling macules or plaques; no itch.

PVA: Mottled slightly (pityriasiform) scaling erythematous patches.

Localisation

SPP: predominantly trunk; skin split lines.

LPP: predominantly trunk and upper extremities.

PVA: trunk or total skin.

Classification

Small plaque parapsoriasis: usually no evolution into CTCL

Large plaque parapsoriasis: potential precursor of CTCL (mycosis fungoides)

Poikiloderma atrophicans vasculare: potential precursor of CTCL (mycosis fungoides)

Laboratory and Other Workups

No special; biopsy.

Dermatopathology

Subtle eczematous changes of the epidermis with a few lymphocytes in the dermis and the epidermis. No band-like infiltrate in the papillary dermis. No lymphocyte microabscesses in the epidermis.

Course

Chronic over years or decades. Follow-up mandatory because of potential development into mycosis fungoides.

Complications

LPP and PVA may develop to CTCL, preferentially mycosis fungoides (after years or decades).

Diagnosis

Clinical picture, histopathology and course.

Differential Diagnosis

Atopic or seborrheic eczema, CTCL subtypes in particularmycosis fungoides, tinea corporis, pityriasis versicolor.

Prevention and Therapy

Prevention not possible. Topical therapy: photo-(helio-) or photochemotherapy. Glucocorticosteroid-cream temporarily.

Cutaneous Lymphoma [15, 6, 22, 5, 8, 17, 32]

Figures 13.46, 13.47, 13.48, 13.49 and 13.50

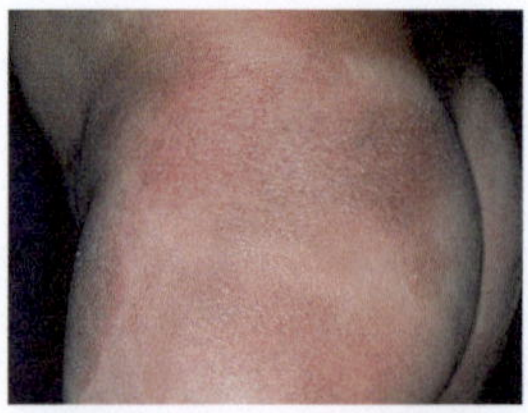

Fig. 13.46 Cutaneous lymphoma: mycosis fungoides, patch stage

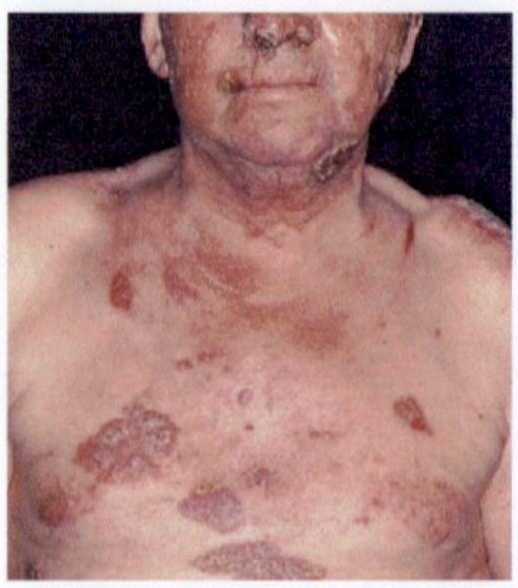

Fig. 13.47 Cutaneous lymphoma: mycosis fungoides, plaque stage

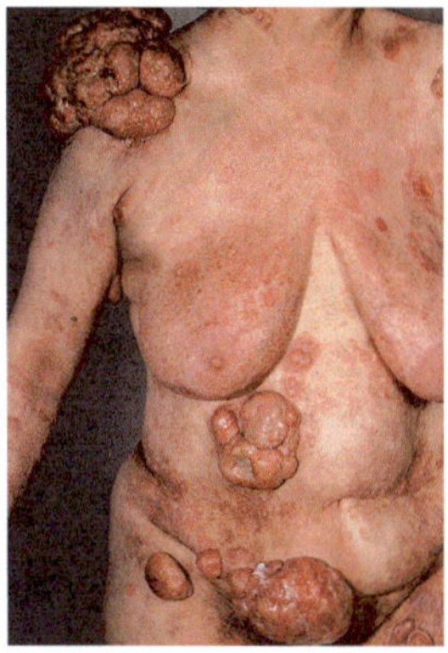

Fig. 13.48 Cutaneous lymphoma: mycosis fungoides, tumor stage

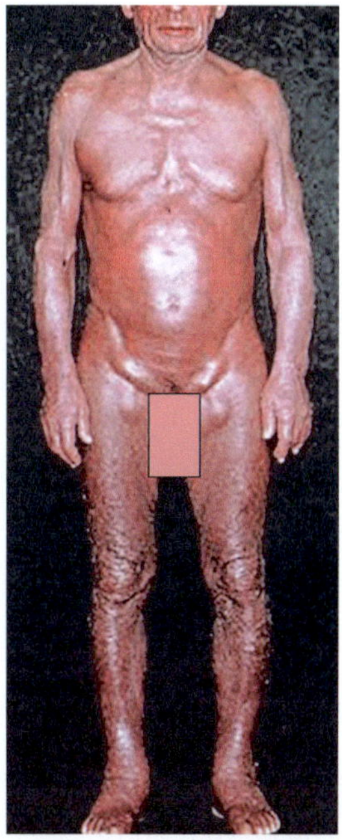

Fig. 13.49 Cutaneous lymphoma: Sézary syndrome

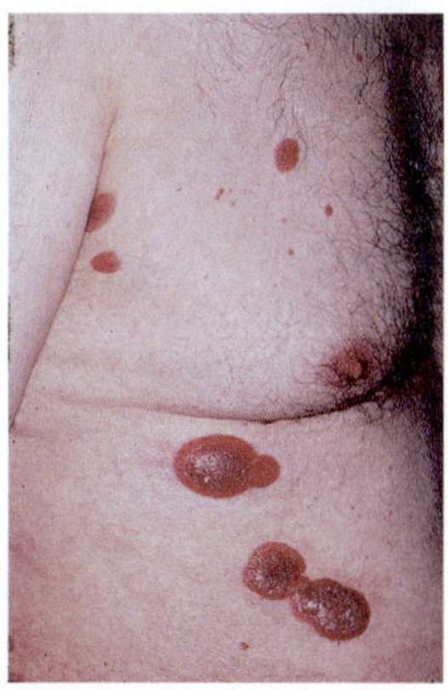

Fig. 13.50 Cutaneous lymphoma: cutaneous B-cell lymphoma

Grading of Importance

C

Level

Advanced

ICD-11

2B33.5

Synonyms

Cutaneous T-cell lymphomas (CTCL), cutaneous B-cell lymphomas (CBCL).

Epidemiology

Rare diseases (1/100000).

Definition

Cutaneous lymphomas are a heterogeneous group of non-Hodgkin lymphomas that primarily involve the skin.

Aetiology and Pathogenesis

Unknown in most cases. Older age, viral infection in some cases (HTLV-1, EBV). Antigen persistence.

Signs and Symptoms

Symptoms of primary cutaneous lymphomas vary depending on the subtype.

Erythematous, hypopigmented or poikilodermic macules or patches with mild scaling can be found in mycosis fungoides (the most frequent CTCL). In advanced stages nodules develop. Pruritus is frequent. Erythroderma is characteristic for Sézary syndrome.

B-cell lymphomas characteristically appear with dome-shaped red papules and nodules, which may become large aggregates.

Localisation

Cutaneous lymphomas can appear anywhere on the body; localisation may depend on the subtype of lymphoma. Early mycosis fungoides is located on sun-protected areas.

Classification

Primary cutaneous lymphomas are classified by the WHO-EORTC classification system. CTCL account for approximately 75% of the cases, of which mycosis fungoides is the most frequent one. The remaining 25% are CBCL or some other rare subtypes of lymphoproliferative diseases.

Laboratory and Other Workups

Serologic testing for lymphotropic viruses (HIV, EBV, HTLV-1), LDH, flow cytometry (CD3, CD4, CD8, loss of CD26 and CD7), T- or B-cell clonality in skin and blood by PCR tests or high throughput sequencing. Staging should be according to the TNMB (tumour node metastasis blood) classification.

Dermatopathology

Cutaneous lymphomas are a proliferation of lymphocytes with variable size, atypia, architecture and immunophenotype, depending on the subtype.

CTCL: infiltrate of small to medium mononuclear cells with mild to moderate atypia in the upper dermis with epidermotropism (T-cell pattern). Immunohistochemistry is used to describe the cell of origin (e.g. anti-CD3 for T cells, CD20 for B cells) and the histological subtype.

CBCL: mostly circumscribed nodular lymphocytic infiltrates in the dermis without epidermotropism (B-cell pattern) and with or without follicular structure.

Course

Prognosis of primary cutaneous lymphomas depends on the subtype and stage and is generally considered better than primary nodal lymphomas. The majority of mycosis fungoides and CBCL cases have an indolent evolution.

Complications

Many cutaneous lymphomas show no or slow evolvement. Erythroderma types are accompanied with severe pruritus and often loss of protein and trace elements via desquamation. Large nodular aggregates at groin or axillary regions can stop lymph drainage. In case of advanced-stage or aggressive form, immunosuppression may lead to cutaneous and systemic infections. Extracutaneous, systemic lymphoma progression (nodal involvement, visceral involvement) may occur.

Diagnosis

The precise diagnosis of cutaneous lymphomas is always obtained by clinical-histological correlation.

Differential Diagnosis

Differential diagnoses for patch stage mycosis fungoides: contact dermatitis, atopic dermatitis, psoriasis, parapsoriasis, pseudolymphomas. In tumour stage CTCL or CBCL: other primary or secondary lymphomas or other tumours.

Prevention and Therapy

The treatment should be adjusted to the subtype (indolent or aggressive), topical or systemic, and stage (early or advanced).

Skin-directed treatments (topical corticosteroids, phototherapy, topical chlormethine/carmustine/nitrogen mustard) in early stage mycosis fungoides.

Systemic treatments (methotrexate, bexarotene, peg interferon), radiotherapy, HDAC (histone deacetylase) inhibitors, immunotherapies (photopheresis in erythrodermic subtypes, monoclonal antibodies) or chemotherapy in advanced stage.

Indolent, localised B-cell lymphomas may be treated by surgical excision, radiation therapy, topical steroids; rituximab (anti-CD20 antibody) in disseminated cases. Aggressive B-cell lymphomas usually require rituximab and polychemotherapy.

Special

Early aggressive treatment modalities must be avoided, unless systemic involvement has been documented (blood, lymph nodes, internal organs).

Lymphomatoid Papulosis [19]

Figure 13.51

Grading of Importance

C

Level

Basic

ICD-11

2B03.1

Synonyms

Continuing self-healing eruption, clinically benign, histologically malignant

Epidemiology

Prevalence 0.1–0.2/100,000; all age groups; predominantly young adults; M > F.

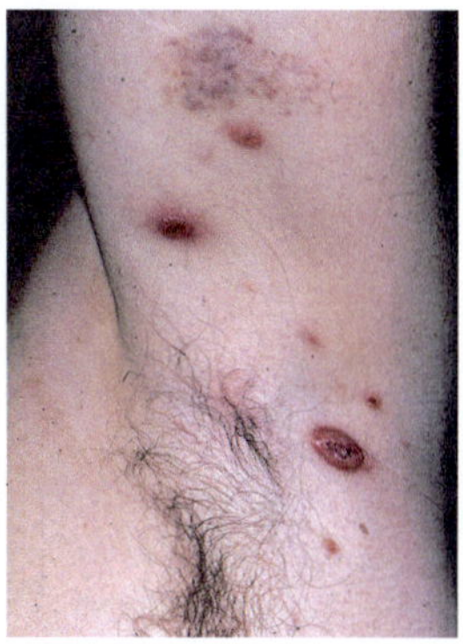

Fig. 13.51 Lymphomatoid papulosis: self-regressing papules and nodules

Definition

Chronic recurrent, self-healing papulo-nodular skin eruption with histologic features of a malignant anaplastic lymphoma; CD30 (Ki-1) positive.

Nosologic relationship to pityriasis lichenoides et varioliformis acuta (PLEVA), to other CD30-positive malignant T-cell lymphomas and to Hodgkin's disease.

Aetiology and Pathogenesis

Unknown.

Signs and Symptoms

Disseminated papules and/or small nodules, which within days or a few weeks become red-brown, haemorrhagic or pustular and finally undergo ulceration, followed by complete spontaneous regression of the lesions, occasionally leaving behind hyper- or hypopigmented varioliform scars.

Localisation

Trunk, buttocks, extremities.

Classification

Histological and immunocytochemical subtypes: Types A-E and Type 6p25.3 (genetic).

Laboratory and Other Workups

Biopsy; immunocytochemistry (CD30).

Dermatopathology

Broad spectrum with variably dense infiltrates of medium-sized to large atypical pleomorphic CD30+ cells are the hallmarks of the disease. Depending on the lesion's stage of evolution, the histological presentation is different. In fresh lesions, there is a wedge-shaped infiltrate of tumour cells with ulceration.

Various subtypes (see Classification).

Course

Chronic recurrent over decades.

Complications

Transformation to Hodgkin's disease. Threat of overtreatment due to confusion with malignant anaplastic lymphoma.

Diagnosis

Clinically; typical spontaneous regressions and recurrences of lesions.

Differential Diagnosis

Malignant anaplastic T-cell lymphoma (CD30 positive); CD30-positive pseudolymphomatous reactions (scabies); Hodgkin's disease (histology).

Prevention and Therapy

Prevention not possible. The prognosis is quoad vitam excellent; permanent healing not possible, only temporary clearing. Follow-up with respect to possible transformation to Hodgkin's disease (very rare).

Temporary clearing: Methotrexate (10–20 mg/week); photo- or photochemotherapy.

Skin care and prevention of superinfection; erosive lesions may be treated with antibiotic weak glucocorticosteroid crème.

Special

It is important to avoid aggressive systemic (cytostatics, bone marrow transplantation) therapy, based on misdiagnosis.

Pseudolymphoma (Not *Borrelia* Induced) [21]

Figure 13.52

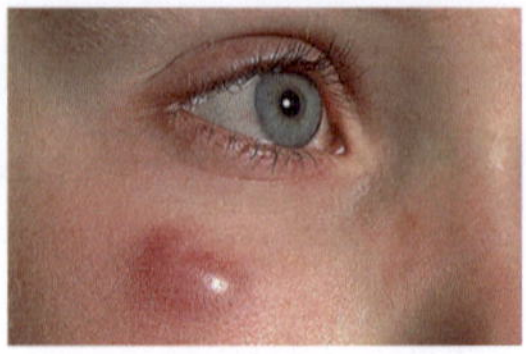

Fig. 13.52 Pseudolymphoma: nodular lesion on the cheek 3 weeks after tick bite

Grading of Importance

B

Level

Basic

ICD-11

4A43.0

Synonyms

Lymphocytic infiltration, lymphoid hyperproliferation.

Epidemiology

Clear epidemiological data lacking.

Definition

Reactive pseudolymphomatous infiltrate of B-, T-, and combined T-/B-cell type with or without follicular structures in the dermis and subcutis, mimicking malignant lymphoma.

Aetiology and Pathogenesis

In pseudolymphoma B and T lymphocytes and other inflammatory cells accumulate in the dermis and subcutis as a reaction to various stimuli: reactions to tattoo dyes, arthropods, systemic medications, infections (syphilis) or vaccinations.

A specific subset of B-cell pseudolymphoma is *Borrelia burgdorferi* subsp. *afzelii* and *garinii* induced lymphocytoma, primarily in Europe in areas endemic for the vector tick *Ixodes ricinus* (see section "Lymphadenosis Cutis Benigna" in Chap. 7).

Signs and Symptoms

Different forms: localised erythematous macules sometimes confluent, nodules, plaques; occasionally with lymphadenopathy.

Localisation

Sites of predilection depending on the underlying trigger: localised (facial), single or multiple, disseminated.

Classification

No international classification.

B -, T-, and B–/T-cell-dominated subtypes.

Laboratory and Other Workups

Borrelia IgG and IgM titres raised in *Borrelia* lymphocytoma. In lymphocytic infiltration immunoserology to exclude lupus erythematosus and blood count for leukaemic infiltrate.

Dermatopathology

Most important to differentiate the subtypes of pseudolymphomas and to exclude primary or secondary malignant B-or T-cell lymphomas, eosinophils and plasma cells in a polymorphous pattern suggest pseudolymphoma.

Course

Spontaneous regression in most cases after cessation of drugs or underlying cause (e.g. scabies, syphilis).

Complications

None.

Diagnosis

Clinical features, serology, histology, PCR.

Differential Diagnosis

Malignant primary and secondary B–/ T-cell lymphomas, disseminated cutaneous sarcoidosis, stage II syphilis.

Prevention and Therapy

Depending on subtype.

Cessation of responsible drugs, removal of causative agent or treatment of infection (syphilis, scabies). Topical mid and high potency corticosteroids. Occasionally intralesional steroids.

Paraneoplastic Disorders [31]

Figures 13.53, 13.54, 13.55 and 13.56

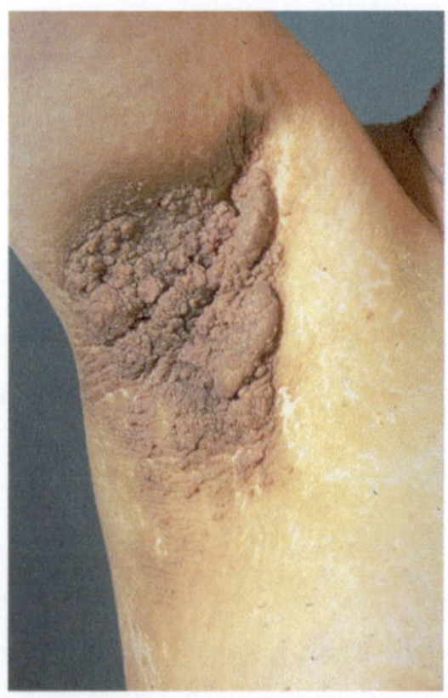

Fig. 13.53 Paraneoplastic disorders: malignant acanthosis nigricans

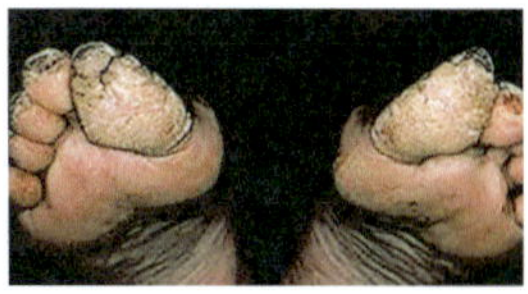

Fig. 13.54 Paraneoplastic disorders: acrokeratosis paraneoplastica of Bazex

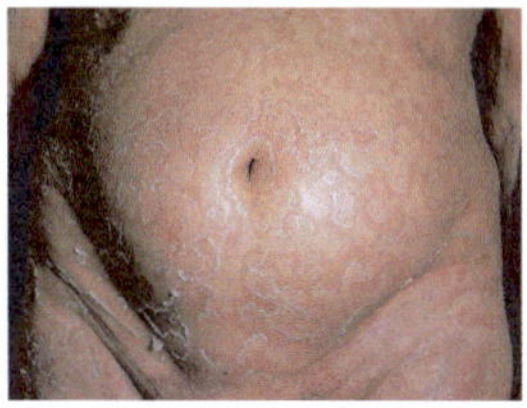

Fig. 13.55 Paraneoplastic disorders: erythema gyratum repens

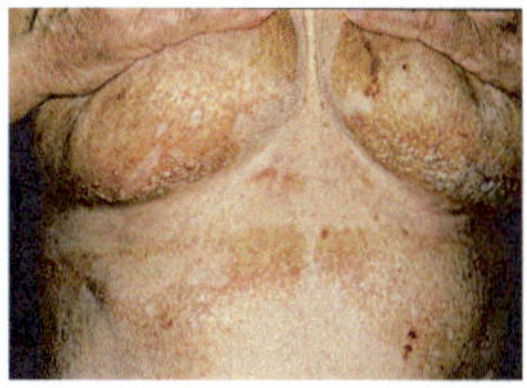

Fig. 13.56 Paraneoplastic disorders: Nazzaro-syndrome in plasmacytoma

Grading of Importance

C

Level

Advanced

ICD-11

EL10

Synonyms

Cutaneous markers of internal malignancy.

Epidemiology

No clear data in general; however, prevalence of association of skin signs with the individual neoplasm exists.

Definition

Cutaneous markers for underlying malignancies (not including metastases). Simultaneous improvement when neoplastic proliferation is removed or treated and recurrence with tumour progression.

Aetiology and Pathogenesis

- Genetically determined syndromes with a cutaneous component (genodermatoses) that predispose individuals at-risk for developing cancer
- Paraneoplastic syndromes which occur as a result of circulating factor(s) or presumed factors produced by the underlying cancer
- Factors related to neoplastic disorders are: immune reaction and production of tumour-associated antibodies from tumour or lymphoma cells or certain cytokines, enzymes, embryonic or foetal or other growth factors / proteins, hormones or precursors substances

Signs and Symptoms

Different depending on the underlying disease.

Localisation

The localisation may be localised or generalised, mostly symmetrical.

Classification

- Obligate paraneoplastic disorders/syndromes (almost 100% tumour-associated): Necrolytic migratory erythema (glucagonoma syndrome), acrokeratosis paraneoplastica of Bazex, acanthosis nigricans maligna, paraneoplastic pemphigus, erythema gyratum repens, hypertrichosis lanuginosa acquisita, Nazzaro syndrome in plasmacytoma
- Obligate paraneoplastic genodermatoses/syndromes: Birt–Hogg–Dubé syndrome, Cowden disease, Gardner syndrome, basal cell naevus syndrome, Peutz-Jeghers syndrome, Torre-Muir syndrome.

- Facultative paraneoplastic disorders (less reliable markers, but still deserve investigation): Ichthyosis acquisita, thrombophlebitis migrans, dermatomyositis in adults, bullous pemphigoid, Sweet's syndrome, paraneoplastic pruritus, endocrine flushing (carcinoid).

Laboratory and Other Workups

The laboratory workup is depending of the suspected tumour which includes skin biopsy, immunofluorescence, immunoblotting and tumour markers; haematological screening.

Dermatopathology

Depends on various types (see Classification)

Course

Depending on type of paraneoplastic disorder. Removal of tumour can lead to complete resolution of symptoms.

Complications

Depending on underlying neoplasm.

Diagnosis

Clinical picture (see Classification).

Differential Diagnosis

The clinical picture resembles the picture of a skin disorder; therefore, a great variety has to be excluded.

Prevention and Therapy

No prevention possible despite early detection by regular tumour prevention programs. Family members of some syndromes with genetical background need to be regularly checked.

Therapy depends on underlying tumour or haematological disease.

Special

Interdisciplinary workup.

References

1. Abbas O, Miller DD, Bhawan J (2014) Cutaneous malignant melanoma: update on diagnostic and prognostic biomarkers. Am J Dermatopathol 36(5):363–379
2. Bhawan J (2007) Squamous cell carcinoma in situ in skin: what does it mean? J Cutan Pathol 34(12):953–955
3. Burg G, Dummer R (1995) Small plaque (digitate) parapsoriasis is an 'abortive cutaneous T-cell lymphoma' and is not mycosis fungoides. Arch Dermatol 131(3):336–338
4. Burg G, Dummer R, Haeffner A, Kempf W, Kadin M (2001) From inflammation to neoplasia: mycosis fungoides evolves from reactive inflammatory conditions (lymphoid infiltrates) transforming into neoplastic plaques and tumors. Arch Dermatol 137(7):949–952
5. Burg G, Kempf W (eds) (2005) Cutaneous lymphomas. Boca Radon, London, New York, Singapore, Marcel Dekker, Taylor & Francis
6. Burg G, Kempf W, Cozzio A, Feit J, Willemze R, Jaffe ES, Dummer R, Berti E, Cerroni L, Chimenti S, Diaz-Perez JL, Grange F, Harris NL, Kazakov DV, Kerl H, Kurrer M, Knobler R, Meijer CJ, Pimpinelli N, Ralfkiaer E, Russell-Jones R, Sander C, Santucci M, Sterry W, Swerdlow SH, Vermeer MH, Wechsler J, Whittaker S (2005) WHO/EORTC classification of cutaneous lymphomas 2005: histological and molecular aspects. J Cutan Pathol 32(10):647–674
7. de Oliveira ECV, da Motta VRV, Pantoja PC, Ilha CSO, Magalhaes RF, Galadari H, Leonardi GR (2019) Actinic keratosis – review for clinical practice. Int J Dermatol 58(4):400–407
8. Dummer R, Vermeer MH, Scarisbrick JJ, Kim YH, Stonesifer C, Tensen CP, Geskin LJ, Quaglino P, Ramelyte E (2021) Cutaneous T cell lymphoma. Nat Rev Dis Primers 7(1):61
9. Habermehl G, Ko J (2019) Cutaneous metastases: a review and diagnostic approach to tumors of unknown origin. Arch Pathol Lab Med 143(8):943–957
10. Hao X, Billings SD, Wu F, Stultz TW, Procop GW, Mirkin G, Vidimos AT (2020) Dermatofibrosarcoma protuberans: update on the diagnosis and treatment. J Clin Med 9(6)
11. Hartman RI, Lin JY (2019) Cutaneous melanoma-a review in detection, staging, and management. Hematol Oncol Clin North Am 33(1):25–38
12. Hoffmann C, Sabranski M, Esser S (2017) HIV-associated Kaposi's sarcoma. Oncol Res Treat 40(3):94–98
13. Kallini JR, Jain SK, Khachemoune A (2013) Lentigo maligna: review of salient characteristics and management. Am J Clin Dermatol 14(6):473–480
14. Kasprzak JM, Xu YG (2015) Diagnosis and management of lentigo maligna: a review. Drugs Context 4:212281
15. Kempf W, Zimmermann AK, Mitteldorf C (2019) Cutaneous lymphomas—an update 2019. Hematol Oncol 37(Suppl 1):43–47
16. Kim DP, Kus KJB, Ruiz E (2019) Basal cell carcinoma review. Hematol Oncol Clin North Am 33(1):13–24
17. LeBoit P, Burg G, Weedon D, Sarasin A (eds) (2006) Tumors of the skin. WHO Books. WHO IARC, Lyon
18. Lopes Filho LL, Lopes IM, Lopes LR, Enokihara MM, Michalany AO, Matsunaga N (2015) Mammary and extramammary Paget's disease. An Bras Dermatol 90(2):225–231
19. Martinez-Cabriales SA, Walsh S, Sade S, Shear NH (2020) Lymphomatoid papulosis: an update and review. J Eur Acad Dermatol Venereol 34(1):59–73
20. Marzuka AG, Book SE (2015) Basal cell carcinoma: pathogenesis, epidemiology, clinical features, diagnosis, histopathology, and management. Yale J Biol Med 88(2):167–179

21. Mitteldorf C, Kempf W (2020) Cutaneous pseudolymphoma—a review on the spectrum and a proposal for a new classification. J Cutan Pathol 47(1):76–97
22. Olsen E, Vonderheid E, Pimpinelli N, Willemze R, Kim Y, Knobler R, Zackheim H, Duvic M, Estrach T, Lamberg S, Wood G, Dummer R, Ranki A, Burg G, Heald P, Pittelkow M, Bernengo MG, Sterry W, Laroche L, Trautinger F, Whittaker S, Iscl/Eortc (2007) Revisions to the staging and classification of mycosis fungoides and Sezary syndrome: a proposal of the International Society for Cutaneous Lymphomas (ISCL) and the cutaneous lymphoma task force of the European Organization of Research and Treatment of Cancer (EORTC). Blood 110(6):1713–1722
23. Que SKT, Zwald FO, Schmults CD (2018) Cutaneous squamous cell carcinoma: Incidence, risk factors, diagnosis, and staging. J Am Acad Dermatol 78(2):237–247
24. Rastrelli M, Tropea S, Rossi CR, Alaibac M (2014) Melanoma: epidemiology, risk factors, pathogenesis, diagnosis and classification. In Vivo 28(6):1005–1011
25. Rubin AI, Chen EH, Ratner D (2005) Basal-cell carcinoma. N Engl J Med 353(21):2262–2269
26. Safai B, Good RA (1981) Kaposi's sarcoma: a review and recent developments. CA Cancer J Clin 31(1):2–12
27. Samaniego E, Redondo P (2013) Lentigo maligna. Actas Dermosifiliogr 104(9):757–775
28. Siegel JA, Korgavkar K, Weinstock MA (2017) Current perspective on actinic keratosis: a review. Br J Dermatol 177(2):350–358
29. Smalberger GJ, Siegel DM, Khachemoune A (2008) Lentigo maligna. Dermatol Ther 21(6):439–446
30. Waldman A, Schmults C (2019) Cutaneous Squamous Cell Carcinoma. Hematol Oncol Clin North Am 33(1):1–12
31. Wick MR, Patterson JW (2019) Cutaneous paraneoplastic syndromes. Semin Diagn Pathol 36(4):211–228
32. Willemze R, Jaffe ES, Burg G, Cerroni L, Berti E, Swerdlow SH, Ralfkiaer E, Chimenti S, Diaz-Perez JL, Duncan LM, Grange F, Harris NL, Kempf W, Kerl H, Kurrer M, Knobler R, Pimpinelli N, Sander C, Santucci M, Sterry W, Vermeer MH, Wechsler J, Whittaker S, Meijer CJ (2005) WHO-EORTC classification for cutaneous lymphomas. Blood 105(10):3768–3785

Part IV

Diseases of the Appendages and of the Mucous Membranes

Various glands, hair and nails represent the skin appendages, which are the morphologic basis for various types of diseases and changes. Diseases of mucous membranes are confined to the nose, mouth and genito-anal regions.

Diseases of Sebaceous and Apocrine Glands

14

Harald Gollnick and Christos C. Zouboulis

Contents

H. Gollnick (✉)
Department of Dermatology & Venereology, Otto-von-Guericke University, Magdeburg, Germany
e-mail: Harald.Gollnick@med.ovgu.de

C. C. Zouboulis
Departments of Dermatology, Venereology, Allergology and Immunology, Staedtisches Klinikum Dessau, Brandenburg Medical School Theodor Fontane and Faculty of Health Sciences Brandenburg, Dessau, Germany
e-mail: christos.zouboulis@mhb-fontane.de

H. Gollnick et al. (eds.), *Dermatology Cyberderm WebBook*,
https://doi.org/10.1007/978-3-031-78491-0_14

Test your learning and check your understanding of this book's contents: use the "Springer Nature Flashcards" app to access questions using ▶ https://sn.pub/1rhh6k.

To use the app, please follow the instructions in Chap. 1.

Acne

Figures 14.1, 14.2, 14.3, 14.4, 14.5, 14.6, 14.7, 14.8, 14.9 and 14.10

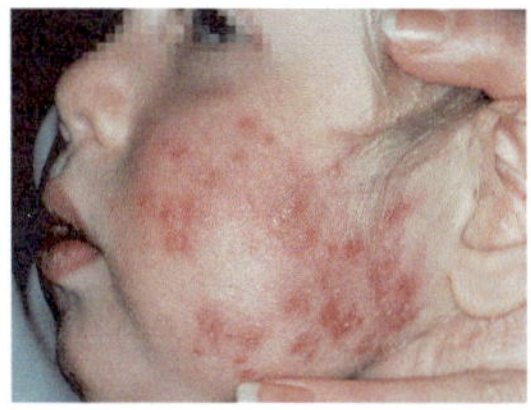

Fig. 14.1 Acne: infantum type

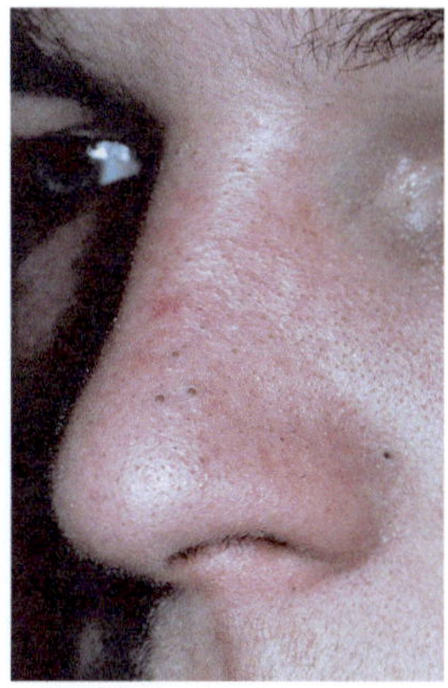

Fig. 14.2 Acne: nose involvement with some black heads

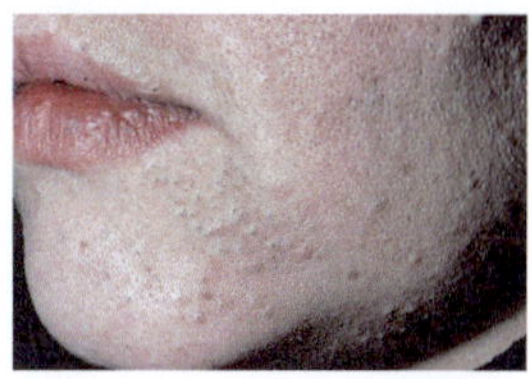

Fig. 14.3 Acne: comedonica, white and black heads

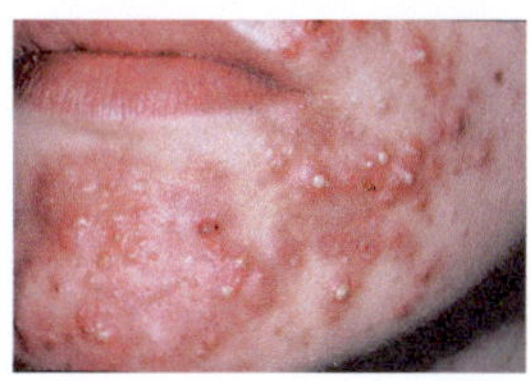

Fig. 14.4 Acne: papulo-pustulosa with small nodules

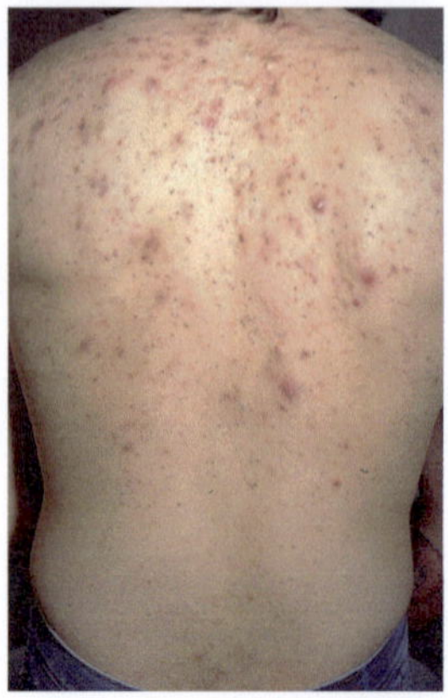

Fig. 14.5 Acne: conglobate type, back, nodes and cysts ,fistular comedones

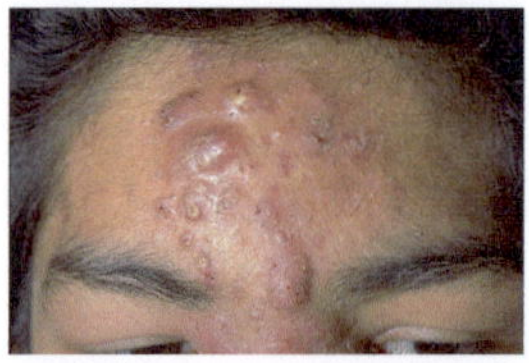

Fig. 14.6 Acne: conglobate, forehead, confluent sinuses

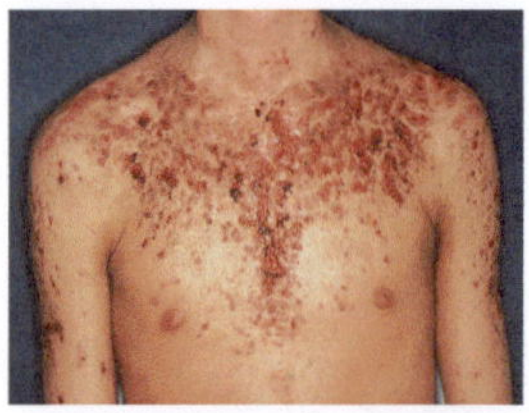

Fig. 14.7 Acne: fulminans type with hemorrhagic crusting

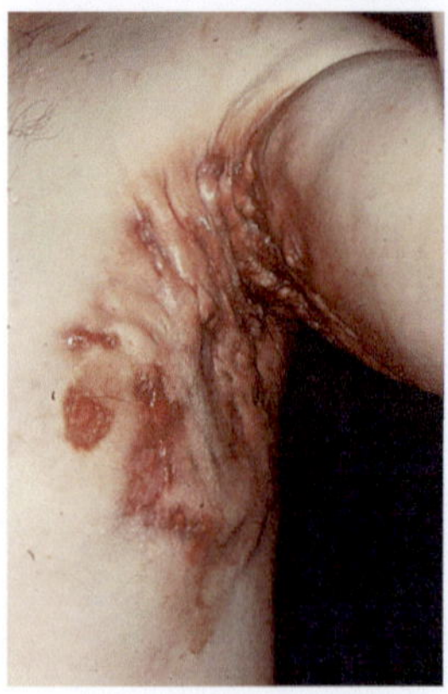

Fig. 14.8 Acne: tetrade, hidradenitis suppurativa Hurley grade III

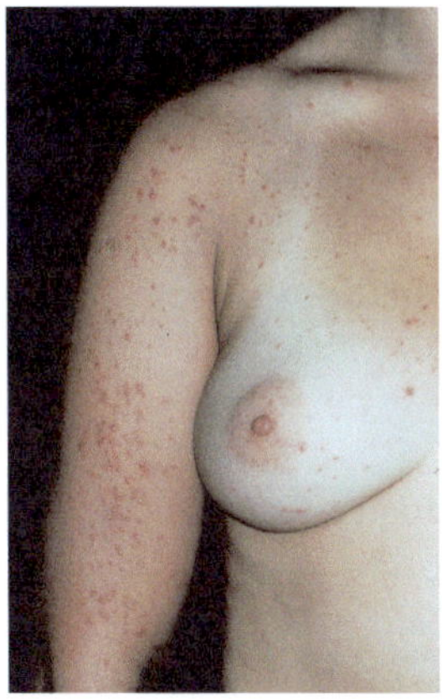

Fig. 14.9 Acne: "Mallorca"-Acne

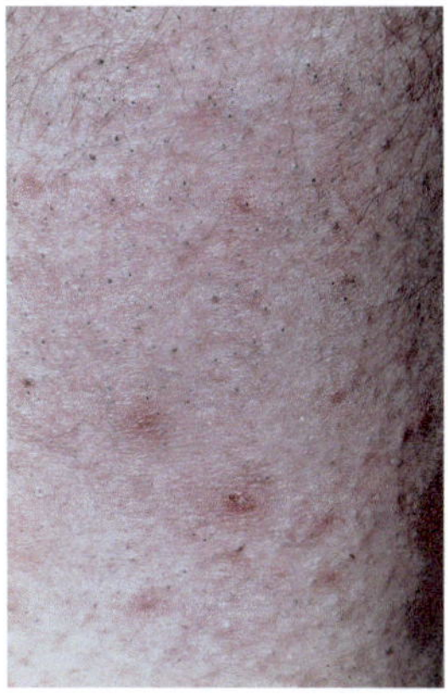

Fig. 14.10 Acne: due to tar

Grading of Importance

B

Level

Advanced

ICD-11

ED80Z

Synonyms

Pimples, spots.

Epidemiology

Very common; highest prevalence in the 16- to 18-year-old adolescents with about 85%. It may sometimes occur in small children and adults (30%) in the third and fourth decade of life.

Definition

Chronic, highly heritable inflammatory disease of the sebaceous follicles appearing in puberty. One can distinguish between physiological acne (60–70%) as an almost normal variant from clinical acne (30–40%) that needs medical care.

Aetiology and Pathogenesis

Genetic predisposition and hormonal stimulation (androgens) lead to:

- Seborrhoea as a result of increased proliferation and change of differentiation of sebocytes caused by androgens and insulin growth factor followed by increased production of sebum including ceramides, squalenes and cholesterol. Release of inflammatory mediators.
- Proliferation of follicular keratinocytes (response to androgen and growth signals), retention hyperkeratosis, keratin- and integrin-pattern disturbance.
- Low oxygen saturation and sebum components promote the proliferation of *Cutibacterium acnes* in the infra-infundibulum. Specific *C. acnes* strains drive the inflammation. Increased expression of TLR-2 and 4 and other danger signals. IL-1 α and *C. acnes* mediators drive inflammation and corneocytes to hyperproliferate.
- Innate immune system reacts strongly. CD 4 and CD 17 T cells accumulate and invade the follicular wall. Later macrophages.

Nutritional factors can play a role: increased carbohydrate load with stimulation of IGF-1 and stimulation of androgens via nuclear factors (Fox O1) symptoms.

Signs and Symptoms

Precursor lesion is a microcomedo, which is not visible for the naked eye.

Primary lesion is a comedo: open comedones (blackheads), closed comedones (whiteheads). Papules, pustules, nodules, nodes, abscesses, fistulas, different types of scars, keloids.

Localisation

Face, chest, upper back.

Classification

Forms

- Acne comedonica: primarily comedones.
- Acne papulo-pustulosa: primarily papules and pustules mixed with comedones.
- Acne papulo-pustulosa nodosa: stronger inflamed and additionally with small nodules.
- Acne conglobata: nodular lesion predominate, scars, abscesses, fistulas, typical localisation (mid-face, shoulders, chest, upper back).

Special Forms

- Late-onset acne (a) persisting or (b) relapsing or (c) first onset. Most prominent in females. Often mild endocrinological dysfunctions. Sometimes evident with PCOS (polycystic ovary syndrome) and androgenic signs.
- Acne fulminans: fever, leukocytosis, arthralgias, immune-mediated vasculitis, sterile abscesses of bone, elevated CRP.
- Acne venenata: can be an occupational induced subtype. Induction, maintenance or aggravation of acne often by medications (e.g. corticosteroids), cosmetics, chlorinated organic compounds, iodine, oil, tar.
- Acne cosmetica: overwashing and overuse of cleansers. Occlusive cosmetics, Vaseline/petrolatum.
- Acne excoriée des jeunes filles: artefactual disorder with excoriations and papules around the mouth and chin, often marked emotional component, sometimes obsessive compulsion disorder.
- Acne neonatorum (common, relative hyperplasia of the adrenals in newborns).
- Infantile acne (after 1 year of age, uncommon, LH/FSH-induced raise in testosterone). Primary manifestation of adrenogenital syndrome.

The special acneiform-type acne inversa (Hidradenitis suppurativa) is discussed under diagnosis 4.1.4. It is characterised by inflammation of terminal hair follicles in intertriginous regions, which are rich in apocrine glands.

Acne tetrade = acne conglobata, acne keloidalis nuchae, pilonidal sinus and acne inversa.

Laboratory and Other Workups

In therapy-refractory acne, causes of elevated androgen levels (hormone-producing tumours, late onset adrenogenital syndrome, polycystic ovarian syndrome) should be excluded.

Dermatopathology

Usually not necessary. In comedonal and papulo-pustular acne sebaceous hyperplasia with infundibular widening and perifollicular lympho-mononuclear cells. Some cells invading the follicular wall. Depending on severity degree stronger perifollicular inflammation and microabcesses and scarring.

Course

Self-limited with downsizing at the end of the second life decade. Late type acne; see above.

Complications

Often marked emotional reaction. Increased risk for suicidal intention.

Scars (atrophic, keloids), fistulas, pigmentary changes, sometimes skin picking as an obsessive compulsory disorder and long-term psychiatric problems.

Diagnosis

Clinical findings.

Differential Diagnosis

Rosacea papulo-pustulosa, folliculitis of face and trunk, beard folliculitis. Gram-negative folliculitis. Ulerythema ophryogenes. Prurigo-type of atopic dermatitis.

PRIDE syndrome: following therapy with EGF receptor agonists.

Acne aestivalis ("Mallorca acne"): is not an acne, but an acneiform reaction in predisposed persons who develop follicular irritation from sun creams and UV exposure, itchy; comedones are lacking.

Prevention and Therapy

Basic topical therapy in comedonic acne with retinoids (comedolytic, anticomedogenic and anti- inflammatory). Alternatively azelaic acid.

Papulo-pustular acne grades I or II: treat sequentially or with combined preparations containing retinoids, benzoyl peroxide, and azelaic acid. Never use topical antibiotics as monotherapy (development of bacterial resistance).

Papulo-pustular acne with nodules: treat always combined topically and systemically (oral tetracycline such as doxycycline which has strong anti-inflammatory effects).

Acne conglobata: Isotretinoin as first choice. Systemic tetracycline combined with retinoids and benzoyl peroxide; in women consider antiandrogens (e.g. cyproterone acetate, or drospirenone combined with estrogens).

Treatment of atrophic and hypertrophic scars: chemical peels (TCA peels 20–30%), dermabrasion, microneedling, CO-2 laser, fillers, surgical defect elevation for depressed scars. Maintenance treatment to prevent relapses essential, above all topical retinoids for the prevention of the development of microcomedones.

Rosacea [2, 5]

Figures 14.12, 14.13, 14.14 and 14.15

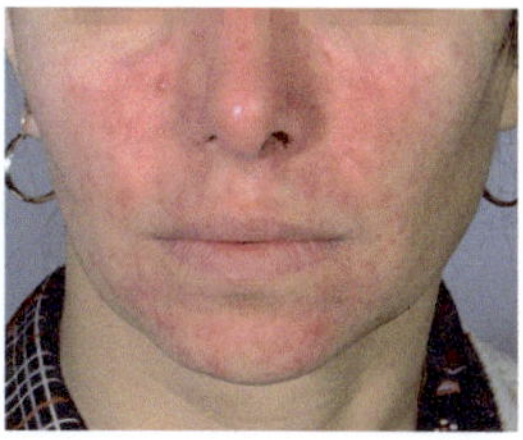

Fig. 14.11 Rosacea: facial erythema

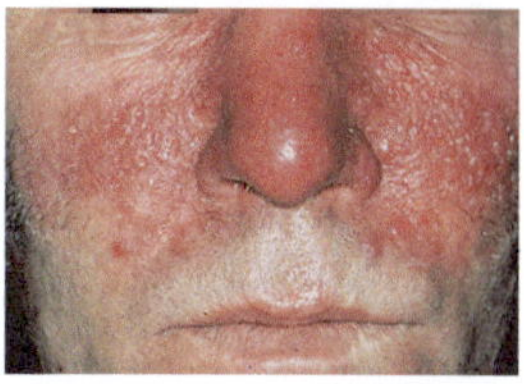

Fig. 14.12 Rosacea: centrofacial papules (butterfly distribution)

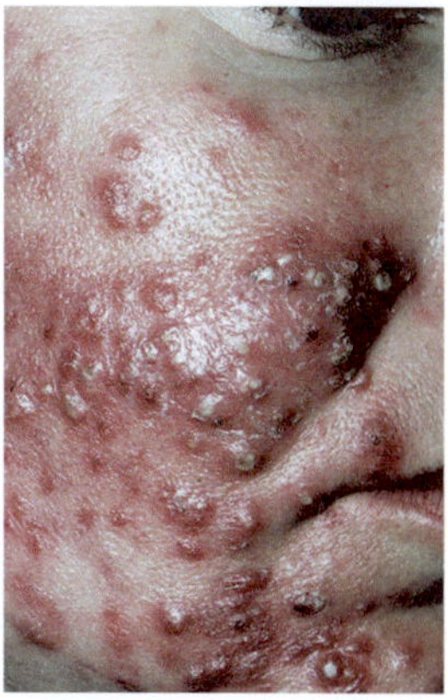

Fig. 14.13 Rosacea: pustular eruptions with confluence

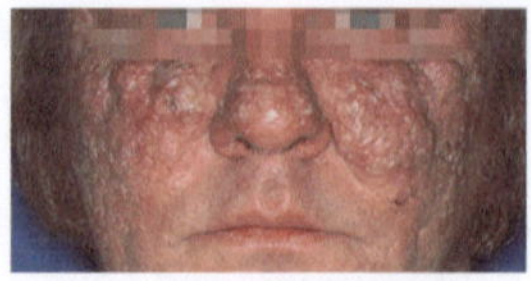

Fig. 14.14 Rosacea: conglobate type , chronic type with cysts and scars

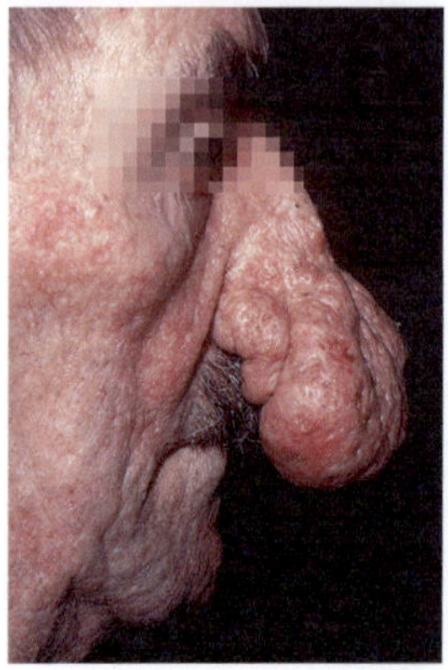

Fig. 14.15 Rosacea: rhinophyma grade III

Grading of Importance

B

Level

Advanced

ICD-11

ED90

Synonyms

Couperose.

Epidemiology

Incidence: 165/100000 per year, prevalence: 1–22% (great variation).

Individuals with fair skin type have an increased risk.

Age of onset 30 to 50 years.

Definition

Chronic, inflammatory disease.

Aetiology and Pathogenesis

Multifactorial aetiology: Environmental trigger factors, demodex, nutritional factors (alcohol, histamine releaser), exercise, acute psychological stress, menstruation, drugs.

Pathogenesis: Impaired permeability barrier in the stratum corneum, antimicrobial peptides, overexpression of Toll-like receptors, inflammatory cells, reactive oxygen species, capillary blood flow dysbalance, neoangiogenesis, sensory nerve activation.

Signs and Symptoms

Centrofacial transient erythema (flushing), teleangiectatic erythema, papules and pustules without comedones, phymas (rhinophyma, gnathophyma, metophyma, otophyma), bilateral conjuctivitis and blepharo-conjunctivitis, stinging and burning sensations.

Localisation

Mid-face, forehead, nose, conjuctiva, V-area of chest.

Classification

Type I (teleangiectatic)
Type II (papulopustular)
Type III (phymatous)
Ocular rosacea
Morbihan's disease

Laboratory and Other Workups

Skin biopsy for ruling out other facial dermatoses. Cyanoacrylate tapestrip for demodex detection.

Dermatopathology

All subtypes show dilated lymph and blood vessels in the upper and mid-dermis and a superficial perivascular and perifollicular mononuclear lympho-histiocytic infiltrate plus plasma cells. Widened follicles. Oedema and thickened elastic fibres may be seen. Type III: hyperplastic sebaceous glands, granuloma formation.

Course

Progressive and chronic.

Complications

Proliferation of connective tissue and sebaceous follicles: rhinophyma (enlarged nose), otophyma (ears), metophyma (forehead), gnathophyma (chin). Rosacea fulminans and rosacea conglobata = maximal variants of rosacea. Keratitis in ocular rosacea.

Diagnosis

Clinical findings.

Differential Diagnosis

Major: Late-onset acne, corticosteroid-induced acne, periorificial dermatitis. In stage I also lupus erythematosus. If lupoid: sarcoidosis (lupus pernio), erysipelas.

Prevention and Therapy

Elimination of triggers.

Type I: Topical, brimonidine tartrate

Procedures: Nd:YAG LASER, pulsed dye LASER, intense pulsed light (IPL).

Type II: *Topical*, metronidazole, azelaic acid, ivermectin 1%, permethrin 5% pimecrolimus, retinoids. *Systemic*: Low-dose doxycycline, low-dose isotretinoin.

Type III: Systemic, isotretinoin. Procedures: dermabrasion, ablative LASERS (for phymas).

Ocular rosacea: Systemic doxycycline.

Periorificial Dermatitis (POD) [4]

Figure 14.16

Grading of Importance

B

Level

advanced

ICD-11

ED90.1

Synonyms

Perioral dermatitis; rosacea-like dermatitis.

Epidemiology

In the USA around 0.5 to 1%, often misdiagnosed.

Definition

Acneiform dermatosis with small papules and tiny pustules without comedones and with almost exclusively perioral and periorbital involvement. F 70% > 30% M. 20–40 years of age.

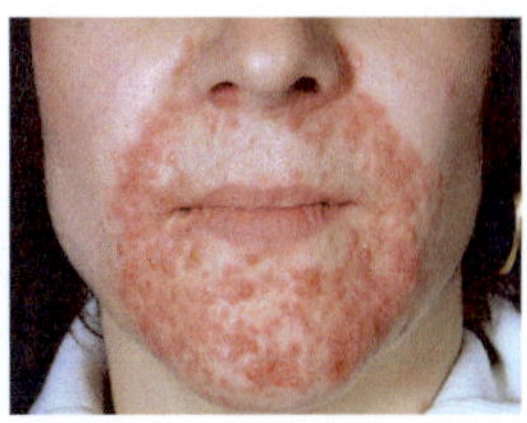

Fig. 14.16 Perioral dermatitis: papules and erythema

Aetiology and Pathogenesis

Some evidence exists that a hyperhydration of the follicular epithelium and steroid induced atrophy of the epithelium can support the release of inflammatory mediators into the surrounding superficial dermis and acroinfundibulum.

- Long-term use of topical steroid preparations
- Daily cosmetics: skin care with high water content ointments and creams including sunscreens and fluorinated toothpastes
- Physical factors: high humidity
- Microbiologic factors: fusiform spirilla bacteria from the oral microbiome settling in the perioral region. Often induction or worsening after long lasting dental procedures. Superinfection by *Malassezia furfur* and *Candida* species may occur.

Signs and Symptoms

Inflammatory small papules with tiny pustules, erythema and small scales are dominant lesions. The patients often complain of burning and tight sensation. No comedones.

Localisation

Perioral, periorbital, nasolabial, glabella. Genital.

Laboratory and Other Workups

Not necessary. Sometimes bacterial and mycologic swab, biotin,folic acid and zinc in serum to check.

Dermatopathology

Usually not necessary. In granuloma-like lesions a biopsy to exclude rosacea, acne agminata, or sarcoidosis and histiocytic diseases may be indicated. Mostly perifollicular and dermal oedema and prominent lymphomononuclear infiltrates with slight spongiosis of the acroinfundibular and interfollicular epithelium.

Course

It mostly starts slowly over 2–3 weeks. Flares can be seen whilst tappering application of corticosteroid creams.

Complications

Granulomatous type of POD.

Diagnosis

Clinical features and localisation. Exclude acne and rosacea.

Differential Diagnosis

Rosacea of papulo-pustular type. Gram-negative folliculitis. Corticosteroid acne, PRIDE syndrome.

Prevention and Therapy

Slow down corticosteroids to every other day or every third day. Change from strong moisturiser to less water containing galenics. Apply initially overnight zinc lotion. Metronidazole lotion, fucidin cream, topical ketoconazole help to reduce spirilla microbes. Systemic: low-dose doxycycline (anti-inflammatory, not for antibiotic effects).

Never use topical corticosteroids as first treatment.

Hidradenitis Suppurativa [1, 3]

Figures 14.17 and 14.18

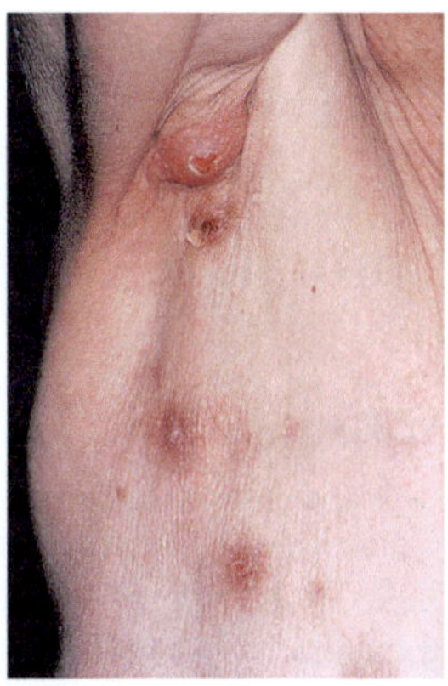

Fig. 14.17 Hidradenitis suppurativa: some pustules and nodes

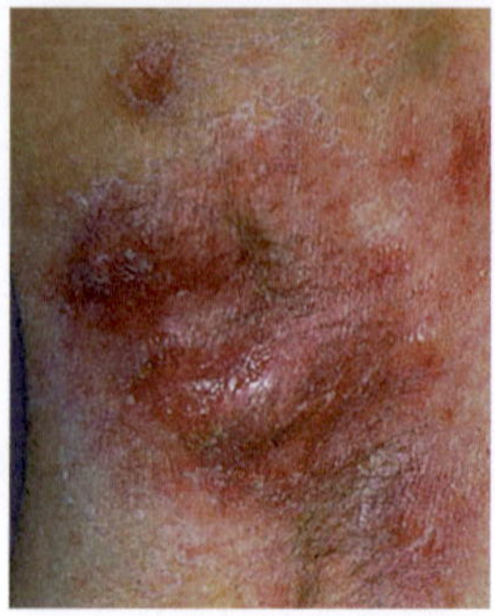

Fig. 14.18 Hidradenitis suppurativa: inflammatory abscesses formation

Grading of Importance

C

Level

Advanced

ICD-11

ED92.0

Synonyms

Acne inversa; pyoderma fistulans sinifica.

Epidemiology

Prevalence 0.03–4% (average 1%), annual age- and sex-adjusted incidence 6.0 per 100,000. Male/female ratio 1:3.

Definition

Chronic, inflammatory, recurrent, debilitating skin disease (of the terminal hair follicle) usually presenting after puberty with painful, deep-seated, inflamed lesions in the apocrine gland-bearing areas of the body, most commonly the axillary, inguinal and ano-genital regions.

Aetiology and Pathogenesis

The exact pathogenetic mechanism of hidradenitis suppurativa remains unclear. Smoking, obesity and metabolic syndrome are major predisposing factors.

Signs and Symptoms

Chronic recurrent inflammatory nodules, abscesses, draining tunnels (sinuses, fistulae and double comedones) and scars.

Localisation

Mostly major intertriginous areas with apocrine glands (axilla, groins).

Classification

Combination of anatomical classification, Hurley I, II, III, and severity classification, mild, moderate, severe.

Syndromic hidradenitis suppurativa diseases.

Laboratory and Other Workups

C-reactive protein, erythrocyte sedimentation rate.

Dermatopathology

Heterogeneous histological pattern with hyperplasia of hair follicular epithelium and subepidermal and deep cellular inflammatory infiltrate.

Course

Acute and chronic.

Complications

Squamous cell carcinoma in chronic ano-genital lesions, deep scars, depression, unemployment, change of profession.

Diagnosis

Outbreak of boils during the last 6 months with a minimum of two boils in one of the following six locations: axilla, groin, genitals, buttocks, under the breasts and perianal area, neck and abdomen regions.

Differential Diagnosis

Staphylococcal infection (furuncle, carbuncle), cutaneous Crohn's disease, primary or metastatic tumors, lymphogranuloma venereum, apocrine abscess.

Prevention and Therapy

Active inflammatory stage

Mild: Topical benzoylperoxide, topical antimicrobials.

Moderate: Oral clindamycin plus rifampicin; tetracycline; adalimumab, secucinumab; acitretin.

Severe: Adalimumab +/− clindamycin/doxycycline.

Chronic including inactive (non-inflammatory) and ative stage.

Local or wide excision completetly removing apocrine gland areas.

Prevention

Weight loss and tobacco abstinence, mediterrenian diet, pain management, treatment of secondary infections.

Special

Comorbid disorders: Inflammatory bowel disease, spondyloarthropathy, increased cardiovascular risk.

References

1. Alikhan A, Lynch PJ, Eisen DB (2009) Hidradenitis suppurativa: a comprehensive review. J Am Acad Dermatol 60(4):539–561; quiz 562–533
2. Marson JW, Baldwin HE (2020) Rosacea: a wholistic review and update from pathogenesis to diagnosis and therapy. Int J Dermatol 59(6):e175–e182
3. Saunte DML, Jemec GBE (2017) Hidradenitis suppurativa: advances in diagnosis and treatment. JAMA 318(20):2019–2032
4. Searle T, Ali FR, Al-Niaimi F (2021) Perioral dermatitis: diagnosis, proposed etiologies, and management. J Cosmet Dermatol 20(12):3839–3848
5. van Zuuren EJ (2017) Rosacea. N Engl J Med 377(18):1754–1764
6. Gollnick HP, Zouboulis CC. Not all acne is acne vulgaris. Dtsch Arztebl Int. 2014;25;111(17):301–12. https://doi.org/10.3238/arztebl.2014.0301. PMID: 24828100; PMCID: PMC4098044

Diseases of Hair and Nails

15

Jonathan M. White and Veronique del Marmol

Contents

J. M. White (✉)
Ecole de Santé Publique, Université libre de Bruxelles, Brussels, Belgium
e-mail: Jonathan.White@ulb.be

V. del Marmol
Département of Dermatology, Hôpital Erasme-HUB, Université Libre de Bruxelles, Brussels, Belgium
e-mail: veronique.delmarmol@hubruxelles.be

H. Gollnick et al. (eds.), *Dermatology Cyberderm WebBook*,
https://doi.org/10.1007/978-3-031-78491-0_15

Test your learning and check your understanding of this book's contents: use the "Springer Nature Flashcards" app to access questions using ▶ https://sn.pub/1rhh6k.
To use the app, please follow the instructions in Chap. 1.

Alopecia Areata [2]

Figures 15.1, 15.2 and 15.3

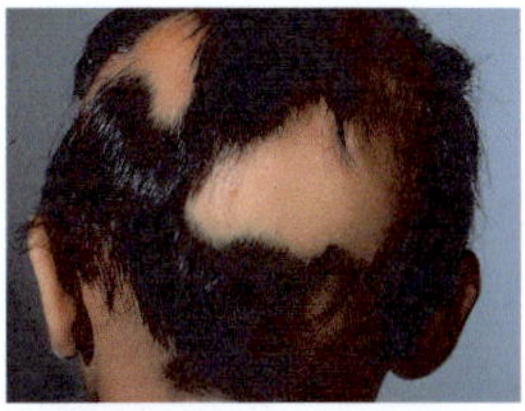

Fig. 15.1 Alopecia areata: capillitium

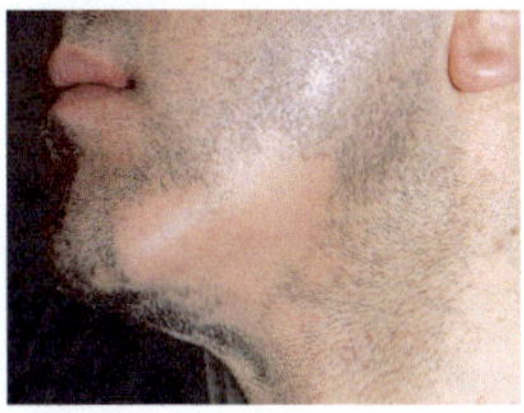

Fig. 15.2 Alopecia areata: beard

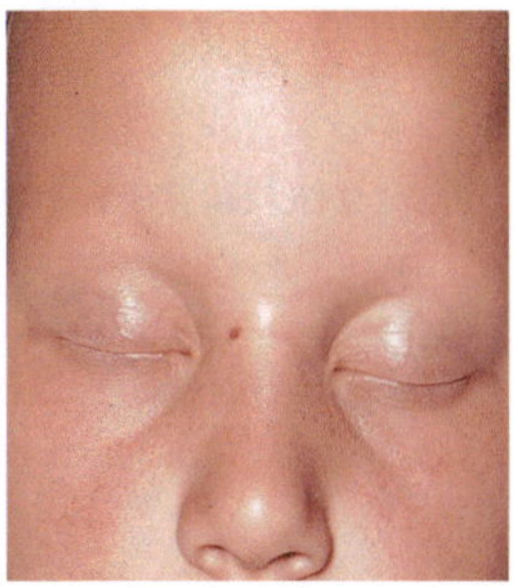

Fig. 15.3 Alopecia areata: alopecia totalis (maligna)

Grading of Importance

B

Level

Advanced

ICD-11

ED70.2

Synonyms

Spot baldness, patchy alopecia, autoimmune hair loss.

Definition

Reversible, non-scarring usually localised but also generalised hair loss.

Epidemiology

Present in all ethnic populations. May affect 0.1% of the population; nearly 2% of the general population is affected somewhen during their lifetime. Patients with atopic diathesis or with autoimmune disorders are at higher risk.

Aetiology and Pathogenesis

Autoimmune process with lymphocytic T-helper and T-cytotoxic cell subsets infiltrate around anagen hair bulb. Association with other autoimmune diseases; Down syndrome.

Signs and Symptoms

Macroscopically non-inflamed, non-scarring loss of hair in circular shapes with solitary, multiple or diffuse patterns. Exclamation mark hairs. Sometimes associated nail changes (pitting) or complete nail loss.

Localisation

Most easily identified in hairy areas such as the scalp or beard region or body hair.

Classification

According to extent of hair loss:

- Alopecia areata: solitary or multiple areas of hair loss
- Alopecia totalis: loss of all scalp hairs
- Alopecia universalis: loss of all scalp and body hairs

Laboratory and Other Workups

Association with atopy with increased IgE (worse prognosis) and autoimmune thyroiditis (TAK /MAK). Syphilis serology (where there are multiple small patches clinically) to exclude moth-eaten alopecia of secondary syphilis. Fungal culture if diagnostic doubt. Anti-streptokinase titre.

Dermatopathology

Not usually required. Perifollicular lymphocytic infiltrate around anagen follicles with apoptosis of follicular keratinocytes and formation of dystrophic hair shafts.

Course

Focal lesions have a high spontaneous remission rate (30% within 6 months, 50% with 1 year, 80% within 3 years). Widespread disease has low spontaneous remission rate. Factors conveying a poor prognosis include positive family history, involvement of occipital scalp hairline (ophiasis type), widespread disease, longer duration (onset in childhood) and atopy.

Complications

Loss of eyebrows and eyelashes with chronic conjunctivitis, nail involvement (20-nail dystrophy), association with autoimmune thyroiditis, vitiligo, pernicious anaemia (other autoimmune disorders less common), psychosocial problems with persistent alopecia are common.

Diagnosis

Clinical diagnosis in most cases.

Differential Diagnosis

Alopecia specifica in secondary syphilis, trichotillomania, early stage of scarring alopecias (such as deep trichophyton infections).

Prevention and Therapy

Await spontaneous regrowth. Small lesions can be treated with high-potency topical corticosteroids or intralesional corticosteroids. More widespread forms may respond to topical immunotherapy with diphenylcyclopropenone. In severe cases, systemic corticosteroid pulsed therapy can be considered. Other evidence-based treatments are not available, but third-line treatments may include methotrexate, zinc and phototherapy. Wigs, permanent make-up for eyebrows and self-help groups.

Androgenetic Alopecia [2]

Figure 15.4

Grading of Importance

B

Level

Advanced

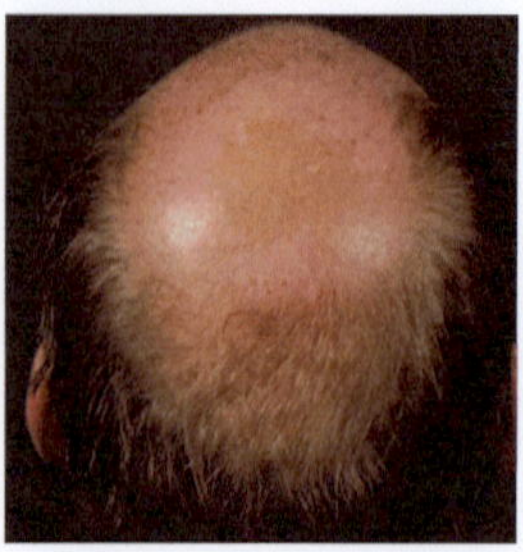

Fig. 15.4 Androgenetic alopecia: male baldness

ICD-11

ED70.0

Synonyms

Male pattern hair loss; common balding; male-pattern baldness; hormone-related alopecia.

Epidemiology

30–40% of women will have thinning hair by the age of 70 or older.

50–60% of men have a bald scalp by 70 years (but may start earlier, especially with a positive family history).

The condition is less commonly seen in men of East Asian ancestry.

Definition

Progressive androgen-dependent hair loss in typical locations associated with genetic predisposition and natural aging. In women, early aggressive disease or specific pattern (Hamilton-Norwood) of hair loss may indicate an endocrine disorder.

Aetiology and Pathogenesis

Polygenic inheritance. Abnormalities of local follicular androgen metabolism, especially increased activity of 5α-reductase, lead to increased levels of dihydrotestosterone.

Signs and Symptoms

Progressive and persistent asymptomatic hair loss in symmetrical pattern.

Localisation

Women—thinning of centro-parietal scalp, with widened parting but retained anterior hair line. The clinical pattern is variable and can be diffuse. Never complete hair loss on vertex.

Men—bi-temporal symmetrical regression, thinning of the vertex, later more complete loss leaving a residual parietal-occipital band.

Classification

Female pattern androgenetic alopecia: Ludwig scale I-III.

Male pattern androgenetic alopecia: Hamilton-Norwood scale (typical pattern; anterior pattern or vertex pattern) I-VII.

Laboratory and Other Workups

Usually not required. Consider endocrinologic evaluation in women with other signs of androgen excess (irregular menses, hirsutism, virilisation). Consider testing for concomitant causes of hair loss (e.g. low ferritin, thyroid dysfunction, lupus erythematosus, etc.).

Dermatopathology

Usually not required. Miniaturisation of the hair follicle with pseudohypertrophy of the associated sebaceous glands, increase in telogen hair follicles.

Course

Progressive but with highly variable course.

Complications

Chronic UV damage to the exposed scalp. Long-standing androgenetic alopecia can lead to micro-scarring. Psychosocial problems.

Diagnosis

Typical clinical findings. Consider a hair pull test and scalp dermoscopy. In women with early androgenetic alopecia, a trichogram (or automated videotrichogram) may be helpful. Excessive androgen production in women must be excluded by history and clinical findings; if other clues of androgen excess are present, endocrine evaluation is needed.

Differential Diagnosis

Other causes of hair loss, e.g. diffuse alopecia areata or especially telogen effluvium in women, long-standing malnutrition with trace elements and vitamins.

Prevention and Therapy

Minoxidil 2 and 5% solutions, oral finasteride (strict avoidance of pregnancy in women of child-bearing years as finasteride is teratogenic), hair transplantation. Also oral contraceptives with anti-androgens in women. Consider wigs.

Hirsutism [4]

Figures 15.5 and 15.6

Grading of Importance

B

Level

Advanced

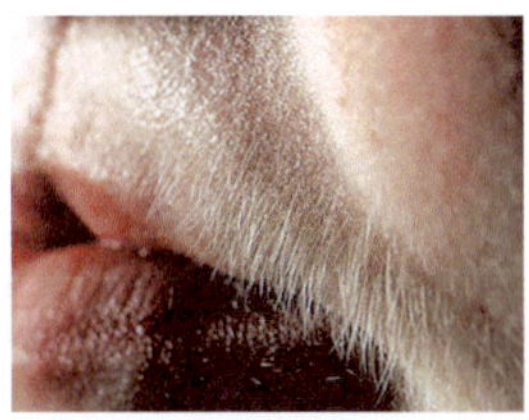

Fig. 15.5 Hirsutism: vellus hair on the upper lip

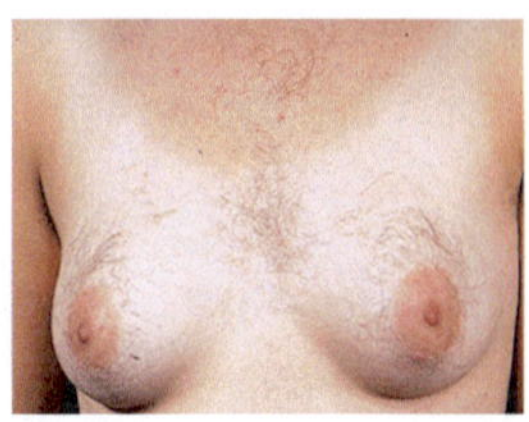

Fig. 15.6 Hirsutism: hair on breast and mammae

ICD-11

ED72

Synonyms

Hirsutes, excessive hair, endocrine hypertrichosis.

Definition

Excessive terminal hair in a male pattern in a woman.

Aetiology and Pathogenesis

Around 5–10% of women may show signs of hirsutism.

There are many different causes.

Endocrine hirsutism: polycystic ovary syndrome; androgen-producing ovarian tumours; congenital adrenal hyperplasia (adrenogenital syndrome); acanthosis nigricans in insulin resistance; adrenal tumours; ACTH-cell hyperplasia; pituitary adenomas (Cushing's disease); hyperprolactinaemia; acromegaly.

Other causes: postmenopausal hirsutism; idiopathic hirsutism; ethnic; medication-induced hirsutism (e.g. anabolic steroids); paraneoplastic.

Signs and Symptoms

Growth of terminal and vellus hairs in woman on upper lip, chin, temples, between breasts, around nipples, on shoulders, linea alba and interior aspects of thighs. Can vary from discrete excess hairs to obvious male pattern with involvement of different locations that are highly variable.

Localisation

Upper lip, chin, temples, breast, abdomen, pubic area, arms, legs, back, buttocks.

Classification

Modified Ferriman-Gallwey system with 19 locations, min 0 to 36 max points. A score of more than 8 indicates androgen excess hirsutism.

Laboratory and Other Workups

Hormone status (FSH/LH ratio, DHEAS, free testosterone, SHBG, 17-hydroxyprogesterone, prolactin), transvaginal ultrasound evaluation of ovaries.

Dermatopathology

Usually not required.

Course

Persistent, if an underlying cause cannot be found or treated adequately.

Complications

Psychosocial problems, tendency toward folliculitis after shaving, diabetes and cancer in polycystic ovarian syndrome.

Diagnosis

Typical hair pattern, endocrine screening with more detailed evaluation if hyperandrogenism is present.

Differential Diagnosis

Ethnic variability. Hypertrichosis. Virilisation. Genetic syndromes causing hypertrichosis (consider especially in children).

Prevention and Therapy

Treat causes of hyperandrogenism.

Mechanical removal of hairs includes shaving, waxing, epilation, electroepilation, laser or light-assisted hair removal. Chemical agents to slow/stop hair growth (e.g. eflornithine). Consider spironolactone, finasteride, cyproterone or oral contraceptives.

Psychosocial support.

Nail Dystrophies [1]

Figures 15.7, 15.8, 15.9, 15.10 and 15.11

Grading of Importance

B

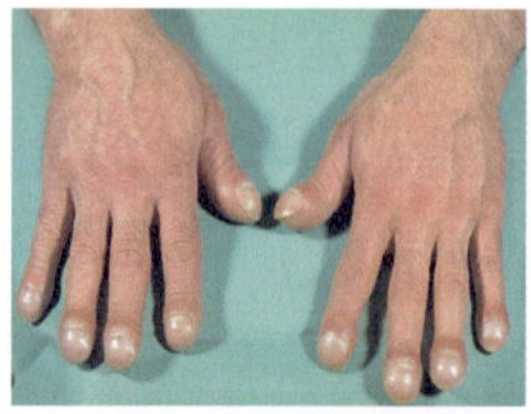

Fig. 15.7 Nail dystrophy: drumstick fingers in cardiovascular disorder

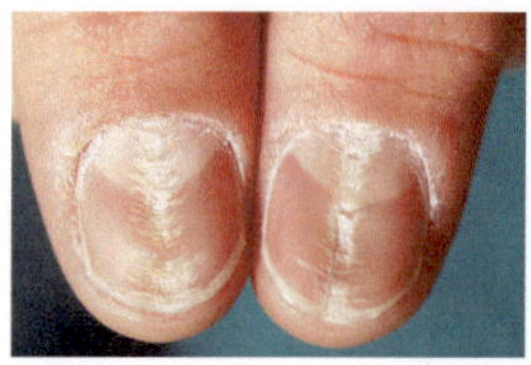

Fig. 15.8 Nail dystrophy: dystrophia canaliformis following trauma of the matrix

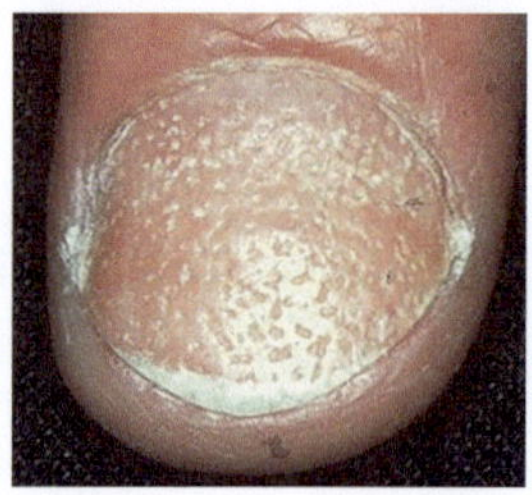

Fig. 15.9 Nail dystrophy: pits in psoriasis

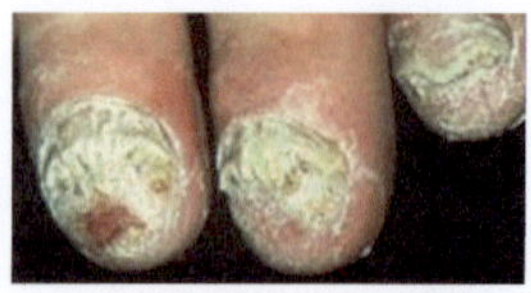

Fig. 15.10 Nail dystrophy: psoriasis

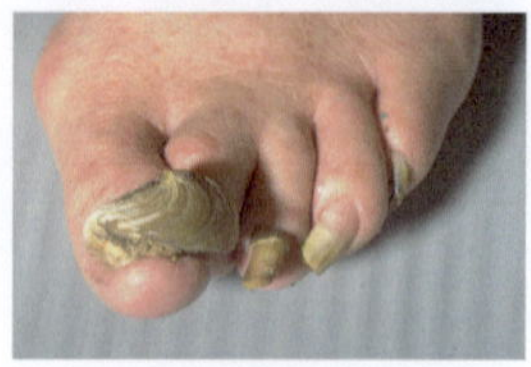

Fig. 15.11 Nail dystrophy: onychogryphosis

Level

Advanced

ICD-11

EE10.5

Synonyms

Onychodystrophy.

Definition

Disturbances in nail growth (proliferation, differentiation and maturation).

Aetiology and Pathogenesis

Often idiopathic, may reflect manifestations of other diseases, e.g. psoriasis, lichen planus, alopecia areata, GVHD, genetic disorders including 20-nail syndrome, different types of eczemas, metabolic disorders, toxic damage, infections, medications (e.g. chemotherapy). May also be due to mechanical irritation including nail manicure.

Signs and Symptoms

Changes in colour, structure and growth pattern of nails.

Localisation

Finger- or toenails. Examine the skin and hair for further signs.

Classification

- Onychoschisis: transverse separation of nail plate
- Onychorrhexis: coarse nails due to longitudinal thickening and ridging
- Onycholysis: lysis of the nail plate
- Onychomadesis: proximal separation of the nail plate from the nail matrix

Laboratory and Other Workups

Microbiological specimen to exclude onychomycosis, *Pseudomonas aeruginosa*.

Dermatopathology

Not usually required.

Course

Varies according to underlying cause. Often chronic.

Complications

Secondary fungal infections possible.

Diagnosis

Clinical findings in context of associated findings.

Differential Diagnosis

Wide. Consider infections, psoriasis, atopic dermatitis, allergic or irritant contact dermatitis, lichen planus, hereditary causes, etc.

Prevention and Therapy

Treatment of underlying disease. Podiatry review for severe toenail involvement impinging on walking.

Nail Colour Changes [3, 5]

Figures 15.12, 15.13, 15.14, 15.15, 15.16 and 15.17

Grading of Importance

B

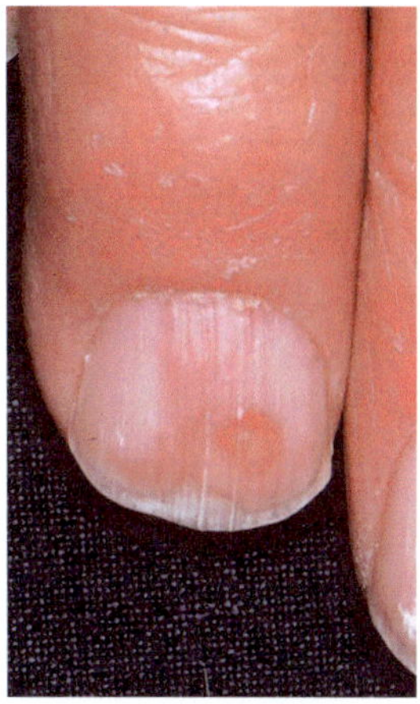

Fig. 15.12 Nail colour changes: psoriasis of the nail bed (oil spot)

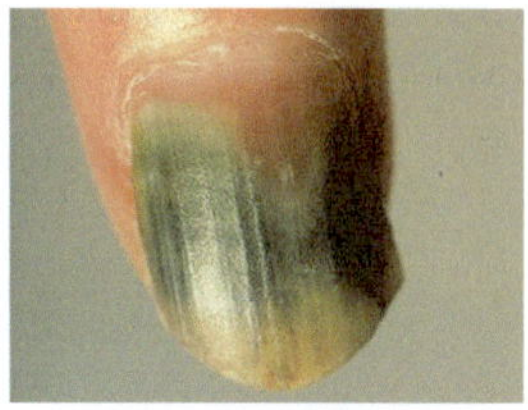

Fig. 15.13 Nail colour changes: pyoceaneus infection

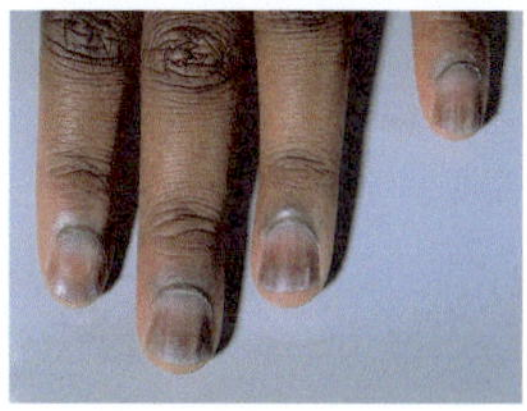

Fig. 15.14 Nail colour changes: Amiadarone discoloration

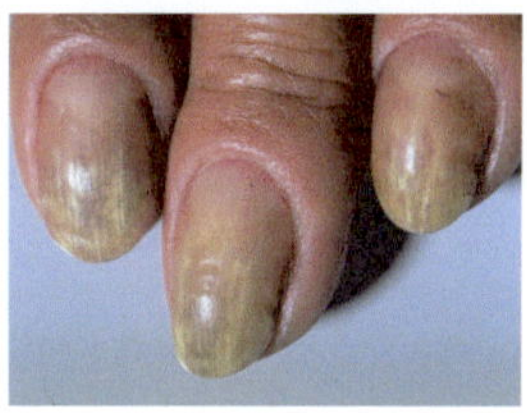

Fig. 15.15 Nail colour changes: yellow nail syndrome

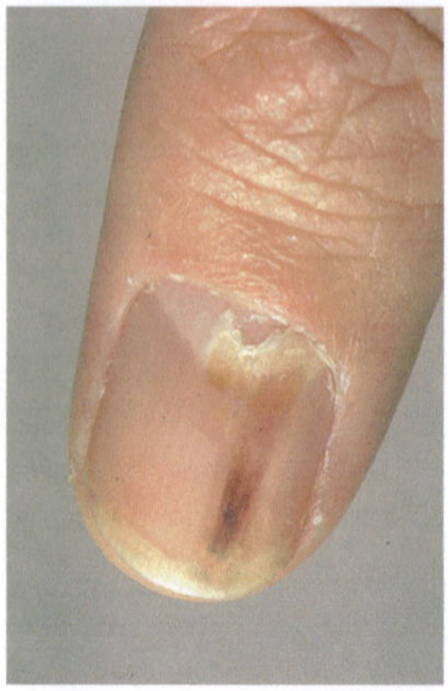

Fig. 15.16 Nail colour changes: pigment nevus in the matrix

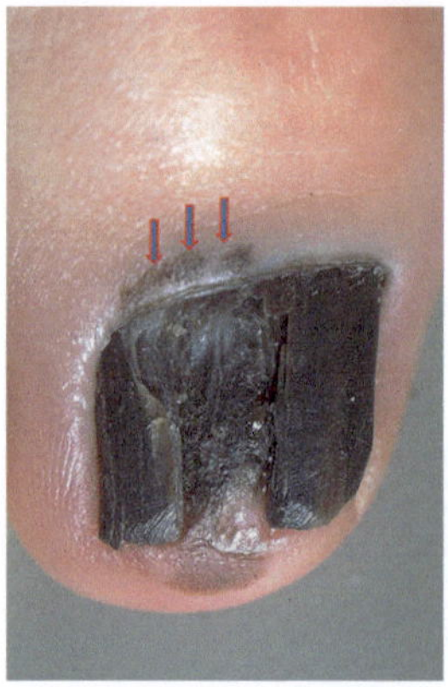

Fig. 15.17 Nail colour changes: acral melanoma

Level

Advanced

ICD-11

EE1Z

Synonyms

Not available.

Definition

Abnormal colours (e.g. black, brown, green, yellow, blue-red, white) in nail plate or nail bed.

Aetiology and Pathogenesis

Vary according to colour.

Brown-Black
- Medications: anti-malarials, cytostatic agents, antibiotics, psoralens, zidovudine in HIV infection
- Melanocytic: ethnic, melanocytic nevus, malignant melanoma
- Endocrine: Addison disease, Cushing disease
- Iron: haematoma, haemochromatosis
- Lupus erythematosus

Yellow-Brown
- Psoriasis
- Onychomycosis
- Lichen planus

Green
- *Pseudomonas aeruginosa*

Yellow
- Onychomycosis
- Yellow nail syndrome (often associated with chronic sinusitis, bronchitis, pleuritis, pulmonary fibrosis, bronchiectases)

Blue-Red
- Glomus tumour
- Nail bed cyanosis (central circulatory problems, methemoglobinaemia)

White
- Deficiency in certain minerals or vitamins. The deficiencies most commonly include zinc and calcium

Signs and Symptoms

Usually asymptomatic discolouration of nails.

Localisation

Finger- or toenails.

Classification

No specific classification.

Laboratory and Other Workups

Depends on suspected underlying disease. Consider clipping of nail for microbial analysis. Histology may be required in brown/black discoloration (mandatory if melanoma suspected).

Dermatopathology

Depends on cause of discoloration.

Course

Acute, sub-acute to chronic, relapsing.

Complications

Depending on cause, often nail destruction.

Diagnosis

Clinical findings, mycology, bacteriology, histology.

Differential Diagnosis

See above.

Prevention and Therapy

Directed at underlying cause.

References

1. Bloom A, Blanken B, Schlakman B, Arena T, Mironov Z, Vlahovic TC (2020) A review of nail dystrophies for the practitioner. Adv Skin Wound Care 33(1):20–26
2. Gilhar A, Etzioni A, Paus R (2012) Alopecia areata. N Engl J Med 366(16):1515–1525
3. Gurcharan S, NayeemSadath H, Uday A (2005) Nail changes and disorders among the elderly. Indian J Dermatol Venereol Leprol 71(6):386–392
4. Matheson E, Bain J (2019) Hirsutism in women. Am Fam Physician 100(3):168–175
5. Ramos-e-Silva M, Chaves Azevedo-e-Silva M, Carneiro SC (2008) Hair, nail, and pigment changes in major systemic disease. Clin Dermatol 26(3):296–305

Diseases of Mucous Membranes

16

Christos C. Zouboulis, Günter Burg, Eija Hiltunen-Back, John A. McGrath, Annamari Ranki, and Alexander Salava

Contents

Annamari Ranki has died before the publication of this book.

C. C. Zouboulis (✉)
Departments of Dermatology, Venereology, Allergology and Immunology, Staedtisches Klinikum Dessau, Brandenburg Medical School Theodor Fontane and Faculty of Medical Sciences Brandenburg, Dessau, Germany
e-mail: christos.zouboulis@mhb-fontane.de

G. Burg
Dermatology, Zurich, Switzerland
e-mail: g.burg@access.uzh.ch

E. Hiltunen-Back · A. Ranki · A. Salava
Department of Dermatology and Allergology, Helsinki University Hospital, Helsinki, Finland
e-mail: eija.hiltunen-back@hus.fi; alexander.salava@hus.fi

J. A. McGrath
St John's Institute of Dermatology, King's College London, London, UK
e-mail: john.mcgrath@kcl.ac.uk

H. Gollnick et al. (eds.), *Dermatology Cyberderm WebBook*,
https://doi.org/10.1007/978-3-031-78491-0_16

Test your learning and check your understanding of this book's contents: use the "Springer Nature Flashcards" app to access questions using ▶ https://sn.pub/1rhh6k.

To use the app, please follow the instructions in Chap. 1.

Leukoplakia [2]

Figures 16.1 and 16.2

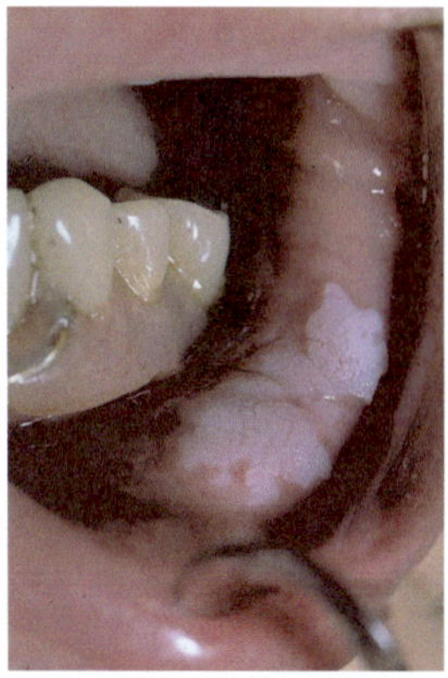

Fig. 16.1 Leukoplakia: gingiva

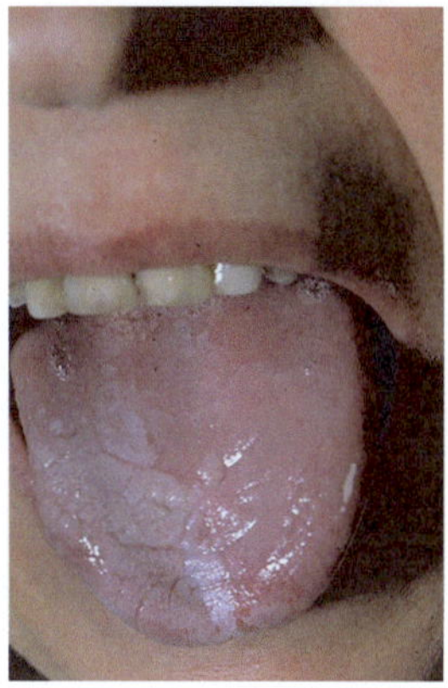

Fig. 16.2 Leukoplakia: tongue

Grading of Importance

B

Level

Advanced

ICD-11

DA01.00

Definition

White adherent mucosal changes, reflecting increased or abnormal keratinisation of the stratified squamous (normally not keratinised) mucosal epithelium of the mouth or transitional epithelium (lips, penis, labiae, anal mucosa)

Aetiology and Pathogenesis

Based on cause. Exogenous: chemical (tobacco) or mechanical irritation (abnormal teeth, dentures), also hereditary

Signs and Symptoms

Asymptomatic white plaques

Localisation

Anywhere in the mouth, especially buccal or sublingual mucosa; also genital or anal mucosa

Laboratory and Other Workups

Unremarkable

Dermatopathology

Epithelial hyperplasia with or without atypia

Course

Chronic, can evolve into carcinoma

Diagnosis

Clinical features; if persistent or infiltrated histology is mandatory.

Differential Diagnosis

Candidiasis (thrush), lichen planus, squamous cell carcinoma

Prevention and Therapy

Clinical follow-up, eliminating irritating factors, in some instances oral retinoids or excision

Aphthae/Mucosal Disease [1]

Figures 16.3, 16.4 and 16.5

Grading of Importance

B

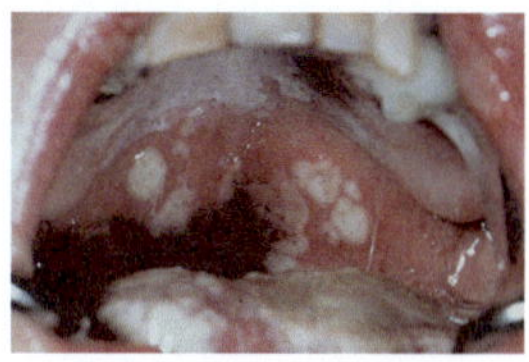

Fig. 16.3 Aphthae: inflammatory ulcerations on the palate

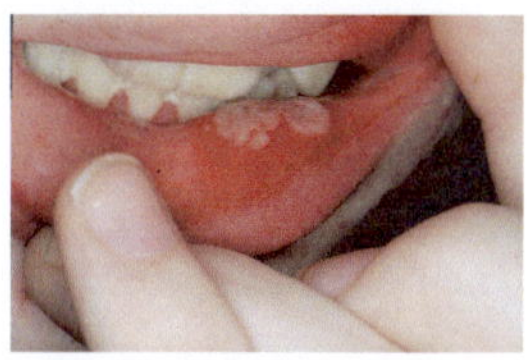

Fig. 16.4 Aphthae: erythema and superficial white necrosis on the lip

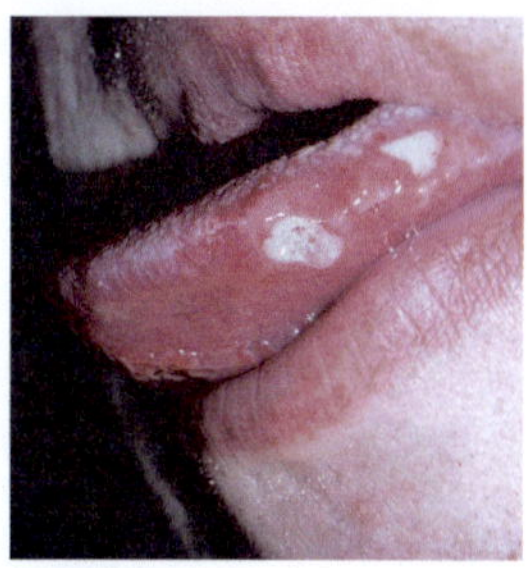

Fig. 16.5 Aphthae: necrotic ulcera of the tongue

Level

Advanced

ICD-11

DA01.10

Synonyms

Recurrent aphthous stomatitis (RAS), aphthous stomatitis, recurrent oral ulcers (ROU), recurrent bipolar(oral/genital) aphthosis

Epidemiology

Common disease with 2–10% of people with a 3-month recurrence rate of 50% and a lifetime prevalence of >35%. More common in females. Recurrent genital aphthous ulcers are much less common. Family history in 24–46%.

Definition

Recurrent, multiple, small, round, or ovoid ulcers with yellow floor and surrounded by erythematous halo.

Aetiology and Pathogenesis

The aetiology of recurrent benign aphthae is unclear.

Signs and Symptoms

- *Minor oral aphthae*: anterior part of the mouth, superficial, <1 cm, healing within 10–14 days.
- *Major oral aphthae*: >1 cm, deep, last for weeks: small (1–2 mm), multiple lesions (5–100). Grey-yellow and without a delineating erythematous border inducing pain in eating and speaking.

A single crop of ulcers may last for approximately 7–14 days; the period of remission between attacks is variable.

Localisation

Non-keratinised mucosa of the oral cavity or genital mucosa

Classification

- Minor: Most common form (85%; do not result in scarring)
- Major: Approx. 10–15% (may leave a scar)
- Herpetiform: 5–10%

Laboratory and Other Workups

None specific

Dermatopathology

Small focal ulceration above the excretory duct of minor salivary glands, mononuclear cells and neutrophilic acute inflammatory infiltrate surrounding the ulcer.

Course

Obligatory recurrent with varying frequency (2–12x/year up to intervals of few days). Relation to menstrual cycle, pregnancy, and dysmenorrhea in females. Usually improve during pregnancy.

Complications

Occurrence at sites of trauma (e.g. from brushing teeth), anaesthetic injection and dental treatment. Certain drugs may induce oral aphthae.

Diagnosis

Clinical picture, personal and family history

Differential Diagnosis

High number/in particular Adamantiades-Behçet's disease, different gastrointestinal inflammatory diseases, viral infections, candidiasis, autoimmune diseases, bullous and lichenoid dermatoses, allergic contact stomatitis, drug-induced ulcerative stomatitis, geographic like stomatitis, traumatic ulcers

Prevention and Therapy

Registered therapies only include topical corticosteroids, topical antiseptics (reduction of new aphthae) and topical anaesthetics (pain relief).

In severe cases, topical treatment can be combined with systemic therapy, e.g. colchicine, pentoxifylline or prednisolone. Also apremilast in oral aphthae of Adamantiades-Behçet's disease.

Hard, acidic and salty food, alcohol and carbonated beverages should be avoided.

Balanitis [3]

Figure 16.6

Grading of Importance

B

Level

Null

ICD-11

GB06.01, 02, 0Z, 0Y: balanitis/balanoposthitis
1F23.11 Candida balanoposthitis
2E67.4 Carcinoma in situ of penis (penile intraepithelial neoplasia (PeIN))

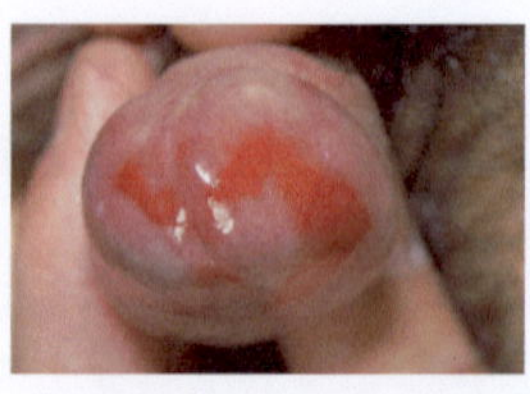

Fig. 16.6 Balanitis: bizarre erythema

Synonyms

Inflammation of the glans penis and/or prepuce (foreskin)

Epidemiology

Balanitis/balanoposthitis is one the most frequent male genital skin problems affecting both, paediatric patients and adults. Prevalence in males of all ages is between 12% and 20%. In adult men, uncircumcised males with diabetes mellitus have the highest prevalence of 35%. Circumcision considerably decreases the prevalence of inflammatory conditions of the glans penis.

Definition

Inflammation of the glans penis and/or the prepuce (posthitis)

Aetiology and Pathogenesis

The most common aetiology of balanoposthitis is poor hygiene. Preputial dysfunction and diabetes are promoting factors. Circumcision considerably decreases the risk.

Spectrum of possible pathogenetic factors: see symptoms and classification, respectively.

Signs and Symptoms

The symptoms and signs vary according to the aetiology.

- **Candidal balanoposthitis**: blotchy erythema with small papules.
- **(Anaerobic) bacterial infection**: uniform erythema with exudative preputial foul-smelling discharge.
- **Irritant/allergic balanitis-balanoposthitis**: mild erythema with or without pruritus, resulting from frequent genital washing, atopy, delayed hypersensitivity to common allergens (e.g. latex condoms, preservatives, fragrances).
- **Fixed drug eruptions** (tetracyclines, phenolphthalein, phenacetin, NSAIDs, barbiturates or sulfa-drugs): round, erythematous patches, turning dark upon healing. Vesicles may occur.
- **Non- specific balanoposthitis:** no evidence of underlying cause.
- **Lichen sclerosus:** white patches on the glans, often with involvement of the prepuce; haemorrhagic vesicles, purpura and rarely haemorrhagic blisters and ulceration; itching. Blunting of the coronal sulcus, destruction of the frenulum,

phimosis or 'waisting' of the prepuce (constrictive posthitis) and meatal thickening and narrowing may develop.

- **Lichen planus**: purplish, well-demarcated plaques or erosive, annular lesions on the glans and prepuce.
- **Psoriasis**: red plaques without scaling.
- **Zoon's (plasma cell) balanitis**: in uncircumcised males aged 40 years or older. It presents with well-circumscribed orange-red glazed areas on the glans and the inside of the foreskin, with multiple pinpoint redder spots—'cayenne pepper spots'.
- **Premalignant lesions**
  - Erythroplasia of Queyrat: red, velvety, well-circumscribed area on the glans or visceral prepuce (45%), glans (38%) or shaft of the penis (3%).
  - Bowen's disease: scaly, discrete, erythematous patches or plaques
  - Bowenoid papulosis: firm papules to plaques, often grouped and pigmented or erythematous

Localisation

Glans penis and/or prepuce (foreskin)

Classification

The balanitis/balanoposthitis is classified in the following main groups based on the etiopathogenesis.

- **Infective balanoposthitis**
  - Viral infections: Human papillomavirus (HPV)
  - Herpes simplex virus (HSV)
  - Fungal infections *Candida* spp.
  - Bacterial infections: *Staphylococcus* spp.; *Streptococcus* spp. Sexually transmitted infections (*Trichomonas vaginalis*, syphilis; *Mycoplasma genitalium*)
- **Inflammatory balanoposthitis:** lichen sclerosus, lichen planus, psoriasis and circinate balanitis, Zoon's balanitis, eczema (irritant, allergic or seborrheic), allergic reactions (including fixed drug eruptions).
- **Penile intraepithelial neoplasia (PeIN**) is a premalignant precursor lesion of invasive penile SCC, a SCC in situ (Bowen's disease, Bowenoid papulosis and erythroplasia Queyrat).
- **Skin diseases** affecting the glans penis and genitalia (psoriasis, erythema multiforme, immuno-bullous disorders (e.g. pemphigus), dermatitis artefacta).

Laboratory and Other Workups

Sub-preputial swab for *Candida* and bacterial cultures (e.g. *Gardnerella vaginalis* as a facultative anaerobe), urinalysis for glucose (if Candida infection suspected), *Trichomonas vaginalis* nucleic acid amplification test (NAAT), full routine screening for other STIs. Testing for HLAB27 in case of circinate balanitis. Patch testing with common allergens.

A penile biopsy should be performed if features are atypical or do not resolve with treatment.

Dermatopathology

Not needed for infectious balanoposthitis patients.

- Lichen sclerosus: atrophic epidermis with follicular hyperkeratosis. Band of hyalinisation with loss of the elastin fibres in the upper dermis with an underlying perivascular lymphocytic infiltrate
- Lichen planus: irregular saw-toothed acanthosis, increased granular layer and basal cell liquefaction and a band-like dermal lymphocytic infiltrate
- Fixed drug eruptions: hydropic degeneration of the basal layer and epidermal detachment and necrosis with pigmentary incontinence
- Zoon's plasma cell balanitis: epidermal thickening, followed by epidermal atrophy. Predominantly plasma cell infiltrate in the dermis with haemosiderin deposition and extravasated red blood cells
- PeIN: dysplastic changes of the squamous epithelium

Course

Most balanitis cases recover with changes in hygiene and therapy with emollients within 1 to 2 weeks.

Complications

Severe balanitis may be complicated by phimosis and urinary retention. Impact on the patient's sexual life and psychosocial problems.

Diagnosis

Clinical features and laboratory workup (see above).

Differential Diagnosis

See classification.

Prevention and Therapy

Exclusion or treatment of predisposing factors (poor hygiene, diabetes mellitus). Good personal hygiene, washing daily, avoiding irritants; keeping the foreskin retracted

- **Nonspecific balanoposthitis:** gentle cleaning of the area two to three times per day by retracting the foreskin and cleaning with gentle use of cotton swab.
- **Candida balanoposthitis:** clotrimazole or miconazole cream, twice a day for 7–14 days. Topical imidazole with 1% hydrocortisone is a choice if marked inflammation is present.
- **Aerobic bacterial**: topically mupirocin cream twice a day or with clobetasone butyrate/oxytetracycline/nystatin cream once or twice daily for 7–10 days. Severe cases may require systemic antibiotics while awaiting culture results: flucloxacillin 500 mg x4/d or clarithromycin 250 mg x2/d for 7 days.
- **Anaerobic sub-preputial infection**: improved genital hygiene, topical or oral metronidazole 400–500 mg x2/d for 1 week. Alternatively, amoxiclav 375 mg x3/d for 1 week or clindamycin cream twice daily until resolved.
- **HSV, *Trichomonas vaginalis*, *Mycoplasma genitalium* or syphilis** is treated as per specific guidelines for these diseases.
- **Irritant/allergic balanitis-balanoposthitis**: avoidance of precipitants like soaps, use of low-allergy products, emollients (used as a soap substitute), hydrocortisone once or twice daily until resolution of symptoms. Avoidance of potential allergens (latex condom, lubricants).
- **Lichen sclerosus**: Topically, ultrapotent topical steroids (e.g. clobetasol propionate) twice daily for a month.
- **Zoon's (plasma cell) balanitis**: good hygiene, topical steroid creams and antibacterial creams (e.g. mupirocin) applied twice daily. Alternative topical calcineurin inhibitors and imiquimod 5% cream.
- **Premalignant penile lesions, PeIN**, should be referred to specialists in dermatology and urology/andrology. For topical therapy imiquimod 5%, fluorouracil cream 5%, fluorouracil 0.5%/salicylic acid 10% combination and podophyllotoxin 0.5% are alternatives. Local surgical excision, cryotherapy, photodynamic therapy or laser treatment.

Special

Lichen sclerosus may be complicated by phimosis and paraphimosis, urethral stenosis, penile intraepithelial neoplasia (PeIN) or even malignant transformation to squamous cell carcinoma (about 50%).

References

1. Akintoye SO, Greenberg MS (2014) Recurrent aphthous stomatitis. Dent Clin N Am 58(2):281–297
2. Akrish S, Eskander-Hashoul L, Rachmiel A, Ben-Izhak O (2019) Clinicopathologic analysis of verrucous hyperplasia, verrucous carcinoma and squamous cell carcinoma as part of the clinicopathologic spectrum of oral proliferative verrucous leukoplakia: a literature review and analysis. Pathol Res Pract 215(12):152670
3. Dayal S, Sahu P (2016) Zoon balanitis: a comprehensive review. Indian J Sex Transm Dis AIDS 37(2):129–138

Part V

Diseases of Blood and Lymph Vessels, Ulcers and Panniculitis

This nosologically heterogeneous group of diseases has in common pathogenetic processes and destructions in the dermis and subcutaneous tissue.

Vascular Diseases

17

Martine Bagot and Christos C. Zouboulis

Contents

M. Bagot (✉)
Service de Dermatologie, Université Paris Cité, Hôpital Saint-Louis, Paris, France
e-mail: martine.bagot@gmail.com

C. C. Zouboulis
Departments of Dermatology, Venereology, Allergology and Immunology, Staedtisches Klinikum Dessau, Brandenburg Medical School Theodor Fontane and Faculty of Health Sciences Brandenburg, Dessau, Germany
e-mail: christos.zouboulis@mhb-fontane.de

H. Gollnick et al. (eds.), *Dermatology Cyberderm WebBook*,
https://doi.org/10.1007/978-3-031-78491-0_17

Test your learning and check your understanding of this book's contents: use the "Springer Nature Flashcards" app to access questions using ▶ https://sn.pub/1rhh6k.

To use the app, please follow the instructions in Chap. 1.

Allergic Vasculitis [1]

Figures 17.1, 17.2, 17.3, 17.4 and 17.5

Grading of Importance

B

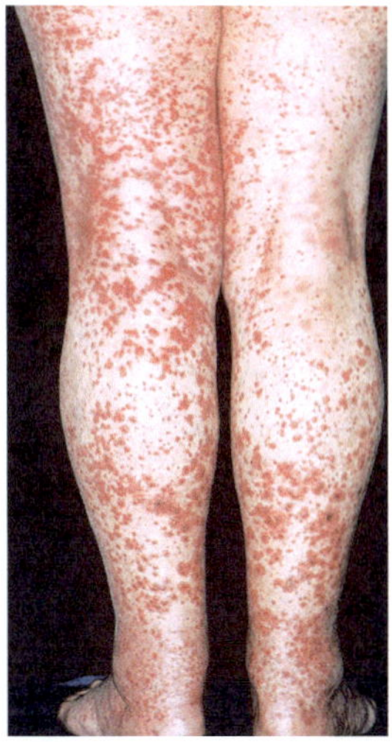

Fig. 17.1 Allergic vasculitis: purpura on the legs

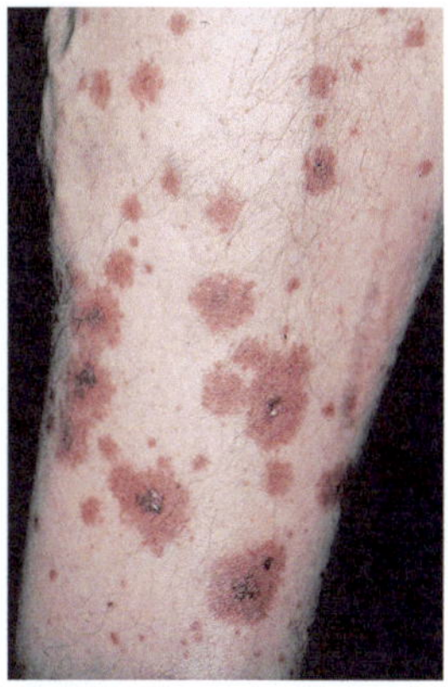

Fig. 17.2 Allergic vasculitis: hemorrhagic patches with central papules and blisters

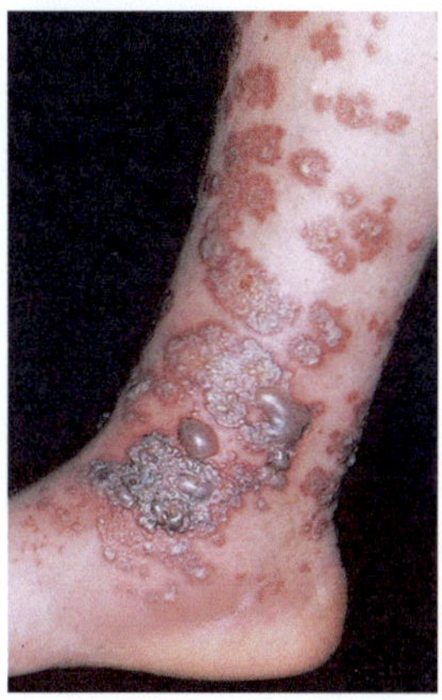

Fig. 17.3 Allergic vasculitis: hemorrhage with bullae

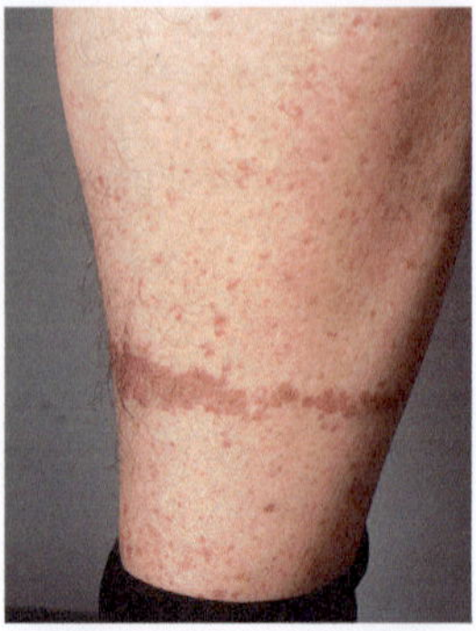

Fig. 17.4 Allergic vasculitis: circular hemorrhage on pressure line from socks

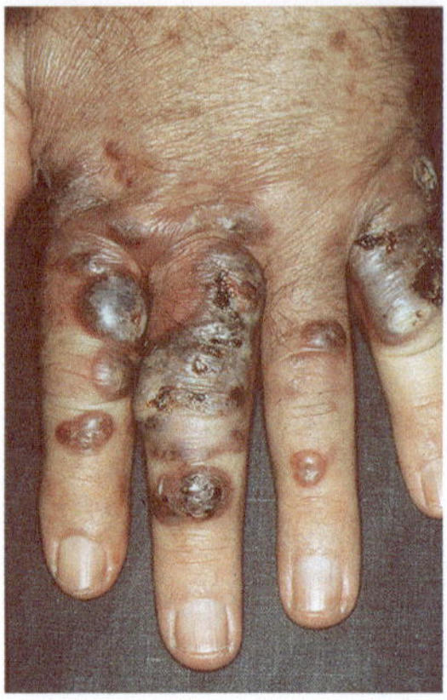

Fig. 17.5 Allergic vasculitis: bullous reaction in myelomonocytic leukemia

Level

Advanced

ICD-11

Leucocytoclastic vasculitis: 4A44.B

Synonyms

Hypersensitivity vasculitis; immunologic type III vasculitis; Schönlein-Henoch purpura

Epidemiology

Allergic vasculitis is one of the most frequent forms of vasculitis.

Schönlein-Henoch purpura has an incidence of 70/100 000 in those in children under 10 years of age.

Definition

The vasculitides are a heterogeneous group of uncommon diseases due to small vessel damage, usually via immune complex deposition in post-capillary venules, leading to blood vessel inflammation and necrosis.

Aetiology and Pathogenesis

Deposition of immune complexes (variable proportions of antibodies and antigens) in small vessel walls leads to complement activation, granulocyte activation and extravasation (leucocytoclasia) and finally microthrombosis of the small vessels. **Triggers** include infections (HIV, Hepatitis-C-Virus (HCV), bacteria), autoimmune and inflammatory diseases (connective tissue disease, anti neutrophil cytoplasm antibodies (ANCA)-associated vasculitis, inflammatory bowel disease), medications, tumour-associated antigens (solid tumours, haemotological). In almost 50% of the cases no trigger is found.

Signs and Symptoms

Initial symptoms of allergic vasculitis include purpuric, palpable, later necrotic lesions, including urticarial and nodular lesions. Internal organ involvement (kidneys, GI tract, joints, nervous system) may occur.

Localisation

Lesions generally predominate on the distal extremities, preferentially on the legs.

Classification

Allergic vasculitis can be separated into purely cutaneous forms (single organ vasculitis) and systemic forms (multi-organ vasculitis).

Laboratory and Other Workups

Histology, screening for blood parameters of inflammation

Dermatopathology

Early stages may show perivascular lymphocytes, macrophages and apoptotic leucocytes ("leucocytoclasia", nuclear dust), fibrin deposition in the vessel wall and sometimes microthrombosis of the small vessels. Usually erythrocyte extravasation occurs. IgG and IgM deposition may be found by direct skin immunofluorescence. IgA deposition is more characteristic of Schönlein-Henoch purpura.

Course

The course of allergic vasculitis may be acute, subacute, chronic or recurrent.

Complications

Allergic vasculitis may affect internal organs depending on the underlying cause. Renal and digestive involvement may characteristically occur in Schönlein-Henoch purpura.

Diagnosis

Allergic vasculitis is diagnosed based on the clinical manifestations and skin histology. Laboratory tests (renal and aetiological workup) are also required depending on the clinical presentation.

Differential Diagnosis

Differential diagnoses of allergic vasculitis include thrombotic diseases (cryoproteinaemia, antiphospholipid syndrome, cold agglutinins), thrombocytopenia clotting factor deficiency, including anticoagulants, embolic disorders (cholesterol emboli, atrial myxoma) and septic-embolic diseases (endocarditis).

Prevention and Therapy

Avoidance of triggers, bed rest, medication (systemic corticosteroids) depending on the aetiology and internal organ involvement. Anticoagulants in some specific cases.

Varicose Veins and Chronic Venous Insufficiency (CVI) [3, 4]

Figures 17.6, 17.7 and 17.8

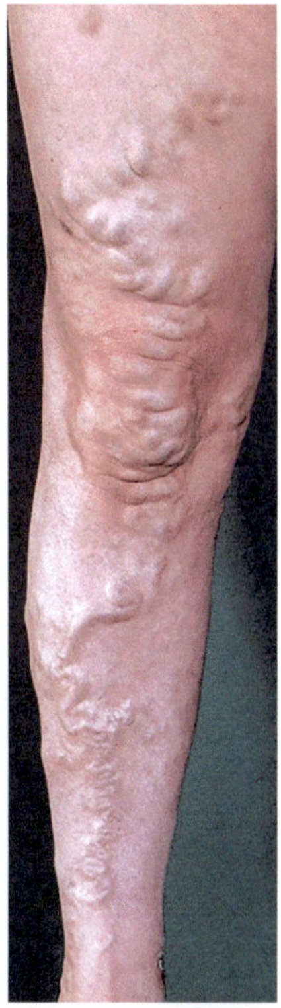

Fig. 17.6 Varicose veins: leg

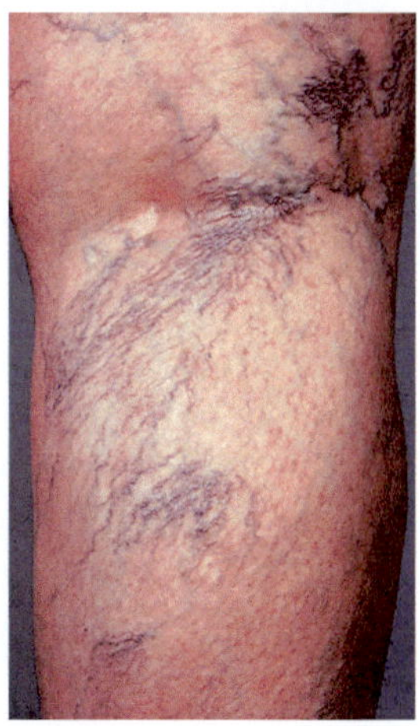

Fig. 17.7 Varicose veins: spider veins

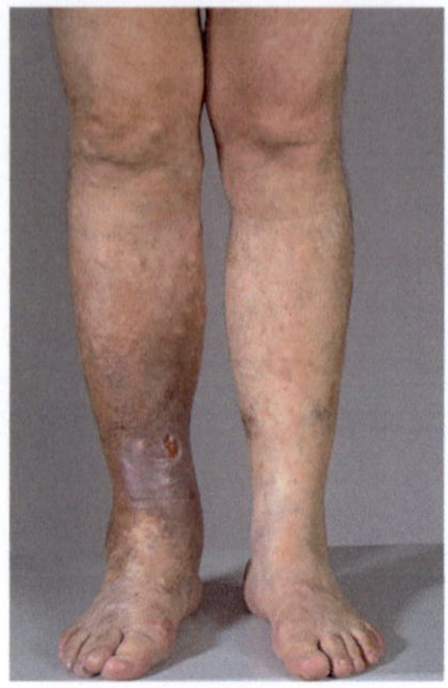

Fig. 17.8 Chronic venous insufficiency: dermatosclerosis, purpura and leg ulcer

Grading of Importance

B

Level

Advanced

ICD-11

BD74.1

Synonyms

Varicosis, varicosity, chronic venous disease, chronic peripheral venous insufficiency

Epidemiology

17% of adults and 37% of those over the age of 70 have chronic venous insufficiency (CVI).

Varicose veins: 37% in females, 19% in males.

CVI: 20% in females and 17% in males.

Definition

Ectatic changes in the superficial veins due to insufficient valves.

Aetiology and Pathogenesis

Primary varicosities (95%): Familial predisposition, prolonged (occupational) standing, multiple pregnancies, obesity and smoking all lead to dilatation of the veins and incompetence of the venous valves with reflux and increased venous stasis.

Secondary varicosities (5%): Post-inflammatory or post-thrombotic changes.

Signs and Symptoms

Stages of chronic venous insufficiency (by Widmer):

- **Stage I**: corona phlebectatica paraplantaris (prominent dilated vessels along sides of foot)
- **Stage II**: atrophie blanche, deposition of haemosiderin, hyperpigmentation, dermatoliposclerosis, stasis dermatitis, eczema, indurated oedema
- **Stage III**: ulcer (active or healed)
  Further clinical symptoms: pain, itching and leg heaviness

Localisation

Venous system of the lower legs:

Truncular

- Epifascial varices

Cutaneous varices with cosmetic relevance

- Reticular varices
- Spider veins

Classification

International standard classification for chronic venous disease (CEAP, clinical aetiology anatomy pathophysiology)

Grading of truncal vein incompetence of the greater and lesser saphenous vein according to Hach Widmer's classification of varicose veins

Laboratory and Other Workups

Imaging techniques: Duplex sonography, Doppler sonography, photoplethysmography, hyperspectral imaging, infrared thermography

Dermatopathology

Usually not necessary, except in situations like capillary convolutes mimicking Kaposi sarcoma.

Course

Chronic over years

Complications

Ulcer, stasis dermatitis and/or contact dermatitis, superficial thrombosis, bleeding, deep vein insufficiency

Diagnosis

Clinical findings. Palpation of the insufficient visible veins, imaging techniques

Differential Diagnosis

Congenital vessel malformation; dermatitis of different causes; lower leg eczema: allergic contact dermatitis, asteatotic, nummular dermatitis, skin mycosis, psoriasis

Prevention and Therapy

Leg training programme with activation of the foot, lower leg and upper leg muscle system. Movement at working place. In the evening resting legs by moving up.

Compression therapy: 90% of venous ulcers heal with adequate compression therapy.

Note: If arterial disease is also present, compression may be contraindicated.

- Truncal varicosities: surgery
- Accessory varicosities: surgery or sclerotherapy
- Spider veins: Sclerotherapy or laser destruction

Special

In young men with CVI, think of Klinefelter's syndrome (47, XXY).

Lymphangitis [2]

Figures 17.9 and 17.10

Grading of Importance

B

Level

Advanced

ICD-11

BD91

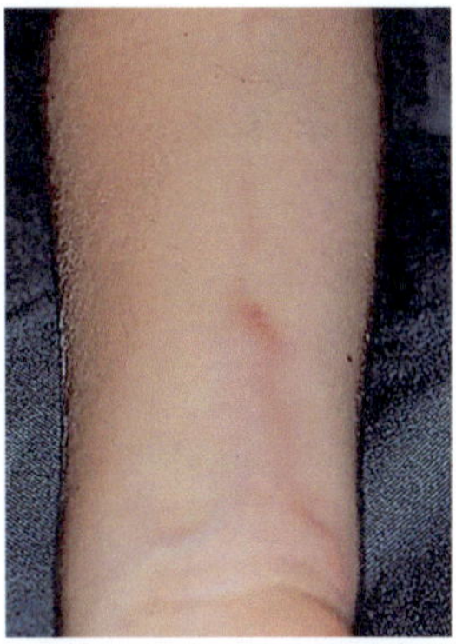

Fig. 17.9 Lymphangitis: inflammation along a lymphatic vessel

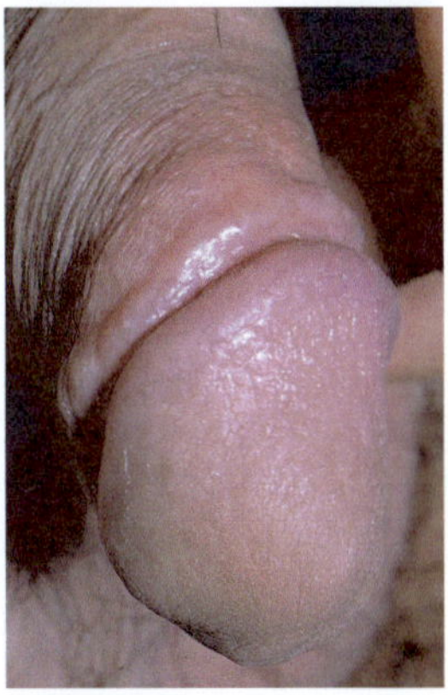

Fig. 17.10 Lymphangitis: sclerosing lymphangitis

Synonyms

None

Epidemiology

No clear statistical data available due to multifactorial pathogenesis

Definition

Inflammation along the lymphatic vessels

Aetiology and Pathogenesis

Most common causes are bacterial and mycotic leading to ascending infection of lymphatics draining to regional lymph nodes. Noninfectious inflammatory processes, such as an arthropod bite or sting (filariasis and onchocerciasis), can also cause lymphangitis/lymphadenitis. Tumour cell invasion causes lymphangitis carcinomatosa.

Signs and Symptoms

Linear, tender erythema between the primary skin lesion (entry point for infection, site of bite or sting, tumour invasion) and the regional lymph nodes

Localisation

Could appear elsewhere, mostly on extremities, sometimes trunk

Special location: sulcus beneath glans penis (sclerosing lymphangitis)

Classification

- Bacterial lymphangitis
  - Infestation-induced lymphangitis
  - Sclerosing lymphangitis (of the penis)
  - Lymphangitis carcinomatosa
- Mycotic lymphangitis: sporotrichosis

Laboratory and Other Workups

Markers for inflammation, bacterial and fungal swabs of entry site, regional lymph node sonography, tumour staging

Dermatopathology

Depending on cause, widening of vessels and accumulation of neutrophils and positive staining for bacteria or nodular lymphatic vessels like in sporotrichosis (PAS stain). In cancerous lymphangitis the lumen of vessels is filled with tumour cells which can be stained by immunohistochemistry according to suspected tumour origin.

Course

Acute. Usually responds rapidly to antibiotic therapy. In tumour association chronic progressive. Lymph vessels may become occluded and lymphedema occurs.

Complications

The primary site can evolve into an abscess. Development of cellulitis or sepsis. Chronic lymphedema (filariasis, relapsing erysipelas)

Diagnosis

Clinical findings, microbiology. Possibly duplex sonography to exclude superficial thrombophlebitis or tumour

Differential Diagnosis

Superficial thrombophlebitis, Mondor disease (inflammation of a superficial vein under the breast or the chest wall)

Prevention and Therapy

Antibiotic and antimycotic therapy, intravenously in severe cases. Start with empiric regimen based on likely causes and adjust with culture results. Treat the entry site (incision, debridement, drainage, disinfection). In severe cases: bed rest, thromboprophylaxis with fractionated heparin. Topical: cool compresses.

Treatment of infestation, tumour surgery (primary tumour) or systemic antitumor therapy (metastases)

References

1. Frumholtz L, Laurent-Roussel S, Lipsker D, Terrier B (2021) Cutaneous vasculitis: review on diagnosis and clinicopathologic correlations. Clin Rev Allergy Immunol. 61(2):181–193
2. Kostman JR, DiNubile MJ (1993) Nodular lymphangitis: a distinctive but often unrecognized syndrome. Ann Intern Med 118(11):883–888
3. Santler B, Goerge T (2017) Chronic venous insufficiency – a review of pathophysiology, diagnosis, and treatment. J Dtsch Dermatol Ges 15(5):538–556
4. Youn YJ, Lee J (2019) Chronic venous insufficiency and varicose veins of the lower extremities. Korean J Intern Med 34(2):269–283

Ulcers

18

Andreas Altenburg, Günter Burg,
and Christos C. Zouboulis

Contents

A. Altenburg (✉)
Staedtisches Klinikum Dessau, Brandenburg Medical School, Dessau, Germany
e-mail: andreas.altenburg@klinikumdessau.de

G. Burg
Dermatology, Zurich, Switzerland
e-mail: g.burg@access.uzh.ch

C. C. Zouboulis
Departments of Dermatology, Venereology, Allergology and Immunology, Staedtisches Klinikum Dessau, Brandenburg Medical School Theodor Fontane and Faculty of Health Sciences Brandenburg, Dessau, Germany
e-mail: christos.zouboulis@mhb-fontane.de

H. Gollnick et al. (eds.), *Dermatology Cyberderm WebBook*,
https://doi.org/10.1007/978-3-031-78491-0_18

Test your learning and check your understanding of this book's contents: use the "Springer Nature Flashcards" app to access questions using ▶ https://sn.pub/1rhh6k.
To use the app, please follow the instructions in Chap. 1.

Venous Leg Ulcers [3, 4]

Figures 18.1 and 18.2

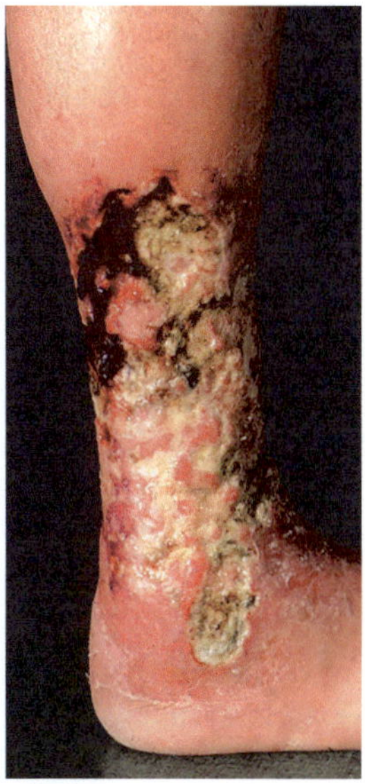

Fig. 18.1 Venous leg ulcer: chronic ulcer on the lower leg covered with fibrin

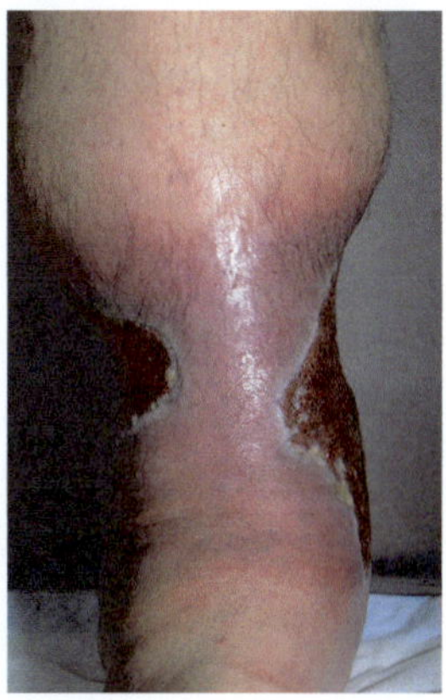

Fig. 18.2 Venous leg ulcer: chronic ulcer with hyperpigmentation and dermatosclerosis

Grading of Importance

B

Level

Advanced

ICD-11

BD74.3

Synonyms

Varicose ulcers

Epidemiology

Prevalence of all leg ulcers: 1–2% in the general population, 4–5% of individuals older than 80 years. 60–70% occur due to chronic venous insufficiency (CVI).

Definition

A chronic ulcer on the lower leg between knee and ankle joint resulting from improper functioning of venous valves and advanced chronic venous insufficiency (CVI).

Aetiology and Pathogenesis

The common denominator of vein ulcers is ischaemia of the upper dermis.

Signs and Symptoms

Moderate pain, which improves on elevation (unlike in arterial/mixed ulcers).

Irregular edges, associated oedema, atrophie blanche, pigmentation, associated superficial CVI.

Localisation

Perimalleolar and almost always medial

Classification

CEAP: clinical class 5, inactive (healed) ulceration; clinical class 6, active ulceration
CVI stage III by Widmer: active or healed ulceration

Dermatopathology

Biopsies from the edge of the wound should be considered if an ulcer does not respond or responds inadequately to therapy and has an atypical appearance.

Course

Chronic, recurrent

Complications

Cellulitis (erysipelas) with an ulcer as the entry site. Recurrent cellulitis is often relatively asymptomatic.

Diagnosis

Additional clinical findings: oedema, atrophie blanche, varicose vein(s)
Identification of CVI: duplex sonography

Differential Diagnosis

Vascular, haematological diseases, infections, traumatic/physical, autoimmune, metabolic/endocrine, iatrogenic, neoplasia, congenital

Prevention and Therapy

Improve general factors, nutrition and physical activity.
Compression therapy, stripping of varicosities, selective vein surgery.
Moist/semi-moist ulcer treatment.

Special

Costs: Venous leg ulcers account for about 1% of healthcare budgets in western countries.

Arterial Leg Ulcers [2]

Figures 18.3 and 18.4

Grading of Importance

B

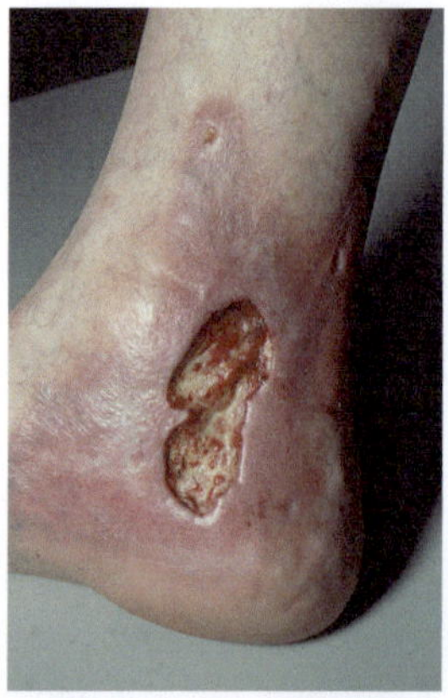

Fig. 18.3 Arterial leg ulcer: typical malleolar localization

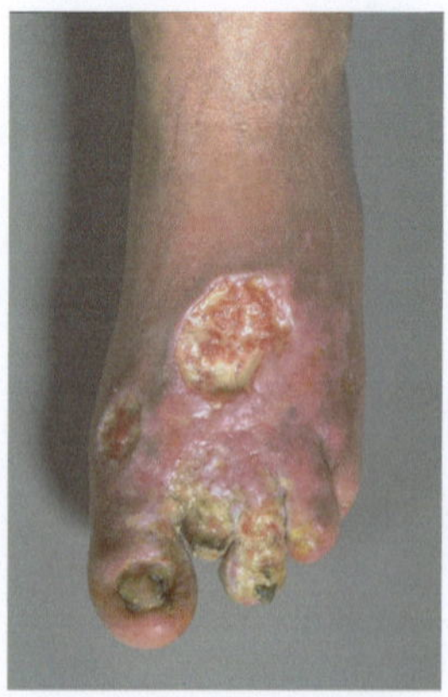

Fig. 18.4 Arterial leg ulcer: loss of a toe due to arterial occlusion

Level

Advanced

ICD-11

BD52.Y
Martorell's ulcer: BD41.Y

Synonyms

None

Epidemiology

Prevalence of all leg ulcers: 1–2% in the general population, 4–5% of individuals older than 80 years. Peripheral arterial occlusive disease (PAOD): the cause of 5–10% of leg ulcers, mixed CVI (chronic venous insufficiency) PAOD in 20%. Ulcus hypertonicum Martorell: 5%.

Definition

A chronic ulcer due to peripheral arterial occlusive disease (PAOD)

Aetiology and Pathogenesis

Chronic limb ischemia due to atherosclerosis of small, middle-sized and large arteries. Frequent trigger is a minor trauma. Martorell's ulcer combines PAOD with hypertensive arteriopathy and skin infarction in patients with essential arterial hypertension.

Signs and Symptoms

Severe local pain
Clinical description of ulcer

Localisation

Lateral side of the lower leg, proximal from (or including) the lateral malleolus or pretibial

Classification

Fontaine stage IV and Rutherford stages III and IV define ulceration with distal necrosis.

Laboratory and Other Workups

None

Dermatopathology

Biopsies from the edge of the wound should be considered if an ulcer does not respond or responds inadequately to therapy or has an atypical appearance, in order to exclude malignancy and to differentiate squamous cell carcinoma from pseudocarcinomatous hyperplasia.

Course

Chronic, progressive

Critical ischemia: poor prognosis without revascularization

Complications

In addition to loss of function, cellulitis (erysipelas) with an ulcer as the entry site and necrotizing fasciitis, amputation and increased mortality

Diagnosis

Clinical examination: Absent foot pulses, cold extremities, severe wound pain, claudicatio intermittens, rest pain, distal necrosis

Apparative examination: Systolic ankle and toe pressure, ankle brachial index (ABI): 0.9 or less, transcutaneaous oxygen pressure (tcPO2), duplex sonography, angiography

Differential Diagnosis

Other vascular diseases, haematological diseases, infections, traumatic/physical, autoimmune, tumour, metabolic/endocrine, iatrogenic, neoplasia

Prevention and Therapy

Prevention: healthy lifestyle, muscle activities, smoking cessation, reduction of metabolic disorder-related factors (hyperlipedaemia, diabetes).

Topical treatment: Appropriate phase-adjusted therapy of chronic wounds: Debridement (surgical, enzymatic), enhance granulation in moist milieu, encourage re-epithelialisation in non-occlusive, semi-moist milieu.

Medications improving arterial flow by infusion (PGE1, vasodilators)

Angioplasty stents, bypass surgery

Martorell's ulcer: necrosectomy and split skin transplantation.

Special

5–10% of ulcers on lower leg are neuropathic (metabolic disorders [diabetes mellitus], alcoholism, leprosy, neurosyphilis, traumas in polyneuropathy).

Neuropathic Ulcers [5]

Figures 18.5, 18.6 and 18.7

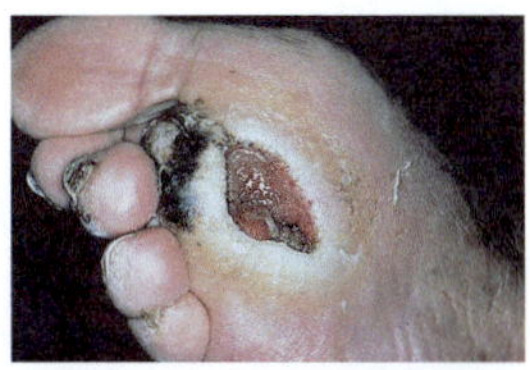

Fig. 18.5 Neuropathic ulcer: diabetic foot

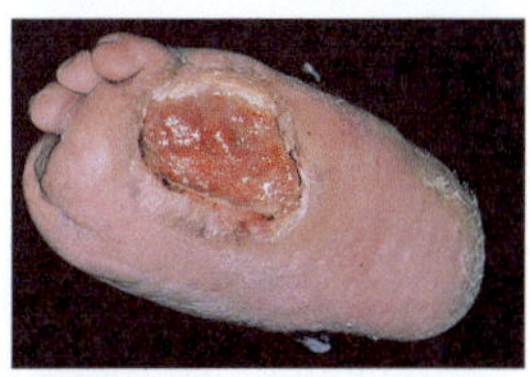

Fig. 18.6 Neuropathic ulcer: acro-osteopathia ulceromutilans in an alcoholic

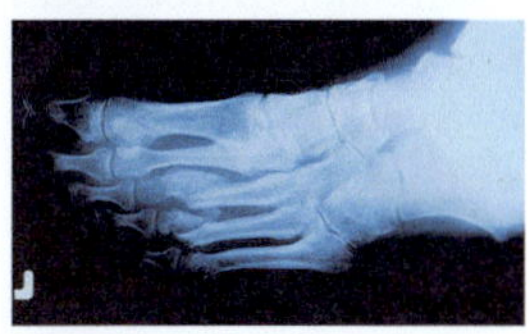

Fig. 18.7 Neuropathic ulcer: x-ray of fractures of the middle phalanx

Grading of Importance

C

Level

Basic

ICD-11

ED30.0

Synonyms

Neurotrophic ulcer, acroosteopathia ulceromutilans, malum perforans

Epidemiology

Prevalence up to 50 (6–51) % of patients with diabetes during their lifetime. There are no published statistics on the epidemiology of malum perforans in late-stage syphilis, leprosy or nerve injuries. The alcohol-induced malum perforans occurs exclusively in males with a distinct genetic disposition.

Definition

Ulceration in areas of physical/mechanical pressure on the basis of poly-aetiologic sensory polyneuropathy. Disturbance of the "trophic of the tissue", not of the venous or arterial circulation.

Aetiology and Pathogenesis

Sensory polyneuropathy with preference of thin nerve fibres on the basis of a genetic predisposition. Dissociated sensation deficit with loss of thermo-, pressure- and pain sensation. Potential causes are:

- Metabolic disorders: diabetes; rarely amyloidosis
- Alcohol (Bureau-Barrière syndrome)
- Infectious
- Syphilis (III/IV)
- Leprosy

- Nerve trauma (ischias)
- Hereditary (Thevenard syndrome)

Signs and Symptoms

Loss of thermo- and pressure sensitivity and of pain. Formation of a localized hyperkeratosis with a haemorrhagic bulla and finally ulceration. Fractures of the underlying bones (foot or toes) (acroosteopathia ulceromutilans). Hyperthermy of the involved limb with an- (diabetes) or hyperhidrosis (alcoholic polyneuropathy).

Localisation

Areas of mechanical pressure; preferentially heel and ball of the foot and toes

Classification

According to aetiology

Laboratory and Other Workups

Search for underlying disease. Imaging methods (X-ray; MRI). Determination of the (severely reduced) nerve conduction velocity. Neurologic status. Orthopaedic counselling

Dermatopathology

Not indicated.

Course

Chronic; depending on the underlying disorder

Complications

Superinfection; (painless) fractures; mutilation

Diagnosis

Clinical picture of painless ulcer in conjunction with an underlying disorder (see aetiology).

Differential Diagnosis

Venous or arterial ulcers

Prevention and Therapy

Prevention: avoidance and treatment of the aetiopahogenetic background.

Since the polyneuropathy is irreversible (vitamin B complex may be supportive in some instances), the only effective treatment is avoidance of pressure by appropriate orthopaedic shoes. Plastic reconstructive surgery must be an exception, since the benefit is only temporary.

Special

Cooperation with internal medicine and orthopaedics

Pressure Sore [1]

Figure 18.8

Grading of Importance

B

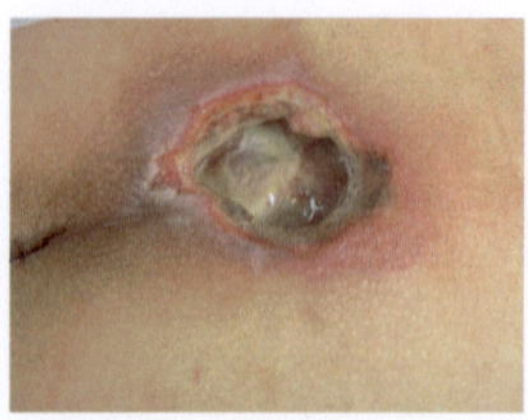

Fig. 18.8 Pressure sore: deep ulcer in the coccyx area

Level

Advanced

ICD-11

EH90.Z

Synonyms

Pressure ulcer, decubitus

Epidemiology

Prevalence: 10% of hospitalized patients, 5% of patients requiring nursing care at home

Definition

Pressure-induced defect of skin and subcutis.

Aetiology and Pathogenesis

Ischaemia caused by prolonged pressure over bony prominences in patients who are unable to move. Two hours of ischaemia is sufficient to induce a pressure sore. Diabetes mellitus, post-cerebral infarct reduced mobility, polyneuropathies, severe obesity and cachexia are risk factors.

Signs and Symptoms

Initial livid or bruise-like colour changes over the pressure points, reduced capillary refill. This stage is reversible. Later ulcers develop, involving skin, subcutis, muscles and often extending to the bones. Fetid odour.

Localisation

Typical sites: sacrum, trochanters, scapulae, heels, vertebral column, elbows, hands, back of head

Classification

Stage I: Livid erythema (macule or patch), some capillary refill

Stage II: Ulcer to dermis

Stage III: Ulcer with full thickness skin loss to subcutaneous fat

Stage IV: Ulcer with exposed or directly palpable fascia, muscle, tendon, ligament, cartilage or bone

Laboratory and Other Workups

Imaging studies, possibly nutritional evaluation, exclusion of diabetes and polyneuropathy

Dermatopathology

Biopsies of the ulcer margin and base should be taken after 8 to 12 weeks of ulcers without tendency to heal, primarily to rule out tumours. Biopsy should be taken especially before invasive measures.

Course

If pressure is not relieved, relentlessly progressive. Risk of cellulitis and sepsis.

Complications

Progression, superinfection with mixed bacterial flora, often with anaerobes, cellulitis, sepsis, osteomyelitis

Diagnosis

Clinical findings, assessment of depth with probe. Debridement. Imaging studies. Assessment of risk factors

Differential Diagnosis

Neuropathic pressure ulcer, ulcerated tumours, chronic infections with fistula formation, artefacts and injuries.

Prevention and Therapy

Prevention is most important.

In stage I the tissue damage is reversible. Immediate institution of pressure-relieving measurements. Protection of damaged skin. In stage II superficial tissue damage has occurred. Debridement of necrotic tissue and standard moist wound therapy. Appropriate antibiotic coverage.

In stages III and IV, the actual extent of the tissue damage is often underestimated. Extensive debridement, resection of the overhanging wound edges, vacuum-assisted wound therapy, standard moist wound therapy. Pressure sores in stages III and IV often require reconstructive surgery.

Special

Consider the potential impact of impaired nutritional status.

References

1. Cushing CA, Phillips LG (2013) Evidence-based medicine: pressure sores. Plast Reconstr Surg 132(6):1720–1732
2. Kirsner RS, Vivas AC (2015) Lower-extremity ulcers: diagnosis and management. Br J Dermatol 173(2):379–390
3. Nelson EA, Adderley U (2016) Venous leg ulcers. BMJ Clin Evid 2016:1902
4. Tan MKH, Luo R, Onida S, Maccatrozzo S, Davies AH (2019) Venous leg ulcer clinical practice guidelines: what is AGREEd? Eur J Vasc Endovasc Surg 57(1):121–129
5. Urso B, Ghias M, John A, Khachemoune A (2021) Neuropathic ulcers: a focused review. Int J Dermatol 60(10):e383–e389

Panniculitis

19

Jonathan M. White and Veronique del Marmol

Contents

J. M. White (✉)
Ecole de Santé Publique, Université libre de Bruxelles, Brussels, Belgium
e-mail: Jonathan.White@ulb.be

V. del Marmol
Départment of Dermatology, Hôpital Erasme-HUB, Université Libre de Bruxelles, Brussels, Belgium
e-mail: veronique.delmarmol@hubruxelles.be

H. Gollnick et al. (eds.), *Dermatology Cyberderm WebBook*,
https://doi.org/10.1007/978-3-031-78491-0_19

Test your learning and check your understanding of this book's contents: use the "Springer Nature Flashcards" app to access questions using ▶ https://sn.pub/1rhh6k.
To use the app, please follow the instructions in Chap. 1.

Panniculitis [1]

Figure 19.1

Grading of Importance

B

Level

null

ICD-11

EF00

Synonyms

None.

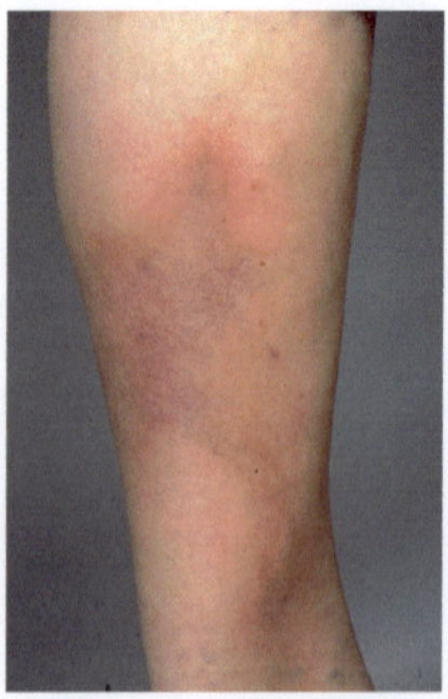

Fig. 19.1 Panniculitis: contusiform lesion on the leg

Epidemiology

Rare depending on underlying cause.

Definition

A heterogeneous group of diseases showing inflammation of subcutaneous adipose tissue.

Signs and Symptoms

Can be asymptomatic or affected areas tender on pressure. Fever, joint pains, systemic upset and ulcers may be present. Signs on examination of other systems may be helpful to make a clinical diagnosis.

Localisation

Varies according to underlying cause. Lupus panniculitis: upper torso and hips. Alpha$_1$-antitrypsin deficiency-associated panniculitis: pelvic girdle. Erythema induratum and lipodermatosclerosis: lower legs.

Classification

Predominantly septal panniculitis:

- As part of morphea or scleroderma
- Due to alpha$_1$-antitrypsin deficiency
- Erythema nodosum

Lobular and mixed septal/lobular panniculitis: all other types listed above

Laboratory and Other Workups

Depending on the underlying diagnosis.

Dermatopathology

Usually not necessary. Isolated pure forms of panniculitis are rare, and clinical and other laboratory features should be considered.

Course

Depending on the underlying cause. Some forms will burn out leaving hard permanent scars. Longstanding and migrating subtypes exist.

Complications

Depending on the underlying cause.

Diagnosis

Clinical features. Occasionally biopsy may be required.

Differential Diagnosis

Polyarteritis nodosa, nodular vasculitis and cellulitis, cutaneous T-cell lymphoma.

Prevention and Therapy

Depending on aetiology.

Special

None.

Pathogenesis

Various underlying causes of suppurative and non-suppurative panniculitis:

- As part of morphea or scleroderma
- Due to alpha$_1$-antitrypsin deficiency
- Post trauma
- Post infection
- Subcutaneous panniculitis T-cell lymphoma
- Lupus profundus

In association with:

- Tuberculosis (erythema induratum)
- Pancreatic disease
- Perinatal asphyxia or hypothermia (sclerema neonatorum and subcutaneous fat necrosis of the newborn)
- Post-steroid therapy
- Autoimmune dermatoses (systemic lupus erythematosus; dermatomyositis)
- Post-trauma including surgery
- Post-infection
- Chronic venous insufficiency (lipodermatosclerosis).

There may be overlapping causes of panniculitis (e.g. lupus erythematosus and trauma).

Reference

1. Requena L, Yus ES (2001) Panniculitis. Part I. Mostly septal panniculitis. J Am Acad Dermatol 45(2):163–183. quiz 184–166

Part VI

Genodermatoses, Metabolic Diseases and Pigmentary Disorders

There are no common features between these groups of diseases.

Genodermatoses

20

Martina Maurelli, Günter Burg, Giampiero Girolomoni, Paolo Gisondi, Ramon María Pujol Vallverdú, and Christos C. Zouboulis

Contents

M. Maurelli (✉) · G. Girolomoni · P. Gisondi
Department of Medicine, Università degli Studi di Verona, Verona, Italy
e-mail: martina.maurelli@univr.it; giampiero.girolomoni@univr.it; paolo.gisondi@univr.it

G. Burg
Dermatology, Zurich, Switzerland
e-mail: g.burg@access.uzh.ch

R. M. Pujol Vallverdú
Dermatology and Venereology, Universitat Autònoma de Barcelona, Hospital del Mar. IMIM, Barcelona, Spain
e-mail: rpujol@psmar.cat

C. C. Zouboulis
Departments of Dermatology, Venereology, Allergology and Immunology, Staedtisches Klinikum Dessau, Brandenburg Medical School Theodor Fontane and Faculty of Health Sciences Brandenburg, Dessau, Germany
e-mail: christos.zouboulis@mhb-fontane.de

H. Gollnick et al. (eds.), *Dermatology Cyberderm WebBook*,
https://doi.org/10.1007/978-3-031-78491-0_20

Test your learning and check your understanding of this book's contents: use the "Springer Nature Flashcards" app to access questions using ▶ https://sn.pub/1rhh6k.

To use the app, please follow the instructions in Chap. 1.

Neurofibromatosis [5]

Figures 20.1, 20.2 and 20.3

Grading of Importance

B

Fig. 20.1 Neurofibromatosis: soft fibromas on the trunk

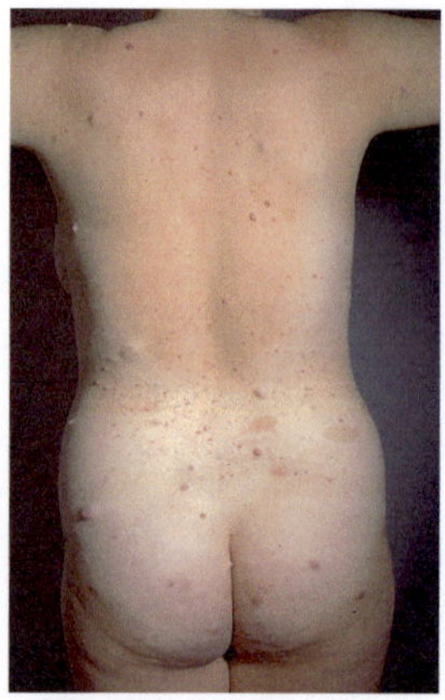

Fig. 20.2 Neurofibromatosis: café-au-lait spot and pigmented macules on the trunk

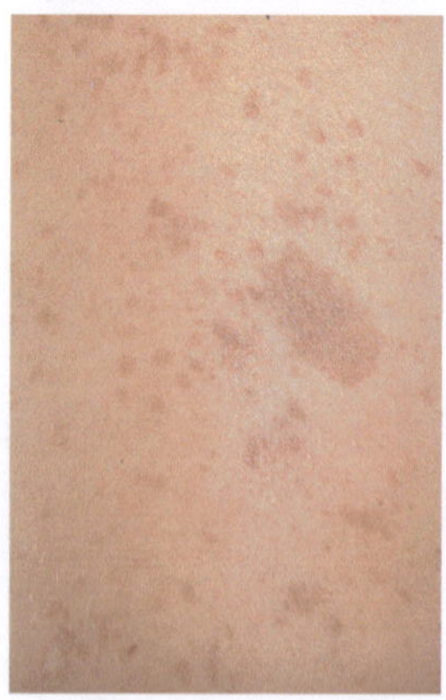

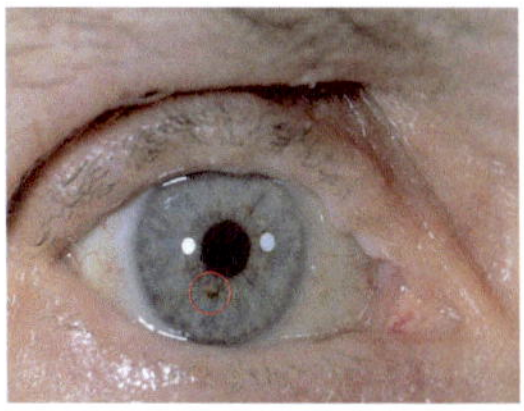

Fig. 20.3 Neurofibromatosis: pigmented iris hamartoma (Lisch nodule)

Level

Advanced

ICD-11

LD2D.1Z

Synonyms

Von Recklinghausen disease

Epidemiology

Rare diseases. Neurofibromatosis Type 1 (NF1); prevalence 1:2000–3500; incidence, 1:2000–3000—male/female ratio approx. 1:1

Neurofibromatosis Type 2 (NF2): Prevalence 1:100,000, incidence 1:33,000–40,000

Definition

Genetic disease, autosomal dominant inheritance, sporadic appearance in 43%. Neurocutaneous disease with multiple benign neurofibromas and potentially multi-organ involvement.

Etiology and Pathogenesis

Mutations in suppressor genes

NF1: Neurofibromin (chromosome 17q11.2)

NF2: Merlin (schwannomin) (chromosome 22q12)

Signs and Symptoms

NF1:

- Skin: café-au-lait macules (>5, larger than 1.5 cm, 86%), axillary and inguinal freckling (84%), cutaneous neurofibromas (localized, buttonhole phenomenon, 75–99%), plexiform neurofibromas (large nodular or diffuse tumors, 30%)
- Eyes: pigmented iris hamartomas (Lisch nodules) (40%)
- Skeletal system: kyphoscoliosis (25%)
- CNS: optic pathway glioma (13%)
- Other organs: hydrocephalus (3%)

NF2:

- Vestibular schwannomas (usually bilateral; 95%)
- Schwannomas on other intracranial nerves and in the spinal compartment
- Meningiomas, ependymomas, and gliomas

Localization

Generalized

Classification

Molecular classification

- NF1: skin findings, neurofibromas, Lisch nodules
- NF2: bilateral acoustic schwannomas

Laboratory and Other Workups

Genetic analysis

Examinations via radiological and other imaging techniques for detection of organ involvement and complications

Dermatopathology

Cutaneous neurofibroma: Nonencapsulated proliferation of all elements of peripheral nerves

Plexiform neurofibroma: Tumor growth within and beyond a nerve bundle

Course

The course of the disease is not predictable. Cutaneous neurofibromas and café-au-lait macules can increase with progressing age (always benign). Plexiform neurofibromas have a potential for malignant transformation. Half of the patients with optic pathway glioma will develop visual symptoms. Long-bone dysplasia can result in pseudarthrosis.

NF1 life time risk for malignant nerve sheath tumor-associated mortality 8–13%.

Complications

Diagnosis

Clinical findings, family history, genetic analysis

Differential Diagnosis

Clinical: lentigines, phakomatoses, neurofibrosarcoma
Histopathological: Schwannoma, perineuroma, dermatofibrosarcoma protuberans

Prevention and Therapy

Genetic counseling, excision of disturbing or painful neurofibromas

Xeroderma Pigmentosum [2, 9, 10]

Figures 20.4, 20.5, 20.6 and 20.7

Grading of Importance

C

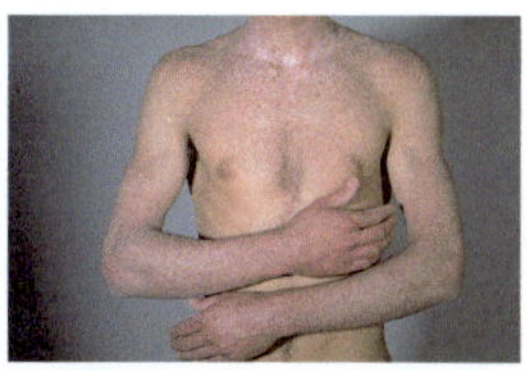

Fig. 20.4 Xeroderma pigmentosum: pigmentation in sun exposed areas

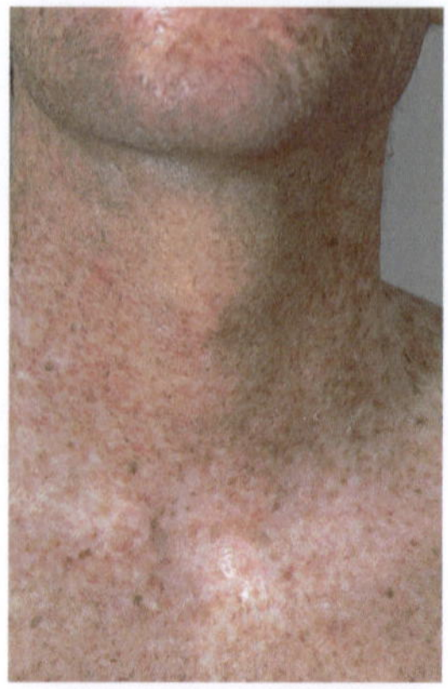

Fig. 20.5 Xeroderma pigmentosum: "dirty" looking de-and hyperpigmentation

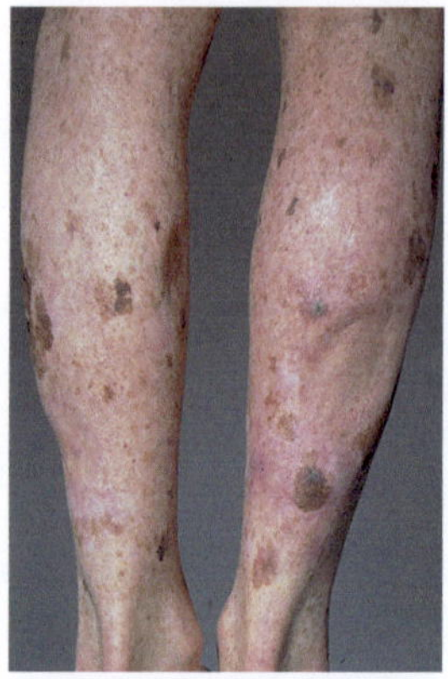

Fig. 20.6 Xeroderma pigmentosum: multiple carcinomas on the legs

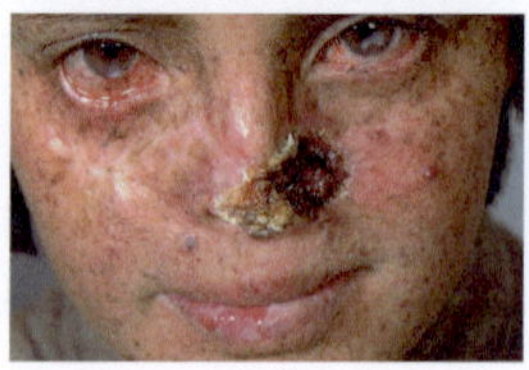

Fig. 20.7 Xeroderma pigmentosum: mutilating carcinoma of the nose

Level

Advanced

ICD-11

LD27.1

Synonyms

XP

Epidemiology

From about 1 in 500,000 live births in Western Europe to much higher frequencies in Japan and North Africa.

Definition

Group of uncommon genodermatoses with markedly increased light sensitivity and tendency toward developing actinic damage and malignant skin tumors.

Etiology and Pathogenesis

Autosomal recessive inherited defects in DNA excision repair enzymes. Cells cannot repair UV-induced damage.

Signs and Symptoms

Marked photosensitivity with acute photodermatitis and marked actinic damage, multiple lentigines, including actinic keratoses, squamous cell carcinomas, basal cell carcinomas, malignant melanomas, poikiloderma, skin atrophy. Eyes also suffer UV damage. Some types (DeSanctis-Cacchione syndrome) have neurological findings.

Localization

Generalized; visible symptoms in UV light-exposed areas

Classification

Types A–G dependent on type of gene defect

Laboratory and Other Workups

Identification of endonuclease and other repair enzyme defects in cultured fibroblasts, DNA sequencing of known genes

Dermatopathology

According to light induced skin damage and type and stage of tumor

Course

Reduced life expectancy starting already in the first life decade and depending on defect. Development of multiple malignant skin tumors, especially squamous cell carcinomas and malignant melanomas.

Complications

Development of malignant skin tumors (squamous cell carcinoma, basal cell carcinoma, malignant melanoma) before 20 years of age.

Diagnosis

Clinical findings (photosensitivity, early actinic damage), genetic analysis, family history.

Differential Diagnosis

Xeroderma pigmentosum variants with same phenotype, later onset, no genetic defects (pigmented xerodermoid).

Prevention and Therapy

Consequent avoidance of UV exposure. Early use of high-potency broad-spectrum sunscreens, close clinical control, prompt tumor excision. Systemic retinoids for prophylaxis. Vitamin D supplementation. Genetic counseling.

Epidermolysis Bullosa [3, 6, 7]

Figures 20.8, 20.9 and 20.10

Grading of Importance

C

Level

Advanced

ICD-11

EC30, EC3Z, EB43

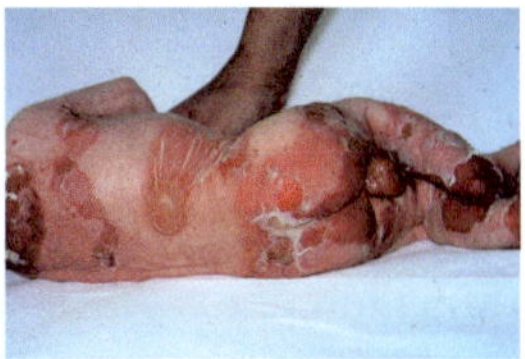

Fig. 20.8 Epidermolysis bullosa: bullae and loss of skin in a newborn

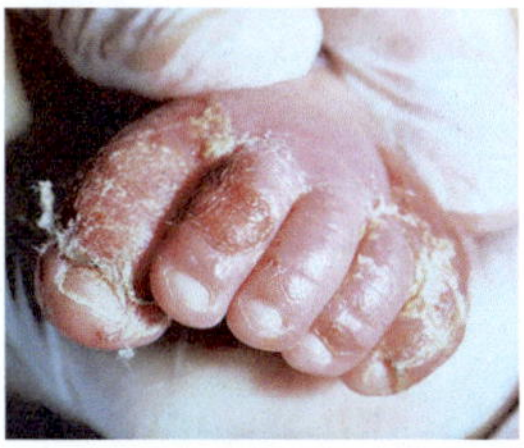

Fig. 20.9 Epidermolysis bullosa: bullae on exposed area of toes

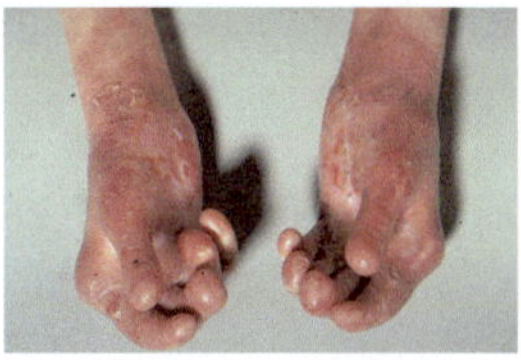

Fig. 20.10 Epidermolysis bullosa: sclerodactyly (scarring) in dystrophic EB

Epidemiology

0.2 in 100000 live births worldwide; estimated 500000 cases worldwide. (Orphan disease). Epidermolysis bullosa simplex the most common subtype of epidermolysis diseases (>90%).

Definition

Group of genetic diseases with skin fragility in which minimal trauma leads to the formation of blisters; autosomal dominant and autosomal recessive inheritance.

Etiology and Pathogenesis

Mutations in structural proteins and adhesive complexes of the epidermis and the epidermal-dermal junction.

Signs and Symptoms

Blisters heal with or without scars, depending on the level of the defect (mutilations). With widespread disease, disturbances in electrolyte, water, and protein balance. With oral and gastrointestinal tract involvement with life-threatening scarring, difficulties for eating and failure to thrive.

Localization

Every part of the body can be involved, predilection to areas exposed to pressure and friction.

Classification

Several subtypes depending on location of defective protein and level of blister formation in the skin. Clinically mild and severe forms of:

- Epidermolysis bullosa simplex
- Junctional epidermolysis bullosa
- Dystrophic epidermolysis bullosa

Laboratory and Other Workups

Dermatopathology, immunofluorescent antigen mapping, electron microscopy, DNA sequencing of candidate genes

Dermatopathology

Epidermolysis bullosa simplex: intraepidermal cleavage (keratin 5 and 14 defects)

Junctional epidermolysis bullosa: cleavage at the dermo-epidermal junction (lamina lucida)

Dystrophic epidermolysis bullosa: subepidermal cleavage (collagen VII)

Course

Depending on variant, ranging from mild nuisance to fatal disease. Life-long disabling disease, continuous wound care, marked psychosocial problems, and reduced quality of life. Epidermolysis bullosa simplex improves with age.

Complications

Variable—none in mild forms; infections, scarring with mutilations and with development of squamous cell carcinomas in more severe variants. Early death possible.

Diagnosis

Clinical findings and laboratory investigations, family history

Differential Diagnosis

Other blistering disorders (pemphigoid, pemphigus, linear IgA bullous dermatosis, epidermolysis bullosa acquisita), peeling skin syndrome, congenital localized absence of skin, suction blisters, and mechanical blisters by friction and trauma.

Prevention and Therapy

Refer severe cases to special centers. Intensive skin care, avoidance of pressure and friction. Prevention of secondary infections. No specific systemic therapy available. Autologous skin transplantation and gene therapy. Patient support groups very helpful.

Ichthyoses [11, 15]

Figures 20.11, 20.12 and 20.13

Grading of Importance

C

Level

Advanced

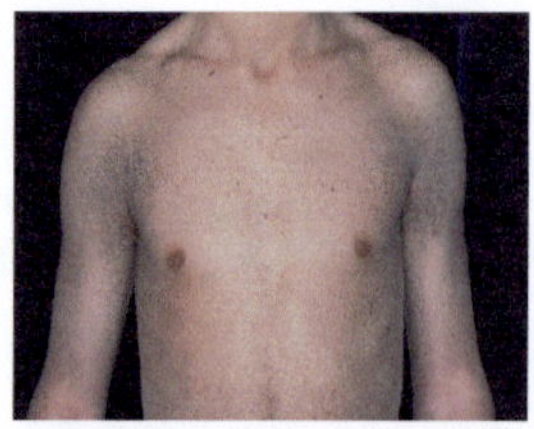

Fig. 20.11 Ichthyosis: "dirty" appearing skin

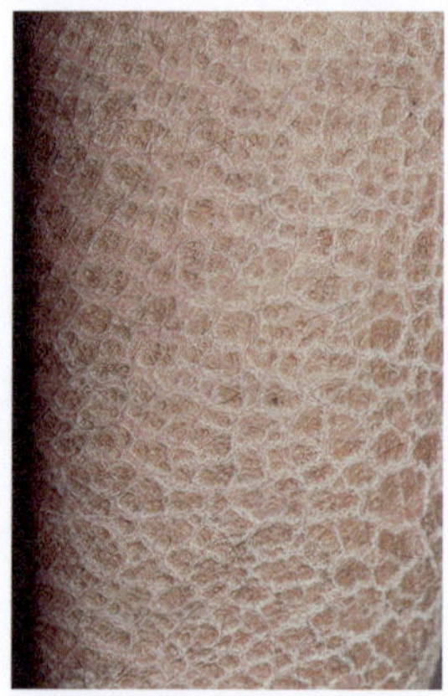

Fig. 20.12 Ichthyosis: hyperkeratotic scales

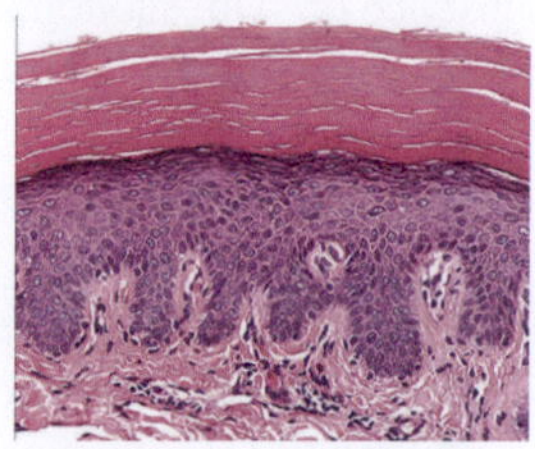

Fig. 20.13 Ichthyosis: histology showing compact hyperkeratosis

ICD-11

ED50.Z

Epidemiology

Ichthyosis vulgaris: prevalence 1:250–1:1000 newborns
X-linked recessive ichthyosis: 1:2000–1:6000 males
Autosomal recessive congenital ichthyosis (ARCI): 1:100000
Acquired ichthyosis: unknown
Syndromic ichthyosis: unknown

Definition

- Group of hereditary disorders of keratinization with different patterns of inheritance and genetic defects
- Group of acquired disorders of keratinization of different origin

Etiology and Pathogenesis

- Ichthyosis vulgaris: autosomal dominant. Loss-of-function mutations in the gene coding profilaggrin (FLG)
- X-linked recessive ichthyosis: hereditary deficiency of the steroid sulfatase (STS) gene deletions
- Autosomal recessive congenital ichthyosis (ARCI): defects in keratin genes, transglutaminase, or other structural proteins
- Acquired ichthyosis: associated with HIV infection, certain drugs, such as, statins, paraneoplastic diseases (see Chap. 12), cutaneous T-cell lymphomas, metabolic disorders
- Syndromic ichthyosis

Signs and Symptoms

Mild to severe scaling and hyperkeratosis:

- Ichthyosis vulgaris: starts in 1st year of life, dry rough scaly skin, symmetrical on the trunk and extremities, sparing of flexural area, hyperlinearity of palms and soles. 50% of cases associated with atopic dermatitis.
- X-linked recessive ichthyosis: similar to ichthyosis vulgaris, but flexures are involved, undescended testes in 30%. Large, dark-brown scales, lesions spread to the whole body.

- Autosomal recessive congenital ichthyosis (ARCI): generalized ichthyosis, present at birth often associated with erythroderma. Occasionally ectropion of eyelids.

Collodium baby: newborn with thick, stiff fissured sheets of stratum corneum; many causes. Initial manifestation of a ARCI.

Localization

- Extremities, especially with or without involvement of flexural areas, groin, palms and soles, lower legs
- All body surface in the extensive forms

Classification

- Non-syndromic: only affecting the skin (ichthyosis vulgaris, ARCI, epidermolytic ichthyosis, acquired ichthyosis, and others)
- Syndromic: involvement of other organ systems in addition to the skin (Chanarin-Dorfman syndrome, Comèl-Netherton syndrome, keratitis. Ichthyosis and deafness syndrome, Refsum's disease, Sjögren-Larsson syndrome, trichothiodystrophy).

Laboratory and Other Workups

Complete blood count, electrolytes, hepatic panel, immunoglobulin levels (including IgE). Peripheral blood smear to evaluate for vacuoles in leukocytes. Hearing screening. Ophthamologic examination. X-rays to evaluate epiphyses. Skin biopsy and genetic test. Transepidermal water loss.

Dermatopathology

Main features: Mild orthokeratotic hyperkeratosis, diminished or thickened granular layer. Immunohistochemistry demonstrates diminished or absent filaggrin. Specific subtypes exist by histology.

Course

Severity and symptoms (itch) depend on the season and the climate, improving in the summer and with high humidity. Ichthyosis vulgaris is usually progressive during childhood, and improves with age.

Complications

Bacterial super-infections. Psychosocial problems. Reduced sweating, compromised thermo regulation, hair loss.

Diagnosis

- Clinical
- Histology
- Blood and molecular tests

Differential Diagnosis

Asteatotic skin (e.g., in higher age or in alcoholics), exsiccation eczema, erythroderma in lymphomas, erythrodermic psoriasis, erythrodermic atopic dermatitis.

Prevention and Therapy

Prenatal diagnosis for congenital ichthyosis. Reference centers for severe cases. Daily application of emollients. Keratolytic agents, such as urea, salicylic acid, lactic acid ointments, topical retinoids. Systemic retinoids (isotretinoin, acitretin).

Palmoplantar Keratoderma [1, 12, 13]

Figures 20.14 and 20.15

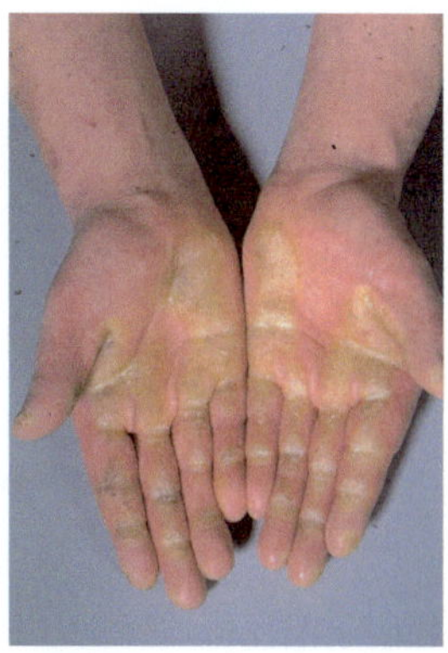

Fig. 20.14 Palmoplantar keratoderma: palmar hyperkeratosis

Fig. 20.15 Palmoplantar keratoderma: plantar hyperkeratosis

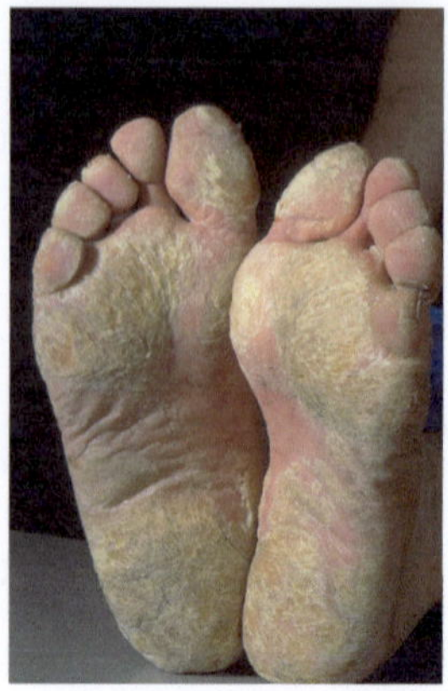

Grading of Importance

C

Level

Advanced

ICD-11

ED55

Synonyms

Keratosis palmoplantaris

Epidemiology

Includes genetic as well as acquired forms. Uncommon disorders. Autosomal dominant (1:100 000) and autosomal recessive disorders. Genetic "hotspot" in the kration island of mijet (name giver).

Definition

Persistent thickening of the epidermis of palms and soles

Etiology and Pathogenesis

Hereditary palmo-plantar keratodermas (PPK) include a high number of genodermatoses with different prognoses with multiple associated cutaneous and extracutaneous features.

Many different genes have been identified in diffuse PPK secondary to keratin mutations (epidermolytic and non-epidermolytic) in an autosomal dominant and recessive pattern of inheritance. Many different clinical variants with multiple implicated genes in focal, striated complex and syndromic hereditary PPKs.

In acquired PPKs, a spectrum of disorders of different etiology may be involved: occupational, irritative, contact allergies, keratoderma climatericum, chemicals, drugs, systemic diseases, malignancies, infectious disorders, inflammatory dermatoses, lymphomas, paraneoplastic.

Signs and Symptoms

Onset usually in infancy, symmetrical, palms and soles thickened, yellow and fissured with diffuse or focal symmetrical lesions, often hyperhidrosis. Some variants may worsen by age and may show involvement of back of the hands and lower arms (transgrediens). Association with other ectodermal defects possible.

Acquired PPK may also be focal, diffuse or punctate.

Localization

Palms and soles. In some cases may extend to the dorsal surfaces of the hands and feet, wrists and Achille's tendons. Different disorders may present associated hyperkeratotic cutaneous or mucosal lesions, often involving the extensor surfaces of the extremities (knees, elbows), hair, nail and teeth abnormalities.

Classification

Depending on Etiology: Hereditary or acquired PPK

- Hereditary PPK: Diffuse or focal hyperkeratosis, with or without associated findings, exact classification based on molecular genetic identification of mutations. Hereditary PPK can be divided into:
  - Non-syndromic isolated PPK: Predominant or unique palmo-plantar involvement
  - Complex PPK: Non-syndromic PPK with additional distinctive cutaneous and adnexal manifestations
- Syndromic PPK: PPK associated with specific extracutaneous manifestations

  - PPK associated with sensorineural deafness
  - PPK associated with prominent mucosal involvement
  - PPK associated with cardiomyopathy and woolly hair
  - PPK associated with other systemic signs

- Acquired PPK: Classification according the observed **clinical patterns**:

  - Diffuse PPK: Generalized epidermal thickening involving the entire palmoplantar surfaces.
  - Focal PPK: Multiple callosities (soles)
  - Striate PPK: Linear hyperkeratotic bands in correspondence with the underlying tendons
  - Punctate PPK: Multiple papular lesions with epidermal thickening (with a central pit or spiny projection)

Laboratory and Other Workups

No abnormalities are usually detected. For certain forms of hereditary PPK molecular profiling has to be done, and in acquired PPK individual workup necessary depending on the underlying disease is needed.

Dermatopathology

Non-epidermolytic PPK: acanthosis, hypergranulosis, hyperkeratosis, orthokeratosis.

Epidermolytic PPK variants: Perinuclear vacuolization, granular degeneration of keratinocytes, large, irregular keratohyaline granules. Subcorneal intraepidermal cleavage.

In acquired PPK the histopathological features are nonspecific: hyperkeratosis with orthokeratosis or parakeratosis and different amount of inflammation.

Course

Chronic

Complications

Secondary fungal infection. In syndromic PPK the associated features (cardiomyopathy) may have prognostic implications. Psychosocial problems.

Diagnosis

Clinical history and features combined with histopathological findings. Positive family history and onset in infancy or childhood may be helpful to distinguish between hereditary and acquired PPK. The clinical pattern (diffuse, striate/focal or punctate) along the presence with other cutaneous or extracutaneous manifestations may also be helpful. In some cases, the genetic study may confirm the diagnosis. In acquired PPK a systematic search for an underlying cause is mandatory.

Differential Diagnosis

The different acquired etiologies that may lead to PPK. Other causes of palmoplantar keratoses: Hand dermatitis (hyperkeratotic, fissured), Psoriasis and hyperkeratotic lesions in secondary syphilis, cutaneous T-cell lymphoma (especially Sézary syndrome), dyskeratosis folLicularis (Darier).

Prevention and Therapy

Topical keratolytics: salicylic acid (5–10%), urea, lactic acid, vitamin A acid, abrasive soaps, mechanical removal. Customized footwear.

Systemic: low-dose retinoids (acitretin) or 9-cis retinoic acid.

In the acquired variants of PPK: To identify (if possible) and treat the underlying etiology.

Dyskeratosis Follicularis (Darier) [14]

Figures 20.16, 20.17, 20.18 and 20.19

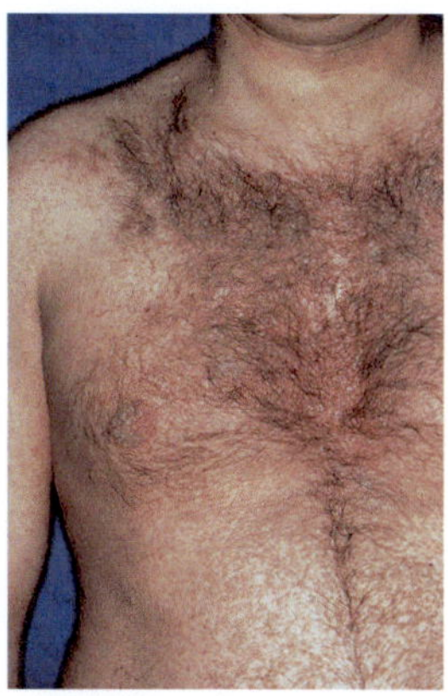

Fig. 20.16 Dyskeratosis follicularis (Darier): small grayish-brown hyperkeratotic tiny papules on the trunk

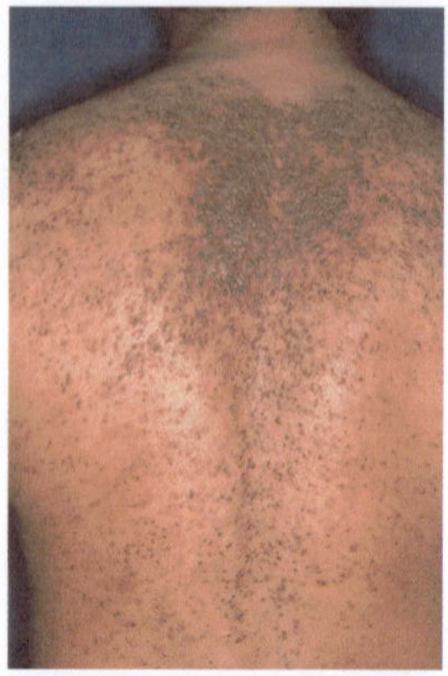

Fig. 20.17 Dyskeratosis follicularis (Darier): hyperkeratotic papules on the back

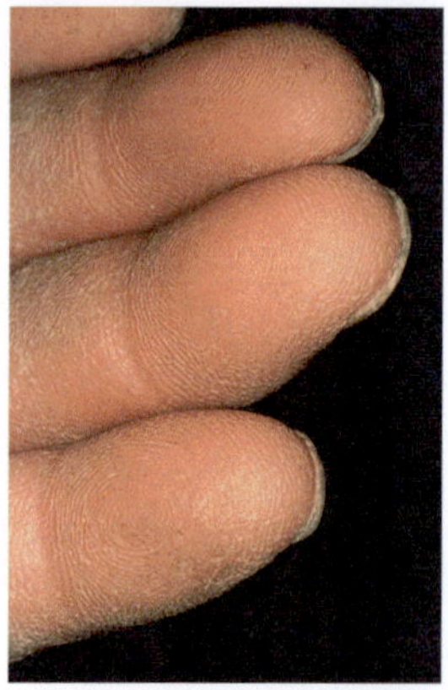

Fig. 20.18 Dyskeratosis follicularis (Darier): punctiform interruptions of the papillary strip structure on the fingers

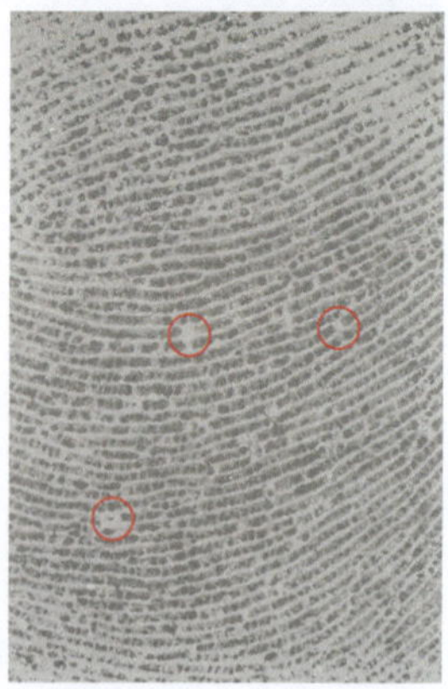

Fig. 20.19 Dyskeratosis follicularis (Darier): imprint of the papillary structure of fingertips

Grading of Importance

C

Level

Basic

ICD-11

EC20.2

Synonyms

Darier's disease, Morbus Darier, Morbus Darier-White

Epidemiology

Incidence 1:30,000–100,000. Men are more severely affected than women. Start in early life or adolescence. Life expectancy normal.

Definition

Autosomal dominant inherited, acantholytic cornification disorder of epidermis, hair follicles, and nails.

Etiology and Pathogenesis

A mutation on chromosome 12 leads to disruption calcium ATPase. The formation of desmosomal tonofilaments and the differentiation of keratinocytes is disturbed, resulting in acantholysis. Trigger factors: UV light, sweating, virus infections (herpes simplex), caffeine, alcohol, stress.

Signs and Symptoms

- Skin: small grayish-brown, itchy keratotic papules; occasionally confluent, weeping, foul-smelling. Punctiform interruptions of the papillary strip structure on the fingers and toes. Verrucous papules on the back of the hand are also known as Acrokeratosis verruciformis Hopf.

- Oral mucosa and hard palate: leukoplakia-like changes with small papules.
- Nails: dystrophy with formation of grooves and subungual hyperkeratosis.

Localization

Seborrheic regions: centrofacial, scalp, axillary region, central breast and back regions, inguinal region, anogenital

Classification

Special form: Verrucous papules on the back of the hand are also referred to as Acrokeratosis verruciformis Hopf.

Laboratory and Other Workups

Skin biopsy

Dermatopathology

- Dyskeratosis: defective differentiation of keratinocytes with corps ronds (eosinophilic cells in str. spinosum) and corps grains (granular nuclear residues in str. granulosum). Verrucous hyperkeratosis, especially in acrokeratosis verruciformis Hopf.
- Acantholysis: suprabasal cleft formation with numerous eosinophilic granulocytes.

Course

Chronic; worsening in the first years of illness

Complications

Superinfection

Diagnosis

Clinical and histological picture

Differential Diagnosis

Seborrheic dermatitis, pemphigus benignus familiaris (Hailey-Hailey), transient acantholytic dermatosis (Grover's disease), pemphigus vegetans (intertriginous), acanthosis nigricans, verrucous epidermal nevi.

Prevention and Therapy

Prevention: Avoidance of direct exposure to the sun (UV; sweating)
Topical: Retinoids, antiseptic baths, short-term weak glucocorticosteroids
Systemic: Acitretin; antibiotics if needed (superinfection)
Surgical: Exceptionally dermabrasion, laser

Special

Grover's disease (transitory acantholytic dermatosis) is an important differential diagnosis predominantly in older men with a tendency to relapse after transient phases of regression.

Pseudoxanthoma Elasticum [4, 8]

Figures 20.20, 20.21 and 20.22

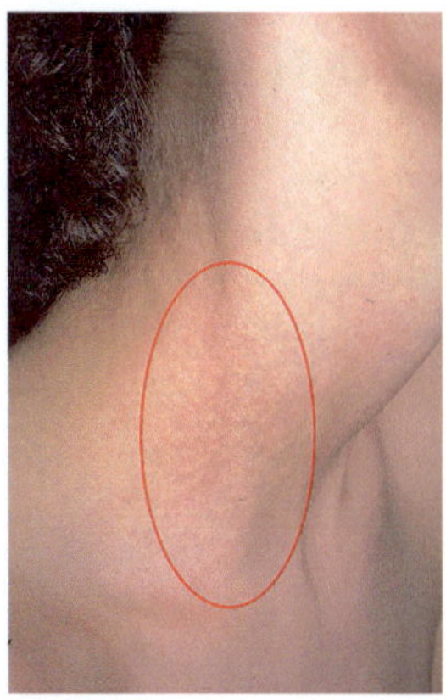

Fig. 20.20 Pseudoxanthoma elasticum: small yellow papules on the neck

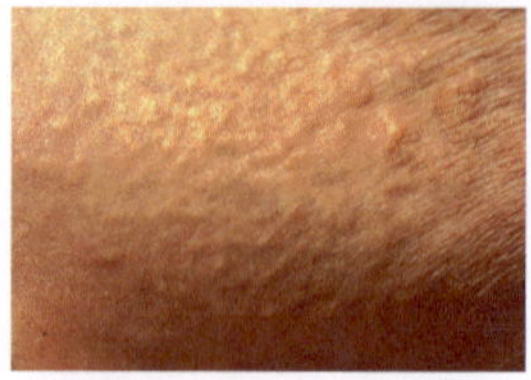

Fig. 20.21 Pseudoxanthoma elasticum: wrinkling structure of the skin

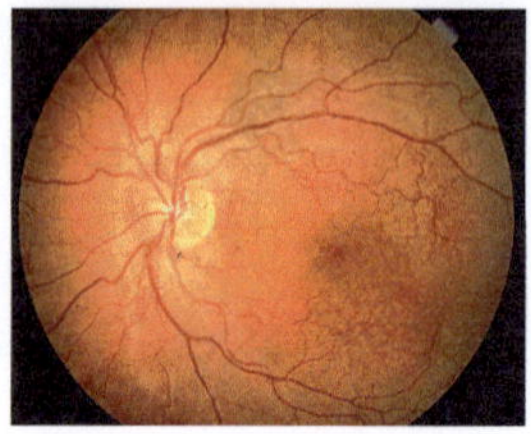

Fig. 20.22 Pseudoxanthoma elasticum: angioid streaks of the eye

Grading of Importance

C

Level

Basic

ICD-11

Q82.8

Synonyms

Grönblad-Strandberg syndrome

Epidemiology

Prevalence: 0.25–1 per 100,000 of the general population; slight female predominance. Cutaneous alterations develop during childhood; ocular and cardiovascular complications manifest in the third and fourth decade of life.

Definition

Autosomal recessive disorder; elastic fibers of the skin, eyes, and cardiovascular system become progressively calcified leading to a spectrum of manifestations with a variable phenotype.

Etiology and Pathogenesis

Various gene mutations on the short arm of chromosome 16, resulting in impairment of the proper function of elastin and elastic fibers in the mid and deep dermis, the media and the intima of mid-sized arteries, and Bruch's membrane in the eye, with the clinical and histological typical pathologic alterations.

Signs and Symptoms

- Skin: small yellow papules (diameter up to 10 mm) on the nape and sides of the neck and in flexural areas, coalescing into reticulated plaques as the disease progresses, giving a cobblestone aspect. Skin becomes loose and wrinkled.
- Mucosal involvement: yellow papules in the inner aspect of the lower lip.
- Eyes: angioid streaks, prevalence of 100% after the age of 30 years, results from breaks in the calcified elastic lamina of Bruch's membrane, which is derived from the retina and the choroid plexus.

Extracutaneous symptoms are associated with complications: loss of visual activity, claudication, hypertension, angina, and myocardial infarction.

Localization

PXE affects the elastic fibers of the skin, eyes, and cardiovascular system.

Skin: papules cobblestone-like plaques in flexural areas: lateral neck, antecubital and popliteal fossae, wrists, axillae, and groin.

Classification

According to sites of involvement: skin, eyes, mucosal, cardiovascular

Laboratory and Other Workups

There are no specific or generally laboratory or biochemical assays for PXE.

Clinical examinations, exploration of the vascular vessels with MR angiography and ultrasound, fundus examination of the posterior pole of both eyes. Molecular biology: screening for ABCC6 mutations.

Dermatopathology

The mid-dermal elastic fibers (Verhoeff-van Gieson stain) in PXE are short, fragmented, clumped, and calcified (von Kossa stain).

Complications

Systemic involvement: ocular and cardiovascular (see above).

Diagnosis

Clinical and histologic features. Additional workup (see above).

Differential Diagnosis

Actinic damage, late-onset focal dermal elastosis, elastoderma, white fibrous papulosis of the neck, perforating periumbilical calcific elastosis and fibroelastolytic diseases of the skin. Treatment with D-penicillamine, longstanding end-stage renal disease, L-tryptophan-induced eosinophilia myalgia syndrome, beta-thalassemia, or sickle cell anemia

Prevention and Therapy

Prenatal diagnosis in families with known mutations.

No treatments available. Antioxidant therapy: daily doses of tocopherol acetate and ascorbic acid.

Ophthalmologic exams: biannual or annual fundoscopy, prevention of retinal hemorrhage through avoidance of head trauma, and smoking. Use of sunglasses. Bevacizumab to stop choroidal neovascularization.

Cardiovascular prevention to avoid calcification of blood vessels: regular exercise, weight control, avoidance of smoking and alcohol consumption, treatment of hypercholesterinemia and hypertension. Low dose of acetylsalicylic acid may be indicated to prevent myocardial infarction in some cases. Pentoxifylline, cilostazol, and clopidogrel are used in patients with intermittent claudication.

References

1. Dev T, Mahajan VK, Sethuraman G (2019) Hereditary palmoplantar keratoderma: a practical approach to the diagnosis. Indian Dermatol Online J 10(4):365–379
2. DiGiovanna JJ, Kraemer KH (2012) Shining a light on xeroderma pigmentosum. J Invest Dermatol 132(3 Pt 2):785–796
3. Fine JD, Bruckner-Tuderman L, Eady RA, Bauer EA, Bauer JW, Has C, Heagerty A, Hintner H, Hovnanian A, Jonkman MF, Leigh I, Marinkovich MP, Martinez AE, McGrath JA, Mellerio JE, Moss C, Murrell DF, Shimizu H, Uitto J, Woodley D, Zambruno G (2014) Inherited epidermolysis bullosa: updated recommendations on diagnosis and classification. J Am Acad Dermatol 70(6):1103–1126
4. Germain DP (2017) Pseudoxanthoma elasticum. Orphanet J Rare Dis 12(1):85
5. Hirbe AC, Gutmann DH (2014) Neurofibromatosis type 1: a multidisciplinary approach to care. Lancet Neurol 13(8):834–843
6. Kridin K, Kneiber D, Kowalski EH, Valdebran M, Amber KT (2019) Epidermolysis bullosa acquisita: a comprehensive review. Autoimmun Rev 18(8):786–795
7. Laimer M, Prodinger C, Bauer JW (2015) Hereditary epidermolysis bullosa. J Dtsch Dermatol Ges 13(11):1125–1133
8. Legrand A, Cornez L, Samkari W, Mazzella JM, Venisse A, Boccio V, Auribault K, Keren B, Benistan K, Germain DP, Frank M, Jeunemaitre X, Albuisson J (2017) Mutation spectrum in the ABCC6 gene and genotype-phenotype correlations in a French cohort with pseudoxanthoma elasticum. Genet Med 19(8):909–917
9. Lehmann J, Seebode C, Martens MC, Emmert S (2018) Xeroderma pigmentosum—facts and perspectives. Anticancer Res 38(2):1159–1164
10. Natale V, Raquer H (2017) Xeroderma pigmentosum-Cockayne syndrome complex. Orphanet J Rare Dis 12(1):65
11. Oji V, Tadini G, Akiyama M, Blanchet Bardon C, Bodemer C, Bourrat E, Coudiere P, DiGiovanna JJ, Elias P, Fischer J, Fleckman P, Gina M, Harper J, Hashimoto T, Hausser I, Hennies HC, Hohl D, Hovnanian A, Ishida-Yamamoto A, Jacyk WK, Leachman S, Leigh I, Mazereeuw-Hautier J, Milstone L, Morice-Picard F, Paller AS, Richard G, Schmuth M, Shimizu H, Sprecher E, Van Steensel M, Taieb A, Toro JR, Vabres P, Vahlquist A, Williams M, Traupe H (2010) Revised nomenclature and classification of inherited ichthyoses: results of the First Ichthyosis Consensus Conference in Soreze 2009. J Am Acad Dermatol 63(4):607–641
12. Patel S, Zirwas M, English JC 3rd (2007) Acquired palmoplantar keratoderma. Am J Clin Dermatol 8(1):1–11
13. Sakiyama T, Kubo A (2016) Hereditary palmoplantar keratoderma clinical and genetic differential diagnosis. J Dermatol 43(3):264–274
14. Takagi A, Kamijo M, Ikeda S (2016) Darier disease. J Dermatol 43(3):275–279
15. Vahlquist A, Torma H (2020) Ichthyosis: a road model for skin research. Acta Derm Venereol 100(7):adv00097

Cutaneous Manifestations of Metabolic Diseases

21

Günter Burg, Zrinka Bukvić Mokos, Veronique del Marmol, Branka Marinović, and Jonathan M. White

Contents

G. Burg (✉)
Dermatology, Zurich, Switzerland
e-mail: g.burg@access.uzh.ch

Z. Bukvić Mokos · B. Marinović
Department of Dermatology and Venereology, School of Medicine University of Zagreb, Zagreb, Croatia
e-mail: branka.marinovic@kbc-zagreb.hr

V. del Marmol
Département of Dermatology, Hôpital Erasme-HUB, Université Libre de Bruxelles, Brussels, Belgium
e-mail: veronique.delmarmol@hubruxelles.be

J. M. White
Ecole de Santé Publique, Université libre de Bruxelles, Brussels, Belgium
e-mail: Jonathan.White@ulb.be

H. Gollnick et al. (eds.), *Dermatology Cyberderm WebBook*,
https://doi.org/10.1007/978-3-031-78491-0_21

Test your learning and check your understanding of this book's contents: use the "Springer Nature Flashcards" app to access questions using ▶ https://sn.pub/1rhh6k.

To use the app, please follow the instructions in Chap. 1.

Skin Changes in Diabetes Mellitus [7, 8]

Figures 21.1, 21.2, 21.3, 21.4, 21.5 and 21.6

Grading of Importance

C

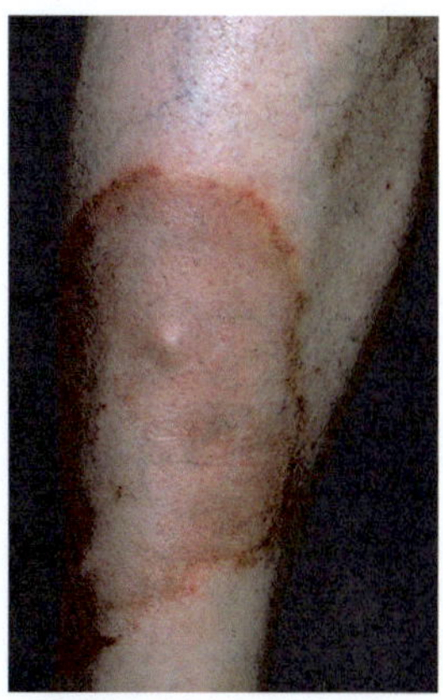

Fig. 21.1 Skin changes in diabetes mellitus: necrobiosis lipoidica

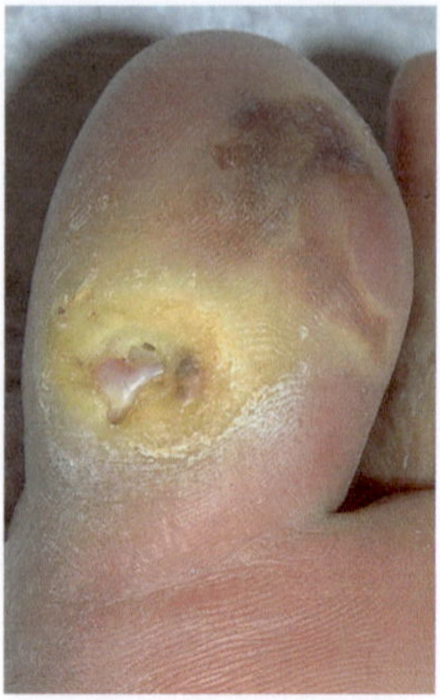

Fig. 21.2 Skin changes in diabetes mellitus: malum perforans

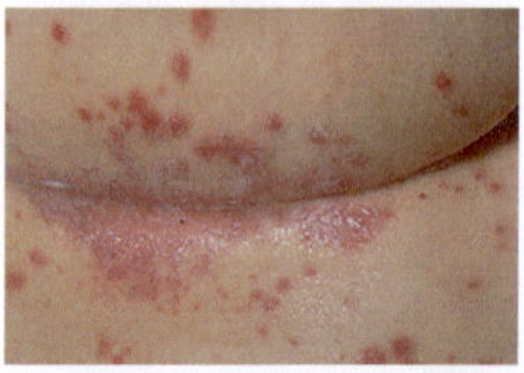

Fig. 21.3 Skin changes in diabetes mellitus: intertriginous candida infection

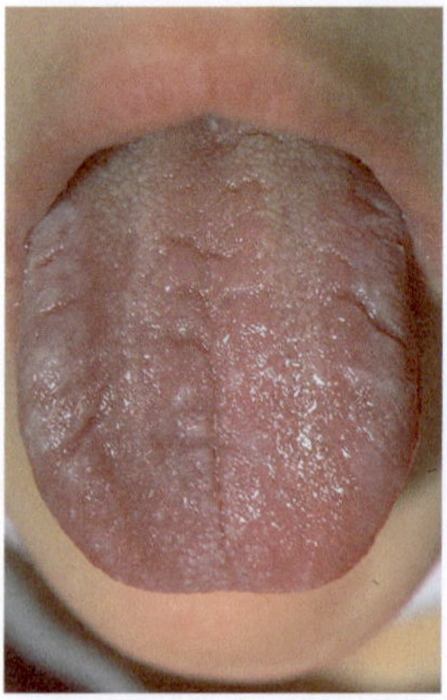

Fig. 21.4 Skin changes in diabetes mellitus: oral candida infection

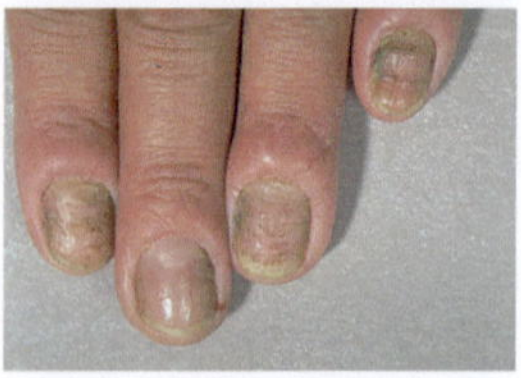

Fig. 21.5 Skin changes in diabetes mellitus: candida paronychia

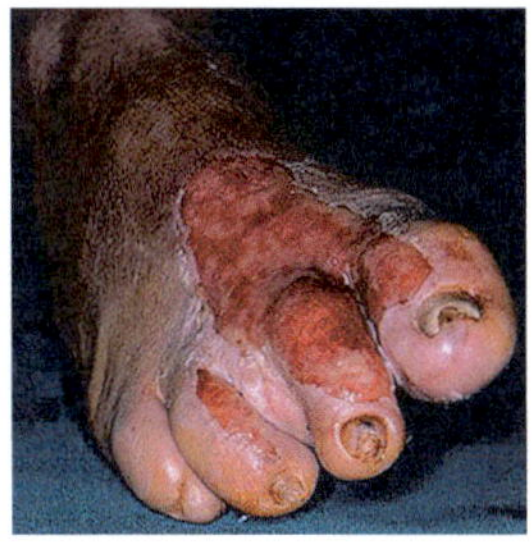

Fig. 21.6 Skin changes in diabetes mellitus: acral bullosis diabeticorum

Level

Advanced

ICD-11

EL3Y

Synonyms

None

Epidemiology

80% of patients with diabetes mellitus have skin changes.

Definition

The spectrum of skin changes seen as a result of hyperglycemia and its multiple effects on the body.

Etiology and Pathogenesis

Due to hyperglycemia, there are pathological changes in the circulation, nerves, and an increased tendency to infection, with reduced wound healing. Depending on the duration of the disease in type 1 vs type 2 diabetes.

Signs and Symptoms

Microangiopathy

- Pretibial pigmented patches (PPP): small, poorly defined brown macules over shins
- Rubeosis faciei: persistent facial erythema

Macroangiopathy

- Peripheral arterial occlusion: intermittent claudication, calves and feet pale or livid and cold, absent or reduced pulses in feet, sometimes ulcers or delay in wound healing

Polyneuropathy

- Neuropathic ulceration: indolent painless ulcers with hyperkeratotic border, primarily on heels, tips of toes (diabetic foot; acroosteopathia ulceromutilans; see section "Neuropathic Ulcers" in Chap. 18); pressure sore.

Granulomatous Disorders

- Necrobiosis lipoidica: primarily on shins, oval sharply demarcated yellow-red plaques with central glassy white-yellow area, mostly asymptomatic, may ulcerate
- Disseminated granuloma annulare: primarily on trunk, asymptomatic papules and plaques, sometimes confluent and often with prominent border

Infections

- Candidiasis: most often intertriginous (groins, rima ani, submammary, umbilicus), also involves mouth, genitalia (balanitis, vulvovaginitis), nails
- Overgrowth of staphylococci: folliculitis and furuncles: usually on trunk

Others

- Generalized pruritus: always rule out diabetes mellitus in patients with unexplained diffuse persistent pruritus.
- Nodular prurigo: pruritic papules with central excoriations, usually on shoulders and arms (females more than males).
- Bullosis diabeticorum: large acral blisters.

Localization

See above.

Classification

According to symptoms.

Laboratory and Other Workups

Swabs to exclude an infection (bacterial or mycotic) may be required. Doppler ultrasound. Neurological examination.

Dermatopathology

Usually not necessary and generally to be avoided, due to impaired wound healing. However, granulomatous diseases of the leg and widespread localization needs confirmation.

Course

Depends on the underlying cause. Generalized pruritus tends to persist, even despite good glycemic control.

Complications

Infection, particularly in the context of the diabetic foot. This may even include osteomyelitis. High dose antibiotics according to resistogram. Amputation should be considered as a last resort.

Diagnosis

Always relies on a secure diagnosis of diabetes mellitus.

Differential Diagnosis

Depends on individual condition (see above symptoms).

Prevention and Therapy

Optimize glycemic control. Regular diabetology/dermatology follow-up in high-risk patients. Treat microangiopathy. Necrobiosis diabeticorum difficult to treat (topical tacrolimus, TNF alpha blocker off label). Orthopedic shoes.

Porphyria Cutanea Tarda [3, 9, 10]

Figures 21.7, 21.8 and 21.9

Grading of Importance

B

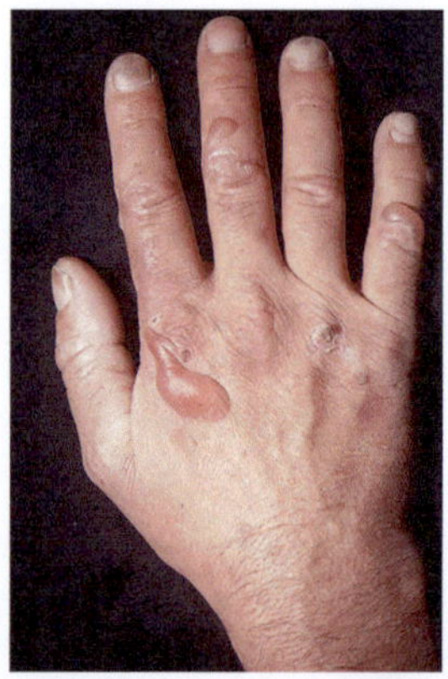

Fig. 21.7 Porphyria cutanea tarda: blisters on the sun exposed back of the hand

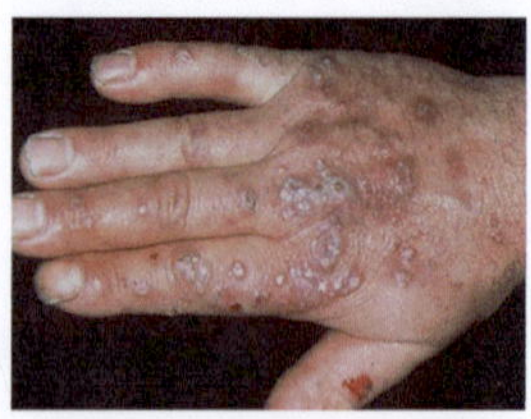

Fig. 21.8 Porphyria cutanea tarda: milia

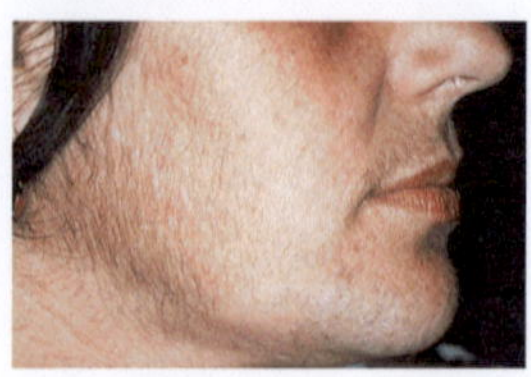

Fig. 21.9 Porphyria cutanea tarda: vellus hair hypertrichosis

Level

Advanced

ICD-11

5C58.10

Epidemiology

The disease typically manifests around the age 40–70 years. It is a rare condition, with less than 1% of the general population affected. However, it accounts for around 1/3 of all cases of porphyria. Males are twice as likely as women to suffer from this disease.

Definition

Porphyria cutanea tarda is a disease caused by a chronic disturbance in hepatic porphyrin synthesis, resulting in accumulation of photosensitive porphyrins in the skin and other organs.

Etiology and Pathogenesis

The etiology is genetic and may be inherited in an autosomal dominant fashion, or acquired. It is characterized by a deficiency in uroporphyrinogen-III decarboxylase. External triggers include alcohol, medications (antifungals, analgesics, barbiturates, contraceptive pill, chloroquine, and many others), and poisoning with heavy metals (such as lead and arsenic). Liver infections such as HIV and/or hepatitis C may cause or unmask the disease.

Signs and Symptoms

Blistering occurs in light-exposed areas and with minimal trauma (e.g., on the face and backs of the hands, bolded scalp). As the blisters are fragile and easily deroofed, commonly only erosions are seen. Skin frequently heals with the appearance of milia and atrophy. Hypertrichosis variably occurs on the cheeks and temples. Pseudoscleroderma is rarely seen. Some patients notice that their urine is discolored.

Localization

See signs and symptoms.

Classification

Hepatic porphyrias

- **Prototype: porphyria cutanea tarda**: sporadic, genetic/familiar, toxic
  - Type 1 (exogenous cause)
  - Type 2 (genetic)

Erythropoietic porphyrias

- Erythropoietic protoporphyria
- Congenital erythropoietic porphyria (Günther)

Laboratory and Other Workups

Laboratory tests are essential for a firm diagnosis, as there can be considerable clinical overlap between different forms of porphyria.

Blood: elevated liver enzymes are usually seen.

Urine: levels of uroporphyrins (I > III) may be measured to confirm the clinical diagnosis.

Dermatopathology

The features on biopsy are not specific but may include subepidermal blisters, thickened basement membrane, and thickened vessels (PAS stain). Biopsy may be helpful to exclude other causes of blistering (e.g., autoimmune blistering conditions).

Course

The course is often chronic. It is important to eliminate as many trigger factors as possible (even in type 2), e.g., reduction of alcohol intake, avoidance of prohibited medications.

Complications

Complications include cosmetically troublesome hypertrichosis and delayed wound healing, pseudoscleroderma causing reduced function/mobility.

Diagnosis

While a clinical diagnosis may be possible in classical cases, the diagnosis should always be confirmed via laboratory tests.

Differential Diagnosis

The differential diagnosis includes other blistering disorders and pseudoporphyrias. Erythropoietic protoporphyria, which however never shows blistering.

Prevention and Therapy

Sun avoidance is important with the use of topical sunscreens (SPF >30).

Avoidance of triggers (such as alcohol, hepatotoxic medications) can be very helpful clinically. If iron stores are very high, regular phlebotomy may be employed. Chloroquine (hepatotoxic) given in very low doses twice weekly may be an effective treatment.

Erythropoietic Protoporphyria (EPP) [1, 6]

Figures 21.10, 21.11 and 21.12

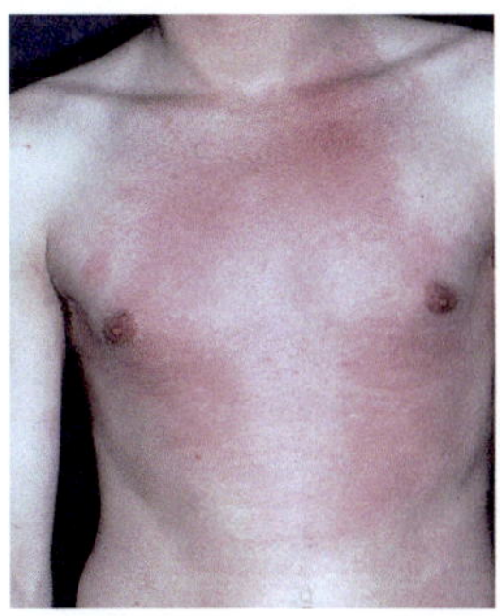

Fig. 21.10 Erythropoietic protoporphyria (EPP): burning erythema after sun exposure

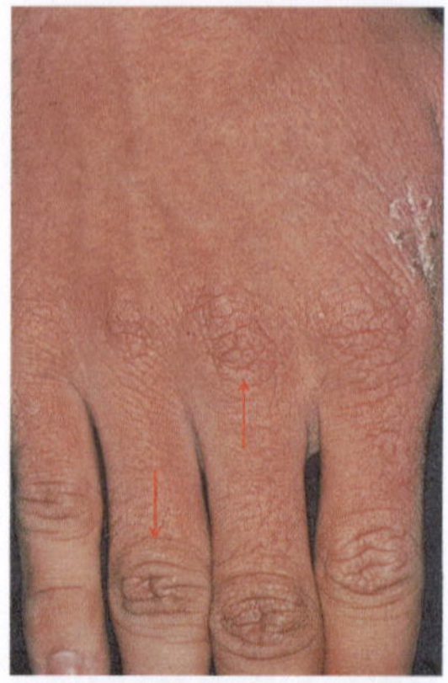

Fig. 21.11 Erythropoietic protoporphyria (EPP): permanent cerebriform lichenification and thickening of the skin

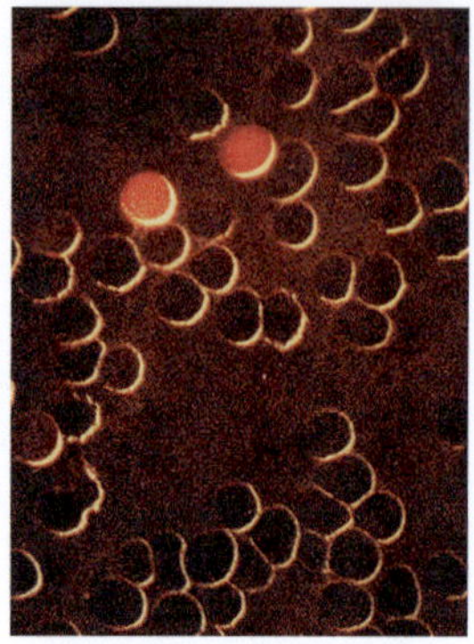

Fig. 21.12 Erythropoietic protoporphyria (EPP): red fluorescence of some erythrocytes in a blood smear under blue fluorescence light excitation

Grading of Importance

C

Level

Null

ICD-11

5C58.12

Synonyms

Disturbance of heme biosynthesis

Epidemiology

Very rare. Symptoms (light sensitivity) starting early in life (<10 years); Incidence 1:100 000

Definition

Chronic polyetiologic disturbance of the heme-(porphyrin) biosynthesis in the erythrocytes, leading to accumulation of photosensitive protoporphyrins in the skin and other organs.

Etiology and Pathogenesis

Autosomal-recessive inherited mutation, usually in the ferrochelatase (FECH) gene

The reduced mounting of iron-ions in the hemoglobin of the erythrocytes leads to accumulation of its precursor protoporphyrin. Light sensitivity in the long wave UVA (400 nm, Soret band).

Signs and Symptoms

Acute: Burning (not itching) of the skin upon sun exposure, also through window glass or front shield of the car, which filters only UVB but not the pathogenetically important UVA.

Acute erythema and edema in the light-exposed areas (face, hands, lower arms). Never blistering.

Permanent chronic changes: cerebriform lichenification and thickening of the skin, especially on the back of the nose, margins of the conch of the ear, back of hands and fingers.

Urine: normal color, since protoporphyrin is not water soluble and therefore is excreted through the stool.

Localisation

Face, back of the nose, margins of the conch of the ear, back of hands and fingers. Sun exposed areas.

Classification

Hepatic porphyrias

- Prototype: porphyria cutanea tarda: sporadic, genetic/familiar, toxic

Erythropoietic porphyrias

- **Erythropoietic protoporphyria**
- Congenital erythropoietic porphyria (Günther)

Laboratory and Other Workups

Diagnostic rapid test: red fluorescence of some (30%) of erythrocytes in a blood smear under the fluorescence microscope (blue light excitation). **Cave**: quick fading. The blood smear should be handled in a dark room.

Urine: negative, since protoporphyrin is not water-soluble.

Stool: qualitative and quantitative determination of protoporphyrin (special laboratory)

Determination of the defective enzymes (special laboratory).

Dermatopathology

Acute: dermal edema; chronic: lichenification; perivascular PAS-positive deposits

Course

Acute and relapsing with chronic sequelae

Complications

Limitation of the open-air mobility; accusation of hypochondriac behavior

Diagnosis

Typical clinical features; confirmation by laboratory tests

Differential Diagnosis

Other photodermatoses without blisters. Never blisters in erythropoietic protoporphyria.

Prevention and Therapy

Topical: Light protection (SPF/LSF >30). **Cave**: Vitamin D deficiency due to lack of vitamin D production in the skin by UV.

Photoprotection against long wave UVA; beta-carotene; afamelanotide.

Congenital Erythropoietic Porphyria (CEP) (Günther) [4, 5]

Figure 21.13

Grading of Importance

C

Level

Basic

ICD-11

5C58.12

Synonyms

Disturbance of the heme biosynthesis

Epidemiology

Very rare. Symptoms (light sensitivity) starting early in life (10 years); Incidence 0.1:100000.

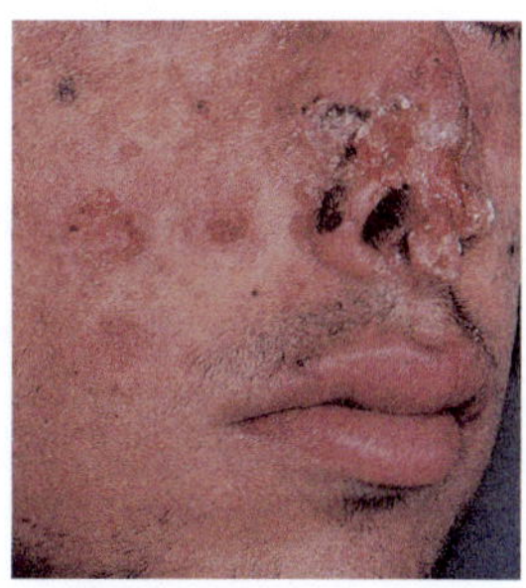

Fig. 21.13 Congenital erythropoietic porphyria (CEP): disfigurement due to scarring mutilations by UV light ("wolf children")

Definition

Chronic polyetiologic disturbance of the heme-(porphyrin) biosynthesis in the erythrocytes, leading to accumulation of photosensitive porphyrins in the skin and other organs.

Etiology and Pathogenesis

Autosomal-recessive inherited mutation of the heme biosynthesis due to reduced activity of the enzyme uroporphyrinogen-III synthase, leading to accumulation of hydroxymethylbilane; accumulation of the hem-precursor uroporphyrinogen I in the skin, bone, teeth, and internal organs.

Signs and Symptoms

Extreme light hypersensitivity, starting at birth. Blister formation and disfigurement due to scarring mutilations by UV light ("wolf children"). Hypertrichosis and poikiloderma. Risk of carcinoma development on scars. Red fluorescence of urine and red teeth (erythrodontia).

Localization

Light-exposed areas

Classification

Hepatic porphyrias

- Prototype: porphyria cutanea tarda: sporadic, genetic/familiar, toxic

  Erythropoietic porphyrias

- Erythropoetic protoporphyria
- **Congenital erythropoetic porphyria (Günther)**

Laboratory and Other Workups

Determination of the defective enzymes and of uroporphyrinogen I in the urine (special laboratory)

Dermatopathology

Subepidermal blisters; scar tissue

Course

Acute with chronic sequelae

Complications

Mutilations; scars

Diagnosis

Typical clinical features; confirmation by laboratory tests

Differential Diagnosis

Other photodermatoses. Porphyria cutanea tarda and other blistering dermatoses

Prevention and Therapy

Topical: Light protection (SPF/LSF > 30). **Cave**: Vitamin D deficiency due to lack of vitamin D production in the skin by UV

To be discussed: gene-therapy; allogeneic stem cell transplantation

Xanthomas [2]

Figures 21.14, 21.15, 21.16, 21.17 and 21.18

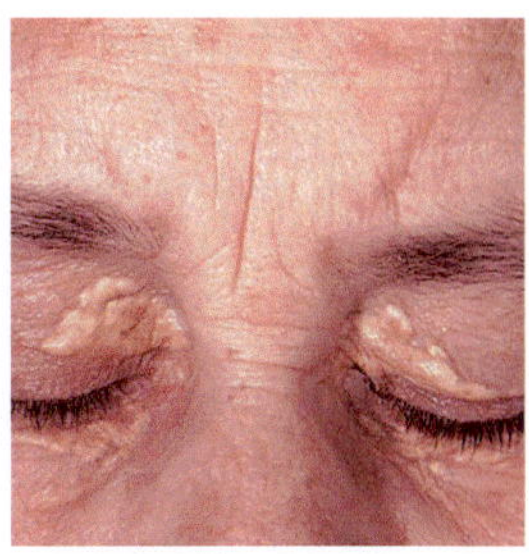

Fig. 21.14 Xanthoma: xanthelasmas

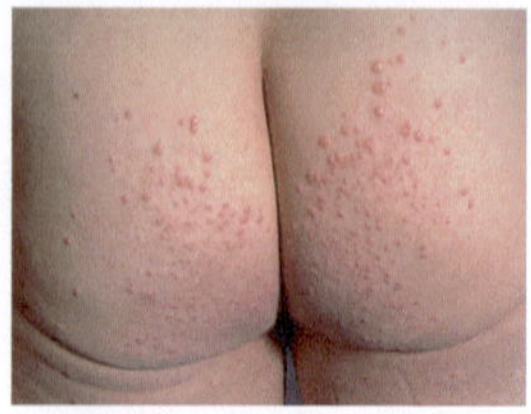

Fig. 21.15 Xanthoma: eruptive xanthomatas on the buttock

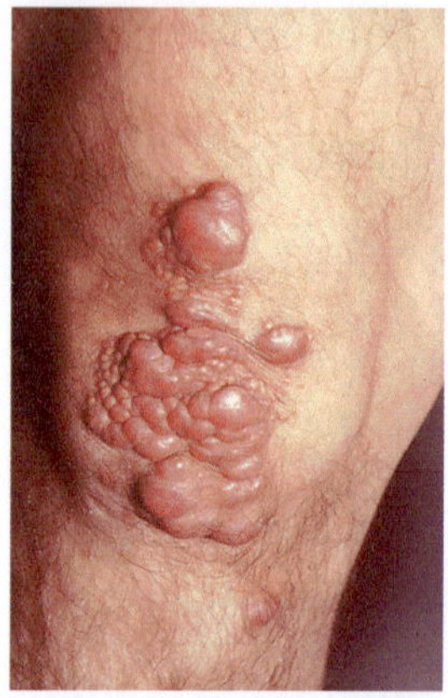

Fig. 21.16 Xanthoma: tuberous xanthomas

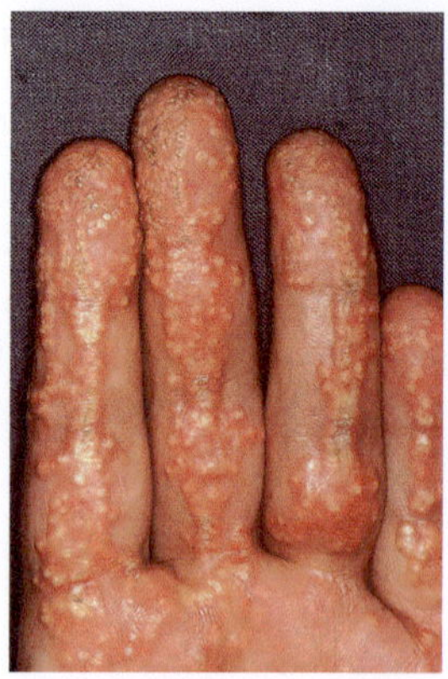

Fig. 21.17 Xanthoma: linear tendinous xanthomas

Grading of Importance

C

Level

Advanced

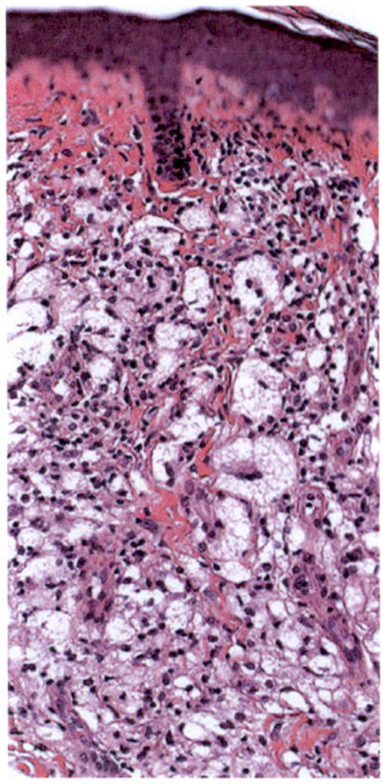

Fig. 21.18 Xanthoma: vacuolated macrophages (foamy macrophages) in the dermis

ICD-11

5C80.0Z; 5C80.2

Synonyms

Lipid deposition disease

Epidemiology

Xanthomas: a common manifestation of hyperlipidemia. Xanthelasmas: the most common type of xanthomas; in persons older than 50 years; 6% of eyelid tumors.

Definition

Tumor-like accumulations of lipid-laden macrophages (foam cells) and accumulation of histiocytes

Etiology and Pathogenesis

In xanthomas: systemic or local disturbance in lipid metabolism (monogenic or polygenic). In eruptive xanthomas: often triglycerides increased. Disseminated plane xanthomas belong to systemic histiocytoses, also juvenile xanthogranuloma. In xanthelasma often normal lipid metabolism.

Signs and Symptoms

Depending on localization; over joints pain may appear. No pruritus.

- Xanthelasmas: soft, flat, yellowish papules
- Eruptive xanthomas: multiple, small yellow papules
- Tuberous xanthomas: firm, yellow nodules
- Tendinous xanthomas: subcutaneous nodules
- Plane xanthomas: yellow macules or plaques

Localization

- Xanthelasmas: eyelids
- Eruptive xanthomas: buttocks, shoulders, extensor sites of the extremities
- Tuberous xanthomas: knees, elbows
- Tendinous xanthomas: along the extensor tendons of the hands, the feet, and the Achilles tendons
- Plane xanthomas: any site; often in palmar creases

Classification

See Symptoms.

Laboratory and Other Workups

Lipid status incl. subtype specification in xanthomas

Dermatopathology

Vacuolated macrophages (foamy macrophages) in the dermis, occasionally with typical multinucleated histiocytes (Touton giant cells)

Course

The lesions are usually slowly enlarging; eruptive xanthomas may resolve spontaneously.

Complications

Patients with hyperlipidemia: atherosclerosis, circulation disorders, cardiac infarction, pancreatitis

Diagnosis

Clinical features and histology

Differential Diagnosis

Syringoma. Nodular and plaque-like localized cutaneous amyloidosis. Lipoid proteinosis.

Prevention and Therapy

Prevention: diet and lipid-lowering drugs

Therapy: treatment of individual hyperlipidemia in xanthomas. In cosmetically disturbing lesions of xanthomas and xanthelasma: electrocautery, surgery or Erbium-/CO_2 laser.

References

1. Balwani M (2019) Erythropoietic Protoporphyria and X-Linked Protoporphyria: pathophysiology, genetics, clinical manifestations, and management. Mol Genet Metab 128(3):298–303
2. Bell A, Shreenath AP (2020) Xanthoma. StatPearls, Treasure Island, FL
3. Bissell DM, Anderson KE, Bonkovsky HL (2017) Porphyria. N Engl J Med 377(9):862–872
4. Erwin AL, Desnick RJ (2019) Congenital erythropoietic porphyria: Recent advances. Mol Genet Metab 128(3):288–297
5. Fritsch C, Bolsen K, Ruzicka T, Goerz G (1997) Congenital erythropoietic porphyria. J Am Acad Dermatol 36(4):594–610
6. Lecha M, Puy H, Deybach JC (2009) Erythropoietic protoporphyria. Orphanet J Rare Dis 4:19
7. Lima AL, Illing T, Schliemann S, Elsner P (2017) Cutaneous manifestations of diabetes mellitus: a review. Am J Clin Dermatol 18(4):541–553
8. Mendes AL, Miot HA, Haddad VJ (2017) Diabetes mellitus and the skin. An Bras Dermatol 92(1):8–20
9. Shah A, Bhatt H (2020) Cutanea Tarda Porphyria. StatPearls, Treasure Island, FL
10. Yasuda M, Chen B, Desnick RJ (2019) Recent advances on porphyria genetics: Inheritance, penetrance & molecular heterogeneity, including new modifying/causative genes. Mol Genet Metab 128(3):320–331

Pigmentary Disorders

22

Veronique del Marmol, Martine Bagot, Günter Burg,
Harald Gollnick, John A. McGrath, and Jonathan M. White

Contents

V. del Marmol (✉)
Département of Dermatology, Hôpital Erasme-HUB, Université Libre de Bruxelles,
Brussels, Belgium
e-mail: veronique.delmarmol@hubruxelles.be

M. Bagot
Service de Dermatologie, Université Paris Cité, Hôpital Saint-Louis, Paris, France
e-mail: martine.bagot@gmail.com

G. Burg
Dermatology, Zurich, Switzerland
e-mail: g.burg@access.uzh.ch

H. Gollnick
Department of Dermatology & Venereology, Otto-von-Guericke University,
Magdeburg, Germany
e-mail: Harald.Gollnick@med.ovgu.de

J. A. McGrath
St John's Institute of Dermatology, King's College London, London, UK
e-mail: john.mcgrath@kcl.ac.uk

J. M. White
Ecole de Santé Publique, Université libre de Bruxelles, Brussels, Belgium
e-mail: Jonathan.White@ulb.be

H. Gollnick et al. (eds.), *Dermatology Cyberderm WebBook*,
https://doi.org/10.1007/978-3-031-78491-0_22

Test your learning and check your understanding of this book's contents: use the "Springer Nature Flashcards" app to access questions using ▶ https://sn.pub/1rhh6k.
To use the app, please follow the instructions in Chap. 1.

Café-au-lait Macules [8]

Figure 22.1

Grading of Importance

B

Level

Advanced

ICD-11

LC1Y

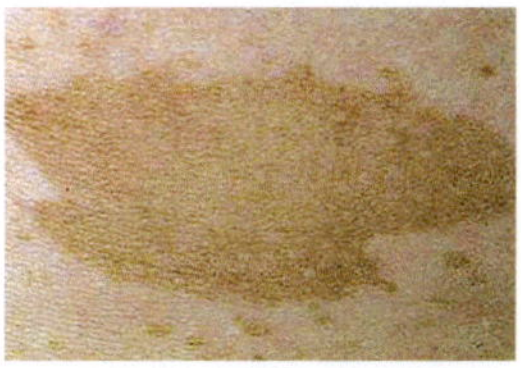

Fig. 22.1 Café-au-lait macules: circumscribed hyperpigmentations

Definition

Homogeneous tan-coloured macules of varying sizes with increased melanin, but no increase in number of melanocytes; often congenital.

Signs and Symptoms

Circumscribed tan macules

Localisation

No favoured sites

Dermatopathology

Increased melanin in basal keratinocyte layer

Course

Stable

Complications

More than five café-au-lait macules may be suggestive of neurofibromatosis.

Diagnosis

Clinical findings

Differential Diagnosis

Lentigo

Prevention and Therapy

None required. Laser destruction possible.

Lentigo [1, 2]

Figures 22.2, 22.3, 22.4 and 22.5

Grading of Importance

B

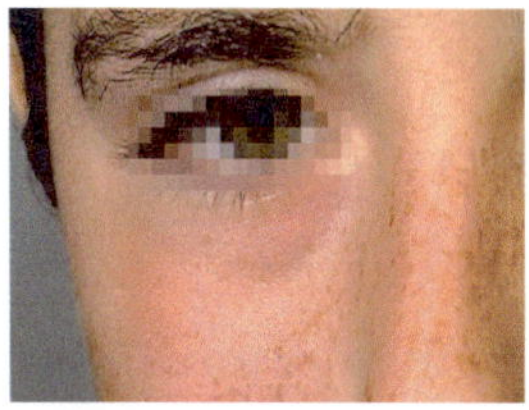

Fig. 22.2 Lentigo: ephelides

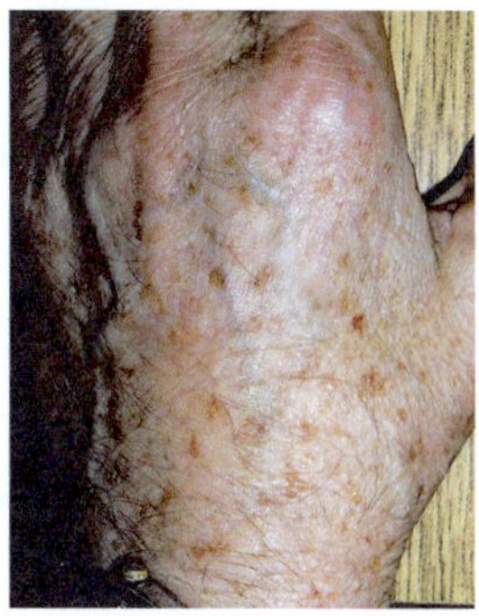

Fig. 22.3 Lentigo: senile lentigines

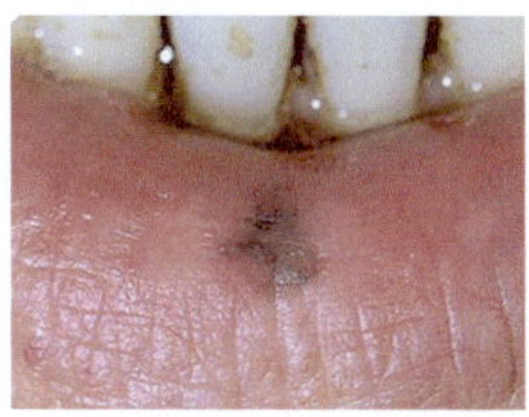

Fig. 22.4 Lentigo: lentigo of the lip

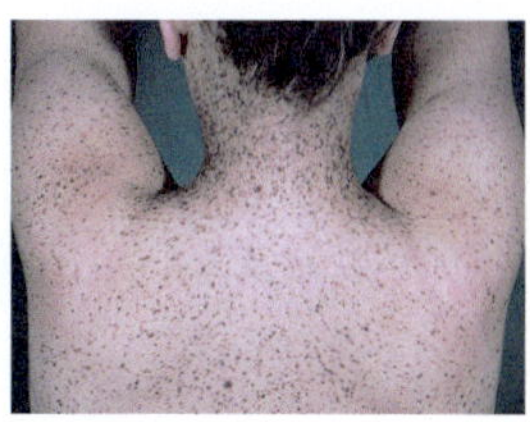

Fig. 22.5 Lentigo: lentigines in LEOPARD-syndrome

Level

Advanced

Definition

General term for small circumscribed macules with increased melanin but no increase in number of melanocytes.

ICD-11

LC1Y

Aetiology and Pathogenesis

Brown macule on skin or mucosa

Signs and Symptoms

Brown macule

Localisation

Most often hands, face, occasionally mucosa

Classification

Mucosal lentigo, ephelides (freckles), sunburn freckles, PUVA freckles, genital lentigo, senile lentigo, solar lentigo

Diagnosis

Clinical findings; skin biopsy not usually needed

Differential Diagnosis

Melanocytic naevus, lentigo maligna and other pigmented skin lesions

Prevention and Therapy

None required

Melasma/Chloasma [7]

Figure 22.6

Grading of Importance

B

Level

Null

ICD-11

ED60.1

Synonyms

Post-inflammatory hyperpigmentation (PIH), chloasma (hormonal), melasma

Epidemiology

Frequent disorder. Mostly appearing due to physical, chemical or drug-induced changes of melanocyte activity or destruction and melanophage accumulation. Chloasma in women during and after pregnancy or under hormonal contraception. Especially in dark-skinned people (South America, Southeast Asia).

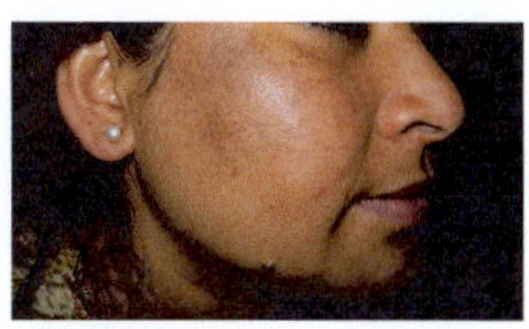

Fig. 22.6 Melasma/chloasma: hyperpigmentation on the cheek

Definition

Troublesome hyperpigmentation of the face, mostly in females

Aetiology and Pathogenesis

Physical (UV-light), chemical (cosmetics), hormones (women, pregnancy, contraceptives) and genetic disposition (coloured skin/phototypes III–VI) play an important role.

Signs and Symptoms

Irregular, "dirty-grey", muddling, poikilodermic, cosmetically compromising, circumscribed hyperpigmentation of the face, forehead and neck. In chloasma distribution in the middle line/front of the lower trunk. PIH may occur elsewhere depending on causative agent or trauma.

Localisation

Face, predominantly cheeks and zygomatic arch, forehead, neck and other areas

Classification

Depending on aetiology: physical, chemical, hormonal, post-traumatic

Laboratory and Other Workups

Not needed. Sometimes endocrinological examination.

Dermatopathology

Usually not needed. In order to determine the localisation of pigment, a biopsy may sometimes be recommended. Increased deposits of melanin in basal keratinocytes and in melanophages of the dermis.

Course

Chronic; depends on aetiology

Complications

Cosmetically compromising; psyche, decreased quality of life index

Diagnosis

Typical clinical pictures

Differential Diagnosis

Phototoxic dermatitis; (exogenous) ochronosis. Pigmentary skin deposits (minocycline).

Prevention and Therapy

Strict UV-protection. Topical bleaching, using a combination of hydroquinone, tretinoin (Vit A-acid) and hydrocortisone (Kligman-formula). Azelaic acid. Superficial chemical peeling and laser treatment have a limited effect and success depends on skin area and depth of pigmentation. Skin pastilla grafts.

Vitiligo [3, 9]

Figures 22.7, 22.8, 22.9 and 22.10

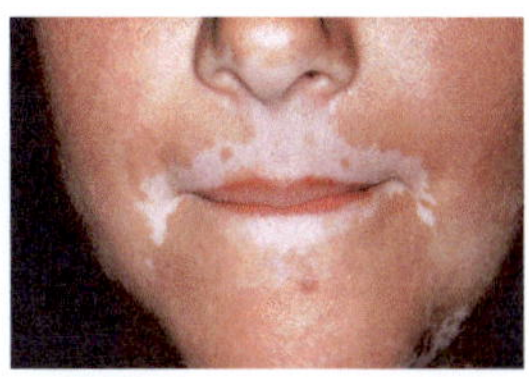

Fig. 22.7 Vitiligo: perioral depigmentation

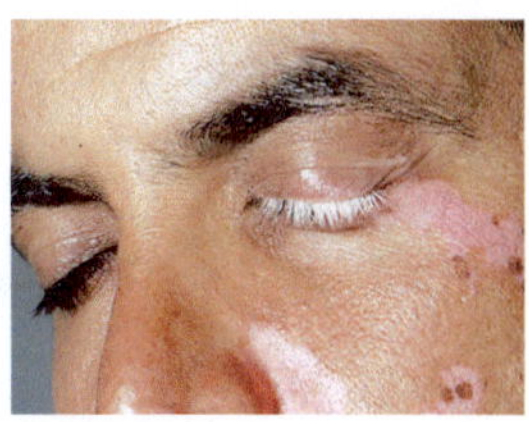

Fig. 22.8 Vitiligo: depigmentation of eyelashes

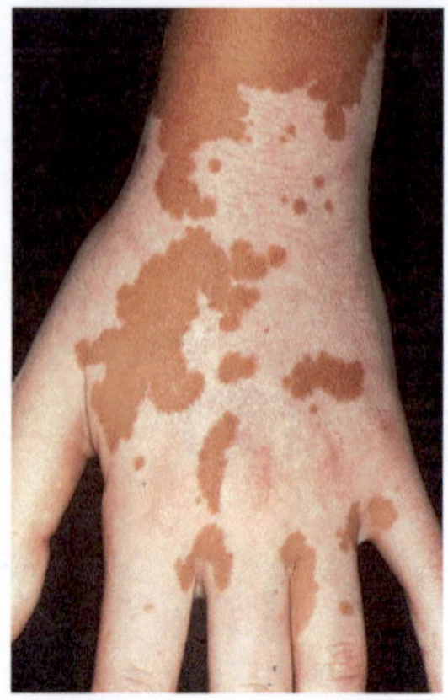

Fig. 22.9 Vitiligo: sun exposed localization

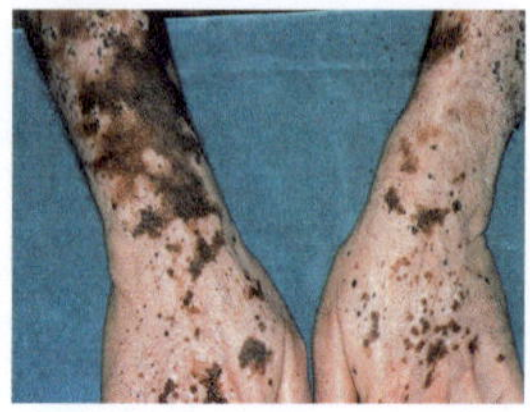

Fig. 22.10 Vitiligo: in an African patient

Grading of Importance

B

Level

Advanced

ICD-11

ED63.0

Definition

Acquired circumscribed depigmentation

Aetiology and Pathogenesis

Autoimmune process affecting, finally leading to destruction of melanocytes. Association with atopy, autoimmune thyroid disease.

Signs and Symptoms

Circumscribed small (confetti-like) macules which may also be confluent to produce larger patches, usually symmetrical; complete depigmentation under Wood's light. Not itchy.

Localisation

Favours face, hands, ano-genital region, peri-umbilical area, but any location possible. Sometimes generalized. May affect hair (poliosis).

Classification

Segmental (affecting only one side of the body).

Non-segmental (affects both sides of the body). Acral and central type.

Laboratory and Other Workups

Screen for other autoimmune diseases, if appropriate.

Dermatopathology

Absence of epidermal pigment, lymphocytic inflammatory infiltrate in early phase, destruction of melanocytes in later chronic phase.

Course

Spontaneous resolution possible. Acral sites (hands, feet and ano-genital areas) are often resistant to treatment; facial vitiligo is often more responsive to treatment than other body sites. Treatment response generally declines with the age of the lesion.

Complications

Because of lack of biological filter (melanin pigment) increased risk of sunburn, and consequent actinic damage. Often severe dysmorphophobia.

Diagnosis

Clinical findings

Differential Diagnosis

Albinism, pityriasis versicolor, naevus anaemicus, naevus depigmentosus, pityriasis alba, dry skin in darker skin types, hypomelanosis pigmentosa, macular form of lichen sclerosus, any cause of post-inflammatory hypopigmentation, other rare, hereditary causes of hypopigmentation (e.g. piebaldism etc.).

Prevention and Therapy

Early treatment.

Topical potent/superpotent corticosteroids; topical calcineurin inhibitors; phototherapy; consider melanocyte-keratinocyte transplants from normally pigmented skin. Consider afamelanotide with UVB photo(chemo)therapy. Cosmetic camouflage with make-up. Bleaching agents for normally pigmented skin if vitiligo is widespread.

Topical sunscreens to prevent sun damage.

Counselling/psychological support especially for those with darker skin types, where the psychosocial impact may be severe.

Albinism and Piebaldism [4–6]

Figures 22.11 and 22.12

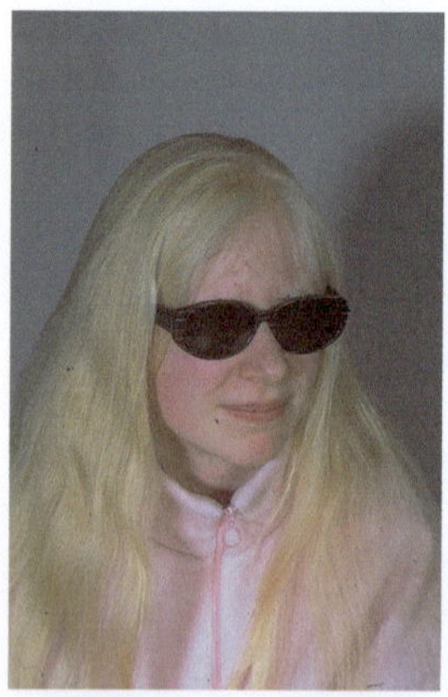

Fig. 22.11 Albinism: blond hair, light skin, protection of eyes

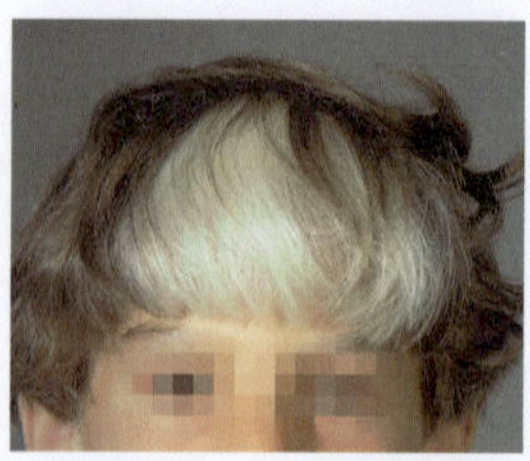

Fig. 22.12 Piebaldism: wight streaks of hair

Grading of Importance

C

Level

Advanced

ICD-11

EC23.20 (oculocutaneous albinism)
EC23.2Y (partial albinism)
LD2H.Y (albinism-deafness syndrome)
EC23.2Y (piebaldism)

Synonyms

None

Epidemiology

Albinism: 1 in 20,000 people; highly variable in different populations. (1 in 1000 people in some genetically isolated communities).

Piebaldism: 1 in 40,000 Caucasians.

Definition

These genetic conditions cause partial or total depigmentation of the skin, hair or eyes.

Aetiology and Pathogenesis

Albinism: Usually autosomal recessive inheritance. Non-inflammatory disease is due to reduced or absent tyrosinase activity, causing reduced or absent melanin pigment, despite normal numbers of melanocytes (unlike vitiligo, where there are fewer melanocytes). This is due to interruption of the synthesis of melanin via enzyme malfunction or absence.

Piebaldism: Usually autosomal dominant inheritance. Mutation in KIT proto-oncogene causing reduced melanocytes. Compare differences to chapter Vitiligo (22.4).

Signs and Symptoms

Albinism: apart from a tendency to sunburn, asymptomatic for the skin, except for potential cosmetic embarrassment. Ocular symptoms may include poor visual acuity, photophobia and nystagmus.

Piebaldism: same as for albinism, but no ocular features. The changes are present from birth, unlike vitiligo.

Localisation

Albinism: the absence of skin pigmentation is usually generalised but more localised forms (i.e. periorificial) exist. In some subtypes, the scalp hair may be a yellow colour and the leg hairs dark.

Piebaldism: A characteristic white forelock of hair is almost always seen in the mid forehead. Depigmented skin is commonly patchy, with typical sites including mid extremities and central trunk.

Classification

Albinism: tyrosinase positive and negative forms

Piebaldism: no classification

Laboratory and Other Workups

Differentiating different types of albinism is not usually of clinical relevance, and such tests are not routinely available apart from specialised centres. One particular test is to incubate a hair bulb with tyrosinase. This test may differentiate tyrosinase positive and negative forms of albinism.

Dermatopathology

This is not required and is not generally helpful, unless to exclude other conditions. Melanocytes present but disturbed function.

Course

The conditions are lifelong.

Complications

The most important cutaneous complication is of skin cancer. The risk of developing skin cancer is greatly elevated as there is no natural sun protection in albinos. They are most prone to develop squamous cell carcinomas, and this may occur at very young ages, particularly in those who live in tropical climates. Decreased quality of life can be observed in both albinism and piebaldism (see **Special**).

Diagnosis

The diagnoses are clinical.

Differential Diagnosis

Vitiligo, post-inflammatory hypopigmentation, idiopathic guttate hypomelanosis, rare genetic syndromes, e.g. Waardenburg syndrome.

Prevention and Therapy

Camouflage. No known effective treatments for the underlying problem. In piebaldism, hair colouring possible.

Limited surgical procedures (skin transplants) are performed in individuals with darker skin.

Effective sun protection (high factor topical sunscreens and clothing, including hats) essential to avoid skin cancers. Ophthalmological review is mandatory in albinism and psychological support should be offered.

Special

In some cultures of the world, body parts from those suffering from albinism are thought to possess magical or medicinal powers. In those situations, albinos may be persecuted and require police protection.

References

1. Byrom L, Barksdale S, Pool L, Weedon D, Muir J (2016a) Reply to unstable solar lentigo is not a defined separate entity. Australas J Dermatol 57(4):332–333
2. Byrom L, Barksdale S, Weedon D, Muir J (2016b) Unstable solar lentigo: a defined separate entity. Australas J Dermatol 57(3):229–234
3. Ezzedine K, Eleftheriadou V, Whitton M, van Geel N (2015) Vitiligo. Lancet 386(9988):74–84
4. Federico JR, Krishnamurthy K (2020) Albinism. StatPearls, Treasure Island, FL
5. Marcon CR, Maia M (2019) Albinism: epidemiology, genetics, cutaneous characterization, psychosocial factors. An Bras Dermatol 94(5):503–520
6. Martinez-Garcia M, Montoliu L (2013) Albinism in Europe. J Dermatol 40(5):319–324
7. Rajanala S, Maymone MBC, Vashi NA (2019) Melasma pathogenesis: a review of the latest research, pathological findings, and investigational therapies. Dermatol Online J 25(10):13030
8. Shah A (2010) The diagnostic and clinical significance of Cafe - au - lait Macules. Pediatr Clin N Am 57:1131–1153
9. Whitton ME, Pinart M, Batchelor J, Leonardi-Bee J, Gonzalez U, Jiyad Z, Eleftheriadou V, Ezzedine K (2015) Interventions for vitiligo. Cochrane Database Syst Rev 2:CD003263

Part VII

Proctologic Disorders and Psychodermatoses

Even though these disorders are put together in this chapter, they have nothing to do with each other except the letter "P."

Proctologic Diseases

23

Annamari Ranki, Eija Hiltunen-Back, Alexander Salava, and Sinikka Salmenkylä

Contents

Annamari Ranki has died before the publication of this book.

A. Ranki · E. Hiltunen-Back · A. Salava (✉) · S. Salmenkylä
Department of Dermatology and Allergology, Helsinki University Hospital, Helsinki, Finland
e-mail: eija.hiltunen-back@hus.fi; alexander.salava@hus.fi

H. Gollnick et al. (eds.), *Dermatology Cyberderm WebBook*,
https://doi.org/10.1007/978-3-031-78491-0_23

Test your learning and check your understanding of this book's contents: use the "Springer Nature Flashcards" app to access questions using ▶ https://sn.pub/1rhh6k.
To use the app, please follow the instructions in Chap. 1.

Anal Fissure [1, 2]

Figure 23.1

Grading of Importance

B

Level

Advanced

ICD-11

DB50

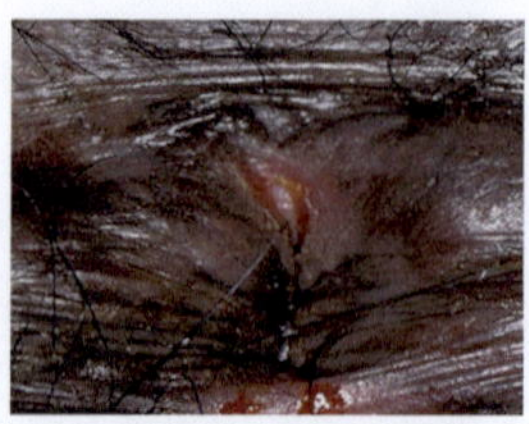

Fig. 23.1 Anal fissure: painful linear tear in the distal anal canal

Synonyms

Fissure of the anus

Epidemiology

Most frequent cause of acute anal pain in Europe; incidence peak is in young adults. Annual incidence in Europe is 0.11 % (1.1 cases per 1000 person-years); due to unreported cases, the true incidence is probably much higher.

Definition

Painful linear tear in the distal anal canal

Etiology and Pathogenesis

The exact etiology of anal fissures is unknown, but usually the initiating factor is a trauma caused by hard or forceful defecation. Obesity, low-fiber diets, hypothyroidism, anal tumors, and chronic constipation have been associated with the development of anal fissures. Anal fissures may infrequently be associated with Crohn's disease, HIV infection, artifacts by manipulation, and tuberculosis.

Signs and Symptoms

The typical symptom is acutely occurring lacerating pain during bowel movements. Mostly the pain recurs with every defecation, which may lead to a cycle of worsening constipation, harder stools, and increase of anal pain and discomfort (vicious cycle). Many patients note bright-red blood on the toilet paper or stool. Small amounts of blood may be visible in the toilet bowl, but unlike hemorrhoids, significant bleeding does not usually occur. Thus, anal fissures do not cause anemia. Symptoms are relatively specific, and the diagnosis can often be made on patient history alone.

Localization

Idiopathic anal fissures are usually localized dorsal in the middle line. If fissures are detected in other localizations, an underlying pathology (e.g., Crohn's disease) should be excluded.

Course

Most frequently anal fissures resolve spontaneously. After a duration of 6–8 weeks, the anal fissure is regarded as chronic.

Complications

Sub-mucous abscess, which impedes wound healing; fistulas of the skin or mucosa surface. More rare complications: anal thrombosis, ulceration, and incontinence.

Diagnosis

The diagnosis is clinical, based on the typical findings of inspection. Proctoscopic rectal examination is painful and often not necessary. If the anal fissure is not visible, the tender wound base of the fissure may be recognizable by gently exploring with the fingertip.

If symptoms are typical and if the fissure is located in the posterior or anterior midline (idiopathic anal fissure), no further tests (biopsy and endoscopy) are necessary.

If fissures are located off the midline, if there are multiple fissures, or if an underlying illness is conceivable (notably Crohn's disease, anal squamous cell cancer, relapsing herpes infection or HIV infection), appropriate tests such as microbiologic swabs, systemic inflammatory parameters, fecal calprotectin, HIV testing, and biopsy should be performed.

Differential Diagnosis

Relevant differential diagnoses include perianal abscess (pain and palpable fluctuation), perianal fistulas of different origin (secret and/or pus draining), and thrombosed hemorrhoids.

Prevention and Therapy

First-line medical therapy includes stool-bulking agents, such as fiber supplementation and stool softeners. Laxatives should be used as needed to maintain regular bowel movements and treat underlying constipation.

Second-line therapy consists of topical medicaments that decrease the muscle tonus of the inner anal sphincter. Nitroglycerin applied in different formulations directly to the internal anal sphincter (e.g., nitroglycerin 0.4 % ointment or anal suppositories). Comparable to the use of nitroglycerin ointment, nifedipine ointment is also available in some European countries. The topical treatment should be continued even after the symptoms subside (e.g., 2 months).

In addition to topical treatments, botulinum toxin has been used to treat acute and chronic anal fissures but poses a small risk of injection site infections. The effect lasts some months, until the regeneration of free nerve endings.

If the anal fissure in unresponsive to conservative treatment and lasts over 2 months, surgical intervention should be evaluated. Symptomatic chronic fissures should be treated operatively because they only rarely heal spontaneously.

Hemorrhoids [3]

Figure 23.2

Grading of Importance

B

Level

Advanced

ICD-11

DB60

Synonyms

Piles

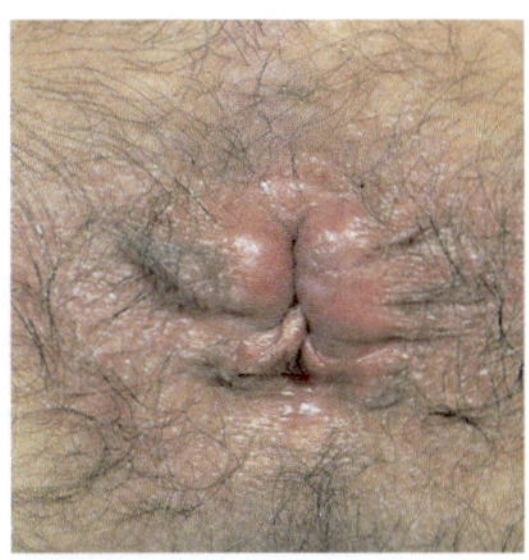

Fig. 23.2 Hemorrhoids: swollen blood vessels in the anus

Epidemiology

Most common anorectal pathology diagnosed in clinical practice. The prevalence of symptomatic hemorrhoids is estimated at 4.4 %. In both sexes, peak prevalence is around the age 45–65 years.

Definition

Symptomatic enlargement and distal displacement of the normal anal cushions resulting from swollen blood vessels in the anus and lower rectum: most common causes of anorectal complaints

Etiology and Pathogenesis

The theory of sliding anal canal lining is widely accepted. Degradation of matrix by matrix metalloproteinases and loss of elastic fibers occurs. Hemorrhoidal venous cushions have therefore a predisposition to dilate and prolapse.

Multifactorial origin: including decreased venous return (low-fiber diets, small caliber stools), straining during defecation and constipation, multiple pregnancies, and more rarely portal hypertension and anorectal varices.

Signs and Symptoms

Symptoms range from mild pruritus to fresh bright rectal bleeding.

Possible other symptoms: pain, burning during or after defecation, weeping, drainage of mucus, feeling of incomplete bowel movement, fecal urgency, and anal venous thrombosis.

Localization

Most common sites (dorsal lithotomy position): 3, 7, and 11 o'clock on the anal ring.

Classification

Four clinical degrees of severity:

- Grade I hemorrhoids project into the anal canal, no prolapse.
- Grade II hemorrhoids protrude beyond anal verge with straining or defecating but reduce spontaneously.
- Grade III hemorrhoids protrude spontaneously and require manual replacement.
- Grade IV hemorrhoids chronically prolapse and cannot be replaced.

Laboratory and Other Workups

Inspection, digital palpation; proctoscopy and rectoscopy

Dermatopathology

Usually not needed. Clusters of vascular tissue, smooth muscle and connective tissue of the normal epithelium of the anal canal. Bleeding is of convoluted arteriovenous communicating vessel with bright color.

Course

Depending on degree, they may consolidate or progress to stages III and IV. Most resolve spontaneously or with conservative medical therapy alone.

Complications

Irritative perianal dermatitis, hemorrhoidal vein thrombosis, secondary infection, ulceration, abscess, and incontinence

Diagnosis

Diagnosis is based on inspection and clinical examination. Proctoscopy or rectoscopy is important to evaluate any bright-red rectal bleeding. Colonoscopy should be considered in the evaluation of any new onset rectal bleeding in patients over 50 years of age or with atypical symptoms.

Differential Diagnosis

Anal fissure, perianal abscess, perianal fistulas and anal prolapse, anal skin tag or fibroma, rectal polyp, condylomata acuminata, vascular tumors including Kaposi sarcoma

Prevention and Therapy

General measures: anal hygiene (soap-free cleansing after defecation), natural regulation of bowel movements (high-fiber diet), adequate fluids, sufficient physical activity, no straining with defecation. Lower pelvis muscle training

The treatment options based on severity and grading:

Grade I: conservative treatments (topical symptomatic treatment, increasing fiber intake, treatment of constipation) and avoidance of nonsteroidal anti-inflammatory drugs, spicy or fatty foods, or fruit juices (orange, grapefruit). Topical treatments include corticosteroids and topical local anesthetics, menthol, astringents (e.g., ichthammol), and sitz baths.

Grade II or III: Initial treatment with nonsurgical procedures (e.g., sclerotherapy, infrared coagulation, rubber band ligation).

Symptomatic grades III and grade IV: surgical hemorrhoidectomy

Treatment of grade IV hemorrhoids or any incarcerated or gangrenous tissue requires prompt surgical consultation.

Special

Severely bleeding hemorrhoids (e.g., due to portal hypertension, coagulopathies) can acutely be treated with rubber band ligation or sclerotherapy.

References

1. Beaty JS, Shashidharan M (2016) Anal fissure. Clin Colon Rectal Surg 29(1):30–37
2. Nelson RL (2014) Anal fissure (chronic). BMJ Clin Evid 2014:0407
3. Reese GE, von Roon AC, Tekkis PP (2009) Haemorrhoids. BMJ Clin Evid 2009:0415

Psychodermatoses

24

Veronique del Marmol, Ana María Giménez-Arnau,
Ramon María Pujol Vallverdú, and Jonathan M. White

Contents

V. del Marmol (✉)
Département of Dermatology, Hôpital Erasme-HUB, Université Libre de Bruxelles, Brussels, Belgium
e-mail: veronique.delmarmol@hubruxelles.be

A. M. Giménez-Arnau · R. M. Pujol Vallverdú
Dermatology and Venereology, Universitat Autònoma de Barcelona, Hospital del Mar. IMIM, Barcelona, Spain
e-mail: rpujol@psmar.cat

J. M. White
Ecole de Santé Publique, Université libre de Bruxelles, Brussels, Belgium
e-mail: Jonathan.White@ulb.be

H. Gollnick et al. (eds.), *Dermatology Cyberderm WebBook*,
https://doi.org/10.1007/978-3-031-78491-0_24

Test your learning and check your understanding of this book's contents: use the "Springer Nature Flashcards" app to access questions using ▶ https://sn.pub/1rhh6k.
To use the app, please follow the instructions in Chap. 1.

Trichotillomania [4, 6]

Figure 24.1

Grading of Importance

C

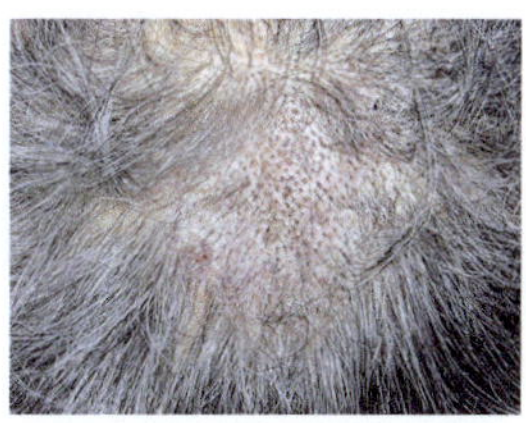

Fig. 24.1 Trichotillomania: broken-off hairs as dark dots on the scalp

Level

Advanced

ICD-11

6B25.0

Synonyms

Hair-pulling disorder; compulsive hair pulling

Epidemiology

Usually seen in adolescence; F>M 3–10:1. It is present in <1:1000 of the general population.

Definition

Compulsive self-manipulation of hairs through pulling, twisting, and plucking (or other mechanisms), leading to localized areas of alopecia.

Etiology and Pathogenesis

The etiology is psychological, and the condition may be considered part of the impulse-control disorder spectrum. Individuals with this disease feel compelled to manipulate the hair to an excessive degree. There may be underlying psychological disease such as body dysmorphic disorder, anxiety, depression, or psychosis.

Signs and Symptoms

The patient is usually distressed by the hair loss. Clinically, solitary (rarely multiple) circumscribed areas of incomplete hair loss with short hairs of varying lengths are seen. Only those hairs reaching 3 mm in length can be removed. The hair shafts often show distal splits and a frayed appearance, especially marked on microscopy. Broken-off hairs may appear as dark dots on the scalp.

Localization

The most common site is the centro-parietal scalp, because the pain tolerance is higher there. This is known as a tonsure trichotillomania, due to the resemblance with a monastic tonsure.

Classification

An imperfect classification is based on the age of the patient.
- The infantile form often results from frustration.
- The adolescent form may reflect obsessive-compulsive disorder.

Laboratory and Other Workups

This is only required to exclude other conditions:
- Trichoscopy may show broken hairs, trichoptilosis (split ends), irregular coiled hairs, empty follicular orifices, etc.
- Trichogram would show an absence of telogen hairs and dystrophic anagen hairs.

Dermatopathology

Not usually required but would show disrupted follicular anatomy without inflammation. In early lesions erythrocytes are found in and around the follicle.

Course

Trichotillomania in young children often resolves spontaneously. In adults, the problem tends to persist.

Complications

Rarely, if the manipulated hair is ingested (a phenomenon known as trichophagia), a trichobezoar (hairball in stomach or intestine) may form. There is a danger of ileus (Rapunzel syndrome) in this situation.

Diagnosis

DSM-5 diagnostic criteria of the American Psychiatric Association for the diagnosis of trichotillomania:

- Recurrent pulling out of one's hair resulting in noticeable hair loss.
- An increasing sense of tension immediately before pulling out the hair or when attempting to resist the behavior.
- Pleasure, gratification, or relief when pulling out the hair.
- The disturbance is not better accounted for by another mental disorder and is not due to a general medical condition.
- The disturbance causes clinically significant distress or impairment in social, occupational, or other important areas of functioning.

Generally, the clinical findings (including trichoscopy) are sufficient for a confident diagnosis, but tests such as a trichogram or biopsy may be required to exclude other conditions. A psychological evaluation is mandatory.

Differential Diagnosis

Alopecia areata, tinea capitis, androgenetic alopecia, adverse effect of medications, post-traumatic

Prevention and Therapy

Best coordinated by a clinical psychologist or psychiatrist (habit reversal therapy and treatment of any underlying psychological disease). It is unclear whether pharmacological treatment is truly helpful or not.

Dermatitis Artefacta [3]

Figure 24.2

Grading of Importance

C

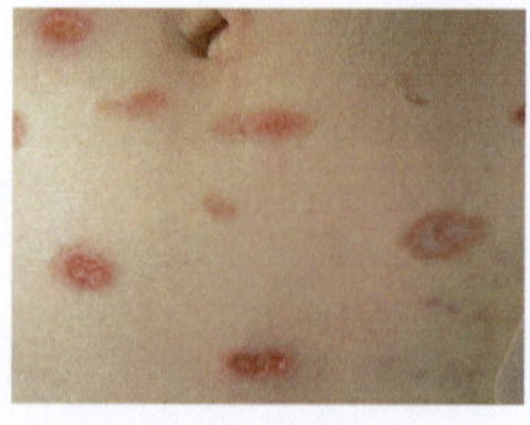

Fig. 24.2 Dermatitis artifacta: excoriations on easy reachable localizations of the trunk

Level

Advanced

ICD-11

ED00

Synonyms

Artifactual dermatitis; self-inflicted skin disorder

Epidemiology

1:23,000 in pediatric populations. Commonest in late adolescence and early adulthood. F>M 8:1.

Definition

A skin condition with no underlying organic cause where skin changes are self-inflicted. The patient invariably denies being the cause.

Etiology and Pathogenesis

Dermatitis artefacta is a cutaneous manifestation of a primary psychiatric disorder. The skin lesions may convey secondary (unconscious) gain for the patient (e.g., attention-seeking). Patients with dermatitis artefacta generally do not want to be hospitalized in order not to be observed during the evolution of the lesions.

Signs and Symptoms

The symptoms are highly variable: atypical skin lesion, ranging from excoriation (scratch) to ulcer to extensive skin damage or loss. May mimic organic diseases. The way the lesions are created may include self-manipulation or the use of tools or chemical substances.

Localization

The disease has a predilection for sites of the body that are easily reached. Locations which cannot be reached are usually spared.

Classification

None

Laboratory and Other Workups

Although medical tests are sometimes required to exclude organic disease (e.g., swab for atypical organisms), unnecessary tests should be generally avoided.

Dermatopathology

The histological findings are highly variable according to the mechanism of injury to the skin.

Course

The disease has a chronic course, even with psychological treatments.

Complications

Secondary infections and scarring of different degrees up to functional disabilities. Unnecessary or inappropriate medical treatments may cause complications.

Diagnosis

Primarily clinical: bizarre-looking lesions in easily reached locations. However, potential organic causes always should be considered and excluded first. Careful psychological evaluation is required. It should be noted that patients with psychological disease may also have concurrent organic diseases.

Differential Diagnosis

Many possibilities, depending on appearance. Consider pyoderma gangrenosum (including superficial forms). Also consider factitious disorder imposed on self, where there is a conscious gain in the self-harming behavior.

Prevention and Therapy

It is unclear whether confronting the patient with the clinical diagnosis is counter-productive or not. A psychological review with therapeutic intervention is often helpful. Occlusive dressings or hospital admission (making further manipulation difficult) may help to confirm the diagnosis or provide treatment.

Special

Analogously to Münchhausen syndrome, dermatitis artefacta may rarely occur by proxy, i.e., the lesions on the patient may be induced by someone else.

Psychogenic Pruritus [2]

Grading of Importance

C

Level

Advanced

ICD-11

EC90.4

Synonyms

Somatoform itch/pruritus; psycho-somatic pruritus; nonorganic itch

Epidemiology

Approximately 6% of dermatology clinic patients suffer with the condition. The frequency in the general population is likely to be lower.

Definition

An itch disorder where organic causes have been excluded and where itch is the primary symptom and where psychological factors affect triggering, intensity, aggravation, or persistence of the itch (modified from the French Psycho-Dermatology Group 2018).

Etiology and Pathogenesis

The etiology of this condition is poorly understood, but there is an interplay of neurological and psychological factors resulting in the symptoms.

Signs and Symptoms

The itch is persistent and often unbearable. Secondary changes such as erythema and erosions/ulcerations and finally scars may occur.

Localization

The condition may be generalized or circumscribed. Localized forms may particularly affect the genitalia or scalp.

Classification

None.

Laboratory and Other Workups

The condition can only be diagnosed by excluding other causes, so laboratory tests are mandatory. Systemic conditions to exclude are diabetes mellitus, thyroid dysfunction, iron deficiency, uremia, cholestasis, Hodgkin and non-Hodgkin lymphomas, and erythropoietic protoporphyria. Primary skin diseases to exclude by examination or tests include dermatitis herpetiformis, scabies, urticaria, atopic dermatitis, and other parasitic infections.

Dermatopathology

Biopsy is seldom necessary, apart from excluding another primary skin condition (e.g., cutaneous lymphoma). Histological findings would be nonspecific, with excoriations and potentially prurigo nodules.

Course

Usually chronic

Complications

Psychogenic pruritus is often accompanied by sleep disturbance, which may further exacerbate the condition. The patient's quality of life is invariably severely reduced. Scarring and secondary infections may also occur.

Diagnosis

Sensitivity should be shown when discussing the diagnosis with the patient.

Compulsory criteria:

- Localized or generalized itch without primary skin lesion
- Rash present for >6 weeks
- No somatic cause

Optional criteria:

- Temporal relation between symptoms and a life event
- Variations in intensity with stress
- Diurnal variation
- Predominance of symptoms at rest
- Associated psychological disorder
- Pruritus improved by psychoactive medications
- Pruritus improved by psychotherapy

Differential Diagnosis

Symptomatic pruritus associated with systemic or cutaneous diseases including scabies, adverse reaction to medications (especially opioids), neuropathic itch, delusional infestations, diffuse mastocytosis, and mast cell activation syndrome.

Prevention and Therapy

Topical antipruritics, e.g., menthol, crotamiton

Systemic antipruritics, e.g., antihistamines (hydroxyzine, cetirizine) or antihistamines with other psychotropic effects (doxepin, mirtazapine)

Psychotherapy and psychopharmaceuticals initiated by a psychiatrist, e.g., fluoxetine and olanzapine

Obsessive-Compulsive Skin Disorders (OCD) [1, 7]

Grading of Importance

C

Level

Advanced

ICD-11

6B20.Z

Synonyms

Obsessive-compulsive neurotic skin disorders

Epidemiology

Estimated prevalence in adults: 2.3%. Age of onset: 20 years.

Persistent disorder for years (mean of 9 years).

Excoriation disorder: 1–5% of the population. Female preponderance.

Onset at adolescence (most common), or adulthood (30–45 years of age).

Body-focused repetitive behavior disorder. Prevalence onychophagia (nail biting): 25–60%.

Definition

Group of dermatoses secondary to a chronic psychiatric disorder characterized by obsessions and compulsions.

Excoriation disorder (neurotic excoriations): Repetitive picking of skin resulting in noticeable tissue damage.

Body-focused repetitive behaviors: onychophagia, dermatophagia, onychotillomania (nail picking), trichotillomania, cheek/lip biting, nose/ear picking, and knuckle cracking.

Etiology and Pathogenesis

Obsessive-compulsive and related disorders (OCRD) is a category of the Diagnostic and Statistical Manual of Mental Disorders (DSM-5).

Body-focused repetitive behaviors are included under "unspecified OCRD" in DSM-5.

Some obsessive-compulsive-related skin and hair disorders, such as trichotillomania (see section "Trichotillomania").

Signs and Symptoms

Excoriation disorders:

- Grouped erosions at easily accessible sites. Picking over areas of acne, scars, scabs, or insect bites.
- Acne excoriee: Acne lesions are scratched and picked.

Body-focused repetitive behavior disorder. Variable clinical features such as:

- Nail biting: paronychia and gingival injuries
- Rubbing of the proximal nail fold: nail matrix damage
- Chronic biting of the skin: localized thickened plaques (lichenification)
- Cheek biting: transverse whitish ridges in the oral mucosa (morsicatio buccarum)
- Repeated attempts to decrease or stop skin picking

Associated psychopathology (depression, anxiety, or stress)

Localization

Acne excoriee: frequent facial involvement.

Body-focused repetitive behavior disorder: nails, fingers, oral mucosa, lips. Accessible skin areas.

Classification

See signs and symptoms.

Laboratory and Other Workups

No abnormalities

Dermatopathology

Cutaneous ulceration without or minor associated inflammatory infiltrates.

Course

Chronic. Waxing and waning evolution

Complications

Secondary infection, bleeding, and inflammation

Diagnosis

DSM-5 diagnostic criteria

Differential Diagnosis

Psychogenic pruritus. Primary psychiatric disorders with secondary excoriations (e.g., delusional infestation or tactile hallucinations).

Skin picking secondary to the physiological effects of a substance (e.g., cocaine) or a medical condition (e.g., scabies).

The differential diagnosis of cheek biting includes oral candidiasis, lichen planus, and white sponge nevus.

In nail biting: nail dystrophy, nail matrix damage, and mycotic infections.

Prevention and Therapy

Cognitive-behavioral therapy (CBT) and habit reversal training.

Antidepressive and antipsychotic agents are helpful by treating underlying anxiety.

N-acetylcysteine 1200–3000 mg/day may reduce skin picking.

In patients with acne excoriee: Additional appropriate acne treatment.

Special

Approximately 90% of individuals with OCD have other psychiatric comorbidities. The most common comorbid disorder in OCD is anxiety disorders, depression, impulse control, and substance use disorders. The comorbidity of OCD and depression significantly increases the risk of suicide.

Body Dysmorphic Disorders [5, 8]

Grading of Importance

C

Level

Advanced

ICD-11

6B21.Z

Synonyms

Dysmorphophobia, dermatologic hypochondriasis

Epidemiology

No gender differences. Global prevalence: 0.7–2.4%.

Symptoms most commonly begin during adolescence (12–13 years of age).

Definition

Complex chronic obsessive-compulsive mental disorder characterized by excessive preoccupation with a perceived defect in physical appearance that is not observable or significant to others and results in repetitive, obsessive behaviors and thoughts.

Etiology and Pathogenesis

Etiology: Unknown

Emotional unconscious displacement causing feelings of shame and embarrassment, persistent feeling of being unloved, insecurity, and rejection

Signs and Symptoms

Broad spectrum of severity, ranging from obsessional worry to frank delusion.

Firm belief that some aspect of his or her appearance is ugly, abnormal, or deformed. Causes severe distress, impairs normal functioning, and decreases quality of life.

Localization

Complete body contour which includes belly, breast, buttocks, and genitalia. Special skin concerns facial contouring, scarring, wrinkles, followed by hair concerns (hair loss, thinning, balding, excessive facial hair or body hair), and nose (e.g., too large or misshapen) and nail concerns.

Classification

Categorized under Obsessive-Compulsive and Related Disorders in the Diagnostic and Statistical Manual of Mental Disorders (DSM-5)

Laboratory and Other Workups

Absence of relevant abnormalities

Dermatopathology

Minor or absent histopathological changes

Course

The condition is chronic and lifelong. Untreated, the prognosis is poor.

Clinical Presentation

Patients constantly seek medical and surgical treatments in order to improve their physical appearance. Distortion of the own physical appearance leads to psychiatric comorbidities: anxiety, stress, depression, and personality disorder.

Complications

Overtreatment. Skin picking is seen in one-third of patients and can exacerbate mild acne, causing scarring.

Major depression, severe anxiety disorders or personality disorders. Suicidal thoughts.

Diagnosis

Careful clinical history. Physical examination. Evaluate the impact on the quality of the patient's life. DMS-5 diagnostic criteria.

Differential Diagnosis

Real dermatological diseases. Invisible dermatoses.

Prevention and Therapy

Psychiatric consultation needed

References

1. Brock H, Hany M (2020) Obsessive-compulsive disorder. StatPearls, Treasure Island, FL
2. Buteau A, Reichenberg J (2018) Psychogenic pruritus and its management. Dermatol Clin 36(3):309–314
3. Chandran V, Kurien G (2020) Dermatitis artefacta. StatPearls, Treasure Island, FL
4. Duke DC, Keeley ML, Geffken GR, Storch EA (2010) Trichotillomania: a current review. Clin Psychol Rev 30(2):181–193
5. Fang A, Matheny NL, Wilhelm S (2014) Body dysmorphic disorder. Psychiatr Clin North Am 37(3):287–300
6. Grant JE, Chamberlain SR (2016) Trichotillomania. Am J Psychiatry 173(9):868–874
7. Mavrogiorgou P, Bader A, Stockfleth E, Juckel G (2015) Obsessive-compulsive disorder in dermatology. J Dtsch Dermatol Ges 13(10):991–999
8. Nicewicz HR, Boutrouille JF (2020) Body dysmorphic disorder. StatPearls, Treasure Island, FL

Part VIII

Special Conditions, Symptoms and Syndromes

Special Conditions, Symptoms, and Syndromes

25

Ramon María Pujol Vallverdú, Martine Bagot, Günter Burg, Adele De Masson, Gabor Dobos, Ana María Giménez-Arnau, Giampiero Girolomoni, Paolo Gisondi, Harald Gollnick, Katariina Hannula-Jouppi, Martina Maurelli, Annamari Ranki, Alexander Salava, and Christos C. Zouboulis

Contents

Annamari Ranki has died before the publication of this book.

R. M. Pujol Vallverdú (✉) · A. M. Giménez-Arnau
Dermatology and Venereology, Universitat Autònoma de Barcelona, Hospital del Mar. IMIM, Barcelona, Spain
e-mail: rpujol@psmar.cat

M. Bagot
Service de Dermatologie, Université Paris Cité, Hôpital Saint-Louis, Paris, France
e-mail: martine.bagot@gmail.com

G. Burg
Dermatology, Zurich, Switzerland
e-mail: g.burg@access.uzh.ch

A. De Masson · G. Dobos
Dermatology and Venereology, Hopital Saint Louis, Université de Paris, Paris, France
e-mail: adele.demasson@aphp.fr; gabor.dobos@charite.de

G. Girolomoni · P. Gisondi · M. Maurelli
Department of Medicine, Università degli Studi di Verona, Verona, Italy
e-mail: giampiero.girolomoni@univr.it; paolo.gisondi@univr.it

H. Gollnick et al. (eds.), *Dermatology Cyberderm WebBook*,
https://doi.org/10.1007/978-3-031-78491-0_25

H. Gollnick
Department of Dermatology & Venereology, Otto-von-Guericke University, Magdeburg, Germany
e-mail: Harald.Gollnick@med.ovgu.de

K. Hannula-Jouppi
Department of Dermatology, Allergology and Venereology, Helsinki University Central Hospital, Skin and Allergy Hospital, Helsinki, Finland
e-mail: katariina.hannula-jouppi@hus.fi

A. Ranki · A. Salava
Department of Dermatology and Allergology, Helsinki University Hospital, Helsinki, Finland
e-mail: alexander.salava@hus.fi

C. C. Zouboulis
Departments of Dermatology, Venereology, Allergology and Immunology, Staedtisches Klinikum Dessau, Brandenburg Medical School Theodor Fontane and Faculty of Health Sciences Brandenburg, Dessau, Germany
e-mail: christos.zouboulis@mhb-fontane.de

Test your learning and check your understanding of this book's contents: use the "Springer Nature Flashcards" app to access questions using ▶ https://sn.pub/1rhh6k.

To use the app, please follow the instructions in Chap. 1.

Red Face [6, 7]

Grading of Importance

B

Level

Advanced

ICD-11

None because the red face is a multifactorial symptom.

Synonyms

Facial erythema.

Epidemiology

Common skin symptom of several diseases, rosacea (81% of the patients with red face), atopic dermatitis, seborrheic dermatitis, and many others

Definition

Fixed or transient (flushing) red coloring of the face of different origins

Etiology and Pathogenesis

Minor temporary facial flushing: exogenous and endogenous physical and chemical stimuli. Major sign of clinically distinct entities, manifestation of particular skin diseases, sign of an internal disease (e.g., endocrine diseases).

Signs and Symptoms

In addition to erythema, other symptoms, such as warmth, edema, infiltration, scaling, exudate, vesicles, crusts, lichenification, and/or purple discoloration may occur depending on the etiology in:

- Inflammatory skin diseases (facial allergic/toxic/irritant dermatitis, seborrheic dermatitis, facial psoriasis, acrodermatitis enteropathica, rosacea, lichen planus actinicus, erythroprosopalgia)
- Infectious dermatoses (erysipelas, acrodermatitis chronica atrophicans, mycobacterial infections, primary herpes simplex, measles, fifth disease, tinea faciei)
- Vascular malformations
- Rare dermatoses (keratosis pilaris atrophicans, ichthyoses, Keratitis-Ichthyosis-Deafness (KID) syndrome, photogenodermatoses, tuberous sclerosis)
- Sign of internal diseases/disorders/conditions (exercise, embarrassment, anger, stress, anxiety, guilt, pregnancy, perimenopause, heatstroke, sunburn, X-ray, UVB, wind, cold/heat exposure, sexual act, fever; cutaneous T-cell lymphoma, Hodgkin's disease, hyperthyroidism, chronic oxygen deprivation, polycythemia, pheochromocytoma, carcinoid tumor, carcinoid syndrome, systemic mastocytosis, collagen disorders, sarcoidosis)
- Drugs and toxins
- Food ingestion

Localization

Entire face or certain pattern

Classification

- Temporary facial flushing
- Persistent red face

Laboratory and Other Workups

Depending on the differential diagnosis

Dermatopathology

Depending on diagnosis

Course

Transient, recurrent, or permanent facial erythema

Complications

Persistent facial erythema may result in several psychiatric disorders.

Diagnosis

Dependent on the facial – and extrafacial – localization and classification of erythema, additional symptoms, history, and results of skin biopsy and clinical and laboratory test.

Differential Diagnosis

See signs and symptoms

Prevention and Therapy

Depends on diagnosis

Erythrodermas [8, 18]

Figures 25.1 and 25.2

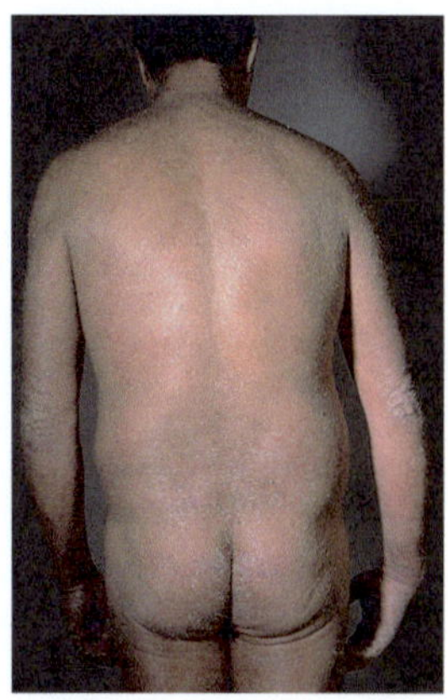

Fig. 25.1 Erythroderma: almost total skin involvement with hyperpigmentation

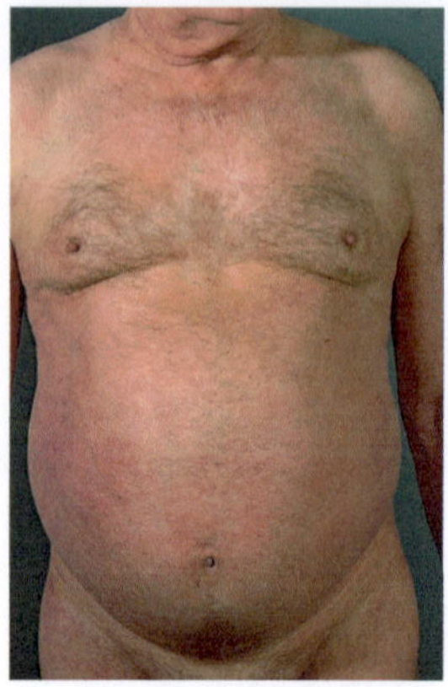

Fig. 25.2 Erythroderma: total redness of the skin

Grading of Importance

B

Level

Basic

ICD-11

EB10; EH40.2; EH64; EC20.03; EC20.0Y; EC20.02

Synonyms

Red man syndrome. Various diagnoses.

Epidemiology

See specific diagnoses. See also chapter Red Face.

Definition

Inflammatory and scaly or exfoliative skin condition with redness and scaling of >90% of the skin, which either is primarily involved or spreads secondarily from a non-erythrodermic dermatosis.

Etiology and Pathogenesis

Depends on underlying diagnosis (see classification).

Signs and Symptoms

Almost complete (>90%) redness and different degree of scaling of the skin, with or without itch. Sparing of the skin in the axila and abdominal folds or on the trunk (nappes claires). Swelling of lymph nodes as a consequence of pruritus scratching, erosions, and superinfections. Due to loss of albumin and electrolytes via the exfoliative scaling edema develops. Sometimes temperature dysregulation and/or fever. Cachexia in some cases.

LocaliZation

Total skin, according to definition

Classification

Primary Erythrodermas

- Sézary syndrome
- Erythrodermic mycosis fungoides
- Staphylococcal scalded skin syndrome (SSSS)
- Erythroderma due to secondary loss of function of the skin (deficiency of vitamins, electrolytes; malabsorption due to alcohol excess with exsiccation)
- Senile-(melano-) erythroderma (with cachexia)
- Congenital ichthyosiform erythroderma
- Severe generalized sunburn
- Ofuji disease

Secondary erythrodermas

- Psoriatic erythroderma
- Pityriasis rubra pilaris
- Atopic eczema
- Drug reaction
- Paraneoplastic
- Generalized cutaneous mastocytosis
- Generalized urticaria

Laboratory and Other Workups

Depending on diagnosis (mostly full blood count, electrolytes, liver enzymes, lymphocyte subpopulations, histamine, IgE)

Dermatopathology

Depending on diagnosis

Course

Can be acute, subacute, and chronic

Complications

Loss of fluid (exsiccation), of proteins and electrolytes (scaling), cardiac insufficiency; thermal loss

Diagnosis

Redness and scaling of the total integument. Specific diagnosis of the underlying disorder is based on the dynamic and follow-up of the dermatosis and the histologic features

Differential Diagnosis

See classification.

Prevention and Therapy

Depending on diagnosis. Because of emergency situations, there may be a necessity of an acute intervention.

Dry Skin [13, 16]

Figures 25.3 and 25.4

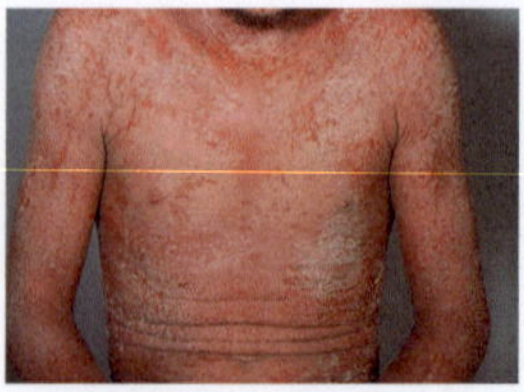

Fig. 25.3 Dry skin: exsiccation in an alcoholic

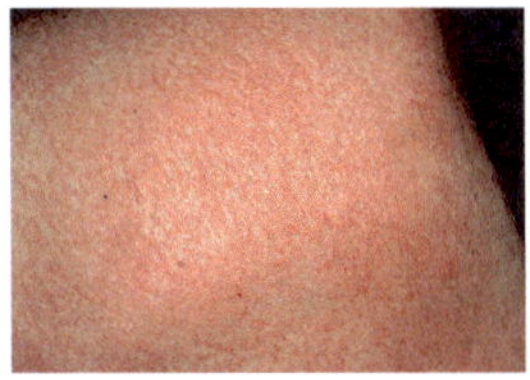

Fig. 25.4 Dry skin: eczema craquelé from obsessive washing

Grading of Importance

B

Level

Basic

ICD-11

ED 54 (ICD-10: L85.3)

Synonyms

Xeroderma, xerodermia, asteatosis cutis, xerosis cutis, exsiccosis, sebostasis

Epidemiology

Dry skin is one of the most common dermatological diagnoses and a symptom present in many dermatological and non-dermatological diseases (prevalence ranging from 35% to 85%). No gender predilection. Affects over 50% of individuals aged ≥65 years.

Frequent symptom in dermatoses characterized by dysfunction of the skin barrier (atopic dermatitis, psoriasis), in individuals with underlying diseases (i.e., diabetes mellitus, renal failure, hypothyroidism, etc.) or taking associated medications modifying the epidermal lipid content and barrier.

Definition

Scaly, rough, cracked, and fissured skin surface showing loss of softness, often accompanied by pruritus, due to decreased quantity and/or quality of lipids and/or hydrophilic substances (natural moisturizing factor) with increase of water loss.

Etiology and Pathogenesis

Dry skin is caused by loss of water from the stratum corneum associated with impairment in the natural barrier function and/or lack of natural moisturizing factors (NMF). Abnormalities in the stratum corneum (intercellular lipids) and/or impaired keratinocyte differentiation along with decreased levels of NMF (degradation products of filaggrin: lactic acid, sugars, amino acids, urea) result in dry skin secondary to transepidermal water loss and dehydration.

Multifactorial etiology. Mediated by genetics, environmental factors, aging, and other factors such as ethnicity.

External Causes

- Intense skin cleansing/overwashing
- Environmental factors: cold weather, low humidity
- Occupational factors: "wet work," contact with irritant agents

Endogenous Causes

Aging, menopause, andropause

Skin diseases

- Inflammatory skin disorders: atopic dermatitis, allergic contact dermatitis, irritant contact dermatitis, etc.
- Infectious skin disorders (in the chronic phase): scabies, bacterial, or fungal infections
- Genodermatoses: ichthyoses, xeroderma pigmentosum
- Neoplasms: Cutaneous T-cell lymphoma

Internal/Systemic Diseases

- Endocrine or metabolic: diabetes mellitus, hypothyroidism, hyperthyroidism, primary biliary cholangitis, cholestasis, hyperparathyroidism, renal failure, and hemodialysis
- Inflammatory: Crohn's disease, ulcerative colitis
- Infections: human immunodeficiency virus (HIV), hepatitis B or C virus
- Hormonal: pregnancy, menopause
- Hematologic: myeloproliferative disorders, multiple myeloma, Hodgkin's and non-Hodgkin's lymphoma, Graft-versus-host disease (GVHD), paraneoplastic
- Neurologic: Autonomic neuropathy

Psychiatric diseases

- Obsessive-compulsive disorders: excess skin washing
- Eating disorders: anorexia with nutrition deficiencies
- Addictions: alcohol or drug abuse, nicotine excess

Dietary

- Dehydration: excess perspiration, insufficient water intake
- Malnutrition

Medication-related

Drugs: Diuretics, beta-blockers, contraceptives, retinoids, long-term use of topical steroids, lipid-lowering agents (statins), radiation therapy (X-ray, UV)

Signs and Symptoms

Dry skin is characterized by a scaly, rough, cracked, and fissured surface and loss of softness. Skin dullness with decreased elasticity, texture coarsening and wrinkling. Often associated with pruritus that may lead to excoriations and hemorrhage.

Erythema may occasionally be present. Rubbing and scratching of the skin can lead to eczematous changes with a reticulate, cracked, or crazy-paving appearance ("eczema craquelé"). Recurrent and intense pruritus may lead to lichenification.

Localization

Could be localized or generalized

Dry skin is more frequently present on the lower legs, dorsal forearms, sides of abdomen, and hands and feet, although any area of the body may be affected.

Classification

Dry skin can develop acutely or be a chronic condition of varying intensity (mild, moderate, or severe dry skin).

Classification according to etiopathogenesis (see above).

Laboratory and Other Workups

Assessment of possible underlying causes: renal and liver function tests, thyroid hormone levels, vitamin levels, blood sugar, hematologic investigations

Measurement of transepidermal water loss (TEWL), corneometry, pH, skin roughness

Dermatopathology

Skin biopsy can be performed in rare instances when needed to distinguish from conditions mimicking dry skin (ichthyosiform dermatoses).

Course

Variable. Although dry skin is often experienced in the winter, in certain individuals may be a lifelong concern. Can be aggravated by environmental factors.

Complications

Increased risk of skin infections (via breaches in the skin surface), skin breakdown from maceration (skin folds), and from pressure in weight-bearing and pressure-prone surfaces. Chronic pruritus and scratching vicious cycle. Secondary impetiginization.

Sensitization: Allergic contact dermatitis (due to compromised skin barrier function).

Diagnosis

Clinical diagnosis with a thorough history and physical examination

Differential Diagnosis

Depending on the cause and course (see above).

Prevention and Therapy

Prevention: Avoidance of possible trigger factors. Treatment of comorbidities.

Therapy: Most cases can be managed conservatively with gentle cleansing and adequate moisturization.

Use of mild cleansers: synthetic detergent cleansers or Syndet cleansers. Avoid traditional soaps.

Skin moisturizers: Oil-based creams better than water-based lotions. Ointments are useful for preventing transepidermal water loss. May include humectants (glycerin, urea 10%, ammonium lactate, hyaluronic acid, gelatin), occlusives (lanolin, paraffin, petrolatum, cholesterol, stearyl alcohol) and emollients (petrolatum, dimethicone). Application immediately after bathing or showering.

In cases with intense itch or associated dermatitis, oral antihistamines, topical corticosteroids, or calcineurin inhibitors may be prescribed.

Prognosis

Dry skin is a benign symptom that can be resolved with avoidance of triggers and incorporating adequate skincare. Some cases may persist or recur for years. When associated with pruritus, it may lead to a considerable impairment in patients' quality of life.

Itching [14]

Grading of Importance

B

Level

Advanced

ICD-11

ME65.1; EC90.6

Synonyms

Pruritus

Epidemiology

Prevalence: most common symptom in dermatology. Chronic itch 12–20% of general population. In particular, about 60% of the elderly complain of chronic itch. According to different dermatoses or non-dermatoses associated itch, no clear data exist.

Definition

Itching is a symptom of many dermatoses or a symptom of a specific physical or psychological sensation. It produces unpleasant feeling of the skin leading to the desire to scratch.

Etiology and Pathogenesis

Different stimuli lead to a provocation of scratching in order to remove a pruritogenic factor, a response likely to have originated when most pruritogens were parasites. Dedicated neural pathway (pruritoceptors) similar but different compared to those dedicated to pain, including unmyelinated C fibers and small myelinated Aδ fibers. Itch mediators include histamine, interleukin (IL)-2, TNF-a, IL-4, IL-13, IL-31, thymic stromal lymphoprotein, proteases, neuropeptides (substance P), and opioid peptides.

Signs and Symptoms

Desire to scratch. Quality of itch: burning, painful, stinging, prickling. Itch may be continuous or intermittent (continuous over the day or may come up at certain times during night or may flare up by stress or when patients go to rest).

Localization

Localized pruritus: usually caused by itchy dermatoses, associated with inflamed skin. Generalized pruritus: can be caused by itchy dermatoses even if the inflamed skin does not show generalized spread or can be caused by extracutaneous disorders or underlying systemic disorders.

Classification

- Acute
- Chronic: Itching lasting 6 or more weeks. Localized or generalized.
- Pruritus with underlying dermatosis (specific skin lesions): atopic dermatitis, eczema, psoriasis, urticaria, scabies, pemphigoid, drug eruptions, cutaneous T-cell lymphoma, insect bite reactions.
- Pruritus associated with excoriated nodules and/or lichenification: prurigo nodularis, lichen simplex chronicus.
- Pruritus in patients with normal skin or minimal scratched lesions (pruritus of unknown origin): neurological diseases, hematological disorders, endocrine diseases, infective diseases, uremic, cholestatic, metabolic diseases, neoplastic, drug-induced, psychiatric diseases, mixed.

Laboratory and Other Workups

Recommended in patients with pruritus of unknown origin certain blood parameters and imaging techniques as well as biopsy.

Dermatopathology

It depends on the type of skin lesions present. In chronic itch an increase of nerve fibers in the upper dermis also reaching epidermis can be found.

Course

The course is depending on the underlying disease and may last months or decades. Itch negatively impacts on the quality of life. Severe itch may be devastating.

Complications

Secondary skin lesions caused by scratching. Usually, secondary skin lesions encompass excoriations, ulcerations, crusts, papules, nodules, lichenification, atrophy and scars, hyper- and hypopigmentation. Sleeping disorder.

Diagnosis

In depth case history, physical examination of skin and lymph nodes, assessment of itch severity, screening lab, and instrumental tests.

Differential Diagnosis

Differentiate pruritus from burning sensations (porphyrias). Specific polyneuropathies.

Prevention and Therapy

Relaxation, mental training, yoga, mindfulness, avoidance of scratching training.

Prevention of dry skin with emollients.

Symptomatic therapy and treatment of underlying disease (where present). Topical treatments: local anesthetics, topical corticosteroids, topical calcineurin inhibitors. Systemic treatments: antihistamines, short term corticosteroids, ciclosporin. Opioid receptor agonists and antagonists, antiepileptics. Antidepressants, neurokinin antagonists, biologics. Ultraviolet phototherapy.

Urticarial Syndromes [5]

Grading of Importance

B

Level

Advanced

ICD-11

EB03

Synonyms

Urticarial eruptions, urticarial rash

Definition

There are many dermatoses mimicking urticaria. In contrast to "urticaria sensu strictu," "urticarial syndromes" is a group of disorders, which reflect or mimic skin lesions that look like wheals or hives.

Etiology and Pathogenesis

There are many dermatoses with an urticarial appearance that correspond to different pathogenic mechanisms such as type 1 or 3 immune reactions or are nonallergic (pharmacologic, toxic, chemical). Many of them with an unknown etiology. They include:

External pathogens

- Insect bites and epizoonoses
- Early stage of contact dermatitis
- Infectious diseases/rashes

Immune dermatoses

- Immunobullous diseases
- Autoinflammatory syndromes
- Neutrophilic dermatosis and autoimmune disorders
- Angioedema

Semantic misnomers

- Urticarial vasculitis
- Urticaria pigmentosa (not primarily urticarial, may evolve urticarial appearance)

Signs and Symptoms

Urticarial lesions last several days; itch is variable; sometimes leave persisting erythema, blood extravasation, hematoma-like or small pigmentation. There may be some scaling.

Localization

Urticarial lesions can develop at any location.

Classification

There is no nosologic classification because of the heterogeneity of the conditions.

Laboratory and Other Workups

There are no specific general laboratory requirements. Some of the diseases need specific diagnostic tests and immunologic and molecular approach.

Dermatopathology

A skin biopsy may be helpful in order to confirm a causative underlying dermatoses.

Course

Depends on the underlying disorder; acute, subacute, or chronic persistent or relapsing

Complications

Depends on the underlying disorder

Diagnosis

The clinicopathological correlation is nearly always essential for the diagnosis of urticarial lesions.

Differential Diagnosis

See etiology and pathogenesis.

Prevention and Therapy

Depends on the underlying disorder

Pregnancy Dermatoses [2, 9, 11]

Grading of Importance

B

Level

Advanced

ICD-11

JA65.1

Synonyms

Disorders of pregnancy. There are several synonyms depending on specific dermatoses.

Polymorphic eruption of pregnancy (PEP): Pruritic urticarial papules and plaques of pregnancy, pruritic eruption of pregnancy, toxemic rash of pregnancy

Pemphigoid gestationis (PG): Gestational pemphigoid, herpes gestationis

Atopic eruption of pregnancy (AEP): Prurigo gestationis, papular dermatitis of pregnancy, pruritic folliculitis of pregnancy

Intrahepatic cholestasis of pregnancy (ICP): Pruritus gravidarum, icterus gravidarum

Pustular psoriasis of pregnancy: Impetigo herpetiformis

Epidemiology

Dermatoses of pregnancy are a group of disorders seen throughout the world. They are usually seen more commonly in late pregnancy and in twin or multiple pregnancies. Some of them may result in an increased fetal risk.

Polymorphic eruption of pregnancy (PEP): Represents the most common specific dermatosis of pregnancy. Incidence: 1:160 pregnancies.

Pemphigoid gestationis (PG): 1 in 40–50,000 pregnancies. Associated with the haplotypes HLA-DR3 and HLADR4.

Pruritic folliculitis of pregnancy: incidence 1:3000 pregnancies

Atopic eruption of pregnancy (AEP) is always causally linked with a personal and/or family atopic background.

Intrahepatic cholestasis of pregnancy (ICP): Geographic pattern. Positive family history > 50% of cases.

Definition

Dermatoses that are specific to pregnancy, resulting from an interaction of multiple factors in the body during pregnancy. Include various types (see classification).

Etiology and Pathogenesis

Polymorphic eruption of pregnancy (PEP): Pathogenesis unknown

Pemphigoid gestationis: Autoimmune response against BP180 (bullous pemphigoid) antigen. Circulating complement-fixing IgG antibodies. Possible occurrence of the disease when using oral contraceptives or during the premenstrual period.

Atopic eruption of pregnancy: May occur in atopic subjects or others without atopy.

Pruritic folliculitis of pregnancy: unknown.

Intrahepatic cholestasis of pregnancy: Not a primary dermatosis but a pregnancy-related liver disorder with secondary cutaneous lesions in particular induced by scratching.

Pustular psoriasis of pregnancy: Impetigo herpetiformis is considered a form of generalized pustular psoriasis.

Signs and Symptoms

Depends on disorder. Skin eruptions usually appear in the third trimester of pregnancy and tend to resolve after delivery.

Polymorphic eruption of pregnancy (PEP): Benign, self-limited, pruritic, papulo-urticarial inflammatory disorder. Clinically polymorphous intensely itchy erythematous papules and plaques within and/or adjacent to striae gravidarum, macules, papulo-vesicules (eczematous), urticarial, targetoid lesions similar to erythema multiforme, annular or polycyclic wheals, and, rarely, small bullae excoriations and crusts:

- Typical onset: last trimester of pregnancy
- Localization: Trunk and extremities

Pemphigoid gestationis (PG): Intensely pruritic. Erythematous urticarial papules and plaques. The lesions progress to tense blisters and bullae:

- Typical onset: second or third trimester of pregnancy
- Localization: Extremities and trunk, mostly on the abdomen (periumbilical)

Atopic eruption of pregnancy (AEP): Generalized pruritic eczematous skin condition in patients with an atopic diathesis:

- Typical onset: anytime during pregnancy
- Localization: classic atopic predilection sites

Prurigo of pregnancy: Excoriated papules and nodules:

- Typical onset: middle of pregnancy
- Localization: limbs and/or trunk

Pruritic folliculitis of pregnancy: Follicular/pustular and papular lesions:

- Typical onset: middle of pregnancy
- Localization: limbs and/or trunk

Intrahepatic cholestasis of pregnancy (ICP): Widespread pruritus. No primary skin lesions, Secondary skin changes due to scratching:

- Typical onset: last trimester of pregnancy
- Localization: widespread, limbs and/or trunk

Pustular psoriasis of pregnancy (PPP)/impetigo herpetiformis: Tiny, superficial, pustules arranged in herpetiform distribution:

- Typical onset: last trimester of pregnancy
- Localization: widespread, limbs and/or trunk; centrifugal spread

Localization

See "Symptoms."

Classification

See "Symptoms."

Laboratory and Other Workups

Polymorphic eruption of pregnancy (PEP): Routine laboratory: normal

Pemphigoid gestationis: Eosinophilia. HG factor. Immune serology (BP180 antigen)

Atopic eruption of pregnancy: Elevated serum IgE levels

Intrahepatic cholestasis of pregnancy: Elevation of the total serum bile acid levels.

Mild abnormalities of liver function tests: (elevated ALT, GGT, hyperbilirubinemia).

Pustular psoriasis of pregnancy: Leukocytosis with neutrophilia, elevated erythrocyte sedimentation rate, hypoalbuminemia, and iron deficiency anemia. Pustules are sterile.

Dermatopathology

Polymorphic eruption of pregnancy (PEP): Nonspecific histologic features: Spongiosis papillary dermal edema; superficial, mid-dermal perivascular lympho-histiocytic infiltrate with occasional eosinophils; DIF and IIF are negative.

Pemphigoid gestations:

- Pre-bullous stage: Perivascular inflammatory infiltrate, composed of lymphocytes, histiocytes, and eosinophils. Spongiosis and focal epidermal necrosis.
- Bullous stage: Subepidermal blister.

Direct immunofluorescence (IF): Linear deposition of C3 along the BMZ (basal membrane zone).

Indirect immunofluorescence/ELISA: Circulating IgG antibodies anti BP180

Intrahepatic cholestasis of pregnancy: Skin biopsy: Nonspecific changes. DIF and IIF: Negative.

Atopic eruption of pregnancy: Corresponding to atopic dermatitis; direct immunofluorescence: negative

Pustular psoriasis of pregnancy: Subcorneal spongiform pustules, corresponding to pustular psoriasis

Course

Most dermatoses of pregnancy resolve after delivery.

Polymorphic eruption of pregnancy (PEP): The lesions usually resolve within 4–6 weeks.

Pemphigoid gestationis: Self-limiting. Spontaneous remission in weeks to months after delivery. Tends to reoccur in all subsequent pregnancies, usually with an earlier onset and increased severity.

Possible recurrences with subsequent pregnancies in **atopic eruptions, intrahepatic cholestasis of pregnancy and pustular psoriasis of pregnancy**.

Complications

Polymorphic eruption of pregnancy (PEP) and atopic eruption of pregnancy: The fetal and maternal prognoses are excellent in almost all cases.

Pemphigoid gestationis, intrahepatic cholestasis of pregnancy [ICP], and pustular psoriasis of pregnancy (PPP) are associated with considerable adverse fetal outcomes such as prematurity, fetal distress, or even stillbirth.

Intrahepatic cholestasis of pregnancy: Increased risk of intra- and postpartum hemorrhage.

Pustular psoriasis of pregnancy: Hypocalcemia, lymphadenopathy, seizures, and malaise, severe dehydration.

Diagnosis

Clinical features, histopathological data, and direct and indirect immunofluorescence studies. Immunopathologic tests (DIF/IIF) play an important role in differentiating pemphigoid gestationis from other bullous disorders. Onset of eruption.

Differential Diagnosis

In many instances should be established with different dermatoses appearing during pregnancy and/or other related or specific dermatoses of pregnancy.

Polymorphic eruption of pregnancy (PEP): Pemphigoid gestationis (pre-bullous) or different dermatoses appearing during pregnancy: Drug eruptions, allergic contact dermatitis, erythema multiforme, scabies.

Pemphigoid gestationis:

- Pre-blistering stage: Polymorphic eruption of pregnancy (PEP)
- Blistering stage: Other autoimmune bullous diseases, bullous drug eruptions, or contact dermatitis coincident with pregnancy

Atopic eruption of pregnancy: Pruritic dermatoses unrelated to and coinciding with gestation scabies, drug eruptions, and possible arthropod bites

Intrahepatic cholestasis of pregnancy: Different dermatologic and/or internal conditions that cause pruritus in the absence of primary skin lesions

Pustular psoriasis of pregnancy: Autoimmune bullous dermatoses, acute generalized exanthematous pustulosis

Prevention and Therapy

Polymorphic eruption of pregnancy (PEP): Symptomatic treatment.

Pemphigoid gestationis: Potent topical corticosteroids. Systemic corticosteroids, to control blister formation, tapered and maintained at the lowest effective dose. Immunosuppressive treatments only used after delivery.

Atopic eruption of pregnancy: Moderately potent topical corticosteroids and oral antihistamines. Emollients or antipruritic additives such as menthol or polidocanol.

Intrahepatic cholestasis of pregnancy: Antipruritic treatments: ursodeoxycholic acid, cholestyramine, antihistamines (nonsedative), anion exchange resins.

Pustular psoriasis of pregnancy: TNF alpha blocker infusions, systemic corticosteroids, ciclosporin. After pregnancy, other agents used in psoriasis could be prescribed: PUVA, oral retinoids. Antibacterials in case of secondary skin infection.

Special

Fetal prognosis: Pemphigoid gestationis, Intrahepatic cholestasis of pregnancy, pustular psoriasis of pregnancy: Increased risk to prematurity fetal distress (22–33%) and fetal abnormalities.

Purpuric Rashes [1]

Grading of Importance

B

Level

Advanced

ICD-11

ME62.1

Synonyms

Purpura, purpuric skin eruptions

Epidemiology

Variable prevalence depending on the etiology

Definition

Purpura is not a specific nosologic or diagnostic term but includes a heterogeneous group of benign, purpuric skin eruptions characterized by red to purple macules, patches, and petechiae secondary to capillary leakage of different mostly unknown causes.

Etiology and Pathogenesis

Purpura is often a symptom indicative of an underlying cause of bleeding (see classification).

Purpuric rashes may be primary (when hemorrhage is an integral part of lesion formation) or secondary (hemorrhage takes place in previously established lesions).

Increase fragility and permeability of vessels in elderly people, venous hypertension, or drugs (glucocorticosteroids, anticoagulants) may be promoting factors.

According to the etiology, different purpuric rashes can be defined:

- Purpuric rashes secondary to coagulation disorders (thrombocytopenic)
- Purpuric eruptions secondary to vascular damage (vasculitis) or vascular damage with thrombosis
- Purpuric eruptions secondary to vascular occlusion (hypercoagulable states, emboli, medium- to large-sized vasculitis)
- Miscellaneous. Secondary to vascular fragility, perivascular inflammation, drug induced purpura, pressure

Signs and Symptoms

Purpuric non-palpable, non-blanchable, red-brown to golden-brown (due to erythrocyte extravasation and hemosiderin deposition) lesions can be divided according their size in:

- Petechiae: capillary, punctiform hemorrhages with a limit of up to 4 mm
- Macular purpura: sized up to a centimeter
- Macular ecchymoses: larger amount of extravasation of erythrocytes

Occasionally confluent or associated with edematous plaques, blisters, or pustules. Can be accompanied by gingival, conjunctival, or gastrointestinal (GI) bleeding, hematuria or by internal hemorrhage depending on the etiology.

In some disorders, fever and a toxic syndrome may be present. Tenderness may suggest an inflammatory process.

Localization

Purpuric rashes can be localized or generalized with variable localizations. Acral areas or dependent areas on the lower extremities preferred.

Classification

Non-palpable and afebrile rash:

- Eczematid-like purpura: pruritic scaly petechial plaques
- Lichen aureus: localized yellow-brown patches
- Purpura annularis telangiectodes: annular macules
- Schamberg disease: multiple patches with pinpoint petechiae on the lower limbs
- Coagulation disorders
- Idiopathic thrombocytopenic purpura
- Hemorrhagic pigmentary dermatoses (Gougerot-Blum, Majocchi)
- Scurvy (follicle bound)
- Genodermatoses (i.e., Ehlers-Danlos syndrome)
- Physical/mechanic by pressure (vomiting, strangulation, coughing)

Non-palpable and febrile rash:

- Infectious coagulopathies
- Virus (i.e., Ebola)
- Meningococci (i.e., purpura fulminans)

Palpable and afebrile rash. Small vessel vasculitis:

- Leukocytoclastic vasculitis
- ANCA-related vasculitis

Palpable or non-palpable and febrile:

Infectious disorders. Potentially life-threatening conditions. Vasculitis meningococcemia, bacterial endocarditis, rickettsiosis, disseminated gonococcal infection, systemic vasculitis, purpuric viral exanthema.

Retiform and afebrile: Embolic conditions. Hypercoagulable states, late stages of Nicolau syndrome; anticoagulant-induced necrosis; calciphylaxis, vasculopathies; anticardiolipin syndrome.

Retiform and febrile: Septic vasculitis, thrombosis, purpura fulminans, disseminated intravascular coagulation.

Senile purpura: Severe dermatoporosis with stasis.

Laboratory and Other Workups

Glass spatula and Rumpel-Leede test. Complete hematological survey. Platelet count and coagulation tests. Biochemistry (liver and renal functional tests, plasma electrophoresis); immunological serum tests, stool guaiac (fecal occult blood test), urinalysis may be performed according the suspected underlying diagnoses. Specific microbiological cultures: in cases of suspected underlying infection.

Dermatopathology

The hallmark of purpuric lesions is extravasation of erythrocytes around the capillaris and venules and interstitial with or without signs of vasculitis. Mixed pattern of purpura and eczema.

Course

Depending on the underlying etiology. Acute, subacute, chronic.

Complications

Depending on the underlying etiology from self-limited to lethal outcome

Diagnosis

Clinical evaluation: All ages: Some purpuric rashes are almost exclusively observed in children (Henoch-Schönlein purpura) or in elderly patients (senile purpura).

Clinical history. Acute or prolonged evolution of lesions. Possible precipitating events (contacts with infectious persons or agents, drugs).

Physical examination: Skin and mucous membranes. Rash distribution and progression. Skin biopsy in cases of palpable purpuric rash or febrile purpuric eruptions.

Associated systemic symptoms (fever, hypotension).

Differential Diagnosis

Exclude secondary hemorrhagic variants of common diseases (e.g., hemorrhagic disseminated zoster, cellulitis). Exclude minor conditions with hemorrhagic lesion (senile purpura, skin areas treated with topical corticosteroids, petechial facial purpura due to vomiting or coughing).

Prevention and Therapy

Depending on the underlying etiology

Red Swollen Legs[15, 17]

Grading of Importance

B

Level

Advanced

Definition

Red swollen legs are characterized by edema and inflammatory erythema due to several underlying disorders.

Epidemiology

Depends on the underlying condition, the most frequent are:

- Erysipelas: prevalence around 1100/100,000 per year
- Deep vein thrombosis: incidence 80 cases per 100,000 annually, prevalence 1 case per 1000 population
- Superficial thrombophlebitis: 125,000 cases a year

Etiology and Pathogenesis

- Erysipelas
- Deep vein thrombosis
- Superficial thrombophlebitis
- Contact dermatitis
- Borreliosis

Increasing age and compounding morbidity, such as reduced mobility following a stroke, arthritic changes, obesity, and generalized frailty are promoting factors. Predisposing factors include potential site of pathogen entry (e.g., ulceration, tinea pedis, and traumatic wounds), chronic edema, lymphedema, and obesity.

Predisposing factors: prolonged standing or sitting with the calf-muscle pump inactive, female gender, obesity, older age, post-thrombotic syndrome

Localization and Symptoms

Redness and swelling due to edema or fibrosis that affects one or both legs and/or feet up to the thighs, accompanied by warmth and tenderness in the area, depending on the underlying condition. Superficial and deep vein thrombosis as well as erysipelas are painful; contact dermatitis is itchy.

Classification

- Acute disorders: erysipelas, necrotizing fasciitis, superficial thrombophlebitis, deep-vein thrombosis (DVT), stasis and contact dermatitis, trauma, and septic arthritis
- Chronic disorders: chronic edema, lymphedema, pretibial myxedema, cardiovascular disease with stasis eczema, venous leg ulcers, and lipodermatosclerosis.

Laboratory and Other Workups

Inflammatory markers: erythrocyte sedimentation rate (ESR), C-reactive protein (CRP), D-dimer, and white cell count for vein thrombosis. Microbiology of any fissures or erosions in the skin should be considered before antibiotics are started. Ultrasound with Echocolor Doppler to confirm or exclude vein thrombosis.

Dermatopathology

It is based on the underlying disorder.

Course

Red swollen legs can be an acute or a chronic disorder depending on the pathological process.

Complications

Age-related poly-morbidity is increasing as people live longer. Complications may result from bacterial or fungal infection, ulceration, traumatic wounds, stage III lymphedema, venous insufficiency, and obesity.

Diagnosis and Differential Diagnosis

- Acute disorders include skin infections (erysipelas, stage I and stage II borreliosis, cellulitis and necrotizing fasciitis), joint infections (arthritis) all of which are associated with fever. Skin infections are detailed in chapter "Erysipelas." The most crucial early characteristic symptom is a disproportionate level of pain compared with the presenting symptoms.
- Deep-vein thrombosis (DVT) manifests with leg pain, swelling, tenderness, increased temperature, pitting edema, and prominent superficial veins. DVT occurs in association with several risk factors, including postoperative immobilization, long-haul travel and age, male gender, genetic or acquired thrombophilia, obesity, cancer, and pregnancy.
- Acute onset allergic contact dermatitis is common, especially in the setting of stasis dermatitis and often related to hypersensitivity reactions to topical medications. There are erythema and vesiculation followed by desquamation and usually severe itch.
- Superficial thrombophlebitis is an inflammation of a superficial vein due to a blood clot and hemostasis. Chronic disorders include cardiovascular disease (CVD) where venous hypertension results in localized edema that traps leukocytes and neutrophils in the tissues. Tissue damage eventually results in the development of fibrosis, dermatitis, and ulceration.
- Lipodermatosclerosis is an inflammation of subcutaneous fat, and presents as fibrosed, rigid, red, or brown skin, typically affecting the medial aspect of the calf. The subcutaneous tissues may become firm and depressed, and circumferential damage that occurs may result in an "inverted champagne bottle" effect.
- Stasis eczema is a consequence of CVD, with skin becoming itchy, red, swollen, dry and flaky, scaly or crusty, and weeping. The severity (edema due to liver cirrhosis, nephrotic syndrome and heart insufficiency or dysbalance of protein metabolism) of these symptoms can fluctuate with periods of improvement and periods of worsening.

Prevention and Therapy

See respective chapters.

Infantile Skin [19, 22]

Grading of Importance

B

Level

Advanced

Definition

- Newborn refers to a baby from birth to 2 months of age.
- Infant denotes children anywhere from birth to 1 year old.
- Children from 1 year to age 4 years old are called toddlers.

Development

- Embryogenesis: epidermis begins to stratify, complete at 34 weeks of gestational age.
- Preterm neonates have decreased epidermal and stratum corneum thickness.
- After birth/newborns: maturation process with adaptation of the skin to a relatively dry environment. Risk of dehydration, hypothermia, and percutaneous absorption of toxic agents.
- Transepidermal water loss (TEWL) decreases along with gestational and postnatal age and TEWL is a good marker of gestational age at birth.

Neonates and infants have a characteristic spectrum of skin problems and associated skin diseases.

Structure and Physiology

- In preterm neonates the epidermis is thin, the dermo-epidermal junction is relatively loose and the anchoring structures susceptible to traumatic or infectious blister formation.
- The skin of newborns is much more permeable than the skin of older children.
- Newborn skin lacks functionally mature metabolic systems, and the superficial microvasculature capillary network is immature and will be accomplished by the age of 3–4 months.
- Relatively high sebum production in the first weeks of life due to mostly maternal androgens.
- Lower amounts of melanin in the epidermis in infants, warranting effective UV protection for prevention of sunburn and melanoma.
- The ratio of body surface to body mass in newborns is more than twice that in adults.

Biochemistry

The acid mantle plays an important role in skin defense and the composition of the microbiome.

In term babies, surface skin acidity (pH) is neutral at birth but drops during the first months to 5 and 5.5. The vernix caseosa is a protective covering, which is lacking in preterm neonates which thus renders them more susceptible for skin infections and hypothermia. Due to the important function of the vernix, bathing of the newborn during the first 6 hours of life is no longer recommended.

Microbiome

Immediately postpartum, skin microbiota is homogeneously distributed across the human body regardless of delivery method or gestational age. The skin of vaginally delivered newborns is colonized by vaginal *Prevotella* and *Lactobacillus* species, while the skin of neonates born by cesarean section show sa diverse community of cutibacteria, corynebacteria, and micrococcae. Anatomically site-specific composition of the microbiome starts to develop between 1 and 3 months but still differs significantly from the adult skin microbiome.

Immunology

The abundant skin-associated immune tissue orchestrates the defense against pathogens, responds to environmental changes, and has also functions in homeostasis. In newborn skin the amount of antimicrobial peptides, lysozyme, and lactoferrin are higher than in adults. Newborn skin contains fewer immune cells than adult skin, but typically anti-inflammatory regulatory T cells (Tregs) occur at higher density than in adult skin.

Sensitivity (Nerves)

The neural network develops early in the fetus, originating from the neural crest and organizing with increasing postnatal age. Neuro-cutaneous responses and sensitivity to touch are important for overall development and skin function but also skin-skin contact and bonding with caregivers.

Risk for Diseases

Due to the immaturity of the innate and adaptive cellular immunity, neonates and infants have a greater risk of skin infections.

Traumatization

The thin skin of a preterm infant is most vulnerable. During admission to neonatal intensive care unit (NICU), skin assessment is an essential part of care to reduce the risk of acquired skin injuries, the main types of which are bruises, blistering, excoriation, erythema, and pressure injuries.

Prevention

Full-term newborns may receive tub baths, while daily cleansing of preterm infant skin is not recommended and swaddle baths are recommended. Particular attention should be devoted to topical agents with excipients due to the increased permeability of neonatal and infant skin and the risk of accumulation of potentially harmful excipients.

Spectrum of Skin Diseases in Neonates and Infants

Most skin problems in the newborn period and infancy are benign and transient: eczematous eruptions (e.g., atopic eczema (AE) and seborrheic dermatitis (SD), reactive pustular rashes (e.g., erythema toxicum neonatorum), and acne (acne infantum) are discussed more in detail in the respective chapters.

Skin infections (e.g., bullous impetigo, staphylococcal scaled skin syndrome) and rare systemic diseases (e.g., Langerhans cell histiocytosis, cutaneous mastocytosis, hyper-IgE syndrome) can also cause skin rashes. Neonatal lupus erythematosus caused by transplacental maternal autoantibodies should be recognized to rule out congenital heart block.

Common Benign and Transient Skin Changes in Newborns

Milia and miliaria in newborns and small infants are based on the immaturity of adnexal structures in newborn skin. Treatment is not needed.

- Milia are characterized by 1- to 2-mm-sized white to yellow papules commonly on the face
- Miliaria are usually red 1- to 2-mm-sized papules concentrated on the trunk and are aggravated by high ambient temperatures.
- Sebaceous hyperplasia on the nose and upper lip.
- Neonatal cephalic pustulosis (neonatal acne) is a facial papulopustular eruption during the first weeks or up to 6–8 weeks which is common and transient.
- Reactive pustular rashes are relatively frequent in the neonatal period.
- The most common transient pustular rash is erythema toxicum neonatorum, which disappears within 1–2 weeks after birth.

- Cutis marmorata is the most common transient skin change in newborns. It consists of a symmetric reticular erythema resulting from a physiological response to cold exposure (vasoconstriction of superficial dermal vessels) in infancy.
- Neonatal jaundice (icterus) is common and physiological and typically peaks at 3–4 days of age or in preterm infants. It is caused by tissue deposition of bilirubin.

Genodermatoses

Most genodermatoses manifest neonatally or during infancy.

- Incontinentia pigmenti manifests neonatally with linear blistering following the lines of Blaschko, turning into linear plaques on the trunk and extremities.
- Café-au-lait macules indicative of neurofibromatosis and hypopigmented macules associated with tuberous sclerosis.
- Genetic mutations in proteins associated with the dermo-epidermal junction and the dermal anchoring cause different genetic blistering diseases (Epidermolysis bullosa).

Collodion baby is a common presentation of several congenital ichthyoses (e.g., lamellar ichthyosis, self-healing collodion baby and Harlequin ichthyosis), and the most severe forms associate with significant morbidity and mortality. Epidermolytic ichthyosis presents with blistering erythroderma.

- Acrodermatitis enteropathica is a very rare disorder of infancy associated with zinc deficiency in zinc absorbance. It presents at the time of weaning with perioral and/or perianal pustular dermatitis.
- Some palmoplantar keratodermas (PPK), especially diffuse PPKs manifest during infancy.

Laboratory and Other Workups

Laboratory investigations are rarely needed in skin diseases of infancy.

- A skin biopsy is warranted if systemic diseases (e.g., Langerhans histiocytosis, mastocytosis) are contemplated.
- In erythrodermic and cases of severe ichtyoses and epidermolysis bullosa intensive care blood tests are mandatory.
- Genetic profiling should be carried out in genodermatoses.

Diagnosis

The diagnosis of skin problems in newborns and infants is usually based on the clinical findings and a thorough history and evaluations of symptoms.

Aged Skin [10]

Grading of Importance

B

Level

Basic

ICD-11

EE40.Y

Synonyms

Dermatoporosis (aged skin)

Epidemiology

Ethnicity-specific aging characteristics
Caucasians: greater skin wrinkle formation and sagging
Asians: Pigment spot intensity
Professional extrinsic characteristic: indoor vs outdoor workers; nutritional and living behaviors

Definition

Natural process of biochemical and immunological events, leading to gradual cell damage accumulation, decreased local immune response, and development of various benign or malignant skin changes or diseases.

Etiology and Pathogenesis

Genetic predisposition, impairment of cellular metabolic and immunologic pathways, qualitative and quantitative hormonal alterations (intrinsic aging), and natural or artificial ultraviolet irradiation, stress, smoking, alcohol, chemicals and toxins, and pollution (extrinsic aging).

Signs and Symptoms

Intrinsically aged skin: macroscopically thin and atrophic skin, exhibits fine wrinkles, subcutaneous fat loss, prominent dryness, and reduced elasticity.

Extrinsically aged skin: deeper wrinkles, thickening of the epidermis varying, dullness, roughness, and mottled discoloration. Telangiectasias (severe photoaging).

Localization

Intrinsic aging: inner side of the upper arm and the gluteal region

Extrinsic aging: UV exposed sites (head and neck, hands)

Classification

- Intrinsic aging
- Extrinsic aging

Laboratory and Other Workups

Photographic severity scales other imagine methods (laser profiling)

Dermatopathology

Light-protected skin: Epidermal thinning (10–50%), decreased mitotic activity, decrease of Langerhans cells, reduction of dermal thickness, atrophy of the extracellular matrix, decrease of skin appendages, thinning of subcutaneous fat.

Light-exposed skin: Epidermal thickening varying, impaired proliferation, and differentiation of keratinocytes, sparce distribution of collagen fibers, broken elastic fibers and accumulation (actinic elastosis) increased mast cells and neutrophils, marked regression, and loss of vascular pattern.

Course

Gradual development in healthy individuals. In women, rapid progression after menopause.

Complications

Increased vulnerability

Diagnosis

Clinical signs, comparison of pictures from various phases of life

Differential Diagnosis

Progeria syndromes, hormonal deficiencies, metabolic disturbances (internal diseases)

Prevention and Therapy

Consequent avoidance of overexposure to extrinsic factors, diagnosis and treatment of underlying internal diseases (the skin is mirror of the body)

Various medico-cosmetic and surgical procedures

Progeria Syndromes [3]

Grading of Importance

C

Level

Basic

ICD-11

LD2B

Synonyms

Progeroid syndrome(s), premature aging syndromes, laminopathy

Epidemiology

Laminopathies are extremely rare disorders. Hutchinson-Gilford progeria syndrome only affects one child per 4,000,000 births worldwide.

Werner syndrome is estimated to occur in 0.5–1 out of 100,000 live births worldwide.

Definition

Syndromes characterized by premature aging signs. Hair loss and alopecia. Skin atrophy, sclerotic skin changes, telangiectasias, poikiloderma, and increased prevalence of skin tumors.

Etiology and Pathogenesis

The majority of progeria syndromes are rare autosomal recessive genetic conditions and show gene defects in DNA replication, recombination, repair, and transcription as well as mitochondrial function. Several of these syndromes are laminopathies (diseases caused by mutations in components of the nuclear lamina due to lamin A (LMNA) gene mutations).

- Hutchinson-Gilford progeria syndrome is mainly caused by a sporadic autosomal dominant point mutation in LMNA gene resulting in differently spliced lamin A protein known as progerin.
- Werner syndrome is caused by a truncating mutation in the WRN gene due to the production of a stop codon from a nonsense or frameshift mutation. The WRN gene plays a role in maintaining proper DNA replication and repair through base excision repair, nonhomologous end-joining, and homologous recombination. It is also involved in maintaining telomere stability, which is pivotal for genomic stability.

Signs and Symptoms

Premature aging only affects certain types of tissues in each syndrome.

Among the typical signs of premature aging in progeria syndromes is the premature onset of the following symptoms or disorders:

- Graying/loss of hair
- Hearing loss
- Cataract
- Scleroderma-like skin changes
- Type 2 diabetes mellitus
- Osteoporosis
- Atherosclerosis and coronary heart disease

- Various malignant tumors

Hutchinson-Gilford progeria syndrome is a systemic disorder that affects the majority of the organs of the body including the skin, bone, skeletal muscle, adipose tissues, heart, and large and small arteries. The children affected start exhibiting the symptoms of the disease at the age of 1–2.

Patients with Werner syndrome develop skin ulcers, cataracts, graying or even loss of their hair, and hypogonadism. The loss of subcutaneous fat and dermal atrophy produces a scleroderma-like appearance. Werner syndrome patients are at an increased risk of tumor formation, with up to 10% of patients developing a malignancy.

Classification

More than 100 syndromes with clinical sign(s) of premature aging have so far been described in the scientific literature, but only in recent years the genetic defects causing these syndromes have been identified. The list of the most prominent progeria syndromes includes:

Congenital progeroid syndromes

- Laminopathies
- Hutchinson-Gilford progeria syndrome (commonly called progeria)
- Restrictive dermopathy
- Mandibuloacral dysplasia
- LEMD2-associated progeroid syndrome
- Atypical Werner syndrome (atypical progeroid syndrome)

Other progeroid syndromes

- Wiedemann-Rautenstrauch syndrome (neonatal progeroid syndrome)
- CAV1-associated neonatal progeroid syndrome
- PYCR1-related cutis laxa syndrome

Juvenile/adult progeroid syndromes

- Werner syndrome (adult progeria)
- Myotonic dystrophy type 1
- Cockayne syndrome
- Néstor-Guillermo syndrome
- Ruijs-Aalfs syndrome
- Lessel-Kubisch syndrome (MDM2-associated progeroid syndrome)

Laboratory and Other Workups

Patients diagnosed with Werner syndrome should undergo regular screening tests for hyperlipidemia, breast and colorectal cancer, diabetes, and thyroid abnormalities. Given the number of musculoskeletal abnormalities and high prevalence of soft tissue sarcomas in Werner syndrome patients, clinicians should perform an X-ray, CT, or MRI studies in the appropriate clinical scenario to evaluate for underlying disorders, infections, or tumors thoroughly. DEXA (specific scans for osteoporosis) scans should also be performed regularly to evaluate and monitor osteoporosis.

Dermatopathology

Skin biopsies from patients carrying *LMNA* or *ZMPSTE24* mutations reveal increased nuclear size and an atrophic epidermis with focal hyperkeratosis and hypoplastic sebaceous glands.

Course

- Hutchinson-Gilford progeria syndrome is characterized by accelerated aging in affected children leading to premature death at an average age of 14.5 years due to cardiovascular complications.
- Werner syndrome patients appear unaffected at birth and develop normally until the adolescent period or second decade of life when, they start to exhibit signs and symptoms of accelerated aging. Werner syndrome patients typically live into the fifth decade of life. Patients usually die of malignancy or cardiovascular disease.

Complications

Werner syndrome patients develop characteristic physical and metabolic abnormalities that result in severe complications more commonly seen in the elderly, including diabetes, hypertension, osteoporosis, myocardial infarction, stroke, and cancer. Caution should be exercised with Werner syndrome patients and chemotherapy treatments. They are at an increased risk of chemotoxicity due to their impaired ability in DNA repair mechanisms.

Diagnosis

Classic Hutchinson-Gilford progeria syndrome is identified on the basis of clinical symptoms and the medical history of the patient. Also, its presence can be confirmed by genetic testing for the mutation (c.1824C>T) in the lamin A gene. However, there is no kit available for its early detection.

Werner syndrome: Genetic testing through nuclear sequencing by reverse transcription-polymerase chain reaction (PCR) with western blot protein analysis can confirm the diagnosis of Werner syndrome. Prenatal testing with amniocentesis and chorionic villus sampling can be performed in patients at high risk for having infants with this disorder.

Differential Diagnosis

All syndromes: Normal aging, hormonal deficiencies, metabolic disturbances (internal diseases)

Werner syndrome: systemic sclerosis, dermatomyositis, and other premature aging syndromes

Prevention and Therapy

Hutchinson-Gilford progeria syndrome: No cure has been found. In several clinical studies, lonafarnib, a farnesyl transferase inhibitor, demonstrated remarkable improvement in weight gain, vascular architecture, and bone structure along with a decreased frequency of headaches and strokes and improvement in the life span.

Werner syndrome: Treatment is aimed at symptomatic relief and control of the secondary organ dysfunction. Treatment of atherosclerosis, hypertension, diabetes, and other diseases is achieved through standard conventional monitoring and medical therapy, but the disorder will continue to progress. Bosentan, an endothelin receptor antagonist, can be used to treat severe cutaneous ulcers. Sodium etidronate can help improve symptomatic calcifications in the soft tissue. Orthotics can be used to manage complications with feet deformities. Cataracts should be managed surgically. Sarcopenia can be treated with diets rich in branched amino acids, exercise, vitamin D supplementation, and hormone therapy, although this is controversial given the increased risk of malignancy.

Special

This group of progeria syndromes should be diagnosed and managed in special centers for orphan diseases and having special interest and expertise in certain types of these rare diseases.

Nutrition Disorders of the Skin [12]

Grading of Importance

B

Level

Advanced

ICD

EB9Y/5C3Y

Synonyms

Skin nutrition deficiency

Definition

Skin disorders which include dermatoses resulting either from disturbed metabolic processes or from defective nutrition.

Epidemiology

Nutritional deficiency is a global problem not only in developing countries. It belongs to the large group of noncommunicable diseases (NCDs), which tend to have of long duration and are the result of a combination of genetic, physiological, environmental, and behavioral factors:

- In developing countries, nutritional deficiency mainly results from insufficient food supply.
- In industrialized countries alcoholism, gastrointestinal disorders and unhealthy and long-lasting diets, including anorexia nervosa, are the main drivers of nutritional deficiencies.
- Higher risk groups include infants, pregnant women, alcoholics, vegetarians, and patients on dialysis, on certain medications, or with a history of malabsorption or gastrointestinal surgery.
- Poverty and low socioeconomic status are closely linked with nutritional deficiency.

Etiology and Pathogenesis and Symptoms

Disorders of essential deficient supply of minerals of trace elements and/or vitamins or their metabolism affecting the skin. Early clinical signs of nutrition deficiency are often visible at the skin, nails, and/or hairs first. Although some signs are characteristic for a specific nutrient deficiency, often an overlap of skin manifestations is observed in multiple deficiency states.

Vitamin Deficiencies

Vitamin A is major factor in the maintenance of epithelial tissues. Deficiency occurs mainly from an inadequate intake, liver disorders, and fat malabsorption. Disturbed keratinization of epidermis and follicles. Phrynoderma is a maximal clinical feature with follicular plugging.

Vitamin B3 (niacin) deficiency (pellagra) arises most commonly in areas where corn is a substantial part of the food intake. Cutaneous manifestations of pellagra include dermatitis, sunlight sensitivity, and hair loss. Supplementation with niacin has a UV light damage protective effect.

Vitamin B6 (pyridoxine) plays a key role as a cofactor in many enzymatic reactions in different metabolic pathways. In the skin, vitamin B6 deficiency leads to seborrheic dermatitis-like eruptions, angular cheilitis, anemia, and atrophic glossitis.

Vitamin B12 (cyanocobalamin) is involved in many metabolic pathways especially the development of red blood cells and function of the nervous system. Vitamin B12 deficiency has become an increasing problem in people having a strict vegan diet without supplemental vitamin B12 in Europe.

Vitamin C (ascorbic acid) is one of the major anti-oxidative factors and plays an important role in collagen synthesis. Skin manifestations of vitamin C deficiency includes rough skin, follicular hyperkeratosis, perifollicular hemorrhage, petechial bleeding, coiled hair, and impaired wound healing. Scurvy represents the extreme of the disease manifestation.

Vitamin D and its active metabolite 1,25(OH)2D3 are decreased when insufficient UVB exposure occurs. Skin types 5 and 6 living in northern European latitudes risk inadequate sun exposure for conversion of 7-dehydrocholesterol in the epidermis. Some evidence exists for low D3 levels aggravating skin aging and xerosis of the skin.

Vitamin H (Biotin) as a coenzyme of carboxylases and acting in signal transduction can be reduced in pregnancy, long-term parenteral nutrition and biotinidase deficiency. Hair loss, brittle nails, periorificial dermatitis of mouth, nostrils, anus, or vulva may appear.

Trace Elements Deficiency

Iron deficiency resulting from reduced delivery via iron-containing food (meat, vegetables) can lead to pale skin due to anemia and via reduced oxygen supply causing disturbed skin, hair, and nail growth (brittle nails). Itchy skin can be another symptom.

Selenium is present in various selenoproteins, including phospholipid hydroperoxide glutathione peroxidase (PHGPx) and thioredoxin reductase (TDR). TDR is associated with keratinocyte cell membranes, and its levels appear to correlate with susceptibility to UVB-induced damage (oxygen radical scavenger). Enzymes that convert the thyroid hormone thyroxine (T4) to triiodothyronine (T3) are selenium-dependent. Hair loss and some skin immune functions result from deficiency.

Zinc deficiency most commonly results from an inadequate dietary intake and imbalanced parenteral nutrition but also from a reduced absorption or increased loss. It is important for protein synthesis and plays a role in wound healing and mucosal barrier. It is needed for constructing keratin and for the formation of structural protein (collagen). In acrodermatitis enteropathica, zinc cannot be absorbed and once breast-feeding stops; erosive inflammatory skin with elevated desquamative margins at the anogenital area, fingers, feet, and perioral area may occur.

Localization

See symptoms.

Classification

Vitamins, trace elements, and combinations.

Laboratory and Other Workups

Laboratory analysis of blood and urine vitamin and trace element levels can be misleading because of the poor correlation with tissue vitamin concentrations. Sometimes genetic counseling because of rare enzymatic deficiency disorders become necessary.

Dermatopathology

Depending on the individual nutritional disorder and symptoms

Course

Depending on type of vitamin or trace elements either alone or in combination

Complications

Depending on severity of malnutrition. The most severe form of protein-energy malnutrition (PEM) is Kwashiorkor. Skin lesions usually first occur where friction or pressure takes place (groin, knees, buttocks, and elbows). In advanced cases, the dermatosis may be almost anywhere on the body. Darkly pigmented patches with desquamation and features like old painting paper are seen.

Diagnosis

Mucocutaneous changes. Difficult in early stages.

Differential diagnosis

Nutritional deficiency disorders of the skin can mimic several dermatoses.

Prevention and Therapy

Individual oral or parenteral supplementation depending on the type of deficiency. Whereas substitution of water-soluble vitamins is without problems, the treatment with fat-soluble vitamins (E-D-K-A) and zinc or selenium should be carefully controlled because of the risk of over-dosage.

Disorders with Primary and Secondary Deposition in the Skin [20, 21]

Grading of Importance

C

Level

Basic

ICD-11

5D00.Z

Synonyms

Amyloidosis, mucinosis, myxoedema, hyalinosis, xanthoma/xanthelasma, gout/hyperuricemia, calciphylaxis, tattoo

Epidemiology

These are rare diseases. AL amyloidosis occurs in about 3–13 per million people per year.

Definition

Disorders with primary and secondary deposition in the skin are a heterogenous group of diseases, characterized by the pathological accumulation of materials in the extracellular matrix of the dermis or subcutis.

Etiology and Pathogenesis

Primary localized cutaneous amyloidosis: idiopathic or mutations in the OSMR or IL31RA gene

Secondary (AL) amyloidosis: light chain deposits that are produced by malignant plasma cells

Mucinosis: thyroid disorders (myxoedema), lymphomas, inflammatory skin diseases

Uric acid deposits (gout): idiopathic or linked to food excess

Calciphylaxis: terminal chronic renal deficiency

Skin calcinosis: connective tissue diseases

Tattoos: trauma, voluntary intradermal pigment injection, or deposition of dust and burned substances

Signs and Symptoms

Primary localized cutaneous amyloidosis: severely itchy patches of thickened, scaly, and reddish-brown skin with multiple small bumps (lichen amyloidosis) or flat and dark brown patches (macular amyloidosis).

Secondary (AL) amyloidosis – vessel fragility with pinch purpura and periorbital purpura, unexplained bleeding or macroglossia.

Mucinosis – flat, shiny erythematous plaques.

Myxoedema – skin-colored flexible plaques, "orange peel" surface, pretibial location frequently, rarely hyperkeratosis.

Xanthoma/xanthelasma – small yellowish soft nodules, grouped.

Connective tissue disorders-associated calcinosis – rock hard subcutaneous nodules that may fistulate.

Calciphylaxis – skin necrosis with accompanying erythematous network like maculae (livedo), extremely painful.

Pathological tattoos – black, grey or brown macules of millimetric size, localized.

Localization

Primary localized cutaneous amyloidosis – lichen amyloidosis: extensor faces of the limbs, and macular amyloidosis: often interscapular.

Secondary (AL) amyloidosis – periorbital or at skin sites exposed to wear and tear/physical trauma.

Mucinosis – depends on the etiology.

Myxoedema – frequently pretibial.

Xanthelasma – periorbital.

Xanthoma – frequently over pressure points.

Calciphylaxis – fatty areas of the body (abdomen, flanks, buttocks, thighs, breasts in women); lower legs.

Tattoos – anywhere.

Gout – hallux (also called podagra) or fingers (also called tophus).

Laboratory and Other Workups

Secondary amyloidosis – blood count, serum electrophoresis and immunofixation, kappa/lambda light chain measurement in blood, eventually bone marrow aspiration

Myxoedema – thyroid hormones

Xanthoma/xanthelasma – lipid profile

Calciphylaxis – calcium, albumin, blood count, renal function

Dermatopathology

Amyloidosis: Congo red stain shows a green birefringence.

Gout: crystal depositions.

Xanthoma and xanthelasma: lipid deposits.

Mucinosis and myxoedema: mucopolysaccharides.

Course

Slow progression followed by a stabilization. The treatment remains difficult in most depositional skin disorders.

Complications

Progression if the underlying disease is not treated.

Diagnosis

Clinical and histological

Differential Diagnosis

All forms of depositional disorders

Prevention and Therapy

Treatment of the underlying disease

Tropical Dermatoses and Travel Medicine [4]

Grading of Importance

B

Level

Advanced

Synonyms

Tropical skin diseases

Epidemiology

Dermatologic and venerologic diseases that are acquired in tropical or subtropical regions.

In nontropical countries most patients diagnosed are immigrants or travellers.

Up to 50% of the local population in the tropics may be affected by skin diseases. Variable incidence and prevalence depend on disease and region. The majority are infections or infestations.

Skin diseases may affect up to 8% of travellers returning from tropical or subtropical climate regions. Frequently common dermatoses such as eczema, acne, psoriasis, or a preexisting skin infection may exacerbate.

Definition

Tropical skin diseases are transmissible or non-transmissible cutaneous diseases that occur principally in tropical and sub-tropical regions.

(Traveler's) Tropical skin diseases: Skin diseases present in travelers, returning from tropical areas.

Relatively rare infections with high impact on the healthcare in tropical and subtropical developing regions of the world are referred to as "neglected tropical diseases (NTDs)." The World Health Organization has focused on a strategy of integrating preventative, investigative, curative, and supportive care for NTDs.

Etiology and Pathogenesis

A significant burden is caused by bacteria, fungi, parasites, protozoa, helminths, and arthropods. Other skin diseases in these areas may be due to environmental (such as heat, humidity, and altitude) and nutritional conditions.

Specific and common tropical skin diseases include:

Infectious disorders

- Fungal infections: Mycetoma, deep fungal infections, dermatophytoses
- Bacterial infections: Staphylococcus aureus, Group A streptococcal infections
- Viral Infections: Yellow fever, Zika disease, dengue, chikungunya
- Treponematosis: Yaws
- Mycobacterial disorders: Leprosy, Buruli ulcer, cutaneous tuberculosis, atypical mycobacteria infections
- Protozoan disorders: Leishmaniasis, trypanosomiasis
- Parasitic diseases: Schistosomiasis, strongyloidiasis, onchocerciasis, tapeworm, trichuriasis, filariasis, tungiasis, scabies, larva migrans
- STI (sexually transmitted infections): HIV infection, chancroid, lymphogranuloma venereum

Noninfectious disorders:

- Insect bite reactions, arthropods, jellyfish

Signs and Symptoms

A wide spectrum of clinical manifestations depending on the etiology. Tropical dermatoses may show some distinctive clinical patterns:

- Cutaneous rashes associated with fever
- Itchy rashes
- Migratory rashes
- Nodular lesions
- Muco-cutaneous ulcers
- Persistent edema of the extremities
- Papular eruptions, maculo-plaques
- Eschars

The lesions may cause pruritus, loss of sensation (hypoesthesia or anesthesia), or changes of the skin pigmentation (hypo- or hyperpigmentation).

Common dermatoses occurring worldwide may show in tropical countries different clinical presentations (e.g., acne, eczema, tinea, insect bites).

Localization

Variable. Localized lesions or generalized eruptions. The lesions often develop on exposed areas (preferentially face, extremities).

Laboratory and Other Workups

Complete blood cell count. Presence of peripheral blood eosinophilia. Complete biochemical survey. Specific serologies in selected cases. Parasitological studies (blood, smears, skin, and stools).

Dermatopathology

Identification (visualization) of the responsible agent. Conventional histology. Specific stains besides HE, i.e., Giemsa, PAS, Fite-Faraco, specific antibody stains (e.g., mycobacterial).

Course

Variable depending on the etiology

Complications

Variable depending on the etiology

Diagnosis

History of travel activities; exposure to fresh or sea water, animals, arthropods, plants, history of previous trauma

Past medical history: Immune status of the host, vaccinations, drugs and prophylaxis

Depending on the clinical context: histopathological evaluation (cutaneous biopsy), bacilloscopy (leprosy), microbiological cultures (swabs and/or skin biopsies); special stains; serology, PCR

Prevention and Therapy

Prevention: Pre-travel counseling; know the local threats. Recommended vaccination for specific tropical infections. Proper clothing, shoes, insect repellents, insecticides, barrier measures, bed netting. Avoiding contaminated water or eating raw or undercooked food.

References

1. Antonov D, Kamarashev J, Kazandjieva J, Neykova T, Tsankov N (2020) The rash that becomes purpuric, petechial, hemorrhagic, or ecchymotic. Clin Dermatol 38(1):3–18
2. Bechtel MA, Plotner A (2015) Dermatoses of pregnancy. Clin Obstet Gynecol 58(1):104–111
3. Burtner CR, Kennedy BK (2010) Progeria syndromes and ageing: what is the connection? Nat Rev Mol Cell Biol 11(8):567–578
4. Cunha PR, Flora TB, Kroumpouzos G (2019) Travelers' tropical skin diseases: challenges and interventions. Dermatol Ther 32(4):e12665
5. Davis MDP, van der Hilst JCH (2018) Mimickers of urticaria: urticarial vasculitis and autoinflammatory diseases. J Allergy Clin Immunol Pract 6(4):1162–1170
6. Dessinioti C, Antoniou C (2017) The "red face": not always rosacea. Clin Dermatol 35(2):201–206
7. Ikizoglu G (2014) Red face revisited: flushing. Clin Dermatol 32(6):800–808
8. Inamadar AC, Ragunatha S (2019) The rash that becomes an erythroderma. Clin Dermatol 37(2):88–98
9. Kroumpouzos G, Cohen LM (2003) Specific dermatoses of pregnancy: an evidence-based systematic review. Am J Obstet Gynecol 188(4):1083–1092
10. Lee H, Hong Y, Kim M (2021) Structural and functional changes and possible molecular mechanisms in aged skin. Int J Mol Sci 22:12489
11. Lehrhoff S, Pomeranz MK (2013) Specific dermatoses of pregnancy and their treatment. Dermatol Ther 26(4):274–284
12. Maarouf M, Platto JF, Shi VY (2019) The role of nutrition in inflammatory pilosebaceous disorders: implication of the skin-gut axis. Australas J Dermatol 60(2):e90–e98
13. Moniaga CS, Tominaga M, Takamori K (2020) Mechanisms and management of Itch in dry skin. Acta Derm Venereol 100(2):adv00024
14. Nowak DA, Yeung J (2017) Diagnosis and treatment of pruritus. Can Fam Physician 63(12):918–924
15. Paulus S, Kirchmayr K (2022) The swollen leg. MMW Fortschr Med 164(17):43–47
16. Proksch E, Berardesca E, Misery L, Engblom J, Bouwstra J (2020) Dry skin management: practical approach in light of latest research on skin structure and function. J Dermatolog Treat 31(7):716–722
17. Reilly DT, Wolfe JH (1991) ABC of vascular diseases. The swollen leg. BMJ 303(6815):1462–1465
18. Rothe MJ, Bialy TL, Grant-Kels JM (2000) Erythroderma. Dermatol Clin 18(3):405–415
19. Schoch JJ, Monir RL, Satcher KG, Harris J, Triplett E, Neu J (2019) The infantile cutaneous microbiome: a review. Pediatr Dermatol 36(5):574–580
20. Touart DM, Sau P (1998a) Cutaneous deposition diseases. Part I. J Am Acad Dermatol 39(2 Pt 1):149–171. quiz 172–144.
21. Touart DM, Sau P (1998b) Cutaneous deposition diseases. Part II. J Am Acad Dermatol 39(4 Pt 1):527–544. quiz 545–526.
22. Visscher MO, Adam R, Brink S, Odio M (2015) Newborn infant skin: physiology, development, and care. Clin Dermatol 33(3):271–280

Part IX

General Dermatology

General dermatology covers basic functions of the skin and diagnostic and therapeutic procedures, which also are mentioned more specifically in conjunction with the respected chapters.

Basic Functions of the Skin

26

Harald Gollnick, Martine Bagot, Adele De Masson, Gabor Dobos, Evelyn Gaffal, and Christos C. Zouboulis

Contents

H. Gollnick (✉)
Department of Dermatology & Venereology, Otto-von-Guericke University, Magdeburg, Germany
e-mail: Harald.Gollnick@med.ovgu.de

M. Bagot
Service de Dermatologie, Université Paris Cité, Hôpital Saint-Louis, Paris, France
e-mail: martine.bagot@gmail.com

A. De Masson · G. Dobos
Dermatology and Venereology, Hopital Saint Louis, Université de Paris, Paris, France
e-mail: adele.demasson@aphp.fr; gabor.dobos@charite.de

E. Gaffal
Department of Dermatology, University of Lübeck, Lübeck, Germany
e-mail: evelyn.gaffal@med.ovgu.de

C. C. Zouboulis
Departments of Dermatology, Venereology, Allergology and Immunology, Staedtisches Klinikum Dessau, Brandenburg Medical School Theodor Fontane and Faculty of Health Sciences Brandenburg, Dessau, Germany
e-mail: christos.zouboulis@mhb-fontane.de

H. Gollnick et al. (eds.), *Dermatology Cyberderm WebBook*,
https://doi.org/10.1007/978-3-031-78491-0_26

Test your learning and check your understanding of this book's contents: use the "Springer Nature Flashcards" app to access questions using ▶ https://sn.pub/1rhh6k.
To use the app, please follow the instructions in Chap. 1.

Cutaneous Anatomy and Physiology [5, 9, 10]

Grading of Importance

No grading

Level

basic

Anatomy

Three layers: the epidermis, the dermis and the subcutis with fascia.

Epidermis: germinative pool of keratinocytes (KC) and differentiating KCs. Substructured into the basal membrane, stratum basale (dividing stem cells), stratum spinosum, stratum granulosum, and stratum corneum. Dendritic cells: Melanocytes, Langerhans cells, and Merkel cells.

Dermis: fibroblasts producing a rich extracellular matrix (collagen and elastic fibers), adnexal structure with associated muscles, dermal dendritic cells, mast cells, Merkel cells, upper and lower vessel pool, apocrine and eccrine glands, and different nerve types.

Subcutis: connective tissue and adipose tissue including vessels and immune surveillance cells. Fascia.

Skin glands: Eccrine sweat glands (palms and soles), apocrine sweat glands (axillae, areola and nipples, perianal region, and genitalia) produce the sweat; sebaceous gland follicles, hair follicles with terminal hair, and vellus hair follicles.

Thermal Regulation

Skin vasculature plays a key role in thermal regulation. Glomus cells help to regulate the diameter of the vessels so that the higher or lower amount of blood can heat or cool down the skin. The eccrine glands produce sweat when stimulated by cholinergic nerves (stress reaction, temperature cooling down the skin), which cools the skin physically by evaporation. An anchoring muscle of the hair follicle (musculus arrector pili) can produce some heat by moving the follicle upward.

Physical Protection

Epidermis (especially the stratum corneum): provides protection from evaporation of water and physical stress.

Dermis: protects the skin against tears and shear forces and provides elasticity.

Subcutis: fat tissue can absorb and distribute physical harm.

Protection Against Chemical Injury

Stratum corneum: corneocytes (keratinocyte envelopes) and sebum help the skin to resist various kinds of chemical injuries and water.

Photoprotection

Melanocytes produce melanin and transfer them in vesicles to the surrounding keratinocytes. Melanin absorbs ultraviolet (UV)-radiation and thereby protect genetic material. KCs produce Radical Oxygen Species (ROS) absorbers and repair enzymes against DNA damage.

Sensory Function

The skin is one of the most important sensory organs: nerves and receptors such as nociceptors (pain and itch receptors) and Merkel cells (mechanoreceptors) are responsible for the touch.

Immune Function

Epidermis: Langerhans cells (antigen-presenting cells); keratinocytes (epithelial cells with immune properties), dendritic epidermal T lymphocytes, resident memory T cells that may serve as a primitive T-cell immune surveillance system; and immunogenic melanocytes. Dermis: most of the lymphocytes in the skin, other leukocytes, dermal dendritic cells, mast cells, and macrophages.

Subcutis: immune surveillance reservoir and progenitor cells for wound healing.

Cutaneous Biochemistry [3, 11]

Grading of Importance

No grading

Level

Basic

Biochemistry of the Epidermis

Keratin Intermediate Filament (KIF) Keratinocytes contain KIF that are fashioned into filament collections (tonofilaments) to construct the cytoskeleton. The different epidermal layers contain varying amounts of keratin (K), ranging from 30% in the stratum basale to 80% in the stratum corneum. Ks occur in acidic (type I) neutral/basic (type II) pairs with more important among them:

- K5 and K14, associated with normal cell proliferation
- K6 and K16, associated with hyperproliferation in the epidermis
- K1 and K10 as well as K2 and K11 indicative of terminal keratinocyte differentiation (maturation).
- Some Ks such as K7 or K20 stain-specific cells like Merkel cells or other benign clear cells or tumor cells (extramammary Paget's disease).

Keratinocyte differentiation: Major proteins involved in keratinocyte differentiation include involucrin, transglutaminase (TGase) and integrins, which lead to keratinocyte detachment from the basement membrane and interruption of proliferation. The transition of keratinocytes from the stratum spinosum to stratum granulosum is mediated by protein kinase C and the induction of the late differentiation markers loricrin and profilaggrin. Stratum granulosum keratinocytes contain protein- and lipid-rich granules (keratohyalin granules). Profilaggrin-containing granules mature to filaggrin (Odland granules), which contain lipids that form the sheets of the epidermal permeability barrier (EPB). EPB function in human epidermis depends on TGase-mediated cross-linking of structural proteins and lipids during the terminal stages of keratinocyte differentiation. Several mutations in genes that encode for the EPB structural components can result in skin diseases.

EPB quality also depends on the presence of epidermal lipids, whereas abnormalities in the following lipids induced disease:

- Ceramides, dominant in atopic dermatitis
- Cholesterol (50% of stratum corneum lipids), dominant in aged and photoaged skin
- Free fatty acids, dominant in psoriasis

EPB repair may be initiated by loss of its regulators Ca^{2+} and K^{+}. There is a fourfold increase in extracellular Ca^{2+} from basal layer to stratum corneum.

Topical application of solvents to the skin removes lipids from the stratum corneum and increases trans-epidermal water loss (TEWL) (please also see chapters aging skin, dry skin, infantile skin), followed by induction of a rapid barrier repair through epidermal metabolic changes.

Skin fatty acids: The permeability of human skin is largely based on the quality and quantity of the lamellar lipids packed between corneocytes and forming the cornified envelope. Both the epidermal cell membranes and the corneocyte layers contain endogenous fatty acids.

Modification of skin fatty acids can lead to disease, like atopic dermatitis. Photoaged and intrinsically aged epidermis exhibit abnormal EPB homeostasis.

Epidermal fatty acids can also derive from the diet. Diet fatty acids (polyunsaturated fatty acids (PUFA)) can be actively metabolized by the skin. PUFA-deficient diets (e.g., linoleic acid) can result in both increased TEWL and scaly skin.

Skin absorption of xenobiotics: Xenobiotics are chemical substances foreign to the biological system (natural compounds, drugs, environmental agents), which can be transported across the stratum corneum in a controlled manner based on their physicochemical traits (partition, diffusion, and solubility). The skin is constantly exposed to xenobiotics by occupational, environmental, therapeutic, and systemic exposure.

Skin-own metabolizing enzymes, like cytochrome P450 (CYP), are involved in their percutaneous penetration. Especially relevant to the skin is the role of CYPs in mediating photosensitivity and reactions to drugs.

Keratinocyte differentiation can be modulated by hormones (thyroid hormone and steroid hormones), vitamins (vitamin D3, retinoic acid, vitamin A/retinol from diet), and electrolytes (mostly calcium and potassium).

Defensins: refer to the chapter on Microbiology and Immunology.

Biochemistry of the Dermis: The main cell type of the dermis is the fibroblast that produces and degrades *extracellular matrix (ECM)* components.

Collagens are the principal ECM component (90% of total dermal proteins), accounting for about 75% of skin total dry weight. At least 25 collagens exist, half are present in skin:

- Collagen type I (85–90%).
- Collagen type III (8–11%.
- Collagen type V (2–4%).
- Collagen type VII forms part of the so-called anchoring fibrils that attach the basement membrane to the ECM of the upper dermis.
- Collagen type XVII contributes to the so-called anchoring filaments that link the basal keratinocytes with the basement membrane.

Collagen abnormalities lead to several scarring or fibrotic diseases, such as congenital bullous diseases, scleroderma, and collagenoma.

Collagen biosynthesis involves the synthesis of procollagen polypeptides followed by both their intracellular and extracellular processing to generate a mature and functional collagen fiber.

Elasticity of skin: The other major ECM fibrous protein is elastin, which is produced by fibroblasts and provides the skin with its elasticity. Elastin is stretchable by more than its full resting length. Elastin is included in an amorphous portion. Elastin changes lead to both genetic and acquired diseases of the skin (cutis laxa and actinic elastosis).

Extrafibrillar matrix: Extrafibrillar matrix, the dermal material lying outside the cells, not consisting of either collagen or elastic fibers, is an amorphous and hydroscopic material consisting of proteoglycans, glycoproteins, water, and hyaluronic acid (mucopolysaccharidosis).

Biochemistry of Adnexal Structures

Eccrine sweat glands: They produce a watery perspiration that serves principally to cool and maintain the body core temperature at 37.5 °C. At maximal output the eccrine glands of an adult human can be up to 2–4 liters per hour or 10–14 liters per day (10–15 g/min·m^2) but is less in children prior to puberty). Eccrine gland activity with secretory and dark cells is regulated through neural stimulation using sympathetic nerve fibers distributed around the gland (neurotransmitter: acetylcholine). Sweat produced by clear cells is a clear, odor-free, colorless, slightly acidic fluid that consists of water (99.0–99.5%); the electrolytes NaCl, K^+ and $HCO3^-$; and lactate, urea, ammonia, calcium, and heavy metals. The dark cells produce macromolecules mixed with the sweat. There are significant regional variations in the composition of sweat, which also is modulated by psycho-emotional and environmental factors.

Apocrine sweat glands: They secrete their sterile, odor-free, weakly acidic product via exocytosis from secretory cells. Its viscous, milky consistency is due to its high content of lipids (fatty acids, cholesterol, squalene, triglycerides), androgens, ammonia, sugars, and Fe^{2+}. Some of these are odoriferous, especially so after their decomposition on the skin surface by bacteria. Myoepithelial cells are arranged spirally along the tubule.

Sebaceous glands: Their product, sebum, is released after sebocytes burst by DNA degradation (holocrine secretion by programmed cell death). There is a remarkable variation in the composition of sebum through human life, and human sebum is unique, with no similarity to other species. Human sebaceous glands not only produce sebum but also regulate steroidogenesis and local androgen synthesis and contribute to skin barrier function, interaction with neuropeptides, potential production of both anti- and pro-inflammatory compounds, and synthesis of antimicrobial lipids (sapienate, oleic acid).

The sebaceous gland contains all enzymes needed for transformation of cholesterol to steroids. Moreover, it expresses beside others the 5α-reductase isoenzymes, needed for the intracellular conversion of testosterone, or even the adrenal androgen dehydroepiandrosterone directly, to the more potent 5α-dihydrotestosterone. Sebaceous glands are part of the skin neuroendocrine system as they produce and release corticotropin-releasing hormone in response to systemic or local stress. Abnormal sebaceous gland function leads to several skin diseases: the most common among them is acne.

Sebum is a yellowish viscous fluid containing lipids, such as triglycerides, free sterols and sterol esters, squalene, wax and free fatty acids, and cell debris.

Hair follicle: Hair fiber growth occurs in a highly time-resolved manner. Glucose (and glutamine) is the principal energy source. The hair follicle can react to most hormones of the human body. Hair follicles in different regions of the body respond differently to androgens. Drug-induced inhibition of the testosterone-metabolizing enzyme to 5α-dihydrotestosterone 5α-reductase type II induces hair regrowth in some balding men.

The hair fiber includes "hard" K, water, lipids, pigment, and trace elements (in order of decreasing amount). Neither the chemical composition of hair proteins nor its amino acid composition shows any difference between different ethnicities.

Hair fibers have a coating of long-chain fatty acids bonded covalently to the protein membrane of the epicuticle (which may be interrupted in disease processes such as Netherton syndrome, ectodermal dysplasia, dystrophic hairs, atopic hair, brittle hair).

Nails: Corneocytes of the nail plate (onychocytes) are also filled with K filaments. Low-sulfur K form α-helical filaments running parallel to the nail surface and are embedded in a non-K matrix of high sulfur, glycine, and tyrosine proteins. Up to 90% of nail Ks are of the hard "hair" K type. Water, lipids, and trace elements including iron, zinc, and calcium are present in the nail plate. The nail low lipid content contributes to their 1000-fold greater water permeability than the epidermis. Exogenous factors, dissolving lipids out of the nail plate lead to brittle nails, onychodystrophy, and superinfection.

Skin Endocrinology

Vitamin D production: Vitamin D3 (cholecalciferol) belongs to the group of fat-soluble secosteroids, which has an important impact in the intestinal absorption of calcium, magnesium, and phosphate. Besides oral ingestion it is photochemically induced in the epidermis through UVB radiation (290–315 nm). Sun exposure to face, arms, and legs for 30 minutes twice per week, or approximately 25% minimal erythema dose (MED) is enough to transform 7-dehydrocholesterol into cholecalciferol (vitamin D3).

Steroidogenesis and neurohormones: Skin and its appendages respond to central hormone regulation but also act as a neuroendocrine organ in a manner largely independent of body central control systems. It includes the production of corticotropin-releasing hormone and downstream proopiomelanocortin peptides.

Pigmentation of skin and hair follicle: Despite the variations in skin and hair color, skin and hair pigmentation is derived from the pigment melanin, synthesized via a phylogenetically ancient biochemical process termed melanogenesis. Synthesis occurs within melanosomes, which are specialized organelles unique to highly dendritic, neural crest-derived, cells called melanocytes.

Melanogenesis starts by the formation of melanosomes, whose size markedly differs between skin types, and continues through the biochemical pathway that converts L-tyrosine into melanin. Both processes are under complex genetic control.

Melanin is a family of polymorphous and multifunctional biopolymers that include:

- Eumelanin: brown-black melanin
- Pheomelanin: red/yellow melanin
- Mixed melanins (containing both eumelanin and pheomelanin)
- Neuromelanin

Both eumelanin and pheomelanin can be produced within the same melanocyte. Pheomelanins are photo-labile with photolysis products including superoxide, hydroxyl radicals, and hydrogen peroxide. Genetic and immunological abnormalities of melanin production can lead to significant diseases such as albinism and vitiligo, respectively.

The conversion of L-tyrosine to melanin follows three steps:

- Hydroxylation of L-phenylalanine/L-tyrosine to L-dihydroxy-phenylalanine (L-DOPA)
- Dehydrogenation/oxidation of L-DOPA to dopaquinone, which is the precursor for both eumelanin and pheomelanin and the limiting step in melanogenesis.
- Dehydrogenation of dihydroxyindole to yield melanin pigment.

The conversion of dopaquinone to leukodopachrome signals eumelanin production, while the addition of cysteine to dopaquinone to yield cysteinyl-DOPA occurs in pheomelanin production.

Cutaneous Immunology [6, 7]

Grading of Importance

No grading

Level

Basic

Introduction

In addition to being a physical barrier that protects the body against external insults, the skin also forms an immunological barrier which is crucial for host defense as well as tissue homeostasis. The cutaneous immune system contains a network of immune cells of the innate and adaptive immune system. Besides skin-resident immune cells, there is also a constant circulation of immune cells between the skin, lymph nodes, and blood stream. It is also referred to as skin associated lymphoid tissue (SALT).

Innate Immune Cells of the Skin

Several cells in the skin are part of the innate (nonspecific, native) immune system.

Keratinocytes

Keratinocytes are the prominent cell type of the epidermis. They form the outermost barrier against potential infection. Damage to the skin leads to the secretion of numerous cytokines and chemokines (e.g., TNF, IL1, CXCL2, CXCL10) by keratinocytes which activate local immune cells and endothelial cells, initiate antigen-specific immune responses, and recruit various immune cells into the skin including T cells and natural killer cells. In addition, keratinocytes secrete antimicrobial peptides (AMPs), such as beta-defensins and cathelicidin, which prevent the invasion of microbes by direct killing of pathogens and activation of the innate immune system. Keratinocytes recognize invading viruses, parasites, bacteria, and fungi in the skin through Toll-like (TLR) and nucleotide-binding oligomerization domain- (NOD)-like receptors.

Epidermal and Dermal Dendritic Cells

Epidermal dendritic cells (Langerhans cells) are important to maintain tissue homeostasis and immune tolerance. In the case of an insult, they can sense microbial antigens via Toll-like receptors. Langerhans cells process and present antigens to naïve T cells thereby inducing an antigen-specific immune response. Dermal dendritic cells are professional antigen-presenting cells (APC, plasmacytoid, and myeloid subtypes) that are also crucial for the induction of adaptive immune responses.

Mast Cells

Mast cells are mostly located in the dermis and around vessels and adnexal structures. They are of major importance for the induction and regulation of immune responses against various allergens as well as bacterial and parasitic infections. Mast cells express a variety of receptors on their surface including, e.g., FcεRI receptors for binding of IgE, Toll-like receptors, IL-4 and IL-5 receptors. Upon stimulation they release a plethora of immune-activating mediators including histamine, heparin, tryptase, or chymase. Consequences of mast cell activation are, e.g., pruritic wheals, vasodilatation, and edema.

Macrophages

Macrophages are the most abundant cell type of skin resident immune cells. They maintain and restore homeostasis of the skin by eliminating invading pathogens (phagocytosis), sometimes resulting in granuloma formation with multinucleated giant cells (sarcoidosis, foreign body granuloma, rheumatism, erythema nodosum). Activated macrophages present antigens to naïve T cells and release cytokines (TNFα, IL1β, IL-6) which further drive inflammation and attract neutrophils to the site of insult.

Eosinophils and Neutrophils

Upon the release of inflammatory cytokines and chemokines from, e.g., keratinocytes or macrophages, neutrophils and eosinophils are recruited to the site of inflammation. Neutrophils release neutrophil extracellular traps (NETs) to immobilize pathogens and directly phagocytose-invading microorganisms (NETosis). They also release chemo-attractants to recruit more neutrophils into the skin.

Eosinophils are of major importance in the defense against parasites. Eosinophilia of the skin is also a typical feature of atopic dermatitis. Besides pro-inflammatory mediators, they are also attracted to immunoglobulins such as IgE. Upon stimulation eosinophils release a wide range of immunomodulatory factors including more than 35 cytokines, growth factors, and chemokines and cytotoxic granules. Thereby they kill parasites and promote Th2 helper T-cell differentiation, recruited also in skin cancer.

Immune Cell Compartment of the Subcutaneous Adipose Tissue

Besides being a mechanical barrier, the subcutaneous white adipose tissue (SWAT) also acts as an immunological barrier. It contains mainly macrophages and T lymphocytes which help to secure tissue homeostasis and integrity.

Adaptive Immune Cells

The adaptive immune response takes longer to develop, and it is highly specific to particular pathogens. It includes both cell-mediated and humoral immunity.

CD8+ and CD4+ T Cells

Cell-mediated immunity is mediated by T cells. Antigen-presenting cells like dendritic cells or macrophages present foreign peptides to naïve T cells which then differentiate into cytotoxic CD8+ T cells or CD4+ T helper (Th) cells. These then antigen-specific T cells migrate into the skin to the site of inflammation, e.g., as seen with, allergic contact dermatitis.

Cytotoxic CD8+ T cells are of major importance in attacking virally infected cells or cancer cells.

CD4+ T helper cells are central for activating B cells thereby inducing humoral immunity. T helper cells can be subdivided in Th1, Th2, Th17, and Th22 cells, with every subtype having a specific cytokine profile and different role in skin immunity.

Th1 cells produce IFN-γ, activate, e.g., macrophages, and induce cell-mediated immune response to kill intracellular pathogens. They play a role in the course of psoriasis.

Th2 cells produce, e.g., IL-4, IL-5, IL-6, or IL-10, and activate B cells as well as eosinophils. They play a role in atopic eczema.

Th17 cells produce IL-17 and IL-22. They regulate bacterial and fungal infections. Th22 cells secrete pro-inflammatory mediators like IL-22 and TNFα. Th17 and Th22 cells are important in the pathogenesis of psoriasis.

Regulatory T Cells

Regulatory T cells (Tregs) are one of the largest immune cell subsets in skin. They play a critical role in regulating the inflammatory immune response, prevent autoimmunity, and support local tissue repair.

Memory T Cells

Memory T cells (TRM) circulate between skin and blood stream or reside in the skin (tissue resident TRM). They are important for mediating a long-lasting protective immunity. See also chapter Drug Reactions and Herpes-Induced Erythema Multiforme.

B Cells

B lymphocytes are central for humoral immunity. Upon activation through cytokines and stimulatory signals from T cells, they produce immunoglobulins that can bind to specific antigens. B cells also present antigens and produce pro- and anti-inflammatory cytokines themselves.

Cutaneous Microbiology [1, 2, 4, 8]

Grading of Importance

No grading

Level

Basic

Definition

Microbes of the skin belong to the microbial ecosystem of the body. The terms microbiota (micro-organisms) and microbiome (includes genetic material) are used interchangeably, despite some differences exist.

Development

The cutaneous microbiome encompasses the microbes that live in and on the skin, including bacteria, fungi, and viruses. It is dynamic, continuously evolving, and diversifying with age, environment (height, latitude, temperature, clothes, skin moisture, pH, sebum), personal hygiene, stress, nutrition status, culture, exposure to skin irritating or protecting agents, UV-light, antibiotics, and/or genetic and epigenetic factors (barrier function, innate and adaptive immune system).

Newborns

In contrast to adults, there are no anatomical differences in the microbiome of the skin in the newborn. However, the type of delivery has an impact on the composition of the microbiome:

- Natural delivery: mother's vaginal flora: predominantly *lactobacilli.*
- Delivery by Caesarean section: mother's skin flora: staphylococci, streptococci, corynebacteria, and cutibacteria.

3rd Week Up to the 3rd Month of Life

- Anatomic site-specific bacterial profiles but still different from adults before adolescence. Colonization interfollicular, intrafollicular, and acrosyringeal.
- Around the 6th week of life: *Staphylococcus* and *Corynebacterium.*
- *Around 1 month: Malassezia* colonization increased with age, becoming adult-like by 1 month of life.

Microbiome and Microbiota

An average healthy human body possesses 10 × 14 microorganisms, including bacteria, fungi, mites, and viruses—tenfold the number of human cells. A single square centimeter of the human skin can contain up to one billion microorganisms.

Immunology

Depending on commensal or pathogenic microbes living on the skin, the local and systemic immune response is different:

- Commensal microbes: homeostatic balance with the host.
- Pathogenic microbes: disruption of the cutaneous "eco-" system and induction of innate and adaptive defense mechanisms responding with pro- and anti-inflammatory mediators and activation of cells depending on the nature of the antigen.

Stress can modulate the composition of the microbiome.

An infection by intracellular pathogens initiates the development of T helper 1 (TH1) cells, whereas extracellular pathogens induce the differentiation of TH2 and TH17 subsets (atopic dermatitis, acne).

At the beginning of life in the late in utero status and after delivery, the vernix caseosa is a key player in the development of early cutaneous innate immunity.

Risk for Diseases

A dysbiosis (dysbacteriosis) occurs when the "healthy" microbiome is altered, for example, by overwashing, humidity, clothes, antimicrobials, and resulting in conditions like erythema toxicum neonatorum, superficial folliculitis, body or feet odor, atopic dermatitis, and acne.

Spectrum of Primary and Secondary Skin Diseases with Change of Microbiota (Examples)

In general, we differentiate primary infections of the skin, skin diseases which become secondary superinfected (impetiginized), and skin diseases in which changes of the microbiota aggravate the course of a disease.

Erythema Toxicum Neonatorum

Macular erythema, papules, and pustules in neonates, mostly self-limited. Most probably related to coccal microbes entering the opening of the follicle.

Superficial and Deep Folliculitis

Overgrowth of staphylococcal species in the acro- and infrainfundibulum of the follicle, showing superficial pustules, infiltrated lesions with papules, and finally abscesses leading to furuncle or carbuncle.

Impetigo Contagiosa

Mostly seen in the first decade of life. Staphylococcal and streptococcal are highly contagious infections, *Staphylococcus aureus* of the intrafollicular epidermis, streptococci of the interfollicular epidermis. For treatment topical disinfectants and antimicrobials are preferred instead of topical antibiotics.

Pityriasis Versicolor

This is a quite common worldwide to diagnose superficial infection with a *Malassezia furfur* species showing multiple asymptomatic scaly hyperpigmented (winter) or hypopigmented (summer) macules. Seborrheic dermatitis is triggered by *M. furfur*. Hot and humid environments, occlusive clothes, increased sweating, immunosuppression, malnutrition, and pregnancy, are precipitating factors. Wood (UVA) light examination for diagnosis.

Atopic Dermatitis (AD)

Barrier dysfunction and microbes contribute to the pathogenesis of AD. 70% of patients with AD are colonized with *Staphylococcus aureus* at lesional sites. Early exposure to *Staphylococcus* may reduce the development of AD (adaptive immune response). AD patients are more prone to suffer from herpes (eczema herpeticatum) or *Malassezia* infections.

Acne

Acne vulgaris originates in the pilosebaceous unit of the skin starting in (pre) puberty. Increased and modified sebum production, disturbance of follicular keratinocyte differentiation, and release of inflammatory mediators are the primary driving forces of acne. The second step in the pathogenic cascade is colonization of this unit by *Cutibacterium acnes*, a commensal bacterium followed by additional triggering of inflammation.

C. acnes produces numerous enzymes and proteinases incl. lipases that altogether alter the sebaceous lipid composition and contribute to the production and release of antimicrobial and immunomodulatory molecules.

Psoriasis

Psoriasis is characterized by hyper-proliferation of keratinocytes with increased desquamation and increased inflammation. The disturbed barrier function of psoriasis gives rise to an altered microbiome. Throat and nasal streptococcal infection have been shown to trigger initiation and exacerbation of psoriasis. Skin microbiota in psoriasis display a higher degree of diversity compared to healthy skin.

Laboratory and Other Workups

- Swaps, scarification (lepra), extraction of follicular material
- Cyanoacrylate stripes
- Wood light (*Malassezia*)
- Biopsy: mycobacteria, deep mycoses, parasites
- Serology, culture, PCR for further specification

References

1. Brüggemann H, Salar-Vidal L, Gollnick HPM, Lood R (2021) A Janus-Faced Bacterium: Host-Beneficial and -Detrimental Roles of Cutibacterium acnes. Front Microbiol 12:673845
2. Byrd AL, Belkaid Y, Segre JA (2018) The human skin microbiome. Nat Rev Microbiol 16(3):143–155
3. Elpa DP, Chiu HY, Wu SP, Urban PL (2021) Skin metabolomics. Trends Endocrinol Metab 32(2):66–75
4. Grice EA, Segre JA (2011) The skin microbiome. Nat Rev Microbiol 9(4):244–253
5. Jiang Y, Tsoi LC, Billi AC, Ward NL, Harms PW, Zeng C, Maverakis E, Kahlenberg JM, Gudjonsson JE (2020) Cytokinocytes: the diverse contribution of keratinocytes to immune responses in skin. JCI Insight. 5(20):e142067. https://doi.org/10.1172/jci.insight.142067. PMID: 33055429
6. Nguyen AV, Soulika AM (2019) The dynamics of the skin's immune system. Int J Mol Sci 20(8):1811
7. Richmond JM, Harris JE (2014) Immunology and skin in health and disease. Cold Spring Harb Perspect Med 4(12):a015339
8. Santiago-Rodriguez TM, Le François B, Macklaim JM, Doukhanine E, Hollister EB (2023) The skin microbiome: current techniques, challenges, and future directions. Microorganisms. 11(5):1222. https://doi.org/10.3390/microorganisms11051222. PMID: 37317196; PMCID: PMC10223452
9. Sun K-L, Liu W, Xiao-Man G, Min Y, Chang J-M A study of normal epidermal melanocyte distribution. Int J Dermatol Venereol 4(1):32–35. https://doi.org/10.1097/JD9.0000000000000125
10. Taylor SC (2002) Skin of color: biology, structure, function, and implications for dermatologic disease. J Am Acad Dermatol 46(2 Suppl Understanding):S41–S62
11. Tobin DJ (2006) Biochemistry of human skinDOUBLEHYPHENour brain on the outside. Chem Soc Rev 35(1):52–67

Diagnostic Procedures

27

Harald Gollnick, Zrinka Bukvić Mokos, Günter Burg, Veronique del Marmol, Branka Marinović, and Jonathan M. White

Contents

H. Gollnick (✉)
Department of Dermatology & Venereology, Otto-von-Guericke University, Magdeburg, Germany
e-mail: Harald.Gollnick@med.ovgu.de

Z. Bukvić Mokos · B. Marinović
Department of Dermatology and Venereology, School of Medicine University of Zagreb, Zagreb, Croatia
e-mail: branka.marinovic@kbc-zagreb.hr

G. Burg
Dermatology, Zurich, Switzerland
e-mail: g.burg@access.uzh.ch

V. del Marmol
Départment of Dermatology, Hôpital Erasme-HUB, Université Libre de Bruxelles, Brussels, Belgium
e-mail: veronique.delmarmol@hubruxelles.be

J. M. White
Ecole de Santé Publique, Université libre de Bruxelles, Brussels, Belgium
e-mail: Jonathan.White@ulb.be

H. Gollnick et al. (eds.), *Dermatology Cyberderm WebBook*,
https://doi.org/10.1007/978-3-031-78491-0_27

Test your learning and check your understanding of this book's contents: use the "Springer Nature Flashcards" app to access questions using ▶ https://sn.pub/1rhh6k.

To use the app, please follow the instructions in Chap. 1.

Bedside Tests [5, 8, 9]

Grading of Importance

No grading

Level

Basic

At the dermatologic examination, several simple bedside tests may help to narrow the differential diagnosis. The most performed bedside tests are listed below. For functional and imaging tests, dermatopathology, and other tests, see sections “Non-invasive Imaging Methods in Dermatology”, “Basics in Dermatopathology” and “Non-invasive Methods in Dermatology: Functional Tests”.

Nikolsky Sign

Nikolsky sign is shearing away the epidermis after gentle lateral or tangential pressure or rubbing the peri-bullous skin. It is positive in patients with pemphigus, staphylococcal scalded skin syndrome (SSSS), and toxic epidermal necrolysis (Lyell’s disease).

Indirect Nikolsky (Nikolsky II) is elicited by the gentle pressure on an intact bulla that results in the spread of fluid in the epidermis away from the site of pressure (the “bulla-spread phenomenon”).

Darier Sign

Darier sign designates the rapid appearance of a wheal or an acute or late persisting erythema when the lesion is stroked. It typically occurs in patients with cutaneous mastocytosis or urticaria factitia.

Auspitz Sign

Auspitz sign is the appearance of punctate bleeding after removing the scales from plaques in psoriasis. The erythematosquamous plaque is gently scraped with a tongue depressor or a glass slide, resulting in the removal of silvery scales. After scraping off all the scales, a glistening transparent membrane (Buckley’s membrane) appears. On removing the membrane, punctate bleeding points are observed. Bleeding comes from the capillaries of the papillary layer beneath a thinner epidermis between broad rete ridges.

Skin Scraping for Diagnosing Fungal Infections and Scabies

For diagnosing fungal infections, scales (squamae) are taken with a glass slide or a metal blade from the border of the lesion and placed onto a glass slide. Afterward, a drop of 10–20% potassium hydroxide (KOH) is added. The fungal infection is confirmed if hyphae or yeast cells are detected.

For diagnosing scabies, scrapings are taken from suspected burrows or inflammatory papules using a metal blade previously dipped into the mineral oil. Scrapings are placed on a glass slide. Scabies is confirmed if mites, feces (scybala), or eggs are seen in the microscopic examination. Dermatoscopy can also help prediagnosing and guiding the site of scraping.

Diascopy

Diascopy is performed by pressing a glass slide on a lesion, causing the compression of small vessels. On diascopy, hemorrhagic lesions (petechiae or purpura) do not blanch; but inflammatory and vascular lesions do. Diascopy may be used in detecting granulomatous diseases such as lupus vulgaris or sarcoidosis, which turn an "apple jelly" color on diascopy.

Köbner Phenomenon

Köbner phenomenon denotes the development of new skin lesions of a preexisting dermatosis within the areas of physical trauma in otherwise healthy skin. Physical trauma includes scratching, friction, rubbing, pressure, incision, laceration, insect bites, etc. Köbner phenomenon may appear 10–20 days (with a range from 3 days to 2 years) after the injury. It is most commonly seen in psoriasis and lichen planus.

Tzanck Smear

Tzanck smear is a very simple and rapid cytologic test that is most commonly used to diagnose viral infections such as herpes simplex and herpes zoster and may help diagnose intraepidermal autoimmune blistering diseases such as pemphigus vulgaris. The blister roof is removed with a sharp blade, and the base is gently scraped with a scalpel or the edge of a spatula. At scraping the base, bleeding should not be provoked, as the inclusion of blood may disable the interpretation of results. The scraping is transferred onto a glass slide, air-dried, and stained with Giemsa stain.

In herpes simplex and herpes zoster, ballooning multinucleated giant cells and eosinophilic inclusion bodies are detected, whereas in pemphigus vulgaris acantholytic cells may be seen.

Dermoscopy

Dermoscopy is a non-invasive diagnostic technique that evaluates colors and microstructures of the skin that are not visible to the naked eye, using a handheld dermatoscope (mostly used), a stereomicroscope, or a videodermatoscope. Often a polarized filter is embedded. The magnification of these instruments may be from

6× up to even 100×. Dermoscopy is mainly used for the assessment of pigmented lesions, i.e., differentiation between melanocytic and non-melanocytic lesions and then evaluation of benign and malignant features of melanocytic nevi and melanoma (see also chapter Imaging techniques).

Non-invasive Imaging Methods in Dermatology [1, 2, 7]

Grading of Importance

No grading

Level

Basic

Although many diagnoses in dermatology are made clinically, sometimes extra help is required. Skin biopsies are still the gold standard if by macroscopy or dermatoscopy a proper diagnoses cannot be made; however, the area and lesion has to be selected carefully and be representative of the whole lesion. Various non-invasive techniques have therefore been developed to close the gap between macroscopy and biopsy to visualize the skin in certain situations. Some of these techniques will not be available in all centers.

Clinical Photography

Photography is very helpful in diagnosing intermittent skin diseases which may not be present on the day of clinical review, e.g., intermittent urticaria. Serial photographs can be very helpful in tracking pigmented lesions to assess the chance of malignant change. In store-and-forward telemedical settings, clinical pictures are pivotal for monitoring the course of diseases (i.e., wound healing, skin cancer, and single or multiple nevi follow-up).

Dermoscopy and Digital Dermoscopy

Examining the skin, hair, follicles, or nails under a magnifying, polarized light (x10–20 the size of normal) can give additional information especially for pigmented lesions but also NMSC and some forms of inflammatory dermatoses, as well as vascular lesions. Digital images (or serial images) may be stored from dermoscopic examination and either reviewed by a clinician, or by artificial intelligence. The original term "dermatoscopy" is still used synonymously with the internationally consented term "dermoscopy."

Diaphanoscopy

Producing anemia of inflamed skin by pressure with a glass spatula may reveal the typical apple yellow color of granulomatous infiltrates, e.g., in sarcoidosis.

Spectrophotometric Intracutaneous Analysis

This machine provides input about the content of melanin, hemoglobin, and collagen in the epidermis and papillary dermis. This technique may be useful especially for nonexperts to calculate risk of melanoma in a clinically atypical pigmented lesion.

Nevisense

This technology relies on the fact that there may be a difference in impedance in skin lesions compared with normal skin and that this can be elicited by a sensitive electrode, such as in the Nevisense machine. It may be a useful adjunct to the clinician in particular for atypical nevi and prior to a biopsy.

Ultrasound

Ultrasound is regularly used in dermatology for measuring depth of lesion (i.e., melanoma or other tumor thickness or mass of a lipoma before dermatosurgery), for lymph nodes or in arterial and venous vessel blood flow diagnostics (i.e., Doppler technique; Duplex-sonography for the assessment of deep thrombosis).

X-Ray/Computerized Tomography (CT) Scan

Sometimes X-ray of other organs may be required for the work-up of certain dermatological conditions (e.g., chest X-ray for cutaneous sarcoidosis). X-ray may be helpful to evaluate some skin problems, e.g., calcinosis cutis. CT or PET-CT (see below) scanning is a mandatory investigation of advanced skin tumors and staging which may have metastasized. It may also be useful for hunting any underlying tumors in conditions such as dermatomyositis or paraneoplastic pemphigus or to find the primary of metastases from an internal tumor.

Positron Emission Tomography (PET)

PET scans involve a radioactive tracer being visualized in vascular or metabolic processes. It may identify neoplasms earlier than other techniques such as CT and can be used to seek an underlying (clinically undisclosed) malignancy, i.e., sentinel lymph node metastasis in malignant melanoma. It may be combined with CT (PET-CT) to enhance sensitivity.

Magnetic Resonance Imaging (MRI)

Similar to CT scanning, MRI can be helpful in certain situations in dermatological diseases, e.g., investigation of neurofibromatosis or Sturge-Weber syndrome and search for metastasis in skin cancer.

Reflectance Confocal Microscopy

This technique focuses light at sequential levels with a spatial pinhole and provides a horizontal image of the skin with high lateral resolution of 1 μm. The maximal penetration of the skin is around 250 μm, which does not allow examination of the deeper part of the dermis at all and does not deliver clear results of the papillary dermis. It is frequently used for assessment of epidermal manifestations of skin malignancies but may also be useful in inflammatory skin conditions.

Vertical Laser Microscopy

This vertical laser technique provides deep penetration in the dermis and can help to close the gap between dermatopathology and reflectance confocal microscopy.

Optical Coherence Tomography (OCT)

Conventional OCT provided both horizontal and vertical sections of the skin and penetrates around 2 mm, with a lateral resolution of around 7.5 μm. High-definition OCT penetrates the skin deeper, but line-field-confocal OCT is the best, with a penetration of 500 μm and a lateral resolution of 1 μm. This can be very useful to delineate margins of tumors in vivo and confirm or exclude malignancy without the need for a skin biopsy. Combination with high resolution ultrasound in one device is possible.

Basics in Dermatopathology [3, 4]

Figures 27.1, 27.2, 27.3, 27.4, 27.5, 27.6, 27.7, 27.8, 27.9, 27.10 and 27.11

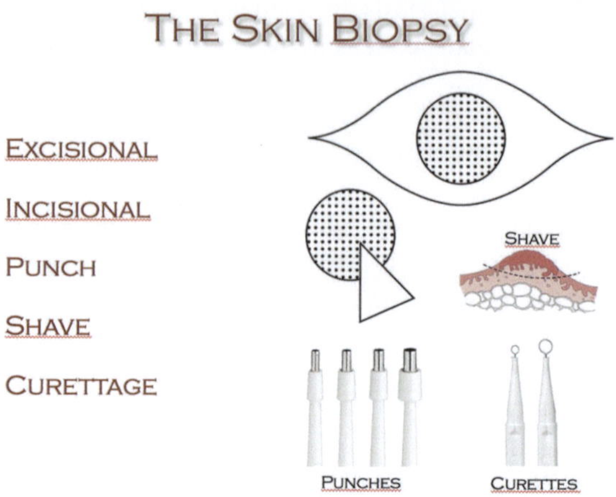

Fig. 27.1 Basics in dermatopathology: skin biopsy techniques

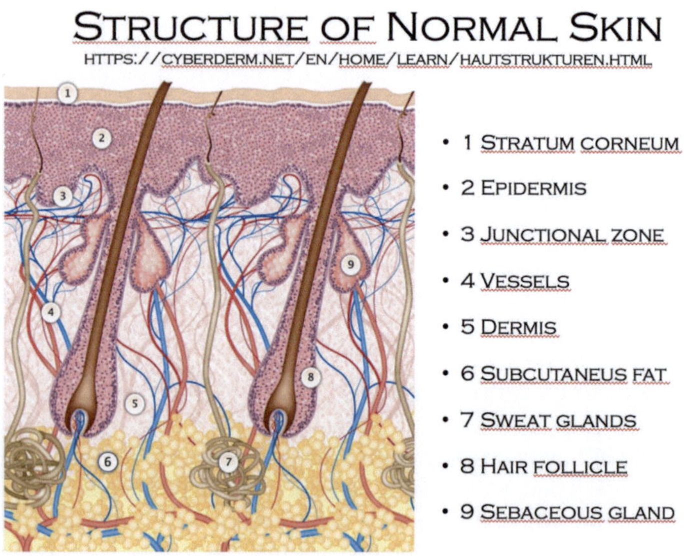

Fig. 27.2 Basics in dermatopathology: structure of the skin

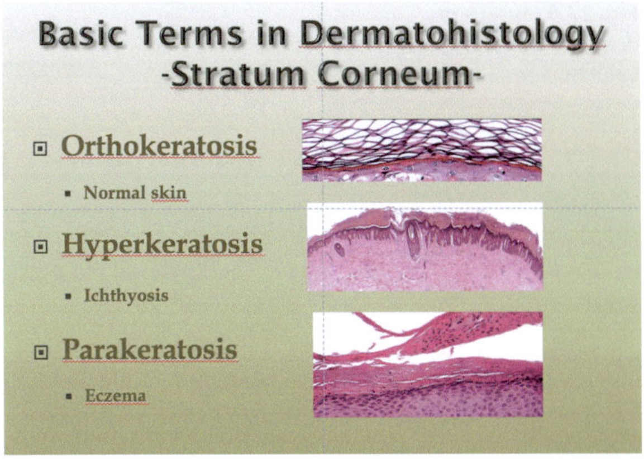

Fig. 27.3 Basics in dermatopathology: epidermis

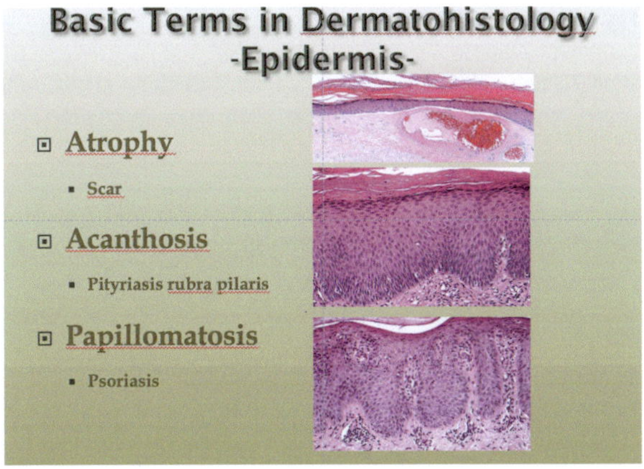

Fig. 27.4 Basics in dermatopathology: epidermis

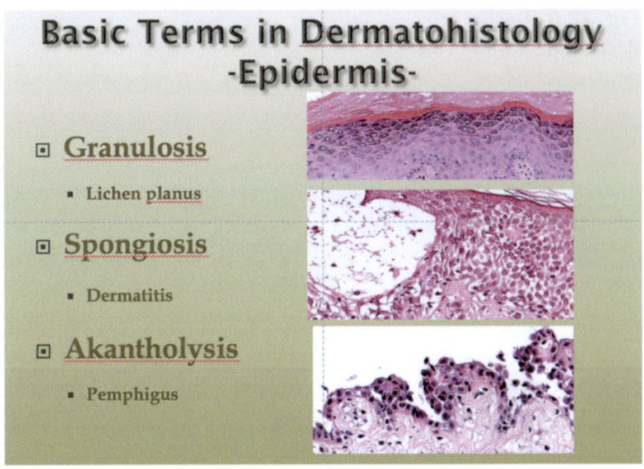

Fig. 27.5 Basics in dermatopathology: epidermis

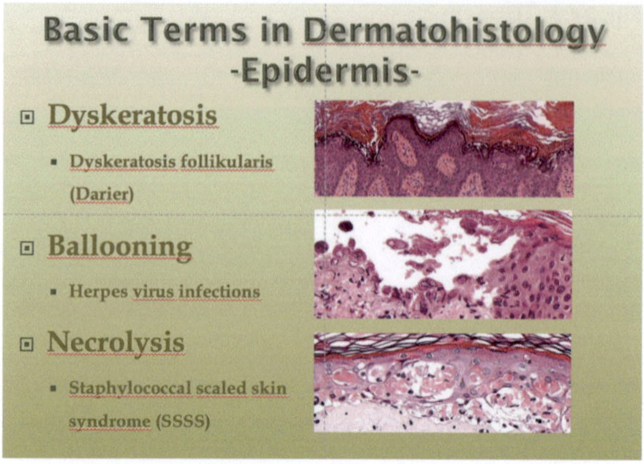

Fig. 27.6 Basics in dermatopathology: epidermis

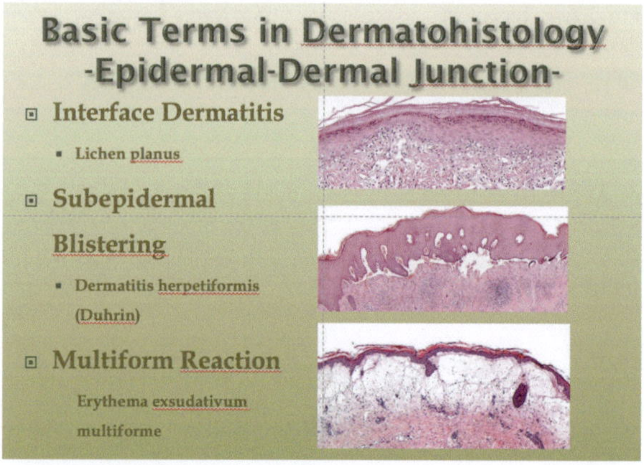

Fig. 27.7 Basics in dermatopathology: epiderma-dermal junction

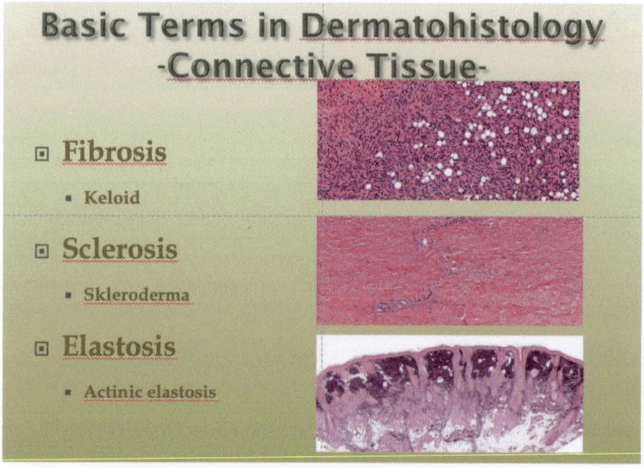

Fig. 27.8 Basics in dermatopathology: connective tissue

Fig. 27.9 Basics in dermatopathology: vessels

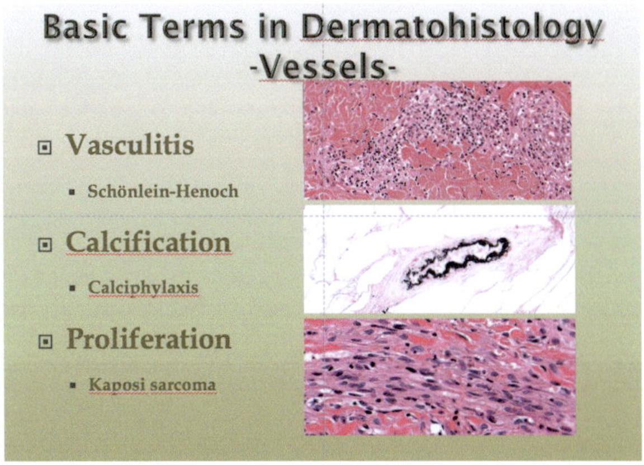

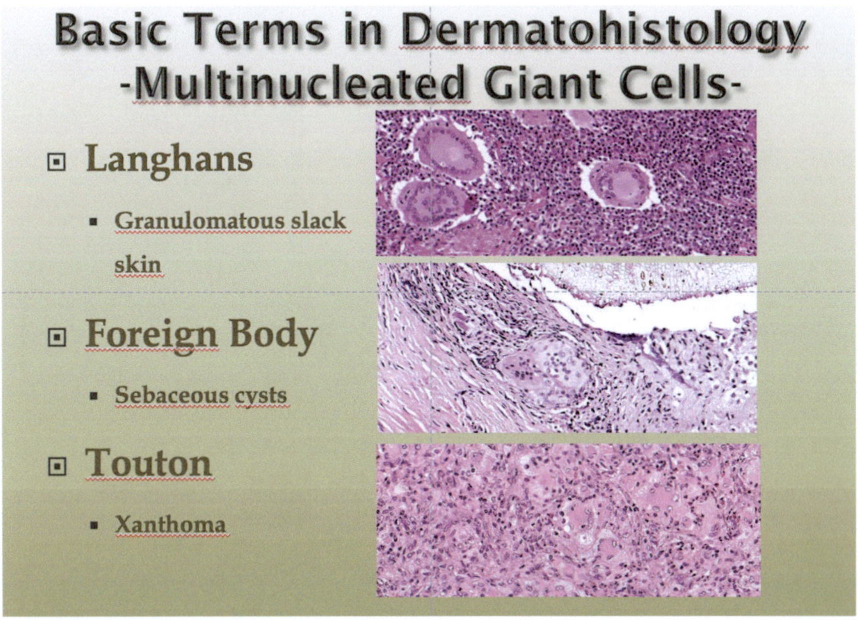

Fig. 27.10 Basics in dermatopathology: giant cells

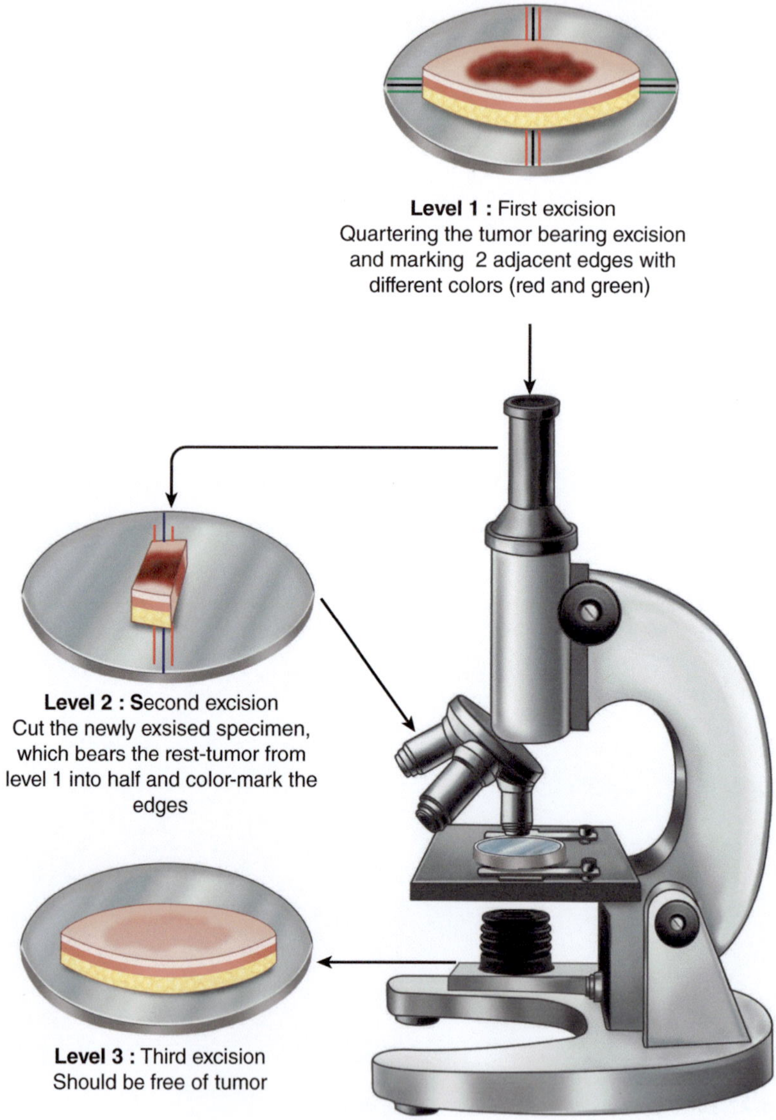

Fig. 27.11 Basics in dermatopathology: Mohs surgery

Grading of Importance

No grading

Level

Basic

The most efficient method in the diagnosis of skin diseases is the combined validation of clinical and histopathological features, i.e., clinicopathologic correlation. The diagnostic impact of histopathology may be decisive or just confirmative of the clinical differential diagnosis. However, there are some dermatoses in which a biopsy is not indicated because typical histopathologic changes are lacking.

Taking a Biopsy

When

When considering clinicopathologic considerations in approaching a diagnosis, there basically are four scenarios, in which the diagnostic impact of histopathology may be high, moderate, low, or none.

Where

In inflammatory processes, infectious or noninfectious, the biopsy should be taken from the border of the lesion, where the initial changes without regenerative, necrotic, fibrous, or secondary granulomatous reactions are found.

In tumors however the biopsy should be taken from the center of the lesion or in some cases from the border, including both normal and neoplastic tissue.

How

It is fundamentally important, that the dermatopathologist, to whom the specimen is referred for microscopic evaluation, can describe his findings in the context of the clinical features. The specimen must include the critical tissue levels and must show the pathologic changes. One of the most frequent mistakes is a superficial biopsy, missing the pathologic changes in the deep dermis or subcutaneous tissue.

In addition, the clinician should provide the pathologist with clinical differential diagnoses.

Depending on the size and the depth of the lesion, it can be either completely excised –especially small tumors – (**excisional biopsy**), or a spindle- or wedge-shaped biopsy is taken from the border (**incisional biopsy**).

In tumorous lesions reaching to the surface of the skin, a flat slice can be removed horizontally with a scalpel (**shave biopsy**).

Punch biopsies can be applied for homogeneous tumor lesions.

Fragmented material from superficial **curettage** may be sufficient in special situations for confirming infectious (mollusca contagiosa) or neoplastic origin, when the morphology of a small cluster of tumor cells is sufficient for making a diagnosis.

Swaps from the nostril area or from the superficially scratched earlobe may provide material for microbiologic investigations under the microscope or in appropriate culture media.

Electroacoustic retrieval of a specimen should be avoided, since important tissue structures may be boiled.

3-D dermatopathology The basic idea of the micrographic controlled surgery (MCS), as invented originally by Frederic Mohs in Madison/Wi, USA, was to confirm by three-dimensional sectioning that the borders of the excised specimens were tumor-free toward the periphery and toward the depth and by serial surgical procedures to completely remove the tumor and saving uninvolved tissue. This technique, originally as pre-fixed, later on as fresh tissue and finally today mostly as post-fixed procedure is indicated for solid tumors with superficially undetermined, "subclinical" borders, not for inflammatory dermatoses.

Sample Processing

The biopsy is trimmed to an optimal size of 1 × 2 × 2 cm and fixed in buffered formalin (4% aqueous solution) for several hours before embedded into a paraffin block. These procedures today can run automatically.

Sections of 2–4 microns perpendicularly from the epidermis to the subcutis are cut with a microtome on to a glass slide, which is transferred to an automatic staining device.

Staining

Routine: Hematoxylin and eosin (HE): blue and red

Special Stains

- Alcian blue: blue. Acid glucosamines
- Berlin blue: blue. Hemosiderin (iron)
- Elastica: black. Elastic fibers
- Fite-Faraco: red. *Mycobacterium leprae*
- Giemsa: violet blue. Mast cells, amastigotes in leishmaniasis
- Gram: blue (Gram-positive bacteriae) or red (Gram-negative bacteriae)
- Grocott: black. Fungi
- Congo red: pink or green in polarized light. Amyloid
- Kossa: black. Calcium
- Masson-Fontana: black. Melanin
- Naphthol-AS-D Chloroacetate esterase: (Leder's stain) red. Mast cells

- Periodic acid-Schiff (PAS): violet, purple. Stains glycogen, fungi, basal lamina
- Sudan (cryosection): orange or yellow. Lipids
- Toluidine Blue: bluish granules. Mast cells
- Van Gieson-Elastica: red (collagen), black (elastic fibers), muscle fibers (yellow)
- Warthin-Starry: black. Spirochetes, fungi
- Ziehl-Neelsen: red. Acid-fast bacteria (tubercle bacilli, leishmania)

Molecular Morphology

Immune histochemistry: Labeling of antigens (epithelial, mesenchymal, vascular, melanocytic, lymphocytic, histiocytic, bacterial, fungal, and proliferation markers) with specific mono- or polyclonal antibodies, which often stain several different cells or structures.

Direct immunofluorescence (DIF): Use of antibodies labeled with a fluorochrome. The most important applications include autoimmune-bullous dermatoses, vasculitis, and lupus erythematosus.

In situ hybridization (ISH): Detection of microorganisms and confirmation of clonality of, i.e., in lymphoproliferative disorders (lymphomas).

Fluorescence in situ hybridization (FISH): Detection of chromosomal aberrations, i.e., in neoplasia.

Polymerase chain reaction (PCR): extremely sensitive for detection of, i.e., microorganisms, clonality (receptor rearrangement), mutations, oncogenes

Structure of Normal Skin

There are striking regional differences with respect to thickness of the skin layers, sensory receptors, vessels, connective tissue, subcutaneous fat, and adnexa.

Epidermis

Multilayer squamous epithelium of 0.3–0.8 mm thick. From the outside to the inside, the following layers are distinguished:

Stratum corneum consists of flat, plate-like, interlocking coreless keratinocytes, which are held together by intercellular “barrier lipids” (e.g., ceramides). Since it is the outermost protective layer of the body, it exerts a mechanical barrier function, prevents excessive water loss, and protects from penetration of microorganisms, chemicals, or allergens.

Stratum granulosum exhibits moisturizing and UV-protective (pyrrolidone carboxylic acid) functions. The granules contain lipids and enzymes, which are released into the intercellular space and lead to the formation of a water-resistant putty substance in the stratum corneum.

Stratum spinosum together with the stratum basale forms the stratum germinativum. The histologic processing of skin samples results in shrinking of the sections, which accentuates their intercellular desmosomal contacts (spiny cell layer). The keratinization process begins in this layer. During their migration to the outermost layer of the epidermis, the cells become flattened and cease to divide, keeping a delegate balance between gain and loss of cells by peeling off the skin surface.

Stratum basale (stratum germinativum). Cells of this layer exhibit qualities of determined stem cells. Following division one cell migrates to the skin surface within the next 4 weeks, whereas the other remains and divides again.

Up to 8% of the cells basal layer of the epidermis are **melanocytes** which produce melanin, a dark pigment blocking UV rays. Ethnic different skin colors are due to the packaging and distribution pattern of the pigment grains (loose fine granules in black people or packed in melanosomes in Caucasians).

Langerhans cells are another type of dendritic cells in the germinative layers of the the epidermis and also present as dendritic reticulum cells (DRC) in the dermis. They derive from the bone marrow and play a pivotal role in the immunological defense and in the recognition of antigens.

Merkel cells are a third type of dendritic cells in the epidermis. Localized in the basal layer, they fulfill sensory receptor functions (pressure).

Dermo-epidermal Junction (Grenz Zone)

The grenz zone comprises a complex PAS-positive basal membrane, which is anchored to the dermis by hemidesmosomes. Metabolic products, dendritic immune cells, and lymphocytes are exchanged between the two compartments. Under the electron microscope, the complex structure of the junction zone is revealed, comprising of (1) the cytoskeleton of the basal keratinocytes with intermediate filaments composed of keratin 5 and keratin 14; (2) the anchor filaments of the hemidesmosomes (lamina lucida), consisting of various molecular structures; (3) lamina densa with collagen IV as the main component besides other components; and (4) the sublamina densa, which is directly adjacent to the lamina densa and consists of collagen types I, III, IV, and VII, anchoring to the papillary dermis. These structural proteins and their antigenic determinants play an important role in the pathophysiology of some autoimmuno- and geno-dermatoses.

Dermis

The **papillary dermis** is the upper part of the dermis, protruding as rete ridges between the epidermal papillae. The capillary loops provide optimal nutrition for the epidermis, and fine nerve endings give sensory protection.

The **reticular dermis** shows a texture of collagen fibers, which is more compact than in the papillary dermis. Moreover it harbors vascular, nervous, and adnexal elements between fibroblasts, histiocytes, macrophages, dendritic, and other cells, permanently migrating through the skin.

Subcutis

This component consists of fat lobuli separated by sepal fibers, connecting it to both the dermis and the deeper tissue. It serves as energy and heat storage, and as mechanical protective pad.

Adnexal Structures

Hairs are found on almost all body surfaces except for soles and palms. They consist of dead, fish-scale-like horn cells produced in the hair follicles of the dermis. The hair follicle consists of an epithelial layer that surrounds the hair root. The lower part of the hair follicle, the hair bulb, is embedded in a net of nerve endings and capillaries.

Sebaceous glands are linked to the hair follicles. They produce lipids (sebum), which protect skin and hair from drying out, water loss, and growth of pathogenic bacteria. Hair growth occurs in a cycle: (1) anagen (growth) phase (2–6 years; 0.3 mm per day) in which 85% of our head hairs are, (2) 2-week catagen (transition) phase, and (3) telogen (resting) phase (3–4 months) in which 50–100 hairs per day are lost.

Sweat glands

- The **eccrine sweat glands** are spread over almost the entire body surface. The twisted part in the deep dermis leads via a straight excretory duct directly to the skin surface and produces an aqueous secretion, which is rich in urea, uric acid, ammonia, salts, and other substances. They are used for temperature regulation and the excretion of metabolic products.
- The **apocrine sweat glands** are found in the axilla, the groin, the anogenital area, and the beard hair in men. The secretory portion lies mainly in the subcutis with the excretory duct duct flowing into the hair follicle.

Pathologic Changes

Epidermis

Orthokeratosis: Basket weave stratum corneum in the fixed tissue section

Example: Normal skin

Hyperkeratosis Thickening of the stratum corneum due to increased epidermal proliferation or retention of horny cells by reduced scaling

Example: Ichthyosis

Parakeratosis: Remnants of nuclei remain in the stratum corneum due to disturbance of the keratinization process (dyskeratosis)

Example: Eczema

Atrophy: Reduced spinal layer and flattening of the basal undulation

Examples: Aged skin; lichen sclerosus et atrophicus

Acanthosis: Thickening of the epidermis to due broadening of the spinal layer following increased proliferation and turnover of keratinocytes

Example: Chronic eczema; psoriasis

Papillomatosis: Hyperplasia of dermal papillae forming an undulating basal lamina

Example: Psoriasis

Granulosis: Broadening of the stratum granulosum due to disturbances in the keratinization process

Example: Lichen planus

Spongiosis: Dehiscence of keratinocytes and intraepidermal blister formation due to intercellular edema; desmosome bridges may be preserved.

Example: Acute dermatitis

Acantholysis: Loss of intercellular desmosomal connections between keratinocytes, resulting in blister formation

Example: Pemphigus vulgaris

Dyskeratosis: Premature or altered (abnormal) keratinocyte differentiation with preservation of nuclei in the stratum corneum

Example: Dyskeratosis follicularis Darier

Ballooning: Intracellular edema, blowing up the cell size

Examples: Herpes virus infections

Complete damage and lysis of the cellular structure and substance

Example: Toxic epidermal necrolysis (TEN)

Dermo-epidermal junction (grenz zone)

Interface dermatitis: Obscuring of the border between epidermis and papillary dermis due to edema (vacuolation) or to cellular infiltrate (lichenoid type)

Examples: Lupus erythematosus; lichen planus

Subepidermal blistering: Supra- or infrabasal blistering separation of epidermis and the papillary dermis

Example: Bullous pemphigoid

Subepidermal edema: Edema in the papillary dermis without blister formation

Example: Erythema exsudativum multiforme

Dermis

Fibrosis: Increased numbers and activity of fibroblasts

Examples: Fibroma; histiocytoma

Sclerosis: Compact densely packed collagen fibers usually paucicellular (reduced number of connective tissue cells)

Example: Scleroderma

Elastosis: Degenerative changes of collagen and elastic tissue with development of coarse fibers

Example: Actinic elastosis

Vessels

Vasculitis: Swelling of endothelia, extravasation of fibrin and erythrocytes, leuko- or lymphocytic perivascular inflammation

Example: Vasculitis allergica

Calcification: Calcium deposits in and around (elastica) vascular endothelial cells

Example: Calciphylaxis

Proliferation: Endothelia cells and vascular spaces

Examples: benign (hemangioma), "semimalignant" (Kaposi) or malignant processes (hemangiosarcoma)

Deposits and Storage

Foreign bodies: Inorganic material (pigment) inserted from outside intentionally (tattoo), or accidentally, into the dermis is ingested by macrophages or – if the particles are too big – leads to enclosure by a granulomatous inflammatory infiltrate with various types of multinucleated giant cells

Examples: Tattoo; foreign body granuloma

Other deposits: Melanin, urate, mucin, iron (hemosiderin), porphyrins, calcium, and other organic or inorganic substances, produced during pathologic disease processes, may be deposited intracellularly (macrophages) or extracellularly between or attached to collagen bundles in the dermis.

Examples: Nevi; xanthoma; gout; mucinosis; pilomatricoma (Malherbe)

Non-invasive Methods in Dermatology: Functional Tests [6]

Grading of Importance

No grading

Level

Basic

A great part of dermato-venereological diseases can be diagnosed by the naked eye, the palpating finger, and the appropriate long-term clinical experience and expertise. However, some situations need invasive techniques such as dermatopathology (see section "Basics in Dermatopathology") and/or non-invasive techniques such as imaging technology (see section "Non-invasive Imaging Methods in Dermatology"). In addition functional tests have been developed to provide measurable objective data.

Epidermal Function Tests

Tests for epidermal function include in particular those measuring desquamation, hydration, and transepidermal water loss, pH, and color including pigmentation. Computer-assisted devices are on the market.

Measuring the epidermal barrier function includes methods such as those written below.

Str. corneum cell desquamation is a permanent and essential physiologic process of normal skin. Different factors may influence via outer and inner environmental signals the degree of desquamation (hyperproliferation of basal layer, dryness, repair signals, wounding, cytokine signals, genetic factors, clothes, profession). There are dermatoses with rapid turnover of cells (e.g., psoriasis) and others with slow turnover (e.g., retention hyperkeratosis in ichthyosis). Age is an important factor.

Chamber techniques are used for measuring desquamation Serial tape strippings can be applied for evaluating the recovery function of the epidermis. Densitometric and light reflectance analysis of the adherent scales together with a specialized software calculates the desquamation index.

Epidermal hydration is essential for skin integrity. If skin becomes dehydrated by increased water loss or by decreased supply, the barrier function is disturbed.

Hydration of the skin can be measured by electrical conductance, impedance, or capacitance. Corneometers (evaporimeter/Tewameter) are used to measure, for example, the loss of hydration due to mechanical stress of the hands in occupational diseases such as hand eczema or the success of external rehydration using a moisturizer. **Trans-epidermal water loss** (TEWL) is measured in g/hcm^2. The system measures the water vapor flow density: JV= g/(m × h) (mass of water vapor (in g) per area (in cm^2) and time (in h)).

The pH value is a biomarker for the skin's natural acid mantle (around pH 5). Hydration from the inside through the capillaries as well as sweat from eccrine and apocrine glands, lipids from the epidermal, and the sebaceous cells are important. A neutral pH value can lead to lower resistance against infections and decreased barrier function.

Oxygen tension is reduced during aging, loss of capillary network in diabetes, chronic renal failure, and sclero- and pseudoscleroderma and may be increased due to vasodilatation in inflammatory disorders.

Skin pigmentation is related to the skin types I to VI. For testing the light protection, e.g., in sun screens Colorimetry **(reflectance methods via chromameter)** is used. The method identifies not only the degree of melanin pigmentation but of other color components.

Tape stripping can be used to measure the recovery time of epidermal basal cells or for allergen testing (see below) and for demonstrating Malassezia spores or hyphae on a tape strip (5–10x) and to glued to a glass slide and stained with a droplet of methylene blue.

Dermal Function Tests

Mechanical properties of the skin depend on the physical function of the dermis.

Twistometry measures the twisting capacity to a given force using a disk glued to the skin and rotated via a small motor. This provides some information on the strength and vitality of elastic fiber and collagen matrix in healthy and diseased skin.

Frictiometry is a method using a constant pressure on the skin by the weight of a rotating disk which is incorporated in handheld device. It gives results on the elasticity and friction related return to normal and disturbances due to loss of elastic fibers, atrophy, or sclerosis.

The **cutometer (identometry)** working with a light source and negative air pressure provides information on the elasticity of the dermis. The light intensity depends on the depth of penetration into the skin. The resistance of the skin to the negative pressure (firmness) and its ability to return into its original position (elasticity) reflect the functional capacity.

Skin temperature depends on body temperature and blood flow.. Thermoregulation detected by thermal imaging devices (e.g., contact thermometry, convection (Schlieren's) photography, thermal infrared cameras) gives an overview on the skin temperature in different areas..

Sebaceous Glands Function Tests

Follicular biopsies are performed to measure the content of the follicular infundibulum and, in particular, to count the number of microcomedones per area. A droplet of cyanoacrylate is applied on a glass slide and then placed with light pressure, for example, on the forehead and removed after 30–60 seconds. Under the microscope one can count on the surface of the glass slide the number of microcomedones. The application is important in acne. It is also used for counting demodex mites in rosacea.

Sebumetry measures the temporary composition of surface lipids and amount of lipids secreted from the follicular canal of the gland in quantity and quality. **Sebutapes** are microporous adherent tapes applied on defatted skin. The lipids are absorbed and can be measured by image analysis. The **results of the gravimetric technique** are more correct by using absorbent paper left on the degreased skin of the forehead for 3 hours and measuring the sebum weight.

Sweat Gland Function Tests

Sweat gland activity may depend on several factors (emotional stress, thermoregulation, paraneoplasia, endocrine disturbances, drugs). Diseases such as cystic fibrosis, scleroderma, congenital ectodermal dysplasia, sympathectomy, or alcohol- and diabetes-induced neuropathy can go along with reduced sweating or even anhidrosis.

Filter paper collection, the quantitative sudomotor axon reflex test (QSART) using iodine-impregnated paper after pilocarpine stimulation. Sweat is visualized by a topical indicator such as iodinated starch or sodium alizarin sulfonate (alizarin Red S).

The **iodinated starch powder** test is prepared by adding 0.5–1.0 g of iodine crystals to 500 g of soluble starch. For smaller body areas, a Minor's starch-iodine test for excessive sweating may be performed by applying Betadine on Q-tips to the affected area. Once the iodine solution has dried, cornstarch can be lightly sprinkled on the area. Deep purple color change will develop over time in the areas affected with hyperhidrosis. The amount of sweat secretion per minute and cm^2 is practicable for definition of hyperhidrosis.

A new **customized camera device** can be used to quantify secretions of individual sweat glands (SGs), following stimulation by pilocarpine in a 2.25 cm^2 skin area. The camera registers sweat from 50 to 400 sweat ducts. The secretion rate of individual SGs, total sweat volume, and number of secreting SGs of different body sites are measured.

Hair Function Test

Different methods exist for evaluation of hair loss and hair growth or the strength and elasticity of hair. Several diseases affecting the hair growth need a biopsy for histological evaluation.

Trichogram is a classical method for studying the type and degree of hair loss, e.g., in androgenetic or androgenic alopecias. After 5 days without washing the hair, hairs are pulled out of its roots using a forceps from the frontal or parietal and from the occipital hair line, moved to a glass slide, imbedded in Corbit balsam, and evaluated under the microscope for the proportion of anagen, catagen, and telogen hairs and for the percentage of dysplastic and dystrophic or broken hairs.

Phototrichogram is a non-invasive and reproducible method to quantify hair density and hair growth parameters. The hairs at a selected site are trimmed for the applied diagnostic optical equipment (0.8–1.5 cm). With a syringe with insulin needle or with a tattoo apparatus basically invisible by bare eye, tattoo marks are set. The test area is covered with a coverslip glass to allow the positioning of the trichoscope lens. An image is analyzed by special computer program evaluation. The program will calculate the total number of hairs/cm^2 as well as the number of terminal and vellus-like anagen and telogen hairs.

Blood Vessel Function Tests

Glasspatel/glass slide. Pressure by a simple glasspatel/glass slide on a lesion can be used to evaluate if erythrocytes are inside or outside capillaries between collagen bundles. Diminishing of the red color or complete bleaching of the erythema speaks is in favor of intact functionality of vessels whereas the color stays unchanged in petechia or purpura.

The glasspatel can also be used to test the capillary reflex related to pressure and friction followed by erythema or whealing. Paradoxical whitening of the irritated skin can be seen in atopy. Whealing is a sign of dermographism of acute and persisting type and needs further evaluation of the skin or other organs (mastocytosis, physical urticaria, desaminoxidase deficiency). With a dermatoscope also the capillary loops are checked at the nail folds at the fingers or toes to diagnose vasculitis or reduction of capacity (scleroderma, Raynaud phenomenon, vasculitis, bleeding). Furthermore specific laser systems can further test flow rate etc.

Immune Function Tests

Test techniques for different test procedures and protocols regarding allergies are highly standardized. Irritant patch testing, standard epicutaneous patch testing, and photo-patch testing or prick testing are the most widely used.

Epicutaneous contact allergy (patch) testing is used to evaluate amount and degree of and to differentiate allergic and irritant eczemas. Standardized or in some cases individualized substances in appropriate vehicles are applied via, for example, Finn chambers with occlusive protection to the back of a patient. They are left there for 48 h and removed for first reading according to a grading protocol. Additional readings follow after 72 and 96 h. Some substances require reading after 120 h or 1 week.

Photo-patch testing is performed if suspicious agents/allergens need photoactivation to become immunologic. In addition to the standard patch test, suspicious allergens are additionally irradiated with UVA light.

Prick testing is used for evaluating type I allergy. Standardized solutions of allergens compared to a NaCl and a histamine control field are applied to the skin in a droplet. Each individual droplet is then separately pierced with a lancet, transporting the substance in the epidermis and papillary. Reading of positive wheals is recorded after 20 minutes.

Other tests not mentioned here in detail include scratch, rubber, prick-to-prick or intradermal testing and systemic provocation tests for drugs, food, food colors, and preservatives.

Tests for Peripheral Nerves

Sensation tests are done in the peripheral nervous system first in a dermatomal pattern. Tests for light touch, sharp/blunt, temperature, and often two-point discrimination are the most common bedside tests (small vs large diameter nerve fibers).

Electromyography and nerve conduction tests are performed by neurologists to evaluate paresthesias and peripheral neuropathy. This concerns in particular dermatologic diseases such as leprosy, scleroderma, chronic graft versus host disease, late borreliosis, late-stage syphilis, patients with neurotrophic ulcers due to diabetes mellitus, deposition disorders such as amyloidosis and traumatic nerve damage, alcohol abuse, and Bureau-Barrière syndrome.

Alloknesis is a specific test of peripheral nerve endings for evaluating of itch signals. With a small brush one sweeps over the skin.

References

1. Chen X, Lu Q, Chen C, Jiang G (2021) Recent developments in dermoscopy for dermatology. J Cosmet Dermatol 20(6):1611–1617
2. Hindelang B, Aguirre J, Schwarz M, Berezhnoi A, Eyerich K, Ntziachristos V, Biedermann T, Darsow U (2019) Non-invasive imaging in dermatology and the unique potential of raster-scan optoacoustic mesoscopy. J Eur Acad Dermatol Venereol 33(6):1051–1061
3. Liersch J, von Kockritz A, Schaller J (2017a) Dermatopathology 101: Part 1—Inflammatory skin diseases. J Dtsch Dermatol Ges 15(1):9–30
4. Liersch J, von Kockritz A, Schaller J (2017b) Dermatopathology 101. Part 2—Skin tumors. J Dtsch Dermatol Ges 15(9):906–929
5. Micheletti RG, Dominguez AR, Wanat KA (2017) Bedside diagnostics in dermatology: parasitic and noninfectious diseases. J Am Acad Dermatol 77(2):221–230
6. Serup J, Jemec G, Grove G (2006) Handbook of non-invasive methods and the skin. CRC Press
7. Tanaka M (2006) Dermoscopy. J Dermatol 33(8):513–517
8. Wanat KA, Dominguez AR, Carter Z, Legua P, Bustamante B, Micheletti RG (2017) Bedside diagnostics in dermatology: viral, bacterial, and fungal infections. J Am Acad Dermatol 77(2):197–218
9. Winsett FT, Patel SG, Kelly BC (2020) Bedside diagnostics for infections: a guide for dermatologists. Am J Clin Dermatol 21(5):697–709

Therapy

28

Branka Marinović, Zrinka Bukvić Mokos, and Alexander Salava

Contents

B. Marinović (✉) · Z. Bukvić Mokos
Department of Dermatology and Venereology, School of Medicine University of Zagreb, Zagreb, Croatia
e-mail: branka.marinovic@kbc-zagreb.hr

A. Salava
Department of Dermatology and Allergology, Helsinki University Hospital, Helsinki, Finland
e-mail: alexander.salava@hus.fi

H. Gollnick et al. (eds.), *Dermatology Cyberderm WebBook*,
https://doi.org/10.1007/978-3-031-78491-0_28

Test your learning and check your understanding of this book's contents: use the "Springer Nature Flashcards" app to access questions using ▶ https://sn.pub/1rhh6k.

To use the app, please follow the instructions in Chap. 1.

Principles of Galenic Formulations for Topical Drugs [4, 8, 10]

Grading of Importance

No grading

Level

Basic

Definition

Topical therapies are a main stay in treatment in dermatology. It involves the external application of a drug on the affected skin. Topical agents consist of one or more active ingredients in a vehicle (non-active base). In topical therapy, choosing a proper vehicle can be as important as choosing a suitable active ingredient.

Main Principles

When using topical therapy, the following factors should be considered:
- Active ingredients
- Vehicle, preservatives, and stabilizers
- Correct mode of application
- Condition of the skin to be treated (acute, subacute, chronic)

The goal of most topical drugs is penetration through the stratum corneum (SC) and upper dermis with direct action to the skin. Penetration through the SC is accomplished by a transepidermal or transappendageal pathway. There are several steps in this process. In each step, it is essential that the active ingredient is more soluble or driven by concentration gradient, enabling the active substance to penetrate the skin.

Glossary of Important Terms

- Liberation – the release of the active ingredient from the vehicle
- Adsorption – binding of the active ingredient to skin structures (i.e., stratum corneum)
- Absorption – uptake of the active ingredient from the vehicle
- Penetration – passage through the stratum corneum
- Permeation – transepidermal and transfollicular passage of active substances throughout the skin
- Resorption – the uptake of topically applied substances with transfer to blood vessels or lymphatics

Factors That Affect Percutaneous Absorption

These include:
- Thickness and integrity of the SC (a thicker SC decreases absorption)
- Anatomic location (the absorption is highest on mucous membranes, scrotum, and eyelids and lowest on palms and soles)
- Skin hydration (increased hydration increases absorption)
- Patient's age (higher absorption in neonates because of their suboptimal skin barrier)

- Occlusion with airtight dressings and greasy ointment bases, which increase percutaneous absorption

Ingredients of Topical Drugs

Topical medications consist of one or more active ingredients combined with a vehicle. The vehicle contains a base to which may be added preservatives, stabilizers, emulsifiers, fragrances, and other products.

Vehicles

The choice of vehicle is one of the critical tasks in topical prescribing, as it is very important for determining the pharmacokinetics (i.e., the active ingredient must be more soluble in the outer layer of SC than in the vehicle, or diffusion will not start).

Vehicles are divided into two groups:

- Liquid (solutions, emulsions, shake lotions)
- Semi-solid vehicles (gels, creams, ointments, and paste)

Most used types of vehicles:

- Cream – two forms: oil in water and water in oil
- Lotion – thin cream, easier to apply
- Solution – alcoholic vehicle
- Ointment – greasy and occlusive
- Gel – semi-solid – converts to liquid when rubbed into the skin
- Paste – ointment + powder – protective
- Shake lotion – water and powder

Ointments are used for dry skin; creams are most commonly used; gels and lotions are used when an easy application is preferred and for the scalp and hairy parts of the body.

Active Therapy

Active ingredients are added to the vehicle. Ideally, the product should contain only one active ingredient, but in some cases, two or more active ingredients can be combined. The most commonly used active substances in dermatotherapy are the following:

- Antiseptics - used against different microbials.
- Antibiotics – used against superficial bacterial infections. As resistance to antibiotics is increasing in recent years, topical antibiotics are not always effective in the treatment of superficial bacterial infections.
- Antifungals – act by attaching to the cellular walls of fungi, inhibiting biosynthesis.

- Antivirals.
- Antiparasitics
- Corticosteroids – very commonly used in dermatology to reduce inflammation, by vasoconstriction, diminution of membrane permeability, inhibition of inflammatory chemical mediators, immunosuppression and inhibition of cell division. Topical steroids are *classified by strength* from high potency steroids to the mild ones. They should be given carefully to avoid *side effects*, i.e., skin atrophy, striae distensae, steroid acne, rosacea-like dermatitis, hypertrichosis, etc.
- Topical hormonal treatments.
- Calcineurin inhibitors.
- Immunosuppressants.
- Immunomodulators.
- Cytostatics.
- Retinoids.
- Vitamin D analogs.
- Keratolytics.

Prescribing

Currently there are many different commercially available products with a standard, fixed combination of active ingredient(s) and vehicle. However, some dermatologists prescribe variable, personalized compound prescriptions which may have some advantage for individual needs of the patient. An advantage of this is the possibility of individualized adjustment of the dose and vehicle.

Application of Topical Drugs

Topical preparations are applied to the skin most commonly once or twice daily. The patient should be prescribed an adequate quantity of the topical drug to be able to follow recommendations. For the entire body, about 30 g of the cream is needed. It can be easily quantified using the measure of "fingertip unit" (the amount of ointment or cream expressed from a tube with a 5 mm diameter nozzle, applied from the distal skin-crease to the tip of the index finger of an adult) which is equal to ca. 0.5 g.

Future Directions

Topical JAK inhibitors have been examined in the treatment of alopecia areata, atopic dermatitis, vitiligo, and psoriasis. Topical phosphodiesterase 4 (PDE4) inhibitors have shown promising results in the treatment of mild to moderate atopic dermatitis.

Pharmacologic Basics of Systemic Therapy in Dermatology [9]

Grading of Importance

No grading

Level

Basic

Introduction

Systemic therapy is required in many dermatological, allergic, and venereal diseases when topical treatment is not sufficient. Use of systemic therapy has increased in the last decades, especially after introducing new agents in dermatological therapy (i.e., biologicals, small molecules). Before introducing therapy, it is mandatory to establish a correct diagnosis, evaluate potential contraindications, and consider possible side effects including drug interactions during the treatment.

Antibiotics

Antibiotics are used to treat infectious skin and venereal diseases and some other diseases due to their antimicrobial, anti-inflammatory, and immunomodulatory effects. In infectious diseases, antibiotics should be prescribed according to the infection type (typing of resistance pattern) and according to the spectrum of action. Antimicrobial resistance development should be avoided whenever possible (definite indication, avoid broad-spectrum antibiotics). *Indications*: primary (i.e., disseminated impetigo contagiosa, Lyme disease) and secondary (i.e., severely impetiginized eczema), deep bacterial infections of the skin as well as venereal diseases (i.e., syphilis, gonorrhea), primarily noninfectious, but pathogen-associated diseases (i.e., severe acne), primarily nonpathogen-associated skin diseases (i.e., nodular rosacea).

Antihistamines

Antihistamines are competitive antagonists acting on the histamine receptor. In dermatology, most commonly used are H1 blockers as they are indicated for the treatment and the prophylaxis of allergic and pseudoallergic reactions. First-generation H1 blockers had sedative side-effects, which has been avoided in the second-generation antihistamines which do not cross the blood-brain barrier. *Indications* include urticaria, allergic rhinitis, and conjunctivitis; intravenously administered antihistamines are the mainstay of the initial treatment of anaphylaxis.

Antimycotics

Systemic antimycotics are used in the treatment of widespread or deep localized dermatomycoses as well as mycotic infections that affect hair and nails. Most commonly used groups of antimycotics are azole-type antifungals (i.e., fluconazole, itraconazole for the treatment of dermatophytes and yeasts) and allylamine derivates (i.e., terbinafine for the treatment of dermatophytoses). Griseofulvin is still used in the treatment of dermatophytoses.

Glucocorticoids

Glucocorticoids are the most widely used drugs in dermatology. Their main *mode of action* are anti-inflammatory, immunosuppressive, and antiproliferative. Glucocorticosteroids are *indicated* in the therapy of inflammatory dermatoses, autoimmune dermatoses, granulomatous dermatoses, and other diseases that are not classified in one of these three groups. They are absolutely contraindicated in active untreated tuberculosis, systemic mycoses, and ocular herpes simplex. The list of relative *contraindications* is much broader, including chronic gastritis, esophagitis and gastrointestinal bleeding, severe osteoporosis, glaucoma, depression, etc. In those patients, glucocorticosteroids can be introduced if needed but with special prophylactic measures. Most common *side effects* are diabetes mellitus, hypertension, increased susceptibility to infections, osteoporosis, aseptic bone necrosis, gastrointestinal bleeding, etc.

Retinoids

Retinoids include derivatives of vitamin A acid and substances with different chemical structures but related biological activities. They belong to the steroids superfamily.

Five groups of retinoids are available for the use in dermatology:

- Acitretin
- Alitretinoin
- Bexarotene
- Isotretinoin and
- Tretinoin

The most common *indications* for use are psoriasis, palmoplantar hyperkeratosis, pityriasis rubra pilaris (PRP), and lichen planus for acitretin; refractory hand eczema for alitretinoin; cutaneous T-cell lymphomas for bexarotene; and severe and refractory forms of acne for isotretinoin. *Contraindications*: familial and clinically relevant acquired lipid metabolic disorders, simultaneous administration of tetracyclines, severe diabetes, pregnancy or plans to become pregnant and breastfeeding due to teratogenicity. Contraceptive care measures should be followed seriously.

Antimetabolites

The two most important antimetabolites in systemic dermatological therapy are methotrexate and azathioprine. *Methotrexate* has a cytotoxic and immunomodulatory function. It is indicated in severe psoriasis, psoriatic arthritis, dermatomyositis, morphea, and some other dermatoses. It is usually prescribed once a week orally or subcutaneously. Contraindications for the therapy are pregnancy and lactation, acute infection, bone marrow depression, and liver diseases. To avoid MTX overdose, folic acid should be given orally in parallel. *Azathioprine* is a cytotoxic agent used as an immunosuppressant. Main indications are autoimmune blistering diseases (in combination with glucocorticoids – as steroid-sparing agents). Other indications include vasculitis, lupus erythematosus, and pyoderma gangrenosum.

Antimalarials

Chloroquine and hydroxychloroquine are most commonly given in dermatology for the treatment of cutaneous and systemic lupus erythematosus. Glucose-6-phosphate dehydrogenase deficiency should be excluded before introducing therapy. *Contraindication* for introducing the drug is retinopathy, visual field restrictions, pregnancy, and lactation. Ophthalmological consultations should be done before starting the treatment and in most patients after five years, in risk groups every year.

Dapsone

Dapsone is an antibacterial and anti-inflammatory drug, in dermatology most commonly used to treat dermatitis herpetiformis, linear IgA dermatosis, and nodular vasculitis. Glucose-6-phosphate dehydrogenase deficiency should be excluded before introducing therapy. Methemoglobin should be checked regularly; hemolytic anemia and agranulocytosis can occur.

Biologics and Small Molecules

Biologics are monoclonal antibodies which target specific proteins involved in the pathogenesis of various dermatological diseases, including psoriasis and metastatic melanoma. Small molecules are agents with a low molecular weight that can pass through cell membranes to modulate intracellular targets. They are most commonly used in the treatment of psoriasis and atopic dermatitis.

Basics of Dermatosurgery Techniques [1, 3, 6]

Grading of Importance

No grading

Level

Basic

Definition

Dermato-surgery refers to surgical procedures involving mainly the skin, its appendages, and the underlying subcutaneous fat and fascia. These may be performed in outpatient or inpatient settings and are mostly performed using local anesthesia.

Indications for Dermato-surgery

Dermato-surgery is indicated for obtaining a skin biopsy for histopathological analysis, for removal of malignant tumors of the skin or for removal of benign skin lesions because of local symptoms including hidradenitis or sweat gland removal or for cosmetic purposes, for therapy of varicosis (stripping), for wound care (transplantation), and for hair transplantation.

Different Types of Procedures (Dermato-surgery Techniques)

Different techniques are used in the surgical management of benign and malignant skin lesions. The most frequently used techniques include incisional biopsy, punch biopsy, shave biopsy, primary excision, with primary closure, shave excision, curettage, electrosurgery (e.g., diathermy, coagulation, cautery). In addition, more advanced techniques comprise Mohs micrographic surgery, complex reconstruction using flap procedures, and skin grafting. A combination of different techniques is often necessary.

The choice of technique depends primarily on purpose (e.g., diagnostic or therapeutic), the diagnosis (benign or malignant), local spread and growth (superficial or infiltrating), and the size and anatomical site of the lesion. Patient profile (age, comorbidity, drugs) and preference combined with the expertise of the surgeon are also very important factors.

Incisional Biopsy (Including Punch Biopsy)

The object is to obtain a diagnostic full-thickness skin specimen for histopathology. It may involve the use of a scalpel (elliptic excisional biopsy; see below) or a cylindrical blade attached to a handle (i.e., punch biopsy). It is best to choose a lesion of recent onset, or the most abnormal-looking edge of an enlarging lesion for a diagnostic biopsy.

Skin lesions suitable for punch biopsy include all kinds of skin tumors and precancerous lesions. It should however not be used for larger melanocytic lesions or those which are showing clinical atypia, which should be excised. The chosen site should be marked and infiltrated with a local anesthetic. Stretch the skin perpendicular to the skin tension lines so that the punch defect will have an elliptical shape. The punch is held vertically over the skin and rotated down until the subcutaneous tissue (visible fat tissue). The specimen is then removed and gently handled to prevent crush artifacts. A separate punch biopsy may be taken from perilesional skin for direct immunofluorescence (e.g., to diagnose autoimmune blistering diseases). Wound closure is usually accomplished by using a single interrupted suture and hemostasis is ensured by pressure and bandage. Skin specimens should always be sent to histopathology.

Shave Biopsy

The technique is similar to shave excision (see below) with the difference that the main purpose is to obtain a specimen for histopathology.

Shave Excision and Curettage

Lesions growing mainly above the skin surface can be shaved off as a tangential excision using a scalpel blade or razor blade. Curettage refers to the use of a sharp spoon-shaped instrument to scrape off a superficial skin lesion. Light cautery or other methods of hemostasis (e.g., iron nitrate solution) are used, and the wound is left to heal by secondary intention. Examples of skin lesions that may be removed this way include skin tags, filiform viral warts and seborrheic keratosis. The technique may result in unsightly scars and lesions may recur. In some cases curettage may be followed by cryotherapy or photodynamic therapy.

Primary Excision

Firstly, it is important to identify the margins of the lesion in good light and to mark out with a surgical pen a fusiform or elliptical shape around the lesion. Its form should be two to three times as long as it is wide and follow the skin tension lines (Langer lines). Thereafter inject a local anesthetic, (usually 1% lidocaine with adrenaline) using a fine needle into the superficial dermis. Wash the surgical area with an antiseptic solution (e.g., alcohol), and apply surgical guards for an aseptic technique. It is important to stabilize the incision area by traction with the fingers. By applying controlled pressure on the scalpel, carry out the cut along marked lines vertically with the angle of the blade. It is usually necessary to cut until the subcutaneous tissue and remove the specimen. The specimen should be placed entirely in a labeled vessel and numbered. It may be necessary to use the scalpel or scissors to undermine the skin edge below the dermis. This will loosen the overlying skin and decrease tension.

Complex Reconstruction Using Flap Procedure

Complex reconstructions using different flap techniques are used in situations where primary closure is not possible, e.g., due to large excisions or anatomical sites where tension may cause functional impairment. Local, regional, or distant flaps can be used, and there are many different techniques available (advancement flap, rotation flap, transposition flap). The basic principle is to reconstruct a skin defect with a lifted skin flap from a donor site and move it to a recipient site with an intact blood supply.

Skin Grafting

Comparable to complex reconstructions using flaps, skin grafts are used to cover large or complex excisional defects. Skin grafting involves the transplantation of skin, usually from the same patient but from another anatomical site. Typical donor sites are the preauricular region or the lateral thigh. The transplanted tissue does not have an intact blood supply and therefore relies on growth of new blood vessels. Principally, there are two types of skin grafts: split thickness skin graft (removal of a thin layer of skin from donor site to close a defect) and full-thickness skin graft (punching or cutting whole skin away from the donor site to close small defects or to treat vitiligo or to transplant hair).

Mohs' Micrographic Surgery

Mohs' micrographic surgery is a surgical technique in which the complete excision of skin cancer is controlled by microscopically controlled margins. The technique is used in situations where high cure rates with maximizing preservation of healthy tissue is needed, e.g., high-risk basal cell carcinomas on the face. Here, the skin cancer is gradually removed in stepwise phases. After each phase of excision, the margins are immediately microscopically examined for remaining cancer cells, and this process is repeated until full removal of all cancer cells. Several other techniques are used for the removal of tissue (fresh versus fixed tissue technique).

Electrosurgery

Electrosurgery is used for hemostasis and desiccation of tissue using high frequency (0.1–1 MHz currents). Methods include electrodesiccation (cautery, contact of electrode with skin, deeper tissue injury), electrocoagulation (diathermy, bipolar forceps, mostly hemostasis), and electrosection (undamped wave, cutting without hemostasis or adjacent tissue injury). Benign lesions can easily be scraped off when light electrodessication is used first. Electrosurgery destroys tissue and prevents accurate histopathological examination. *Cave*: Ask about the presence of a cardiac pacemaker.

Local Anesthesia

Local anesthesia involves the use of topical anesthetics and injections of local anesthetics directly into the tissue (infiltration) or into the vicinity of peripheral nerves (nerve blocks). Topical anesthesia may be useful for small procedures, e.g., scissor snipping of skin tags. The anesthetic cream is applied 1–2 h before the procedure (e.g., eutectic mixture of prilocaine and lidocaine, cream, or plaster). Most skin procedures require an subdermal anesthetic, such as lidocaine (xylocaine). After injection the onset of action is rapid in a few minutes and lasts 1–3 h. The addition of adrenaline 1:100,000 extends duration and may control bleeding (but avoid adrenalin in acral lesions).

Hemostasis

Methods of hemostasis for superficial bleedings include local pressure and hemostatic solutions (e.g., iron or aluminum chloride) applied with cotton tips. In deeper bleeding, typically after excisions with primary closure or more complex reconstructions using flap procedures, pinpoint diathermy is used.

Suturing

For wound closure there are several techniques. The most used is a single-layer closure using simple interrupted sutures tied using the needle holder. The stitches should be arranged equally on each side including at the least the whole dermis. The surgical knot is tightened so that the edges of the wound are lightly in contact to avoid scarring. In some sites a continuous suture may provide more satisfactory cosmetic results. Deeper and larger wounds may require subcutaneous sutures to eliminate dead space (e.g., hematoma and infection risk).

After suturing, light pressure should be applied to ensure that the bleeding has completely stopped. Thereafter the wound should be cleaned and dressings should be applied. In most cases the first dressing should be removed after 1–2 days. Sutures should be removed after the procedure depending on body site, the size of the wound, and the amount of tension on it (e.g., face 5–7 days, arms and trunk 7–10 days, lower legs 10–14 days).

Complications

Typical complications after skin surgery are wound infections, hematoma formation, wound dehiscence, and scarring. Scar formation can cause cosmetic problems but also have functional impairments (contractures of joints, ectropion of the eye lid). In rare cases peripheral nerve damage may lead to paresthesia and impairment of motoric innervation (eye lid ptosis).

Prevention of Complications

Procedures should be performed in aseptic circumstances to avoid wound infections. Based on patient risk factors, prophylactic systemic antibiotics are sometimes administered. Hematoma formation can be prevented by meticulous hemostasis and risk management of possible anticoagulant drugs. Wound dehiscence and scarring is best prevented by minimizing tension of the excisional defect and adequate suturing techniques.

Scarring

To reduce scarring after dermato-surgery excisions should be performed in right angles to the muscle pull directions or parallel to skin tension lines (Langer lines). Scars are at first red and firm, but usually after some months, the induration and erythema reduce leaving a softer scar that is paler than the nearby skin. Scars may stretch if there is wound tension. There is an increased risk of scarring if the patient has had prior hypertrophic scars or keloids (consider ethnic susceptibility), if the direction of the scar is not parallel to natural lines and in some high-risk anatomical sites (upper sternum, shoulders, joints). Visible scarring may also be evident if complications like hematoma formation, wound infection, or wound dehiscence occur after the procedure.

Basics of Ultraviolet Radiation Therapy and Lasers [2, 5, 7]

Grading of Importance

No grading

Level

Basic

Synonyms

- Ultraviolet (UV) radiation therapy: phototherapy
- Photochemotherapy (PUVA)
- Photodynamic therapy: photoradiation therapy
- Extracorporeal photopheresis
- Laser (light amplification by stimulated emission of radiation)

Definition

The following physical radiation methods should be reserved for medical specialists routinely dealing with the diseases described below.

UV radiation therapy (phototherapy) consists in the use of UVB/A light in the treatment of skin diseases.

Photochemotherapy consists in the use of UVA light and oral or topical photosensitizer of the psoralen type.

Photodynamic therapy consists in a photochemical reaction, which requires the presence of a photosensitizing molecule, photoactivating wavelengths of light and tissue oxygen.

Extracorporeal photopheresis consists of extracorporeal exposure of patient's blood immune cells, psoralens and UVA.

Laser therapy consists in the emission of coherent radiations using unique light sources rooted in the process of stimulated emission. Different laser types with different wave lengths emissions.

Radiofrequency consists in an oscillation rate of an alternating electric current or voltage or of a magnetic, electric, or electromagnetic field or mechanical system in the frequency range 20 kHz–300 GHz.

Soft and hard X-rays are X-rays with high photon energies (above 5–10 keV, below 0.2–0.1 nm wavelength) defines hard X-rays and while those with lower energy and longer wavelength, soft X-rays. Hard X-rays are widely used to image the inside of objects for their penetrating ability in medical radiography. Soft X-ray irradiation is usually used to treat skin-related diseases (including non-melanoma skin cancer and cutaneous lymphomas).

Modes of Action

UVB phototherapy (broadband: 290–320 nm; narrowband: 311–313 nm; excimer laser: 308 nm) refers to the use of artificial UVB radiation without the addition of exogenous photosensitizers. The radiation is absorbed by endogenous chromophores, and the subsequent photochemical reactions cause a variety of biologic effects, ultimately leading to the therapeutic effects. The most important chromophore for UVB is DNA photoproducts, in particular pyrimidine dimers. UVB exposure reduces DNA synthesis and induces the expression of the tumor suppressor gene p53, with a subsequent cell cycle arrest or apoptosis of keratinocytes if the damage is too severe to be repaired. In addition, UV radiation exerts immunomodulatory activities.

UVA phototherapy (320–400 nm) is subdivided in UVA1 (340–400 nm) and UVA2 (320–340 nm). UVA2 is similar to UVB in the ability to cause erythema as well as immunomodulation and photocarcinogenesis. UVA1 radiation, because of the longer wavelength, penetrates more deeply into the skin layers, and consequently not only the epidermis but also dermis and blood vessels.

Photochemotherapy with psoralens (PUVA) combines the use of psoralens (P) and long-wave radiation (UVA). Psoralens can be administered orally or topically in solutions, creams, or baths, with subsequent UVA exposure. This combination results in a therapeutic phototoxic and immunomodulating effect.

Extracorporeal photochemotherapy (photopheresis) consists in the induction of an immune response against malignant cells (e.g., circulating cutaneous T-cell lymphoma cells), downregulation of graft vs host reaction on host immune cells and solid organ transplantation reactions. This acts throughout the induction of the generation of antigen-specific regulatory T-cells.

Photodynamic therapy is a photochemical reaction throughout the use of a photosensitizing molecule, which may be administered systemically as intact macrocycles or topically as pro-photosensitizers, which are metabolized to photoactive molecules (protoporphyrin).

Laser therapy can be delivered in continuous and pulsed waves. The specificity of each laser is characterized by a destruction of specific target structured of the skin, with limited damage of surrounding tissues, via utilization of a wavelength of light preferentially absorbed by the target.

Non-ablative radiofrequency is a procedure commonly used in skin aging for the treatment of skin laxity and wrinkles from an increase in tissue temperature. The main physiological effect is to induce thermal damage to thus stimulate neocollagenesis in deep layers of the skin and subcutaneous tissues.

***Soft and hard X-rays*:** hard X-rays are widely used to image the inside of objects for their penetrating ability in medical radiography. Soft X-ray irradiation is usually used to treat skin-related diseases (including non-melanoma skin cancer and cutaneous lymphomas).

Main indications

***nbUVB*:** psoriasis, mycosis fungoides, vitiligo, atopic dermatitis, graft-versus-host-disease (GVHD), pityriasis lichenoides, lymphomatoid papulosis, seborrheic dermatitis.

***UVA1*:** localized scleroderma, chronic sclerodermoid GVHD, urticaria pigmentosa, cutaneous T-cell lymphoma (CTCL).

***PUVA*:** psoriasis, mycosis fungoides, atopic dermatitis, lichen planus, GVHD, miscellaneous dermatoses.

***Photopheresis*:** Sezary syndrome, erythrodermic CTCL, acute and chronic GVHD after allogeneic stem cell transplantation.

***Photodynamic therapy*:** neoplasias, such as actinic keratosis, actinic cheilitis, in situ and invasive squamous cell carcinoma, basal cell carcinoma, mycosis fungoides, Paget's disease, port-wine stains; acne, porokeratosis, leishmanias, photodamage.

***Laser therapy*:** Vascular lesions: pulsed eye, variable-pulsed potassium titanyl phosphate (Nd:YAG), long-pulsed alexandrite, long-pulsed diode, long-pulsed Nd:YAG, intense pulsed light; endovascular application throughout diode laser, Nd:YAG, radiofrequency energy source. Pigmented lesions and tattoo removal: Q-switched lasers such as Q-switched Nd:YAG, frequency-doubled, Q-switched ruby, Q-switched alexandrite, Q-switched Nd:YAG; long-pulsed lasers and intense pulsed light such as long-pulsed ruby, diode, Nd:YAG, intense pulsed light source. Laser hair removal with long-pulsed lasers such as ruby, alexandrite, Nd:YAG (moderate efficacy), and diode (high efficacy); with intense pulsed light source (low efficacy). Laser skin resurfacing superficial (non-ablative): vascular lasers such as pulse dye and pulsed potassium-titanyl-phosphate laser; mid dermis with infrared lasers or intense pulsed light; deep dermis (ablative lasers): carbon dioxide lasers (pulsed and scanned-continuous wave) and erbium:YAG laser.

Adverse Effects

UV light: depending on UVB range, erythema peak with 313 nm. Acute: itchy or painful erythema, burns with blistering, increased recurrence of herpes simplex viral infections.

UVA and UVB can induce persisting cell mutations, skin cancer risk. Chronic: xerosis, photoaging, carcinomas (basal-cell carcinoma).

PUVA therapy: long-term risk of skin cancer, PUVA freckles, gastrointestinal intolerability for psoralens. Photodynamic therapy and laser therapy may be painful depending on area and dosing.

References

1. Ashraf I, Butt E, Veitch D, Wernham A (2021) Dermatological surgery: an update on suture materials and techniques. Part 1. Clin Exp Dermatol 46(8):1400–1410
2. Boord M (2006) Laser in dermatology. Clin Tech Small Anim Pract 21(3):145–149
3. Butt E, Ashraf I, Veitch D, Wernham A (2021) Dermatological surgery: an update on suture materials and techniques. Part 2. Clin Exp Dermatol 46(8):1411–1419
4. Daniels R, Knie U (2007) Galenics of dermal products--vehicles, properties and drug release. J Dtsch Dermatol Ges 5(5):367–383

5. Grimes DR (2015) Ultraviolet radiation therapy and UVR dose models. Med Phys 42(1):440–455
6. Hafner J, Löser C, Roka F (2023) Dermatosurgery - from surgical option to integral part of dermatologic therapy. J Dtsch Dermatol Ges. 21(4):355–358
7. Singer S, Berneburg M (2018) Phototherapy. J Dtsch Dermatol Ges 16(9):1120–1129
8. Straube MD, Zesch A (2004) Current guidelines applicable for the approval of topically applied dermatological drugs in the EU. Fundam Clin Pharmacol 18(5):503–511
9. Wakelin S, Maibach H, Archer C (2023) Handbook of systemic drug treatment in dermatology. CRP Press
10. Wohlrab J (2016) Topical preparations and their use in dermatology. J Dtsch Dermatol Ges 14(11):1061–1070

Part X

Neglected Tropical Dermatoses (NTD'S)

NTDs have been defined by the World Health Organization (WHO). They include bacterial, viral, fungal, and parasitic infections that principally affect over 1 billion people of poor low-income and medically underserved countries in tropical and subtropical regions of the world, where they have a high socioeconomic impact.

Bacterial Infections

29

Günter Burg, Martine Bagot, Veronique del Marmol, Gabor Dobos, Giampiero Girolomoni, Paolo Gisondi, and Martina Maurelli

Contents

G. Burg (✉)
Dermatology, Zurich, Switzerland
e-mail: g.burg@access.uzh.ch

M. Bagot
Service de Dermatologie, Université Paris Cité, Hôpital Saint-Louis, Paris, France
e-mail: martine.bagot@gmail.com

V. del Marmol
Départment of Dermatology, Hôpital Erasme-HUB, Université Libre de Bruxelles, Brussels, Belgium
e-mail: veronique.delmarmol@hubruxelles.be

G. Dobos
Dermatology and Venereology, Hopital Saint Louis, Université de Paris, Paris, France
e-mail: gabor.dobos@charite.de

G. Girolomoni · P. Gisondi · M. Maurelli
Department of Medicine, Università degli Studi di Verona, Verona, Italy
e-mail: giampiero.girolomoni@univr.it; paolo.gisondi@univr.it

H. Gollnick et al. (eds.), *Dermatology Cyberderm WebBook*,
https://doi.org/10.1007/978-3-031-78491-0_29

Test your learning and check your understanding of this book's contents: use the "Springer Nature Flashcards" app to access questions using ▶ https://sn.pub/1rhh6k.
To use the app, please follow the instructions in Chap. 1.

Buruli Ulcer (BU) [3, 12]

Figures 29.1 and 29.2

Grading of Importance

B

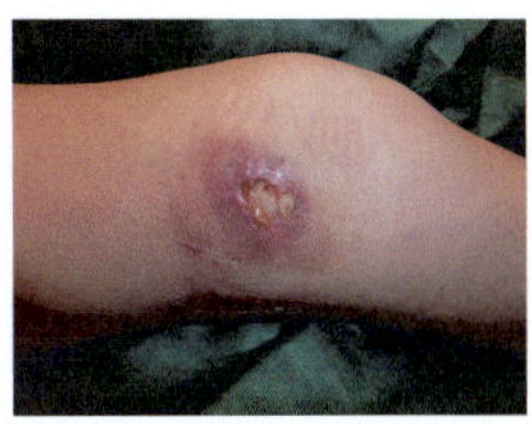

Fig. 29.1 Buruli ulcer: knee (courtesy of Dr DN Friedman, Australia)

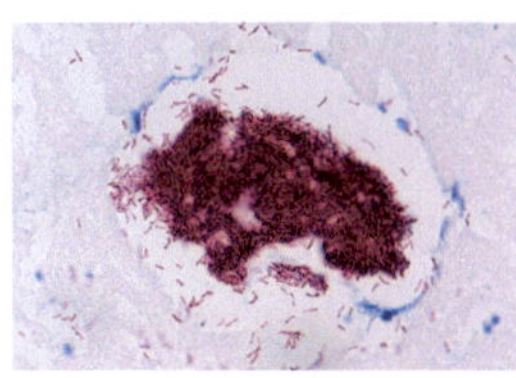

Fig. 29.2 Buruli ulcer: Mycobacterium ulcerans (courtesy of Dr DN Friedman, Australia)

Level

Special

ICD-11

1B21.20

Synonyms

Mycobacterium ulcerans infection

Epidemiology

West Africa (>70% of global incidence; 50% of cases are children) and some other tropical or subtropical countries. Sporadic imported cases in moderate climate zones.

Definition

Necrotizing and disabling cutaneous disease caused by *Mycobacterium ulcerans*

Etiology and Pathogenesis

Infection with *M. ulcerans* probably comes from stagnant or slowly moving water; no evidence for human-to-human transmission. Some evidence for mosquitoes as a potential passive vector for *M. ulcerans* has been reported in some areas. Responsible for the extensive ulceration is an exotoxin called mycolactone, a polyketide-derived macrolide that is synthesized by the *M. ulcerans* bacteria.

Signs and Symptoms

BU starts with a papule, nodule, plaque, or edematous lesion, progressing to extensive painless ulcer with irregular borders. General health is not affected.

The ulcer grows rapidly with undermined borders. Within 3 weeks to 1 year of evolution, tendons and bone can be involved, leading to osteomyelitis. Most of the time, there is a single lesion; however, small satellite lesions can be present.

Localization

Exposed body areas, like limbs or face

Classification

None

Laboratory and Other Workups

Acid-fast bacilli in smears or histopathology. Cultering is difficult. Real-time PCR.

Dermatopathology

Hyperplastic epidermis, necrosis, and inflammation. Staining for acid-fast bacilli.

Course

Chronic leading to disabilities and deformities if not treated. Large scars and contractures leading to functional impairment may further happen due to prolonged ulceration, even under and after adequate treatment.

Complications

Without or delayed antibiotic therapy, patients could be left with life-long disabilities and deformities. Paradoxical reaction is the worsening of symptoms during effective antibiotic treatment. Secondary bacterial infections, producing a foul smell.

Psychosocial sequelae due to disfiguration.

Diagnosis

Diagnosis relies on clinical, socioeconomic, and geographic facts.

Differential Diagnosis

Limb ulcers due to other etiologies.

Prevention and Therapy

Vaccination with *Mycobacterium bovis* bacillus Calmette-Guérin (BCG) vaccination has been tried but mostly is uneffective. The best preventative measures are to be careful in risky environments (swimming, fishing) in endemic areas.

Rifampicin (10 mg/kg orally once daily) and streptomycin (15 mg/kg intramuscularly once daily; cave nephrotoxicity and ototoxicity, especially in children) for 8 weeks.

Thorough wound management.

Leprosy* [1, 7, 11]

Grading of Importance

B

Level

special

ICD-11

1B20.Z
1B20.0 Paucibacillary (tuberculoid)
1B20.1 Multibacillary (lepromatous)
1B20.2 Leprosy reactions
1B20.3 Complications of leprosy

Synonyms

Hansen's disease

Epidemiology

Worldwide, about 720,000 new cases of leprosy are registered each year and about 2 million people suffer from leprosy-related disabilities, predominantly in India, Brazil, Indonesia, Democratic Republic of Congo, Tanzania, Angola, Central African Republic, Myanmar, Madagascar, Nepal, Mozambique, and the Philippines (90% of all new cases).

Age peak between 10 and 20. After puberty, there are twice as many cases in males as in females.

Definition

Leprosy is a chronic minimally contagious, granulomatous disease caused by *Mycobacterium leprae*, primarily affecting the peripheral nerves and skin. Incubation period 3–20 years.

Etiology and Pathogenesis

Mycobacterium leprae, which can survive outside human hosts for many months, is an obligate intracellular gram-positive acid-fast bacillus. *M. leprae* from the nasal mucosa spreads via the recipient's nasal mucosa to skin and nerves. The organism can survive outside human hosts for many months. Household contact with a person with leprosy is a strong risk factor for infection. There seems to be little evidence for the impact of an association with HIV infection, nutrition, or socioeconomic status.

Signs and Symptoms

The clinical picture depends on the individual's immune response to *M. leprae* according to the Ridley-Jopling scale:

- Tuberculoid leprosy: good cell-mediated immunity and few skin lesions
- Lepromatous leprosy: low reactivity for *M. leprae*, causing uncontrolled bacterial spread and skin and mucosal infiltration

  Skin: poorly defined hypopigmented or erythematous macules in early lesions.
- Tuberculoid leprosy: single or very few scaly, dry, and hairless macules or plaques with central flattening and well-defined edges. In dark skin lesions are hypopigmented rather erythematous, which is found in lighter skin. Reduced sensation and loss of sweating.
- Lepromatous leprosy: widely and symmetrically distributed, poorly defined hypopigmented or erythematous macules. Papules and nodules (leproma) may be present. Peripheral edema of the legs and ankles due to increased stasis. The skin of the face and especially at the ear lobes gets thicker due to dermal infiltration, featuring a leonine face. Eyelashes and eyebrows lose their hair.
- Borderline leprosy: skin lesions intermediate between the two polar tuberculoid and the lepromatous forms. They may be macular, papulonodular, plaque-like, annular, or large geographic.

  Nerves: sensory, motor, and autonomic function of peripheral nerves are affected.
- Nerve damage may occur before, during, or after treatment across the total spectrum of the disease. Some people have no nerve damage, while others develop

anesthesia of the hands and feet, putting them at risk of developing neuropathic injuries, with loss of the fingers and toes, due to repeated injury.

- Weakness and paralysis of the small muscles of the hands, feet, and eyes puts people at risk of developing deformity and contractures.
- Palpable thickening of nerves (e.g., ulnar), impaired sensation, motor and sensory problems (muscle atrophy), neuropathic ulcers.
- Eye involvement: lagophthalmia, uveitis, cataract, corneal involvement, optic neuropathy, diffuse involvement (panophthalmia leprosa), which can lead to loss of vision and blindness.

Localization

Hypopigmented macules with sensitivity loss can occur anywhere on the body. Leproma nodules are frequently located on the face, ears or hands.

Most commonly involved are the posterior tibial nerve, leading to anesthesia on the soles of the feet followed by the ulnar, median, lateral popliteal, and facial nerves.

Classification

There are two systems used for classification of leprosy:

- The Ridley-Jopling system is based on clinical (number of skin lesions; the WHO) and histopathological features. It spans from indeterminate leprosy (IL, potential initial stage), tuberculoid leprosy (TT), to lepromatous leprosy (LL) and borderline leprosy (spectrum of transient forms, BT, BL, BB):
  - Single lesion leprosy
  - Two to five skin lesions (paucibacillary leprosy)
  - More than 5 skin lesions (multibacillary leprosy)
- The bacteriologic index of lesions reflects the density of leprae bacilli in the smear. It uses a logarithmic scale and ranges from 0 (no bacilli in any of the 100× oil immersion fields) to 6+ (more than 1000 bacilli, on an average, in each oil-immersion field).

Laboratory and Other Workups

- Determination of the bacteriologic index in smears.
- Skin biopsy.
- A polymerase chain reaction in skin can be used to identify *Mycobacterium leprae* but can be negative in tuberculoid forms without ruling out the diagnosis.

Dermatopathology

- *Tuberculoid leprosy*: granulomas surrounding neurovascular elements and extend into the papillary dermis. Acid-fast bacilli are not seen.
- *Lepromatous leprosy:* atrophic epidermis with loss of the rete ridges. The papillary dermis is free, whereas the deeper dermis is diffusely infiltrated with macrophages (Virchow cells), lymphocytes, and plasma cells. Abundant acid-fast bacilli singly or in clumps.
- *Borderline leprosy*: small granulomas becoming more diffuse from borderline tuberculoid (BT) to borderline lepromatous (BL) disease.
- *Histoid leprosy*: This is a variant of lepromatous leprosy occurring in patients with lepromatous leprosy and inadequate or irregular therapy. Histology shows interlacing bundles of spindle-shaped fusiform histiocytes in the dermis arranged in storiform or crisscross pattern.

Course

Tuberculoid infection may resolve spontaneously, whereas borderline status gradually develop lepromatous infection.

Complications

- Complications of leprosy include nerve damage, immunological reactions, and bacillary infiltration.
- Immune-mediated reactions may induce further nerve damage and neuritis:
  - Type 1: type IV immunologic reaction; flare-up of old skin lesions and neuritis. Occurs during therapy.
  - Type 2: type III immunologic reaction in lepromatous or borderline leprosy. Skin changes known as erythema nodosum leprosum.
- Erythema nodosum leprosum (type 2 reactions, occurring in in 20% lepromatous leprosy) is an immune complex mediated reaction with fever, malaise, and neuritis. It may be superficial or deep, causing panniculitis.
- Secondary impairments like wounds, contractures, malum perforans (osteopathia ulceromutilans), chronic ulcers, mutilations due to digit resorption, and blindness occur in 30–50% of patients with nerve involvement.
- Lucio phenomenon is a vasculitis with inflammatory microthromboembolic occlusion of the dermal vasculature. It rarely occurs in lepromatous leprosy, presenting as painful irregular patches, which become purpuric, bullous, and ulcerative and may be fatal.

Diagnosis

Skin lesions with definite sensory loss and neurological defects. The diagnosis is confirmed by the existence of a specific leproid granuloma histologically and/or by the identification of *M. leprae* (by Ziehl-Neelsen or Fite-Faraco, and immunohistochemistry staining and/or PCR) especially in lepromatous form.

Differential Diagnosis

Hypopigmented lesions: nevus depigmentosus, *eczema, psoriasis*, dermatophytes infection, *seborrheic dermatitis*, mycosis fungoides, *vitiligo*, *pityriasis versicolor*, *dermatophyte infections*, pityriasis rosea, cutaneous tuberculosis, *granuloma annulare*, hereditary sensory motor neuropathy type III, Refsum's disease, amyloidosis.

Nodules: *sarcoidosis*, *cutaneous lymphoma*, *leishmaniasis*, *syphilis*.

Prevention and Therapy

Vaccination is the most efficient method of preventing the contraction of leprosy:

- *Bacillus Calmette-Guerin* (BCG) vaccination.
- *Bacillus Calmette-Guerin* (BCG) vaccination plus killed *M. leprae*.
  Multidrug therapy (MDT) can cure leprosy and prevent disability.
- Paucibacillary leprosy: Rifampicin 600 mg administered once per month and dapsone 100 mg/daily over 6 months.
- Multibacillary leprosy: Rifampicin 600 mg + clofazimine 300 mg administered once per month and clofazimine 50 mg + dapsone 100 mg/daily over 12 months.
  Erythema nodosum leprosum: immunosuppression.

Special

Severe psychologic and socioeconomic impact. Rehabilitation is very important.

*see also section "Leprosy" Chap. 7

Tuberculosis* [8, 10]

Grading of Importance

B

Level

Special

*see section "Skin Tuberculosis and Atypical Mycobacterioses (MOTT)" in Chap. 7.

Anthrax [2, 9]

Figures 29.3 and 29.4

Grading of Importance

B

Level

Special

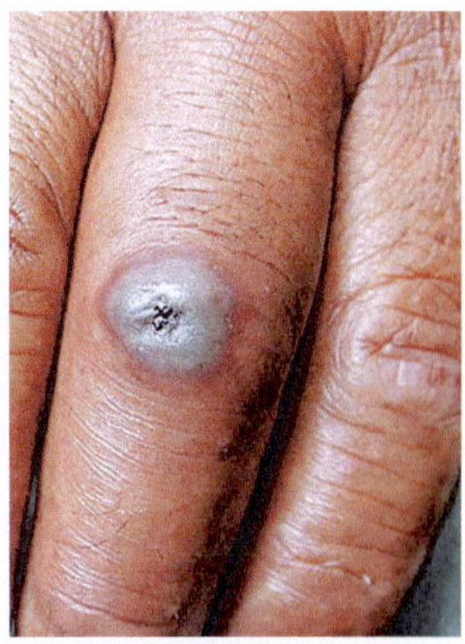

Fig. 29.3 Anthrax: centrally necrotic vesicle

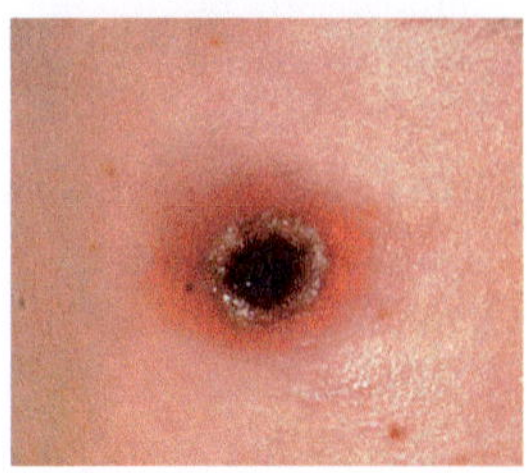

Fig. 29.4 Anthrax: inflamed ulcer with black eschar

ICD-11

1B97

Synonyms

Bacillus anthracis infection

Epidemiology

Rarely occurring in western countries; endemic in the Middle East, Central Asia, and African countries. Annual global incidence is estimated between 2000 and 20,000 cases. Among the three forms (cutaneous, respiratory, and gastrointestinal), cutaneous anthrax accounts for 95% of human cases globally.

Definition

Infection with the gram-positive bacteria *Bacillus anthracis*. Clinical signs depend on the route of infection: inhalation, ingestion, or cutaneous contact.

Etiology and Pathogenesis

Bacillus anthracis is environmentally stable in spore form and may contaminate soil worldwide, resulting in infections of herbivores. Spores can remain dormant and viable in the environment for decades. Transmission is by inhalation, ingestion, or cutaneous contact with *Bacillus anthracis* spores in domestic sheep, goat, cattle, wild deer and antelope, through butchering and working with or ingestion of raw or uncooked meat. Incubation period between 1 and 19 days. *B. anthracis* spores get through the abraded skin into subcutaneous tissues. The toxin produced leads to the characteristic edema and cutaneous ulceration.

Signs and Symptoms

Generally single lesions, sometimes two or more.

Mild cutaneous anthrax lesion (<4 cm in diameter) centrally depressed vesicle, filled with hemorrhagic fluid and surrounded by a narrow erythema, without systemic symptoms.

Severe cutaneous anthrax: large cutaneous lesion with bullous hemorrhagic reaction, extensive, edema, central (black) necrosis.

Toxemic shock: systemic symptoms (fever, tachycardia, and tachypnea).

Localization

Exposed area of the body, mostly on the face, neck, hands, and wrist.

Classification

- Cutaneous *anthrax*: clinical course varies from mild to severe.
- Pulmonary *anthrax*.
- *Anthrax* pneumonia.
- Pneumonia in *anthrax*.

Laboratory and Other Workups

Confirmation is by identification of *Bacillus anthracis* in a sample, or detection of antibodies or toxins and culturing on sheep blood agar. Peripheral blood count, blood biochemistry, and chest X-ray.

Dermatopathology

Hemorrhage, necrosis, and submucosal thrombosis. Staining of the capsule of *B. anthracis* in the capillaries at the infection site with Indian ink.

Course

Hemorrhage, necrosis, and submucosal thrombosis.

Complications

Extensive edema, sepsis, toxemic shock and other organ involvement. Healing with scarring in severe cases. Superinfection.

Diagnosis

A detailed history, including the occupation of the patient, exposure to a sick animal or animal products. Demonstration or isolation of *B. anthracis* or gram-positive bacilli from a lesion.

Clinical feature (pustula maligna).

Differential Diagnosis

Staphylococcal skin abscess, cat scratch disease, tularemia, spider bite, and ecthyma gangrenosum.

Prevention and Therapy

Prevention of contact with infected animals or contaminated animal products.

Intramuscular procaine penicillin, oral amoxicillin or penicillin V for mild uncomplicated.

Cutaneous anthrax. Intravenous penicillin G in severe cases. Doxycycline or Ciprofloxacin are alternatives.

Vaccination.

Special

Bacillus anthracis also has been used as a biologic weapon.

Yaws [4–6]

Figure 29.5

Grading of Importance

B

Level

special

ICD-11

1C.1D (1C1D.0; 1C1D.1; 1C1D.2; 1C1D.3)

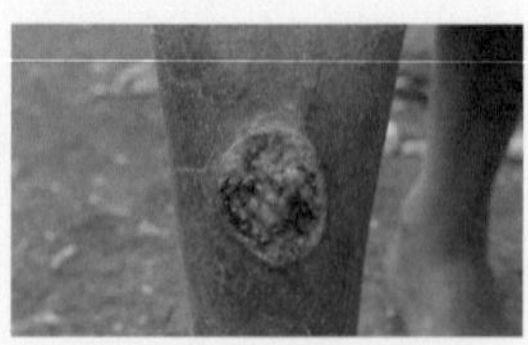

Fig. 29.5 Yaws: ulcer on the leg (courtesy of Dr Yves Thierry and M. Barogui, Gabon)

Synonyms

None

Epidemiology

Most commonly seen among children between 2 and 15 years of age (reservoirs for the spirochete) in endemic tropical regions with warm and humid environments. Infection is spread by direct skin to skin contact. Since the annual incidence fell dramatically over the past years, there is hope that the disease will be eradicated. Poor hygiene, poverty, crowding, rural settings, and a climate of heavy rainfall and high humidity are risk factors for transmission.

Definition

Non-venereal tropical infectious disease caused by *Treponema pertenue*, which is closely related to the syphilitic spirochete, *Treponema pallidum*.

Etiology and Pathogenesis

Unlike syphilis, yaws is neither sexually transmitted nor transmitted from mother to baby. Disease is most commonly seen in children and is transmitted from skin to skin and possibly by fly vectors; there is no evidence of zoonotic transmission.

Signs and Symptoms

Clinical stages, similar to syphilis:

The initial stage ("mother yaw") at the site of inoculation on average 9–90 days after exposure: solitary nodules or multiple ulcerative non-tender exudative papules, 2–5 cm in diameter, showing a distinct red base of granulation tissue with elevated borders, that may degenerate into a single crusted non-tender ulcer. Untreated lesions heal spontaneously over 3–6 months leaving hyperpigmentation.

Second stage ("crab yaws") (2 months up to 2 years after inoculation; may overlap with the initial stage)**:** Lymphatic or hematogenous spread of the organism with progression of the disease. Symptoms include arthralgias, disseminated papillomatous, or ulcerative lesions with macular or hyperkeratotic palmoplantar involvement with painful fissuring and secondary infection, generalized lymphadenopathy and osteoperiostitis (most frequently radius, ulna, and phalanges).

Tertiary disease (5–10 years after inoculation): In 10% of untreated patients. Symptoms are ulcerative necrotic nodules, leading to facial destruction, and juxta-articular nodules (gummas), bowed tibia (saber shins), nasal cartilage destruction (gangosa), or exostosis of the paranasal maxilla (gondou).

Latent periods: Between primary and secondary and tertiary stages, without clinical signs but positive serology.

Localization

The most common location is the lower extremity, but any site of exposure may be involved.

Classification

Stages (see above).

Laboratory and Other Workups

T. pertenue belongs to the group of uncultivable spirochete. They are not viable ex vivo, and therefore, diagnostic methods are limited. Darkfield microscopy – which is not everywhere available – does allow direct visualization of spirochetes. Serologic assays and nucleic acid amplification tests have been used as the primary mode of identification.

Dermatopathology

In early yaws there is marked epidermal hyperplasia and papillomatosis, with focal spongiosis, neutrophilic microabscesses in the epidermis and plasma cells in the dermis, with only little endothelial cell proliferation or vascular obliteration (in contrast to syphilis). With Warthin-Starry silver stains or polyclonal antibodies to *T. pallidum*, the bacteria can be detected in the epidermis.

Course

Slowly progressive through several stages if not treated.

Complications

Superinfection. Progression of the disease through latent stages, if not properly treated.

Diagnosis

Diagnosis is based on the combined clinical picture and serologic testing (see also syphilis section "Syphilis" in Chap. 10)

Differential Diagnosis

Other treponemal diseases and tropical ulcers.

Prevention and Therapy

Benzathine penicillin-G, or single dose of azithromycin for primary and secondary stages.

References

1. Britton WJ, Lockwood DN (2004) Leprosy. Lancet 363(9416):1209–1219
2. Doganay M, Metan G, Alp E (2010) A review of cutaneous anthrax and its outcome. J Infect Public Health 3(3):98–105
3. Guarner J (2018) Buruli ulcer: review of a neglected skin mycobacterial disease. J Clin Microbiol 56(4):e01507
4. Marks M, Mitja O, Solomon AW, Asiedu KB, Mabey DC (2015) Yaws. Br Med Bull 113(1):91–100
5. Mitja O, Marks M, Konan DJ, Ayelo G, Gonzalez-Beiras C, Boua B, Houinei W, Kobara Y, Tabah EN, Nsiire A, Obvala D, Taleo F, Djupuri R, Zaixing Z, Utzinger J, Vestergaard LS, Bassat Q, Asiedu K (2015) Global epidemiology of yaws: a systematic review. Lancet Glob Health 3(6):e324–e331
6. Mitja O, Smajs D, Bassat Q (2013) Advances in the diagnosis of endemic treponematoses: yaws, bejel, and pinta. PLoS Negl Trop Dis 7(10):e2283
7. Patil A, Mishra M, Taiwade P, Shrikhande S (2020) A study of indices in smear positive leprosy in post-elimination era: experience at a Teaching Tertiary Care Centre. J. Med. Sci. 6(3):211–215
8. Scollard DM, Dacso MM, Abad-Venida ML (2015) Tuberculosis and leprosy: classical granulomatous diseases in the twenty-first century. Dermatol Clin 33(3):541–562
9. Simonsen KA, Chatterjee K (2023) Anthrax. StatPearls, Treasure Island, FL
10. van Zyl L, du Plessis J, Viljoen J (2015) Cutaneous tuberculosis overview and current treatment regimens. Tuberculosis (Edinb) 95(6):629–638
11. Walker SL, Lockwood DN (2007) Leprosy. Clin Dermatol 25(2):165–172
12. Yotsu RR, Suzuki K, Simmonds RE, Bedimo R, Ablordey A, Yeboah-Manu D, Phillips R, Asiedu K (2018) Buruli ulcer: a review of the current knowledge. Curr Trop Med Rep 5(4):247–256

Fungal Infections

30

Günter Burg

Contents

G. Burg (✉)
Dermatology, Zurich, Switzerland
e-mail: g.burg@access.uzh.ch

H. Gollnick et al. (eds.), *Dermatology Cyberderm WebBook*,
https://doi.org/10.1007/978-3-031-78491-0_30

Test your learning and check your understanding of this book's contents: use the "Springer Nature Flashcards" app to access questions using ▶ https://sn.pub/1rhh6k.

To use the app, please follow the instructions in Chap. 1.

Chromoblastomycosis [3, 7] [4, 5]

Figure 30.1

Grading of Importance

B

Level

special

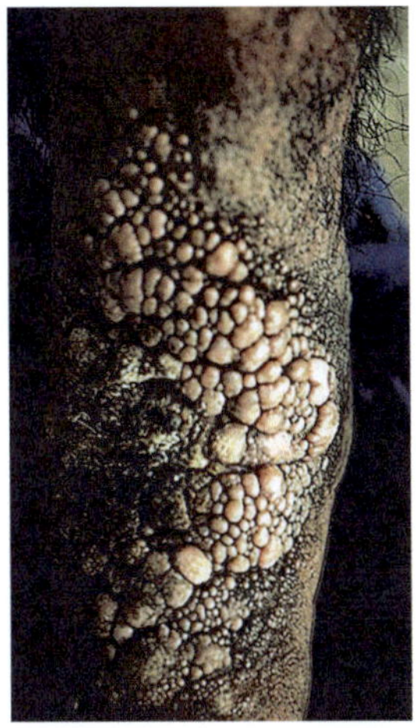

Fig. 30.1 Chomoblastomycosis: popular and nodular proliferations on the leg

ICD-11

1F24

Synonyms

Medlar bodies; muriform bodies; copper pennies

Epidemiology

Affecting mostly adult male agricultural workers in the rural tropical and subtropical areas of the world.

Definition

Chronic granulomatous infection of the skin and subcutaneous tissue caused by several different brown pigment-producing (dematiaceous) fungi.

Etiology and Pathogenesis

A large number of dematiaceous, i.e., brown pigment producing, fungi can cause the disease, the most common of which are *Cladosporium carrionii*, *Phialophora verrucosa*, and *Fonsecaea pedrosoi*, present in wood and soil.

Signs and Symptoms

Localized, slowly growing and peripherally extending, warty cauliflower-like plaques, which may ulcerate. Sclerotic bodies are extruded transepidermally, appearing as black dots. Large hyperkeratotic and ulcerating masses may form. The lesion is usually painless. Sometimes lymphatic spread due to scratching result in the sporotrichoid pattern. Hematogenous dissemination with brain abscesses is very rare.

Localization

Areas exposed to trauma

Classification

None

Laboratory and Other Workups

Microbiology; 10% KOH

Dermatopathology

Marked pseudoepitheliomatous hyperplasia of the epidermis. Transepidermal elimination of fungal cells, which are in the stratum corneum. Foreign body granuloma with isolated microabscesses. In the dermis, a granuloma composed of epithelioid cells and Langhans giant cells is visible. The golden-brown fungal elements are visible as thick-walled, single, or multicelled clusters, forming sclerotic or muriform bodies.

Course

Chronic but curable. The prognosis depends on the size of the lesions and the immune status of the patient. Long-standing cases can spread over joints and lead to lymphatic involvement and elephantiasis. Disseminated disease, with the involvement of the central nervous system, has the worst prognosis.

Complications

Ulceration, secondary bacterial infection, lymphedema resulting in elephantiasis. Malignant transformation to squamous cell carcinoma is rare.

Diagnosis

Clinical feature, histologic and microbial findings

Differential Diagnosis

Other verrucous lesions: tuberculosis verrucosa cutis, verruca vulgaris, blastomycosis, yaws, verrucous hemangioma, hypertrophic lichen planus, lupus vulgaris. Sporotrichosis in sporotrichoid type. Psoriasis.

Prevention and Therapy

Prevention of trauma

Best results are achievable in small lesions with surgery, cryotherapy, or electrodessication in combination with antifungal therapy: itraconazole 200–400 mg/day or terbinafine, 250–500 mg/day given for a period varying from 6 months to 1 year or more. Flucytosine alone or combined with amphotericin and oral supersaturated potassium iodide solution are additional options.

Special

Best management is by an interprofessional team, including an infectious disease consultant, surgeon, emergency department physician, wound care nurse, and a specialist for internal medicine.

Sporotrichosis [2, 5, 6, 8, 9]

Figure 30.2

Grading of Importance

B

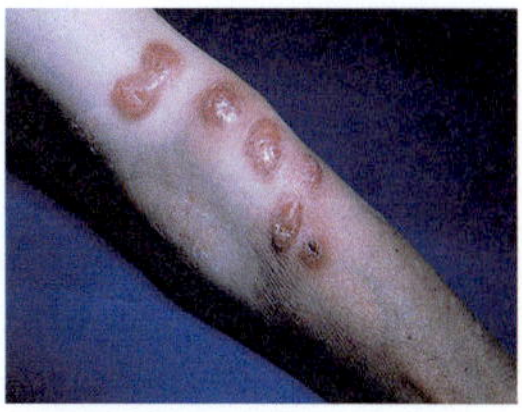

Fig. 30.2 Sporotrichosis: nodules over lymphatic vessel

Level

Special

ICD-11

1F2J.Z; 1F2J.0; 1F2J.1

Synonyms

Lymphocutaneous and fixed cutaneous sporotrichosis

Epidemiology

Worldwide distribution. Preferentially in areas with warm, humid, tropical, or subtropical climates (Africa, Asia, South America). Young adult is the preferred age group; children are rarely affected.

Definition

Sporotrichosis is a polymorphic subacute or chronic infection by dimorphic fungi of the *Sporothrix schenckii* complex, which includes several phylogenetically distinct species of dimorphic fungi.

Etiology and Pathogenesis

Through injury or wounds, inoculation of soil, plants, and decaying material, contaminated with the fungus of the *Sporothrix schenckii* complex in florists ("Gardner's disease"). The respiratory route is less common. Transmission also may occur by various animals (rodents). There are various forms of manifestation (see classification). Average incubation time is 3 weeks. The risk of disseminated disease is increased in immunocompromised patients, or in patients with chronic obstructive pulmonary disease, alcohol abuse, and diabetes.

Signs and Symptoms

Sporotrichosis mostly presents in its *cutaneous-lymphatic* (>90%) form, with papules, pustules, or linearly distributed, painful or pruriginous ulcerated nodules (chancre), which may develop verrucous plaques in chronic forms and spread along lymphatic vessels.

The second form is *cutaneous-fixed sporotrichosis* (30% of cases), which occurs in the same inoculation site (called sporotrichoid chancre), usually consisting of an asymptomatic, sole, vegetative, or slow-growing verrucous lesion, and a squamous, erythematous, or violaceous halo.

The cutaneous-disseminated (hematogenous) sporotrichosis is reported in up to 8% of cases and is usually seen in immunocompromised patients. It can manifest at any part of the body surface and involve even mucous membranes, bones, and joints, producing small granulomatous or extensive lytic lesions and osteomyelitis, associated with joint effusions, edema, and severe pain.

The extracutaneous forms are less commonly seen and include disseminated sporotrichosis, pulmonary sporotrichosis, and various osteoarticular, ocular, and central nervous system disorders.

Localization

Upper and lower limbs and face

Classification

Sporotrichosis is classified into cutaneous, pulmonary, and disseminated, with cutaneous being the most common form of the disease.

Laboratory and Other Workups

Cultures (5–8 days; Sabouraud dextrose agar) from exudative lesions, scale, tissue fragment, sputum, and blood.

Detection of "cigar-shaped" yeast elements (scarce in cutaneous-lymphatic forms; better to be seen in cutaneous-disseminated or pulmonary forms, using PAS or Grocott staining). The two main causative agents are *Sporothrix schenckii* and *Sporothrix brasiliensis*. Determination of species by polymerase chain reaction.

Dermatopathology

Suppurative granulomas with scarce yeasts and asteroid bodies (PAS and Grocott stains). It must be distinguished from histoplasmosis.

Course

Chronic spread and dissemination

Complications

Involvement of extracutaneous organs (see symptoms).

Diagnosis

Clinically ("sporotrichoid") spread along lymphatic vessels. Cave: confusion with histoplasmosis.

Differential Diagnosis

Cutaneous leishmaniasis, histoplasmosis, psoriasis

Prevention and Therapy

Prevention of trauma

Cutaneous-lymphatic and cutaneous-fixed sporotrichosis: potassium iodide in diluted solutions. Drug of choice for both clinical forms: itraconazole at 200 mg/day for 3–6 months.

Cutaneous-disseminated, disseminated, pulmonary, and osteoarticular sporotrichosis: amphotericin B, 3–5 mg/kg/day.

Mycetoma [1, 5, 10–12]

Figure 30.3

Grading of Importance

B

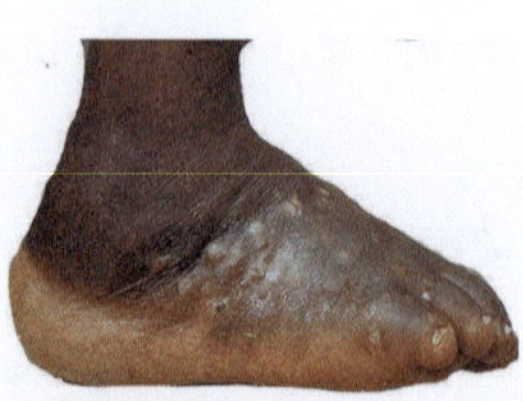

Fig. 30.3 Mycetoma: swelling of the foot due to bacterial infection

Level

Special

ICD-11

1F29 Eumycetoma
1C43 Actinomycetoma
1G60.0 Mycetoma of unknown or unspecified type

Synonyms

Madura foot

Epidemiology

The so-called mycetoma belt (latitude 15°S and 30°N). It is endemic in Sudan, Somalia, Senegal, India, Yemen, Mexico and Venezuela and affects preferentially farmers and poor populations in remote areas with higher humidity.

Males are more frequently affected than females (4:1). Age range: 30–40 years.

Definition

Chronic granulomatous infection of the skin and subcutaneous tissue, either by fungi (60%; eumycetoma) or by bacteria (40%; actinomycetoma)

Etiology and Pathogenesis

- Causative agents of eumycetoma: *Madurella mycetomatis* (most common), *Madurella grisea*, *Pseudallescheria boydii*, and *Leptosphaeria senegalensis*
- Causative agents of actinomycetoma: *Nocardia spp.*, including *Nocardia brasiliensis*, *Nocardia asteroids*, and *Nocardia otitidiscaviarum.*

Signs and Symptoms

The clinical presentation of eumycetoma and actinomycetoma are almost identical. They involve the skin and subcutaneous tissue, presenting the classic triad of hard woody swelling, painless discharging sinuses, and presence of grains (colonies of bacteria or fungi).

Variants:
- Swelling without sinuses
- Cystic type
- Verrucous plaque type

Localization

Mostly foot, but also any other part of the body

Classification

See etiopathology.

Laboratory and Other Workups

KOH
- Fungal hyphae: periodic acid-Schiff, Gomori methenamine silver stain.
- Nocardia species: gram-positive and weakly acid-fast-positive. Actinomadura grains are Gram-positive and acid-fast-negative.
  Ultrasound and radiograph, Magnetic resonance imaging (MRI)
  PCR and grain cultures

Dermatopathology

Chronic fibrosing inflammation with suppurative granuloma and mycetoma grains. Periodic acid-Schiff (PAS), Gomori methenamine silver (GMS), and gram stains.

Course

Chronic; untreated, the infection spreads through the fasciae and may involve the bone and muscle.

Complications

Socioeconomic burden
  Invasion of the periosteum and adjacent bones, leading to osteomyelitis
  Vertebral compression with neurological manifestations when affecting the back
  Rarely lymphatic spread

Diagnosis

Clinically, histologically, investigation of grains

Ultrasound and radiograph, Magnetic resonance imaging (MRI) for recognizing the extension of the disease

Differential Diagnosis

Actinomycosis; aspergillosis; botryomycosis; chromoblastomycosis; coccidioidomycosis; sporotrichosis; tuberculosis; osteomyelitis; neoplasias.

Prevention and Therapy

Surgical treatment is indicated for small, localized lesions and also for large lesions to reduce the organism load. Eumycetoma requires a combination of antifungals and surgery and may still have recurrences.

Note: fungal and bacterial mycetoma respectively needs completely different therapeutic approaches.

- Actinomycetoma responds well to antibiotic treatment: Amikacin 15 mg/kg IM divided into two doses + sulfamethoxazole (35 mg/kg/day) and trimethoprim (7 mg/kg/day) divided into three doses for 21 days.
- Eumycetoma requires a combination of antifungals and surgery and tends to recur: ketoconazole (400 mg/day), itraconazole (200–400 mg/day), posaconazole, (200 mg four times daily), voriconazole 400–600 mg/day, amphotericin B (0.5–1.25 mg/kg per day), and terbinafine (500–1000 mg/day), alone or in any combination.

References

1. Ahmed AA, van de Sande W, Fahal AH (2017) Mycetoma laboratory diagnosis: review article. PLoS Negl Trop Dis 11(8):e0005638
2. Bonifaz A, Tirado-Sanchez A, Paredes-Solis V, Cepeda-Valdes R, Gonzalez GM, Trevino-Rangel RJ, Fierro-Arias L (2018) Cutaneous disseminated sporotrichosis: clinical experience of 24 cases. J Eur Acad Dermatol Venereol 32(2):e77–e79
3. Brito AC, Bittencourt MJS (2018) Chromoblastomycosis: an etiological, epidemiological, clinical, diagnostic, and treatment update. An Bras Dermatol 93(4):495–506
4. Kurien G, Sugumar K, Chandran V (2023) Chromoblastomycosis. StatPearls, Treasure Island, FL
5. Lupi O, Tyring SK, McGinnis MR (2005) Tropical dermatology: fungal tropical diseases. J Am Acad Dermatol 53(6):931–951. quiz 952-934.
6. Morris-Jones R (2002) Sporotrichosis. Clin Exp Dermatol 27(6):427–431
7. Queiroz-Telles F, de Hoog S, Santos DW, Salgado CG, Vicente VA, Bonifaz A, Roilides E, Xi L, Azevedo CM, da Silva MB, Pana ZD, Colombo AL, Walsh TJ (2017) Chromoblastomycosis. Clin Microbiol Rev 30(1):233–276

8. Ramos-e-Silva M, Vasconcelos C, Carneiro S, Cestari T (2007) Sporotrichosis. Clin Dermatol 25(2):181–187
9. Sizar O, Talati R (2023) Sporotrichosis. StatPearls, Treasure Island, FL
10. van de Sande WW, Fahal AH, Goodfellow M, el Mahgoub S, Welsh O, Zijlstra EE (2014a) Merits and pitfalls of currently used diagnostic tools in mycetoma. PLoS Negl Trop Dis 8(7):e2918
11. van de Sande WW, el Maghoub S, Fahal AH, Goodfellow M, Welsh O, Zijlstra E (2014b) The mycetoma knowledge gap: identification of research priorities. PLoS Negl Trop Dis 8(3):e2667
12. Verma P, Jha A (2019) Mycetoma: reviewing a neglected disease. Clin Exp Dermatol 44(2):123–129

Protozoan Diseases

31

Zrinka Bukvić Mokos, Günter Burg, and Branka Marinović

Contents

Z. Bukvić Mokos (✉)
Department of Dermatology and Venereology, School of Medicine University of Zagreb, Zagreb, Croatia

G. Burg
Dermatology, Zurich, Switzerland
e-mail: g.burg@access.uzh.ch

B. Marinović
Department of Dermatology, University of Zurich, Zürich, Switzerland
e-mail: branka.marinovic@kbc-zagreb.hr

H. Gollnick et al. (eds.), *Dermatology Cyberderm WebBook*,
https://doi.org/10.1007/978-3-031-78491-0_31

Test your learning and check your understanding of this book's contents: use the "Springer Nature Flashcards" app to access questions using ▶ https://sn.pub/1rhh6k.
To use the app, please follow the instructions in Chap. 1.

Leishmaniasis* [1–3, 7]

Grading of Importance

B

*see section "Leishmaniasis" in Chap. 9.

Post-Kala-Azar Dermal Leishmaniasis (PKDL) [4–6, 8, 9]

Grading of Importance

B

Level

Special

ICD-11

1F54.0

Synonyms

None.

Epidemiology

Approximately 1 million new cases of cutaneous leishmaniasis worldwide per year. In South Asia (India, Nepal, Bangladesh), 5–10% of the patients with supposedly cured visceral leishmaniasis develop PKDL 2–3 years after treatment. In East Africa (Sudan, Ethiopia, Kenya, and Uganda), the incidence of PKDL is higher (50–60%), and it may appear even during treatment.

Definition

Cutaneous manifestation following visceral leishmaniasis in up to 20% of patients after successful treatment.

Aetiology and Pathogenesis

PKDL lesions are due to interferon (IFN)-gamma-producing cells causing skin inflammation as a reaction to parasites persisting in the skin.

Depending on the geographical region, *Leishmania donovani* parasites are genetically different.

PKDL may develop through reinfection or relapse, genetic susceptibility of the host (polymorphism in the IFN-gamma receptor gene), UV-induced skin damage, organ-specific failure of memory T cell and reinfection or persistence of the parasite.

The skin lesions are a reservoir for *L. donovani* and promote the transmission by the female phlebotomus sandflies.

General immune response:

- Asian PKDL: delayed immune response, associated with CD8+ T-cell infiltration into the cutaneous lesions.
- Sudanese PKDL: early reactivation of the immune response.

Signs and Symptoms

Asymptomatic skin rash, usually starting in the face, around the mouth from where it spreads to other parts of the body, presenting in two different versions:

Polymorphic PKDL (more common; higher burden of parasites): papulonodules (South Asia), or hypomelanotic (macular) lesions (East Africa).

Monomorphous PKDL: only one type of lesion, mostly papulonodes

Localisation

Face, spreading to other parts of the body

Classification

Dependent on geographic region: Sudan vs India

Laboratory and Other Workups

Parasitological (PCR), serological, immunological, cytological, histological biomarkers

Dermatopathology

- Polymorphic PKDL: diffuse dermial cell infiltrate with many macrophages and B cells, but fewer dendritic and Langhans cells.
- Monomorphic PKDL (lower parasitic load): reduction of Leishmania-Donovan bodies.

Course

Immune responses to PKDL in Asia and Africa are different, which may explain the better self-healing tendency in Africa (85%) compared to the worse situation in Asia.

Complications

Persistence of the infection, relapses. PKDL is not life-threating but affects the quality of life and may be a socioeconomic burden.

Diagnosis

Clinical sign and symptoms, along with a previous kala-azar episode and positive antibody tests.

Differential Diagnosis

A variety of papulonodular and macular dermatoses.

Prevention and Therapy

PKDL lesions heal spontaneously in most cases.

Sodium antimony gluconate (SAG) (20 mg/kg per day for 20 days per month for 6 months). However, side effects may include cardiac toxicities and arthralgia.

References

1. Aronson NE, Joya CA (2019) Cutaneous leishmaniasis: updates in diagnosis and management. Infect Dis Clin North Am 33(1):101–117
2. Burza S, Croft SL, Boelaert M (2018) Leishmaniasis. Lancet 392(10151):951–970
3. de Vries HJ, Reedijk SH, Schallig HD (2015) Cutaneous leishmaniasis: recent developments in diagnosis and management. Am J Clin Dermatol 16(2):99–109
4. Diro E, Edwards T, Ritmeijer K, Fikre H, Abongomera C, Kibret A, Bardonneau C, Soipei P, Mutinda B, Omollo R, van Griensven J, Zijlstra EE, Wasunna M, Alves F, Alvar J, Hailu A, Alexander N, Blesson S (2019) Long term outcomes and prognostics of visceral leishmaniasis in HIV infected patients with use of pentamidine as secondary prophylaxis based on CD4 level: a prospective cohort study in Ethiopia. PLoS Negl Trop Dis 13(2):e0007132
5. Gedda MR, Singh B, Kumar D, Singh AK, Madhukar P, Upadhyay S, Singh OP, Sundar S (2020) Post kala-azar dermal leishmaniasis: a threat to elimination program. PLoS Negl Trop Dis 14(7):e0008221
6. Le Rutte EA, Zijlstra EE, de Vlas SJ (2019) Post-Kala-Azar dermal leishmaniasis as a reservoir for visceral leishmaniasis transmission. Trends Parasitol 35(8):590–592
7. Reithinger R, Dujardin JC, Louzir H, Pirmez C, Alexander B, Brooker S (2007) Cutaneous leishmaniasis. Lancet Infect Dis 7(9):581–596
8. Volpedo G, Pacheco-Fernandez T, Holcomb EA, Cipriano N, Cox B, Satoskar AR (2021) Mechanisms of immunopathogenesis in cutaneous leishmaniasis and Post Kala-azar Dermal Leishmaniasis (PKDL). Front Cell Infect Microbiol 11:685296
9. Zijlstra EE (2019) Biomarkers in Post-kala-azar Dermal Leishmaniasis. Front Cell Infect Microbiol 9:228

Helminthic Infections (Parasitic Worms): Nematodes

32

Günter Burg

Contents

G. Burg (✉)
Dermatology, Zurich, Switzerland
e-mail: g.burg@access.uzh.ch

H. Gollnick et al. (eds.), *Dermatology Cyberderm WebBook*,
https://doi.org/10.1007/978-3-031-78491-0_32

Test your learning and check your understanding of this book's contents: use the "Springer Nature Flashcards" app to access questions using ▶ https://sn.pub/1rhh6k.

To use the app, please follow the instructions in Chap. 1.

Filariasis [3, 4]

Grading of Importance

B

Level

Special

ICD-11

1F66.Z Filariasis, unspecified

Synonyms

Elephantiasis

Epidemiology

Tropical and subtropical areas of Asia, Africa, the Pacific Islands, several of the Caribbean Islands, and South America

Definition

Tropical disease, infestation by nematodes, resulting in massive disfiguration by thickening of the skin and underlying tissues

Etiology and Pathogenesis

Infestation mostly by *Wuchereria bancrofti* (90%), which causes, *Brugia malayi* and *Brugia timori.* After a bite of infected mosquitoes, the larvae which have been deposited in the lymphatic system develop into adult worms, blocking the lymphatic vessels, resulting in disfiguring elephantiastic swelling of the extremities, scrotum, vulva, and breasts.

Signs and Symptoms

Hardening of the hyperkeratotic and hyperpigmented, warty skin, which shows folds, fissures, and cracks, is swollen, painful, and foul smelling. Recurring acute lymphadenitis with swelling of lymph nodes in the groin and axillae is an immune response to dying adult worms.

Chronic, initially reversible, lymphedema finally leads to elephantiasis.

Elephantiasis is a disfiguring, chronic manifestation and presents months to years after initial infection as severe swelling of the extremities, scrotum, vulva, and breasts. Following treatment acute filarial lymphangitis with small, tender nodules at the site of the dying worms may be seen.

Localization

Extremities, scrotum, vulva, and breasts

Classification

Early and late (chronic)

Laboratory and Other Workups

Antigen released by adult filarial worms can be detected by immunochromatographic test.

Microfilariae can be detected in peripheral blood during the early stages of filariasis. Blood eosinophilia.

Dermatopathology

Edematous and fibrotic thickening of the skin with dilated lymph vessels. Dense lymphocytic inflammatory reaction with many eosinophils. In advanced stages, edema gradually resolves and is replaced by fibrosis.

Course

Chronic

Complications

Superinfection

Diagnosis

Clinical feature; laboratory findings (see there).

Differential Diagnosis

Podoconiosis ("mossy foot"), which is a noninfectious tropical lymphedema occurring in tropical volcanic highland areas.

Prevention and Therapy

Diethylcarbamazine (DEC; no longer approved by the FDA): 200 mg PO q12h 3 12 days, repeat 10 days later, or 6 mg/kg/day PO 3 12 days (pediatric dose), repeat 10 days later.

Onchocerciasis [3, 4]

Figures 32.1 and 32.2

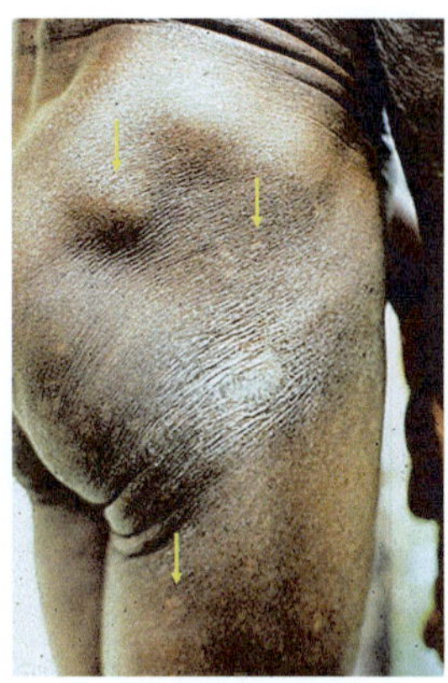

Fig. 32.1 Onchocerciasis: subcutaneous nodules on the buttock

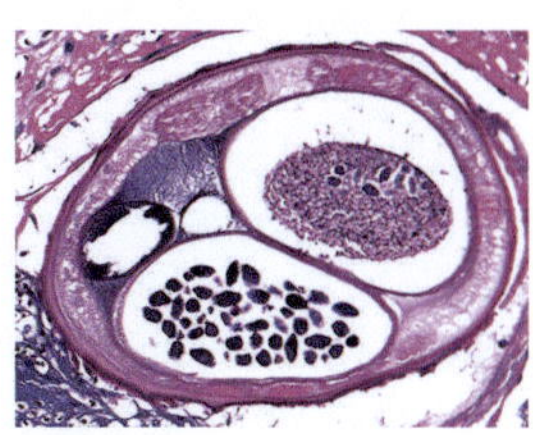

Fig. 32.2 Onchocerciasis: microfilaria

Grading of Importance

B

Level

Special

ICD-11

1F6A

Synonyms

Elephantiasis.

Epidemiology

In tropical and subtropical humid endemic areas, mostly commonly in sub-Saharan Africa. “Imported” cases have been reported from other areas.

Onchocerciasis is one of the most frequent causes of (“river”) blindness.

Definition

Parasitic infectious disease caused by the filarial nematode *Onchocerca volvulus*, causing dermatologic, ocular, and systemic manifestations.

Etiology and Pathogenesis

In endemic areas of Africa and Central America, the black fly (buffalo gnat; which breed near fast-flowing rivers) is the vector for *Onchocerca volvulus*. Subsequent to the bite of a fly, thousands of microfilariae (immature worms) migrate via blood into the subcutaneous tissue and eyes where they mature into adult worms and cause symptoms.

Signs and Symptoms

Painless, freely mobile, subcutaneous onchocercal nodule (1–3 cm; onchocercoma), replete with organisms are most commonly found at bony prominences. There also is severe pruritus, eczematous dermatitis, lichenification, subcutaneous and dermal atrophy, and spotted depigmentation ("leopard skin"); accompanying blindness ("river blindness").

Localization

Extremities, trunk, buttocks, waist, and upper aspect of the thighs

Classification

- Acute papular onchodermatitis
- Chronic papular onchodermatitis
- Lichenified onchodermatitis
- Atrophy
- Depigmentation

Clinical classification and grading system (Murdoch)

Laboratory and Other Workups

Eosinophilia (up to 40%). Microscopic examination of microfilaria, emerging from skin snips and in subcutaneous nodules, respectively.

Dermatopathology

- Multitude of entangled worms of both sexes (paired worms) within encapsulated nodules (onchocercoma).
- Microfilaria in the papillary dermis.
- Subepidermal edema and strong inflammatory response with formation of micro-abscesses around necrotic larvae.
- Mixed cellular infiltrate, with histiocytes, lymphocytes, neutrophils, eosinophils, and plasma cells.

Course

Chronic; see classification.

Complications

In endemic areas, onchocerciasis is one of the most frequent causes of ("river") blindness.

Diagnosis

Clinical, eosinophilia, microscopic identification of microfilaria

Differential Diagnosis

Podoconiosis; other tropical parasitic infestations

Prevention and Therapy

- Ivermectin: 0.15–0.2 mg/kg PO 3 1 dose; may repeat in 3–12 months for the life of an adult worm
- Doxycycline: 100 mg QD PO 3 6 weeks

(Cutaneous) Larva Migrans (CLM) [1, 2, 5]

Figures 32.3 and 32.4

Grading of Importance

B

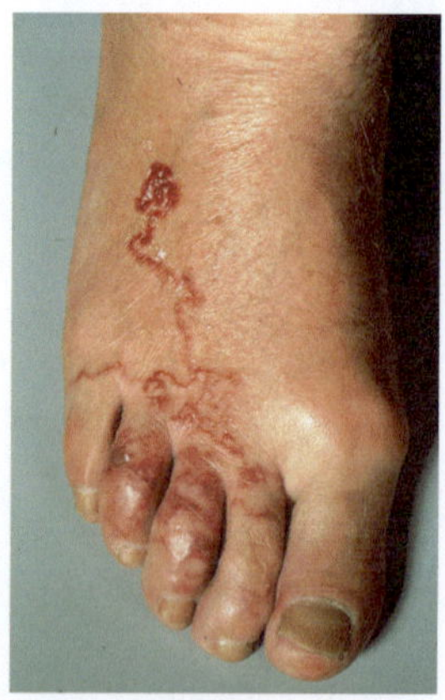

Fig. 32.3 (Cutaneous) Larva migrans: serpiginous snake-like elevated mobile track on the dorsum of the foot

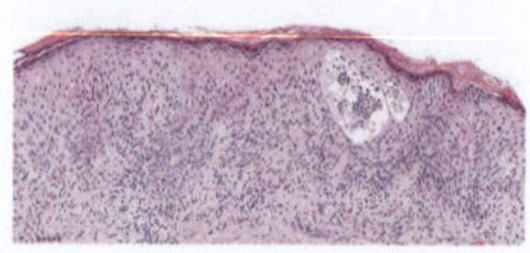

Fig. 32.4 (Cutaneous) Larva migrans: histology showing subcorneal canal

Level

advanced

ICD-11

1F68.2

Synonyms

Creeping disease.

Epidemiology

Cutaneous larva migrans is the most commonly disease transmitted by animal feces through direct contact with skin. It usually affects inhabitants or tourists in wet tropical and subtropical climates (southeastern United States, Latin America, the Caribbean, Southeast Asia, and Africa).

Definition

Infection by multiple types of hookworms

Etiology and Pathogenesis

CLM is caused by animal hookworms (most commonly *Ancylostoma braziliense*, *Ancylostoma ceylanicum*, and *Ancylostoma caninum*), present in sand or soil contaminated with animal feces.

Larvae attach to the skin of their animal host (usually nondomesticated cats or dogs) are swallowed and enter the gastrointestinal tract, where they shed eggs, which are eliminated with the feces in sand or soil. The mature filariform larvae then penetrate the corneal layer by secreting a hyaluronidase and burrow through the superficial cutaneous layers of human skin in a snake-like fashion. Due to the lack of a specific collagenase, they cannot penetrate the basal membrane to enter lymphatic vessels. They die without reproducing and completing their life cycle after approximately 2–8 weeks, and therefore the disease is self-limited.

Signs and Symptoms

Erythematous, pruritic eruption with papules or a linear or serpiginous snake-like elevated mobile track. The hookworm migrates through the skin at about 1 mm to 3 cm per day.

Localization

The most commonly affected areas are the feet, buttocks, thighs, and lower legs, but lesions can appear anywhere.

Classification

None

Laboratory and Other Workups

Not needed; dermatoscopy; biopsy usually not needed. Eosinophilia and increased immunoglobulin E levels may occur.

Dermatopathology

Spongiotic dermatitis with vesicles, containing neutrophils and eosinophils. Larvae may be found in the epidermis or below surrounded by eosinophilic infiltrate.

Course

Resolution without treatment. However, pruritus may persist over weeks or months.

Complications

Superinfection (*Staphylococcus aureus* and streptococcal species) caused by scratching, excoriations, vesiculobullous lesions.

Complications include secondary infection, most commonly with *Staphylococcus aureus* and streptococcal species. Visceral disease has been rarely reported.

Diagnosis

(Travel-) history (walking barefoot and exposure to contaminated sand or soil) and typical clinical feature showing the classic serpiginous rash.

Differential Diagnosis

Scabies, loiasis, myiasis, schistosomiasis, tinea corporis, and contact dermatitis may have some overlapping features. The most similar disease is the migrating lesion of *Strongyloides stercoralis*, moving much faster and termed larva currens. Noninfectious linear or serpiginous, nonmigratory dermatoses: jellyfish stings, lichenoid eruptions, and phytophotodermatitis.

Prevention and Therapy

Prevention: wearing protective footwear

The disease is self-limited.

- Topical thiabendazole 10% solution or 15% ointment, applied two to three times daily for 5–10 days.
- Ivermectin (0.15–0.2 mg/kg QD PO 3 1 or 2 days) can help to shorten the clinical course of the disease and to prevent superinfection.

Local disease has historically been treated with cryotherapy. However, freezing the leading edge of the skin with either liquid nitrogen, solid carbon dioxide, or ethylene chloride spray has been shown to be largely ineffective and should be avoided.

Special

Freezing (cryotherapy) with either liquid nitrogen, solid carbon dioxide, or ethylene chloride spray has been shown to be largely ineffective and should be avoided.

Schistosomiasis (Bilharziasis) [2]

Figure 32.5

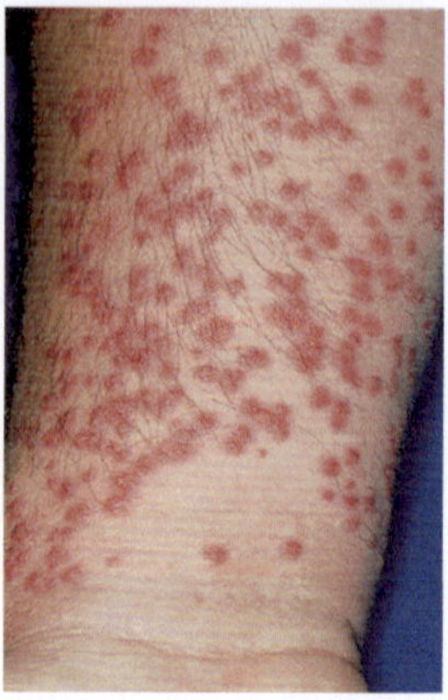

Fig. 32.5
Schistosomiasis: tiny itching papules on the arm

Grading of Importance

B

Level

Special

ICD-11

1F86.Z (1F86.4 Swimmer's itch)

Synonyms

Bilharziasis

Epidemiology

The disease is most commonly affects children (playing in contaminated water) in tropical and developing countries of Africa, Asia, and South America.

Definition

Systemic disease caused by parasitic trematode infection (schistosomes) of the gastrointestinal tract with deposition of the parasites into the perianal region, leading to skin irritation.

Etiology and Pathogenesis

Disease-specific perianal dermatitis, common in freshwater, brackish, and marine habitats in shallow inshore water, along the coasts worldwide.

Contamination of freshwater with human feces or urine containing eggs from *Schistosoma mansoni*, *Schistosoma haematobium*, or *Schistosoma japonicum*. The first intermediate host is a water snail, in which it develops into sporocysts, and finally to cercaria, which penetrates human skin and mature. Adult worms migrate to the intestine (*S. japonicum* and *S. mansoni*) or the bladder (*S. haematobium*) and produce eggs, contaminating water through feces and urine respectively.

Swimmer's itch: genera responsible mostly are *Trichobilharzia* and *Gigantobilharzia*.

Signs and Symptoms

Cutaneous findings vary from a mild pruritus ani to a macular rash and to even severe perianal ulceration from uncontrolled scratching or superinfection. Humans infected develop a short-term immune reaction (cercarial dermatitis) within hours, lasting up to a week.

Pruritic papular dermatitis, preferentially on the legs (early), followed by allergic febrile reaction with accompanying urticaria, edema, arthritis, and eosinophilia (intermediate stage). In chronic stage, internal organs (lungs, liver, bladder, CNS) may be involved. In the skin, often intensive inflammation with verrucous papules and nodules, preferentially at perineal and gluteal sites. These inflamed skin lesions may contain Schistosoma eggs, albeit in very low numbers.

Localization

Perianal region, legs

Classification

None

Laboratory and Other Workups

Identification of parasite eggs in stool or urine. Blood cell count (eosinophilia). Detection of antibodies against Schictosomas.

Dermatopathology

Eggs are rarely found in chronic skin lesions. Leading histopathological changes are dense infiltrates mainly composed of neutrophils and eosinophils. In routine sections, cercariae can be found in exceptionally rare cases.

Course

Depending on visceral involvement. Effective treatment modalities available.

Complications

Systemic symptoms (fatigue, myalgia, diarrhea, hematuria, and abdominal pain) due to immune reactions to the deposition of eggs in the host.

Bilharziasis cutanea tarda showing clusters of granulomas in the dermis may occur in patients with chronic, visceral involvement.

Superinfection.

Diagnosis

(Travel-) history. Clinical presentation. Investigation of stool or urine. Eosinophilia of the blood.

Differential Diagnosis

Arthropod bites; urticaria; other worm infections

Prevention and Therapy

Prevention: topical applications of water-resistant insect repellents

Single dose of oral praziquantel

Antihistamines orally

References

1. Hochedez P, Caumes E (2007) Hookworm-related cutaneous larva migrans. J Travel Med 14(5):326–333
2. Khubchandani IT, Bub DS (2019) Parasitic infections. Clin Colon Rectal Surg 32(5):364–371

3. Lupi O, Downing C, Lee M, Bravo F, Giglio P, Woc-Colburn L, Tyring SK (2015a) Mucocutaneous manifestations of helminth infections: trematodes and cestodes. J Am Acad Dermatol 73(6):947-957; quiz 957-948
4. Lupi O, Downing C, Lee M, Pino L, Bravo F, Giglio P, Sethi A, Klaus S, Sangueza OP, Fuller C, Mendoza N, Ladizinski B, Woc-Colburn L, Tyring SK (2015b) Mucocutaneous manifestations of helminth infections: nematodes. J Am Acad Dermatol 73(6):929–944. quiz 945-926.
5. Maxfield L, Crane JS (2023) Cutaneous larva migrans. StatPearls, Treasure Island, FL

Arthropod: Arachnids

33

Zrinka Bukvić Mokos, Günter Burg, and Branka Marinović

Contents

Z. Bukvić Mokos (✉)
Department of Dermatology and Venereology, School of Medicine University of Zagreb, Zagreb, Croatia

G. Burg
Dermatology, Zurich, Switzerland
e-mail: g.burg@access.uzh.ch

B. Marinović
Department of Dermatology, University of Zurich, Zürich, Switzerland
e-mail: branka.marinovic@kbc-zagreb.hr

H. Gollnick et al. (eds.), *Dermatology Cyberderm WebBook*,
https://doi.org/10.1007/978-3-031-78491-0_33

Test your learning and check your understanding of this book's contents: use the "Springer Nature Flashcards" app to access questions using ▶ https://sn.pub/1rhh6k.

To use the app, please follow the instructions in Chap. 1.

Scabies*[1, 2, 4, 10]

Grading of Importance

A

Level

medium

*See section "Scabies" in Chap. 9.

Scabies crustosa (Norwegica) [6, 8, 9]

Figure 33.1

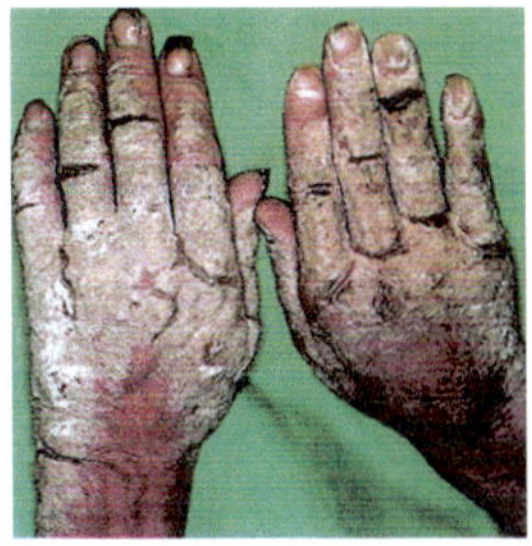

Fig. 33.1 Scabies crustose: hyperkeratotic scales, containing myriads of mites

Grading of Importance

B

Level

Special

ICD-11

1G04.1

Synonyms

Crusted scabies; scabies Norwegica; Norwegian scabies

Epidemiology

Approximately 300 million individuals are affected worldwide each year with scabies. Risk factors for developing crusted scabies include immune deficiency, increased age, dementia, long-term immunosuppression, past history of leprosy, special environmental factors (prison), misdiagnosed eczema, or psoriasis. Population on risk: aboriginal communities in northern Australia.

Definition

Highly contagious infestation with *Sarcoptes scabiei* var *hominis*, mostly seen in immunocompromised patients and showing unhindered proliferation of mites. No special aetiopathogenic or semantic relationship to Norway.

Aetiology and Pathogenesis

Impaired immune status may lead to unlimited spread of mites. *Sarcoptes scabiei* var. *hominis* is a human ectoparasite with marked host specificity. Human-to-human transmission occurs with close personal contact, sometimes via clothing or bedding. Female mites (0.3–0.5 mm) dig a burrow in the stratum corneum of the epidermis to lay their eggs; sexually mature mites develop in 3 weeks. Immunologic reaction to mite antigens causes inflammation and pruritus.

Signs and Symptoms

Erythematous patches develop into thick scaly hyperkeratotic, psoriasiform, fissured, and yellow-to-brown crusted plaques. Unlike classical scabies, pruritus is either mild or absent.

Localisation

Total body. Predilection sites: fingers, under the nails, and diffusely over palms and soles; elbows and knees.

Classification

A grading scale has been proposed, based on four clinical symptoms: the distribution and extent of crusting, the depth of crusting, the degree of skin cracking and pyoderma, and the number of previous episodes.

Laboratory and Other Workups

Investigation of the immune status. Identification of the mite, its eggs, or scybala (faeces) under the dermatoscope or microscope. Blood tests (eosinophilia, antinuclear antibodies).

Dermatopathology

Usually not necessary. Acanthosis and hyperkeratosis. Marked thickening of the stratum corneum, containing numerous parasites. Polariscopic examination (birefringence) may be a helpful clue for the visualization of mites and scybala.

Course

Risk of reinfection due to impaired immune status; increased mortality rate

Complications

Highly contagious. Contamination of contact persons and secondary bacterial infection, due to scratching and fissuring of the skin. Septicaemia with increased mortality rate.

Diagnosis

Clinical feature. Identification of mites, eggs, or scybala (feces) by dermoscopic, skin scraping or de-roofing burrow with scalpel blade, microscopic examination or reflectance confocal microscopy of burrows.

Differential Diagnosis

Pruritic dermatoses, prurigo, psoriasis, hyperkeratotic eczema

Prevention and Therapy

Prevention and topical treatment like in conventional scabies

Systemic treatment: Ivermectin 200 µg/kg (adults and children over 14 kg), together with a fatty meal to improve absorption

Tungiasis [3, 5, 7]

Figures 33.2, 33.3 and 33.4

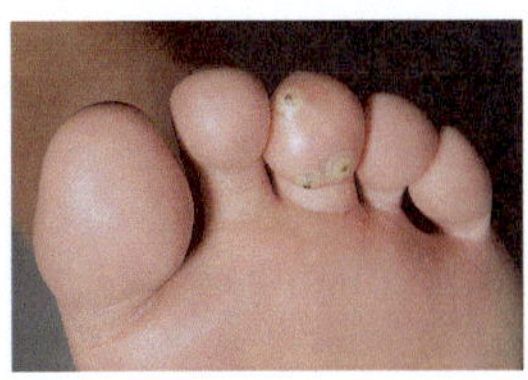

Fig. 33.2 Tungiasis: itchy lesions on the toes

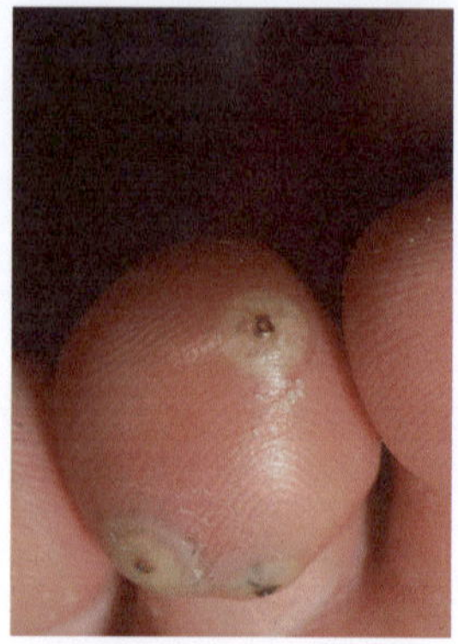

Fig. 33.3 Tungiasis: closeup view

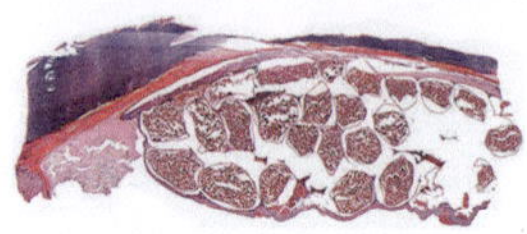

Fig. 33.4 Tungiasis: *Tunga penetrans* filled with eggs

Grading of Importance

B

Level

Medium

ICD-11

1G05

Synonyms

Several popular designations:
Europe: Sandfloh
Mexico, Caribbean islands, Peru: chigoe flea, jigger flea, pico, chique, piroque, nigua *Argentina*: pique
Brazil: bicho dos pe's, pulga de porco, pulga da areia
Sudan: moukardan
South America: puce chique, ogri eye, kuti, suthi-pique, sikka, chica, and piqui

Epidemiology

Occurring preferentially in poor communities, beaches, and farms in the Caribbean, South America and sub-Saharan Africa.

Definition

Ectoparasitosis by the female sand flea *Tunga penetrans*

Aetiology and Pathogenesis

Transmission is through the bite of an infected flea, or by direct contact with an infected animal. The female sand flea *Tunga penetrans* (or less common *Tunga trimamillata*) burrows into the skin, enlarges from 1 mm up to 1 cm, and expels several hundred eggs within 2–3 weeks.

Signs and Symptoms

Mostly on the nail rim: itchy and painful lesions due to fissuring, hindering from normally walking; foreign body sensation. Expelled eggs and the release of brownish threads of faeces are pathognomonic signs.

Localisation

Preferentially but not exclusively on feet, toes, under the toenails, and interdigital sites

Classification

None

Laboratory and Other Workups

Tetanus immune status

Dermatopathology

Not needed. Presence of the parasite, eggs or chitinous fragments of the female flea in the dermis, bearing hundreds of eggs within its body. Accompanying polymorphous round cell infiltrate.

Course

Self-limiting

Complications

Loss of toenails, deformation, and auto-amputation of digits. Risk of superinfection (staphylococci and streptococci), which may lead to formation of pustules, suppuration, and ulcers. Tetanus in unvaccinated patients.

Diagnosis

Travel history and clinical feature in typical localization. Identification of *Tunga penetrans*.

Differential Diagnosis

Subungual warts; pyogenic granuloma, foreign bodies, acute paronychia, cutaneous larva migrans, cysts, dracontiasis, arthropod bites, melanoma

Prevention and Therapy

Prevention: Closed shoes and socks and avoidance of secondary infection

Self-limited infestation. Death of the fleas after 3 weeks

Surgical extraction of the flea (sterile conditions) and treatment of secondary infection

Ivermectin single dose (200 μg/kg body weight)

References

1. Alexander L, Buckley CJ (2020) Chigger bites. StatPearls, Treasure Island, FL
2. Arora P, Rudnicka L, Sar-Pomian M, Wollina U, Jafferany M, Lotti T, Sadoughifar R, Sitkowska Z, Goldust M (2020) Scabies: a comprehensive review and current perspectives. Dermatol Ther 33(4):e13746

3. Cestari TF, Pessato S, Ramos-e-Silva M (2007) Tungiasis and myiasis. Clin Dermatol 25(2):158–164
4. Chandler DJ, Fuller LC (2019) A review of scabies: an infestation more than skin deep. Dermatology 235(2):79–90
5. Coates SJ, Thomas C, Chosidow O, Engelman D, Chang AY (2020) Ectoparasites: pediculosis and tungiasis. J Am Acad Dermatol 82(3):551–569
6. Davis JS, McGloughlin S, Tong SY, Walton SF, Currie BJ (2013) A novel clinical grading scale to guide the management of crusted scabies. PLoS Negl Trop Dis 7(9):e2387
7. Heukelbach J (2005) Tungiasis. Rev Inst Med Trop Sao Paulo 47(6):307–313
8. Palaniappan V, Gopinath H, Kaliaperumal K (2021) Crusted scabies. Am J Trop Med Hyg 104(3):787–788
9. Roberts LJ, Huffam SE, Walton SF, Currie BJ (2005) Crusted scabies: clinical and immunological findings in seventy-eight patients and a review of the literature. J Infect 50(5):375–381
10. Thomas C, Coates SJ, Engelman D, Chosidow O, Chang AY (2020) Ectoparasites: scabies. J Am Acad Dermatol 82(3):533–548

Sexually Transmitted Infections (STIS)

34

Annamari Ranki, Eija Hiltunen-Back, and Alexander Salava

Contents

Test your learning and check your understanding of this book's contents: use the "Springer Nature Flashcards" app to access questions using ▶ https://sn.pub/1rhh6k.

To use the app, please follow the instructions in Chap. 1.

Syphilis* [1, 3]

Grading of Importance

B

https://www.cyberderm.net/en/learn/skin-diseases/syphilis-2
*see section "Syphilis" in Chap. 10.

Annamari Ranki has died before the publication of this book.

A. Ranki · E. Hiltunen-Back · A. Salava (✉)
Department of Dermatology and Allergology, Helsinki University Hospital, Helsinki, Finland
e-mail: eija.hiltunen-back@hus.fi; alexander.salava@hus.fi

H. Gollnick et al. (eds.), *Dermatology Cyberderm WebBook*,
https://doi.org/10.1007/978-3-031-78491-0_34

Gonorrhea* [4]

Grading of Importance

A

https://www.cyberderm.net/en/learn/skin-diseases/gonorrhea
*see section "Gonorrhoea" in Chap. 10.

Ulcus Molle (Chancroid)* [1, 2]

Grading of Importance

C

*See section "Chancroid" in Chap. 10.

References

1. Çakmak S, Tamer E, Karadağ A, Waugh M (2019) Syphilis: a great imitator. Clin Dermatol 37:182–191
2. Irizarry L, Velasquez J, Wray AA (2020) Chancroid. StatPearls, Treasure Island, FL
3. Peeling RW, Mabey D, Kamb ML, Chen XS, Radolf JD, Benzaken AS (2017) Syphilis. Nat Rev Dis Primers 3:17073
4. Unemo M, Seifert HS, Hook EW 3rd, Hawkes S, Ndowa F, Dillon JR (2019) Gonorrhoea. Nat Rev Dis Primers 5(1):79

Glossary

A Glossary of Basic Dermatologic Lesions[1,2,3]

Aberrant Aberrant is an adjective pertaining to a deviation from normal.

Ablation Ablation is the destruction of tissue, often by cautery, cryotherapy, or laser.

Abscess A localized collection of pus in a cavity formed by disintegration or necrosis of tissues.

Acantholysis The separation of keratinocytes of the epidermis by loss of intercellular connections permitting the cells to become round and hyaline. Immunoreactive acantholysis is typical of pemphigus. Acantholysis occurs as a secondary change in viral bullae and in epithelial malignancies.

Acanthoma Acanthoma is a benign tumor located in the prickle cell layer of the epidermis. There are several specific forms of acanthoma.

Acanthosis Acanthosis is a histological term for thickening of the epidermis and elongation of the rete ridges due to thickening of the spinous layer and enlargement of rete pegs.

Achromia Achromia means loss of color. In the skin, achromia is also called leukoderma or depigmentation and means a lack or absence of melanin.

Acneiform Acneiform is an adjective used to describe a resemblance to acne.

Acral Acral is an adjective relating to or involving a distal site, e.g., ear, finger, toe, nose, penis, and nipple.

Acrochordon Acrochordon is a fibroepithelial polyp of the skin, commonly known as a skin tag.

Acrokeratoderma Acrokeratoderma is skin thickening of the hands and feet, usually due to hyperkeratosis.

Actinic Actinic is an adjective pertaining to sun or ultraviolet radiation.

---

[1] Adapted from

- Glossary of Basic Dermatology Lesions. ILDS 1987.
- DermNet NZ https://dermnetnz.org/.
- A Dictionary of Dermatologic Terms. Robert L. Carter. Williams & Wilkins, Baltimore 1992.

[2] Is not intended to include diagnostic terms.

[3] Nast et al. British Journal of Dermatology (2016) 174, pp. 1351–1358.

H. Gollnick et al. (eds.), *Dermatology Cyberderm WebBook*,
https://doi.org/10.1007/978-3-031-78491-0

Actinic keratosis Actinic keratosis is a scaly skin spot showing some atypia of keratinocytes caused by chronic sun exposure.

Acuminate Adjective meaning rendered sharp or pointed.

Adenoma Adenoma is a benign epithelial tumor with glands and gland-like structures.

Adhesion Adhesion is the process of the sticking together of components, e.g., adhesion between keratinocytes.

Adipocyte Adipocyte is a fat cell, also known as a lipocyte or adipose cell.

Adjacent Adjacent is an adjective meaning to be next to or adjoining.

Adjuvant Adjuvant is a noun and adjective meaning helper or helpful. An adjuvant is an extra agent added to improve efficacy, for example, added to immunizations to improve the immune response. Adjuvant therapies are used after the main treatment for cancer to reduce the risk of recurrence and the chance of secondary tumors.

Adnexal Adnexal is an adjective pertaining to an adnexa, an accessory, or appendage. In dermatology, adnexal may pertain to hair, nail, sweat gland, etc.

Aerobe Aerobe is an organism that requires oxygen.

Aetiology Aetiology (American spelling etiology) is the study of causes and causation. Aetiology is also the cause of a situation, e.g., the aetiology of a disease may be an infection.

Aggregation Aggregation is a collection or clustering. For example, aspirin prevents platelet aggregation to form a clot.

Agminate Gathered together in a group.

Albicans Turning or becoming white.

Allele Allele is a variant form of a gene found on the same locus of a chromosome.

Allergen Allergen is a substance capable of inducing an immediate or delayed hypersensitivity reaction (allergy).

Allergy Allergy is a hypersensitivity reaction of which there are several different types; an abnormal reaction of the immune system to an exogenous agent such as pollen or peanuts.

Alopecia Absence of hair from normally hairy areas of skin is termed alopecia. Alopecia can be diffuse or localized.

SYN: baldness (of scalp)

Amelanotic Amelanotic is an adjective pertaining to a lack of melanin, the skin pigment.

Amenorrhoea Amenorrhoea (American spelling amenorrhea) is the temporary or permanent absence of menstruation.

Amiantacea Adjective meaning in the nature of asbestos (amiant; tinea amiantacea).

Amorphous Amorphous is an adjective describing a lack of form or shape.

Amyloid Amyloid is an abnormal aggregate of proteins deposited in tissue with characteristic staining and appearance on microscopy.

Anaerobe Anaerobe is an organism that does not require oxygen. It may be a facultative anaerobe meaning it tolerates oxygen in its environment, or a strict anaerobe meaning it is killed by oxygen.

Anagen Anagen is the growth phase of the hair follicle.

Anaphylaxis Anaphylaxis is an immediate hypersensitive reaction that can be severe, and potentially fatal, in a sensitized individual.

Anaplastic Anaplastic is an adjective used in histology to describe specific features usually indicative of malignancy. Anaplastic cells have irregular dark-staining nuclei and are typically poorly differentiated.

Anetoderma Atrophic skin patches, giving the palpating finger the same sensation as a hernial orifice.

Angiogenesis Angiogenesis is the formation of new blood vessels.

Angioid Adjective meaning like or resembling blood vessels.

Angioma Angioma is a benign collection of dilated congested blood vessels. On the skin, an angioma typically presents as a red papule. The cherry angioma is a common example.

Anhidrosis Anhidrosis is the inability to sweat appropriately; it may be due to an abnormality of the sweat glands or associated with a neurological lesion or disease.

Annular Annular is an adjective describing a ring-like or circular shape. In dermatology, this may be used for lesions grouped in a circle, or a ring-shaped lesion as in granuloma annulare.

Anogenital Anogenital is the adjective pertaining to the area around the anus and genitals.

Anterior Anterior is an adjective to describe being towards the front or before. In anatomy, anterior location means on the front (ventral) surface of a body part, e.g., the anterior eye meaning the front of the eye.

Antigen Antigen (Ag) is any substance that evokes an immediate or delayed immune response.

Aphtha Small ulcers of the mucous membranes are usually termed aphthae.

SYN.: canker sore

Aplasia Aplasia is the failure to develop, as in aplasia cutis.

Apocrine Apocrine is an adjective pertaining to glands that form a secretion by releasing cytoplasm.

Apoptosis Apoptosis is the regulated, normal physiological process by which a cell undergoes self-destruction in response to signals from the cell nucleus.

Appendages Appendages: plural of appendage; additional things or supplements. The skin appendages are things additional to the epidermis and include eccrine (sweat) glands, apocrine (scent) glands, pilosebaceous structures (hair and oil glands), and nails.

Arachnids Arachnids: plural of arachnid; arthropods with four pairs of legs, e.g., spiders, mites.

Arciform Arciform is an adjective to describe an arched or bow shape.

Arcuate Arcuate is an adjective to describe an arched or bow shape.

Areata Limited to a circumscribed area.

Areola Areola is a circular area. In anatomy, the areola is the pigmented circular area around the breast nipple. It is also used in dermatology to mean a red ring around an inflamed spot.

Arthropod Arthropod is an invertebrate animal with a segmented body, jointed limbs, and a hard shell that is shed periodically. Examples of an arthropod include an insect, spider, and crustacean.

Astringent Substance that is binding, contracting, constrictive, or styptic.

Atopy Atopy is a genetic (inherited) tendency to develop allergies such as hay fever (allergic rhinitis), asthma, food allergies, and atopic dermatitis.

Atrichia Atrichia is the absence of hair which can be either congenital or acquired.

Atrophy A diminution of a tissue.

Types:

–Dermal atrophy—e.g., focal dermal hypoplasia

–Elastic tissue atrophy—e.g., anetoderma

–Epidermal atrophy—e.g., lichen sclerosus

–Subcutaneous atrophy—e.g., lipoatrophy

Auspitz's sign Pinpoint bleeding observed when the scale of a lesion of psoriasis is removed. The phenomenon is due to the rupture of capillaries which lie high in the papillary dermis beneath a thinned suprapapillary plate.

Autoantibody Autoantibody is an immunoglobulin directed against a normal component of the host individual producing it (self, auto).

Autoantigen Autoantigen is a normal self-protein targeted by a host antibody.

Autoimmunity Autoimmunity is an immune reaction against "self"; when antibodies are made against a normal body protein resulting in disease.

Autoinflammatory Autoinflammatory is an adjective describing recurrent inflammatory episodes not associated with an autoimmune disease, malignancy, allergy, immunodeficiency, or infection.

Autosomal dominant Autosomal dominant is an adjective to describe a genetic disorder in which only one copy of the abnormal gene is required to cause the condition, and that gene is located on a non-sex chromosome.

Autosomal recessive Autosomal recessive is an adjective to define a genetic disorder that requires both copies of a gene to be abnormal to cause the condition, and that gene is located on a non-sex chromosome.

Axial Axial is an adjective pertaining to the axis, the center or midline of a body about which it rotates; thus, the axial skeleton is the cranium, sternum, and spine.

Baldness Hairlessness, particularly of the scalp.

Balloon cells (degeneration) Intracellular edema.

Basement membrane Basement membrane is the structure between an epithelium (epidermis in skin) and the underlying connective tissue (dermis in skin).

Basophil Basophil is a granulocytic white blood cell (leukocyte) closely related to mast cells and eosinophils and involved in allergic disease. The cytoplasm of a basophil contains granules that stain blue with basic dyes, i.e., basophilic.

Basophilic degeneration Change in tinctorial properties of connective tissue, usually of elastic fibers or collagen.

Bathing trunk nevus Giant congenital nevus.

BCC Basal cell carcinoma.

Biopsy Biopsy is a noun and verb pertaining to a tissue sample, for example, a dermatologist may take a skin biopsy, the dermatologist may biopsy the skin.

Blaschko line Blaschko line is an embryological clonal expansion line in the skin following a roughly linear, segmental pattern. A birthmark may be distributed along a Blaschko line.

B lymphocyte B lymphocyte, also called a B cell, originates in the bone marrow and is normally involved in producing immunoglobulins to detect and combat infection.

Bleb Bleb is a small thin-walled blister containing air or fluid.

Blister Superficial relatively thin-walled structure containing air or fluid.

BRAF BRAF is a proto-oncogene that encodes a threonine protein kinase called B-Raf. It is essential for normal cell development and function; however, mutations in the BRAF gene may result in cancer.

Breslow thickness Breslow thickness, also called Breslow depth, is the thickness of an invasive melanoma in millimeters measured from the granular cell layer to the deepest tumor cell. Breslow thickness is an important prognostic factor so should be measured and recorded on the histology report.

Bromhidrosis Bromhidrosis is an abnormal or offensive body odor.

Bubo Enlarged lymph node.

Bulla A bulla is circumscribed elevation of skin over 0.5 cm in diameter containing a liquid. Also a bleb or a blister. The distinction between vesicle and bulla is arbitrary and depends only on size.

Examples of Bullae:

Dermal bulla: A bulla caused by separation of tissue components of the dermis with collection of serous fluid,

e.g., Dystrophic epidermolysis bullosa

Epidermal vesicle or bulla: A blister formed within the epidermis by pathologic change in epidermal cells or cellular cohesion.

Spongiotic vesicle or bulla: An intraepidermal multilocular vesicle or blister formed by separation of epidermal cells by edema. Lymphocytes predominate in allergic contact dermatitis and neutrophilic leukocytes predominate in irritant dermatitis.

Subcorneal bulla: A bulla formed by exudate beneath the stratum corneum, and above the stratum spinosum, as in bullous impetigo.

Subepidermal vesicle or bulla: A vesicle or bulla formed by cleavage of the dermal–epidermal interface and with the roof of the bulla composed of the epidermis.

Burrow A cuniculus, passage, or tunnel in the skin that houses a metazoan parasite, particularly the acarus of scabies.

Cachexia Cachexia is a state of weight loss associated with anorexia, muscle and fat loss, poor quality of life, and fatigue. It is associated with cancer, AIDS, and chronic organ failure such as congestive cardiac failure or renal failure.

Calcification Calcification is the process of depositing calcium salts in body tissues.

Callus A localized callus is the hyperplasia of the stratum corneum (keratoderma) due to physical pressure.

Canities Gray or graying scalp hair.

Carbuncle A necrotizing infection of skin and subcutaneous tissue composed of a group of furuncles (boils).

Carotenosis Yellowish discoloration of the skin.

Caseating necrosis Caseating necrosis is a histological term for a specific form of collagen destruction typically associated with granulomas; a mix of coagulative and liquefactive necrosis resembling friable cheese.

Catagen Catagen is the short involutional phase of the hair cycle.

Caudal Caudal is an adjective pertaining to the tail. A caudal location is on or near to the tail or base of the spine.

Cautery Destructive procedure employing electricity (electrocautery) and chemicals (chemocautery).

Cavernous Adjective meaning relating to a cave or hollow.

Cellulitis An inflammation of cellular tissue, particularly purulent inflammation of dermis, subcutaneous tissue, and soft tissue.

Centrifugum Means fleeing from the center.

Checkpoint inhibitor Checkpoint inhibitor is a drug or agent that blocks an inhibitory checkpoint molecule protecting a tumor from immune attack. It is a form of immune therapy (immunotherapy).

Chemokine Chemokine is a chemotactic cytokine; a signaling molecule that induces chemotaxis in nearby cells. An inflammatory chemokine, for example, attracts leukocytes (white blood cells).

Chemotaxis Chemotaxis is the movement of organisms, cells, or cellular components, in response to a chemical stimulus.

Chemotherapy Chemotherapy is an adjective and noun pertaining to the chemical treatment of disease, for example, chemotherapy drug, chemotherapy is the drug regime to treat cancer.

Chloasma Patchy hyperpigmentation especially on the face.

Cholinergic Cholinergic is an adjective pertaining to acetylcholine, a neurotransmitter.

Chromatin Chromatin is the DNA and protein packaged to fit into the nucleus of a cell.

Chromosome Chromosome is a long chain of genes; the entity carrying the genetic material of a cell (organism) which is passed to progeny, and is expressed as proteins for cellular functions.

Circumscribed Lesions that are sharply limited to an area by clean borders.

CNS Central nervous system; the brain and spinal cord.

Coagulation Coagulation is the process by which blood forms a clot.

Collagen Collagen is a large family of proteins with a triple helix structure found in most tissues. In the skin, collagen is an important and major component of the dermis.

Comedo A comedo is a plug of keratin and sebum in a dilated pilosebaceous orifice.

SYN.: blackhead

Commensal Commensal is an adjective and noun pertaining to a close relationship between unrelated organisms without harm to either, and sometimes with benefit to one or both.

Complement Complement is a system of glycoproteins important in the innate immune system. Activation of the complement cascade results in enhancement of the cellular immune response.

Compound naevus Compound naevus (American spelling nevus) is a benign melanocytic naevus in which melanocytes are found in both the epidermis and dermis.

Computer tomography (CT) Computer tomography (CT) is a diagnostic radiology test that scans the body to produce cross-sectional images of the part.

Concentric Concentric is an adjective pertaining to arrangement around a central point, e.g., an archery or shooting target is concentric rings around the central bull's eye.

Concomitant Concomitant is an adjective meaning accompanying or at the same time, simultaneous, e.g., concomitant treatments means more than one treatment at the same time.

Confluent Confluent is an adjective pertaining to confluence, flowing or coming together, e.g., confluent pustules.

Congelation Freezing.

Congenital Congenital is an adjective to mean present at birth, born with.

Constriction Constriction is used to mean a narrowing of something, such as a blood vessel.

Contracture Contracture is a permanent shortening of muscle, connective tissue, or skin typically resulting in deformity across a joint.

Corneocyte Corneocyte is an epidermal cell (keratinocyte) in the stratum corneum (outermost layer of the epidermis) which normally lacks a nucleus.

Cornoid Cornoid is an adjective meaning horn-like, e.g., cornoid lamella is a thin horn-like layer.

Corium Portion of the skin that is below the epidermis. The term dermis is used interchangeably with corium.

Craquelé Scaling surface with cracks.

Cream Cream, when used in dermatology, is a semi-solid formulation for topical application. A cream may be water in oil (lipid) emulsion or lipid (oil) in water emulsion. Common usage also makes cream a verb, to apply a cream.

CRP C-reactive protein; a nonspecific inflammatory marker protein produced by the liver and commonly measured in the blood. An elevated CRP in the blood is associated with infection, tumors, and inflammatory diseases.

Crust A crust is an outer layer from the drying of exudate, secretion, or hemorrhagic.

Cryoglobulin Cryoglobulin is an immunoglobulin that precipitates out in the blood on exposure to cold.

Cryotherapy Cryotherapy is treatment using a very cold substance such as liquid nitrogen or dry ice. In dermatology, cryotherapy is often used to treat warts or actinic keratoses.

Crypt Crypt is a chamber or room under the surface. So in dermatology, a crypt is a tube or recess extending down from the skin surface.

CT Computed tomography; a CT scan is a diagnostic radiology test that produces cross-sectional images of the body.

Cubital Cubital is an adjective pertaining to the ulna bone in the forearm. The cubital (also called antecubital) fossa is the elbow crease anterior to (in front of) the elbow.

Cumulative Cumulative is an adjective pertaining to accumulation; describes increasing by successive additions.

Curet, curette, curettage Instrument and procedure that scrapes away tissue.

Cuticle Cuticle is the outermost layer of a hair and is also the transparent layer of dead cells that connects the proximal nailfold to the nail plate.

Cyanosis Cyanosis is the bluish coloration of the skin and mucous membranes due to deoxyhemoglobin in the surface capillaries. This may be seen in either heart or lung disorders causing inadequate oxygenation, or when cold and the peripheral circulation is sluggish.

Cyst A cyst is any closed cavity or sac (normal or abnormal) with an epithelial, endothelial, or membranous lining and containing fluid or semi-solid material.

Cytogenetic Cytogenetic is an adjective pertaining to cytogenetics, the study of chromosomes and their structure.

Cytokeratin Cytokeratin is better known as keratin, a family of cytoplasmic proteins in epithelial cells.

Cytokine Cytokine is a low-molecular-weight molecule that acts as an intercellular messenger. Interleukins, interferons, colony-stimulating factors, and chemokines are examples of specific types of cytokine.

Dandruff Visible scaling of the scalp, not associated with a disease.

Darier sign Darier sign is positive when stroking the skin or lesion induces whealing; typically seen in cutaneous mastocystosis.

Debridement Debridement is the process of removing infected or dead tissue to aid the healing process.

Demarcation Demarcation is a noun meaning the boundary or plane of separation between two areas.

Dendritic cell Dendritic cell has long finger-like processes called dendrites. Examples of a dendritic cell include a neuron, melanocyte, Langerhans cell, and some types of tissue macrophage (immune cell).

Dermal naevus Dermal naevus (American spelling nevus) is a benign melanocytic naevus in which the melanocytes are entirely within the dermis. Dermal nevus is also called an intradermal nevus.

Dermatitis Dermatitis is inflammation of the skin, but is mostly used more specifically as a synonym for eczema, i.e., spongiotic inflammation of the epidermis.

Dermatome Dermatome is the area of skin innervated by a single sensory spinal nerve. A dermatome is also a tool for taking fine slices of skin.

Dermatopathology Dermatopathology is the study of the microscopic appearance of skin diseases.

Dermatoscopy Dermatoscopy, also called dermoscopy, is the use of a dermatoscope, comprising a power source, light, and magnification to examine the skin, hair, and nails.

Dermographism Means "writing on the skin." Dermographism may be black (metallic particles rubbed off) or urticarial (whealing in the precise form of scratching) or white (blanching that occurs upon stroke of skin affected by atopic dermatitis).

Desensitisation Desensitisation (American spelling desensitization) is a process of reversing a hypersensitivity reaction such as an allergy.

Desmoglein Desmoglein is one of a family of molecules involved in forming desmosomes, the intercellular junctions that stick skin cells (keratinocytes) together. There are three main types of desmoglein in the skin.

Desmoplastic Desmoplastic is an adjective used in histology pertaining to desmoplasia, the presence of a fibrous connective tissue reaction typically related to specific tumors.

Desmosome Desmosome is a structure that holds adjacent epidermal skin cells (keratinocytes) tightly together, rather like cement between bricks.

Desquamation Desquamation is the peeling of skin, coming off in scales, loss of squames.

Diascopy Diascopy is a test using pressure from clear glass or plastic to see if a rash or lesion blanches. Diascopy also allows assessment of the underlying color.

Differential diagnosis Differential diagnosis is a list of conditions with similar symptoms or signs needed to be considered as possible diagnoses.

Diffuse Diffuse is an adjective and verb pertaining to spread over a wide area. In dermatology, diffuse is used as an adjective to describe a change that is not localized or patchy, e.g., diffuse alopecia compared to patchy alopecia.

Diploid Diploid is an adjective describing a cell having two sets of chromosomes, as is typically seen in a normal somatic cell.

Discoid Discoid is an adjective to describe being round like a disk. In dermatology, it is used to describe lesions that are circular or oval and often well defined, e.g., discoid eczema and discoid lupus.

Disseminated Disseminated is an adjective to describe being scattered or widespread and derives from the verb to disseminate meaning to scatter. Disseminated is therefore also the past tense of the verb. Examples in dermatology may include an infection that gained entry through the skin disseminated throughout the body; a rash may present as disseminated lesions distributed/scattered widely over most of the body surface.

Distal Distal is an adjective to describe being furthest from the point of origin or closest to the end. Anatomically, this may mean being furthest from the center of the body.

Distribution Distribution is the localization or pattern. The distribution of a dermatosis refers to the pattern or localization of skin lesions, and can be quite characteristic for a specific condition.

DNA Deoxyribonucleic acid, a long nucleic acid chain that can encode genes, the famous double helix.

Dorsal Dorsal is an adjective pertaining to the back or posterior part. A dorsal location means on the upper surface or back of a body part.

Double-blind Double-blind is an adjective used to describe clinical trials in which neither the participants nor the researchers know which treatment or intervention has been selected for the individual, i.e., both the assessor and the participant are blinded to the intervention.

DSM-5 According to the American Psychiatric Association (Book).

Duplex ultrasound Duplex ultrasound is an imaging test combining two types of ultrasound to produce a scan of blood flow in arteries and veins. Traditional ultrasound scans a fixed object (i.e., the artery or vein) and is combined with a Doppler scan of moving objects (i.e., blood flow). Uses of duplex ultrasonography scan include identification of a DVT, incompetent valves in varicose veins, or to map out vessels for sclerotherapy.

Dysaesthesia Dysaesthesia (American spelling dysesthesia) literally means abnormal (dys) sensation (aesthesia) and describes unpleasant, uncomfortable sensations produced by ordinary stimuli. There are many specific types of dysesthesia, e.g., orodynia, pruritus ani, brachioradial pruritus, male genital dysesthesia.

Dyskeratosis Dyskeratosis is a histological term for premature or altered (abnormal) keratinocyte differentiation.

Dysmorphic Dysmorphic is an adjective pertaining to an anatomical malformation.

Dysplasia Dysplasia is a histologic term for an atypical or abnormal appearance of a cell or tissue. In dermatopathology, it is most commonly used to mean atypical cells in the epithelium.

Dysplastic Dysplastic is an adjective pertaining to dysplasia, abnormal or atypical appearance of a cell or tissue.

Dystrophy Dystrophy refers to degeneration or abnormal formation of tissue due to disease or malnutrition. A well-known example is muscular dystrophy caused by a genetic mutation. An example in dermatology is nail dystrophy, meaning a nail that did not develop normally or has become abnormal due to a disease such as tinea.

EASI Eczema Area and Severity Index, a tool used for assessment and monitoring of atopic eczema.

ECG ECG (American terminology EKG) stands for electrocardiogram; graph of the electrical activity of the heart.

Ecchymosis A macular red or purple or colored hemorrhage in skin or mucous membrane more than 2 mm in diameter.

SYN: bruise

Eccrine gland Eccrine gland is the common sweat gland in the skin.

Ectodermal Ectodermal is an adjective pertaining to the ectoderm. An example is ectodermal dysplasia. The ectoderm is the outermost of the three primary germ layers of an embryo (the other two being mesoderm and endoderm). Ectoderm develops into epidermis and neural tissue.

Ectopic Ectopic is an adjective pertaining to not being in the right place, e.g., an ectopic pregnancy has developed somewhere other than inside the uterus.

Ectropion Ectropion is a turned out part. Common usage has ectropion meaning the eversion (turning out) of a lower eyelid resulting in exposure of the inside surface of the eyelid.

Eczema Eczema, also called dermatitis, is an inflammatory condition of the skin defined histologically by the presence of epidermal spongiosis.

Effluvium Effluvium, when used in dermatology, refers to diffuse hair loss of various causes. In general usage, an effluvium is an unpleasant gaseous smell.

Elastic fibre Elastic fibre (American spelling fiber) is composed of elastin and microfibrils of fibrillin, collagen VI, and other proteins and glycoproteins. An elastic fiber demonstrates elasticity, the ability to stretch and return to the original.

Elastolytic Elastolytic is an adjective pertaining to elastolysis, the breakdown and loss of elastic fibers.

Elastosis Elastosis is a histological term for an increase in the elastic fibers in the skin.

Elastotic Elastotic is an adjective used in histology pertaining to elastic tissue and fibers. Due to observed histological changes, elastotic often finds its way into the name of the condition as well.

Electrocoagulation Destroying tissue by curdling (coagulation) with heat generated by a bipolar electrical instrument.

Electrodesiccation Destroying tissue by drying it out (desiccation). The electrical instrument used involves high frequency, unidirectional current that concentrates heat at a point in the form of a spark.

Electron microscopy Electron microscopy is a laboratory tool used to examine extremely thin specimens with a beam of electrons passed through an electromagnetic lens. Electron microscopy allows visualization of much smaller structures than light microscopy.

Electrophoresis Electrophoresis is a laboratory technique to separate molecules by their electric charge and size using an electric field.

Elevatum Adjective meaning raised.

Embolus Embolus is a small particle that has been carried through the bloodstream and blocks a small blood vessel. The particle is foreign to the bloodstream and examples include an air bubble, fat, clump of bacteria, or blood clot.

Emollient Emollient derives from the Latin to soften, so an emollient is a moisturizer that softens the skin.

Enanthem Enanthem, also called an enanthema, is a rash on mucous membranes.

Encapsulated Encapsulated is an adjective and verb pertaining to being within a capsule. A medication may be encapsulated, i.e., in a capsule form rather than a tablet. In histology, encapsulated describes a pathological process being contained by a membrane or wall, e.g., a cyst is encapsulated by the fibrous wall. Microorganisms can also be encapsulated by a protective thick mucoid or polysaccharide layer.

Endemic Endemic is an adjective used to describe being constantly present in a population or region, e.g., an endemic disease may be due to an infectious organism or arthropod that spreads an infection occurring in an area due to climatic factors.

Endocrine Endocrine is an adjective pertaining to the production and release of secretions (hormones) directly into the blood.

Endogenous Endogenous is an adjective to describe an origin from within. In medicine, an endogenous cause for an illness means it has not been caused by an external agent or event, e.g., atopic dermatitis is an example of an endogenous form of eczema.

Endoscopy Endoscopy is the use of an endoscope, an instrument introduced into a body cavity or organ allowing direct visual examination.

Enzyme Enzyme is a biological catalyst involved in biochemical reactions.

Eosinophil Eosinophil is a type of granulocytic white blood cell (granular leukocyte) involved in the innate immune system primarily as defense against parasitic infections. Eosinophils are pro-inflammatory and are found in large numbers in allergic inflammation.

Eosinophilia Eosinophilia is an increase in the number of eosinophils in the peripheral blood.

Eosinophilic Eosinophilic is an adjective pertaining to staining red with the dye eosin on microscopy. Examples include the eosinophilic cytoplasmic granules seen in eosinophils, the eosinophilic stratum corneum of the epidermis, and normal eosinophilic collagen fibers in the dermis.

Ephilides Ephilides: plural of ephelis; freckles.

Epidemic Epidemic is the sudden occurrence of a disease (or other event) in excess of that normally expected. Epidemic can be used as a noun or adjective, e.g., a flu epidemic or epidemic typhus.

Epidemiology Epidemiology is the study of the distribution of a disease and factors involved in the spread of that disease in populations.

Epidermis Epidermis is the outer epithelial layer of the skin overlying in the dermis. It is mainly composed of keratinocytes, but also includes melanocytes, Merkel cells, and other cell types in small numbers.

Epidermolytic Epidermolytic is an adjective used in histology to describe loosening of the epidermis.

Epidermotropism Epidermotropism is movement into or towards the epidermis. It is a histological term for the migration of cells into the epidermis typically seen in mycosis fungoides and Paget disease.

Epigenetics Epigenetics is the study of phenotypic change due to changes in gene expression without changes in the gene itself. An example is modification of DNA methylation.

Epilation Removal of hair.

Epithelioid cell Epithelioid cell is large and round with abundant eosinophilic cytoplasm, prominent vesicular nucleus, and large nucleolus.

Epithelioma Neoplasm or overdevelopment of epithelial tissue.

Eponychium Eponychium is the nail cuticle, the skin attaching the proximal nailfold to the nail plate.

Erosion An erosion is a loss of the epidermis which heals without scarring.

Erythema The redness of the skin produced by vascular congestion or perfusion. Perivascular lymphocytic inflammation.

Erythrocyanosis A condition marked by a red-purple color.

Erythroderma A generalized redness of the skin. It is often associated with desquamation, as in exfoliate dermatitis.

Eschar Eschar is a full-thickness scab that develops in a healing wound. Examples include wounds caused by a thermal burn, cauterization, or chemical burn. An eschar can be typical of some infections particularly rickettsia.

ESR Erythrocyte sedimentation rate, a test of blood viscosity. The ESR is a non-specific test often raised in inflammatory diseases and infections.

Eukaryote Eukaryote is a cellular organism in which the genetic material is contained within a nucleus.

Exacerbation Exacerbation is a noun meaning an aggravation, worsening, or flare up.

Exanthem Exanthem is a widespread skin rash typically caused by a drug or infection, usually accompanied by systemic symptoms such as fever, malaise, and headache.

Excisional biopsy Complete surgical removal of a lesion for microscopic evaluation.

Excoriation An excoriation is any loss of substance of skin produced by scratching.

Exfoliation Exfoliation is the splitting off or separation of the keratin and epidermal skin surface in scales or sheets.

SYN.: desquamation

Excisional biopsy Excisional biopsy is the complete surgical removal of a lesion for diagnosis, treatment or both.

Excoriation Excoriation, also called a scratch mark, is a loss of epidermis and a portion of the dermis due to scratching. An excoriation may be linear or punctate.

Exfoliation Exfoliation is the process of peeling or shedding of the epidermal stratum corneum. It may occur after skin inflammation or be induced by chemicals or abrasion.

Exocrine Secretion to the outside (autonomous to endocrine).

Exocytosis Exocytosis is a histological term for the random migration of inflammatory cells, such as lymphocytes, neutrophils, basophils, into the epidermis. Exocytosis is induced by cytokine release in inflammatory processes of the epidermis.

Exogenous Exogenous is an adjective pertaining to an outside influence or cause. In medicine, an exogenous cause for an illness means the cause is not from within, e.g., contact dermatitis is an example of an exogenous form of eczema.

Extravasation Extravasation is the leakage of fluid or cells from a blood vessel into body tissue, e.g., extravasation of red blood cells results in a bruise.

Exudate Exudate is the ooze typically seen in wounds, derived from blood, and composed of protein and blood cells. An exudate can be described as serous, purulent, sanguineous, or serosanguineous.

Fascicle Bunch of fibers.

Fibril Single fine thread-like structure.

Fibroblast Fibroblast is the most numerous cell type seen in loose connective tissue. In the dermis, fibroblasts produce collagen, elastin, ground substance, and fibronectin.

Fibrosis Fibrosis is the formation of excessive fibrous collagen.

Filament Filament is a thread-like structure or fiber.

Filiform Filiform is an adjective pertaining to filament, a thread-like structure, e.g., filiform wart or filiform papilla of the tongue.

FISH Fluorescent in situ (in-situ) hybridization, a cytogenetic test used to detect chromosomal abnormalities.

Fissure A fissure is any linear gap or slit in the skin surface.

Fistula A fistula is an abnormal passage from a deep structure to the skin surface or between two deep structures. It is often lined with squamous epithelium.

Flexural Flexural is an adjective relating to a bend or fold. In the skin, the back of knees (popliteal fossae), the armpits (axillae), the antecubital (cubital) fossae, and the groin are examples of flexural sites. Atopic dermatitis is described as having a flexural distribution on the limbs as it commonly involves the popliteal and antecubital (cubital) fossae.

Foam cell Histiocyte that has imbibed lipids and thus come to appear bubbled.

Foliaceus Leaflike.

Follicular Follicular is an adjective pertaining to a follicle. In dermatology, this usually means a hair follicle, e.g., a follicular lesion is located within or around a hair follicle. However, in histology, follicular also pertains to lymphoid follicles and ovarian follicles.

Free radical Free radical is an unstable form of an atom with an unpaired electron, for example, a reactive oxygen species.

Fungating Fungating is an adjective pertaining to a fungus. In dermatology, it is typically used to describe a tumor erupting like a mushroom or toadstool.

Furuncle A localized pyogenic infection originating in a hair follicle.

Syn., **boil**

Gamete Gamete is a haploid cell (having one copy of each chromosome instead of two) for sexual reproduction. In the female, this is an ovum (egg) produced in the ovaries, and in the male, sperm produced in the testes (testicles).

Gammopathy Gammopathy is a condition characterized by excessive antibodies (gammaglobulins, immunoglobulins) in the blood. It is typically used for a monoclonal proliferation of gammaglobulins.

Gangrene Gangrene is the death of tissue, associated with loss of blood supply.

Gene Gene is the biological unit of heredity. A gene is encoded in DNA or RNA and is usually located on a chromosome in the genome.

Generalised Generalised (American spelling generalized) is an adjective meaning widespread or extensive. A generalized rash is distributed over most of the body surface area. (generalized/widespread/disseminated).

Genodermatosis Genodermatosis is a genetically determined skin condition.

Genome Genome is an organism's complete set of genetic material. It includes all the genes and information required to construct that organism. In eukaryotes, the genome is stored in the nucleus. Although a genome in a nucleus is constructed of double-stranded DNA, some viral genomes are made from single- or double-stranded RNA.

Genotype Genotype is the genetic message at a specific gene locus or the whole genome. The genotype can be sequenced looking for mutations or identifying alleles at a locus. Mutations in the genotype may or may not affect the phenotype.

Genotyping Genotyping is the process of determining and comparing genetic differences between individuals, using biological assays and nucleic acid sequencing.

Germline Germline is a noun and adjective pertaining to the genetic material passed to offspring, the next generation. The germline is the cells that produce gametes, the cells by which genetic material is passed between generations. In humans, these gametes are the sperm in men and the ova (eggs) in women. Germline as an adjective describes the genetic material passed from a parent, e.g., germline mutation meaning every cell in the offspring carries the same mutation.

Granule Little grain.

Granular layer Granular layer of the epidermis (stratum granulosum) is characterized by flattened cells filled with dark granules containing keratohyalin protein.

Granulocyte Granulocyte is a type of white blood cell (leukocyte) with a cytoplasm filled with microscopic granules containing enzymes and other proteins important in innate immunity. Neutrophils, basophils, and eosinophils are the three most common forms of granulocyte in the blood.

Granuloma Chronic inflammatory tissue composed of macrophages, fibroblasts, and granulation tissue.

Granulomatous Granulomatous is an adjective pertaining to granulomas, a type of chronic inflammation characterized by histiocytes.

Grenz zone Grenz zone is a histological term for an apparently uninvolved area (zone) of papillary dermis separating the epidermis from an inflammatory or tumor cell infiltrate in the dermis.

Ground substance Ground substance is the gel component of the dermis. It contains hyaluronic acid, dermatan sulfate, chondroitin-6-sulfate, anionic polysaccharides, and glycosaminoglycans. It does not include the fibers such as collagen and elastin, or cells.

Gumma A necrotic granuloma of tertiary syphilis.

Guttata Drop-like spots.

Gyrate Gyrate is an adjective meaning spiral-like or rotating. In dermatology, it is used to describe a pattern that is convoluting, winding, or coiled.

Haematocrit Haematocrit (American spelling hematocrit) is defined as the ratio of the volume of red blood cells to the total volume of blood. It is measured by separating red blood cells from plasma by centrifugation.

Haematogenous Haematogenous (American spelling hematogenous) is an adjective pertaining to blood, its production, constituents, dissemination, or derivation, e.g., haematogenous spread of a cancer means cancer cells have been spread via the bloodstream.

Haematoma A localized, tumor-like collection of blood.

Haemolysis Haemolysis (American spelling hemolysis) is the rupture or destruction of red blood cells.

Haemorrhage Haemorrhage (American spelling hemorrhage) is a noun and verb pertaining to a bleed or to bleed.

Hair cycle Hair cycle consists of a growth phase (anagen); a short involutional phase (catagen); a resting phase (telogen).

Hair pull test Hair pull test is used for assessing a patient complaining of hair loss. If more than 10% of hairs in a pulled bundle are removed, the result is considered abnormal (positive). None, one or two hairs removed when gently tugging on a bundle of 50–60 hairs is considered normal.

Hamartoma Hamartoma is a benign overgrowth of a mature cell type normal to the site or organ. In the skin, a hamartoma often presents as a birthmark (congenital naevus), but may first develop, appear, or be noticed in adult life (acquired). Examples include naevus sebaceous, follicular hamartoma, and chondroid syringoma.

Haploid Haploid is an adjective describing a cell with only one set of chromosomes, as is typically seen in gametes (ova and sperm).

Helminth Helminth is a parasitic worm. Examples of a helminth include a tapeworm, liver fluke, roundworm, and leech.

Hemidesmosome Hemidesmosome is a structure in the basement-membrane zone, made by the epidermal basal keratinocytes, and involved in sticking the basal keratinocytes to the dermis.

Hereditary Hereditary is an adjective pertaining to inheritance. In medicine, it is used to describe a genetic (inherited) mutation or condition.

Herpetiform Herpetiform is an adjective meaning to resemble herpes, so is used to describe clustered vesicles and does not imply a viral origin.

Heterogenous Heterogenous refers to a structure having a foreign origin.

Histamine Histamine, 2-[4-imidazolyl]ethylamine, is stored in the granules of mast cells and basophils, and released rapidly via an IgE-mediated mechanism during hypersensitivity and inflammation. Local histamine release causes capillary vasodilation and plasma leakage. In anaphylaxis, large amounts of histamine are released with systemic effects on smooth muscle and blood pressure.

Histiocyte Histiocyte is a tissue macrophage; a phagocytic cell important in granuloma formation.

HIV Human immunodeficiency virus.

HLA Human leukocyte antigen(s), a complex of proteins expressed on human cells that help the immune system to distinguish self. HLA is the human version of the Major Histocompatibility Complex (MHC). HLA typing is also known as tissue typing and is important for matching organ donors and recipients. Specific HLA types can be associated with disease susceptibility risk.

Horn A keratosis which is taller than it is broad.

Homogenous Homogenous describes a thing or things as being the same throughout.

Homozygous Homozygous is an adjective pertaining to homozygosity, identical alleles of a specific gene, e.g., an autosomal recessive condition requires the relevant gene to be homozygous.

Horny layer Horny layer of the epidermis (stratum corneum) consists of stacks of keratinized dead cells without nuclei. The top layer of these cells loosens and falls off.

Human leukocyte antigen Human leukocyte antigen (HLA) is a complex of proteins expressed on human cells that help the immune system to distinguish self from foreign.

Hyalinization Hyalinization is the process of forming hyaline in the dermis resulting in a ground-glass appearance, a word used in dermatopathology.

Hydrophilic Hydrophilic is an adjective pertaining to the ability to combine with or dissolve in water.

Hydrophobic Hydrophobic is an adjective pertaining to the inability or failure to mix with water.

Hyperhidrosis Hyperhidrosis is excessive sweating and be localized to one body site, e.g., palms, or generalized, affecting the whole body.

Hyperkeratosis Hyperkeratosis is a thickening of the stratum corneum, the outermost layer of the skin.

Hyperlipidaemia Hyperlipidaemia (American spelling hyperlipidemia) is a higher than normal blood level of one or more of the lipids (fats) such as cholesterol or triglycerides.

Hyperpigmentation Hyperpigmentation is a darker color than normal for that person or site, due to increased pigment. It can be localized or generalized.

Hyperplasia Hyperplasia is the enlargement of a tissue by an increase in cell numbers.

Hypersensitivity Hypersensitivity is an exaggerated immune reaction to an allergen or antigen following sensitization. There are several types of hypersensitivity reaction: type I (immediate); type II (cytotoxic); type III (immune complex); type IV (delayed, T-cell mediated). Non-allergic hypersensitivity is a pseudoallergy as it does not involve the immune system.

Hypertrichosis Hypertrichosis is excessive hair growth, not in the patterned distribution of hirsutism. Hypertrichosis may be localized or generalized.

Hypertrophy Hypertrophy is excessive growth or enlargement.

Hypohidrosis Hypohidrosis is decreased sweating.

Hypopigmentation Hypopigmentation is color that is paler than normal for that person or site, due to reduced pigment. It may be generalized or localized.

Hypotrichosis Hypotrichosis is a relative lack of hair growth, often congenital or genetic in origin.

Hystrix Lesion with sharp keratotic spines.

Iatrogenic Iatrogenic is an adjective describing an event or outcome as a result of a doctor's action. In dermatology, an example of an iatrogenic illness would be a rash due to prescription of a medicine.

Idiopathic Idiopathic is an adjective pertaining to an unknown cause.

Immunophenotyping Immunophenotyping is the identification of specific antigens or markers expressed by a cell, using antibodies (immunoglobulins).

Immunopathogenesis Immunopathogenesis is the process of disease development involving the immune system.

Impetiginisation Impetiginisation (American spelling impetiginization) is the process of secondary bacterial infection of a rash.

Incarnatus Converted into flesh.

Incisional biopsy Incisional biopsy is the surgical procedure to sample a selected portion of a lesion for evaluation by a pathologist.

Indolent Without significant pain or discomfort.

Infarct An area of coagulation necrosis due to local ischemia.

Infestation Harboring metazoal ("animal") parasites on or in the body.

Inflammasome Inflammasome is an intracellular complex comprising a receptor, a caspase-1 enzyme, and an apoptosis-associated speck-like protein. It is part of the innate immune system involved in binding and eliminating microbes.

Infundibulum Infundibulum is a funnel-shaped passage. In the skin, the hair follicle infundibulum is that part of the follicle above the level of the insertion of the sebaceous gland.

Innate Innate is an adjective pertaining to being present from birth, inborn, is not acquired later in life.

Inoculation Inoculation is the process of introducing microorganisms or cells to grow in culture medium or a living body. Inoculation is often used synonymously with immunization (vaccination) using a live vaccine through abraded skin as was done for smallpox prophylaxis.

In situ In situ means "in place"; an adjective and noun pertaining to being confined to the site of origin or placement, e.g., preinvasive phase as in melanoma in situ; the dressing remains in situ.

Intercellular Intercellular is an adjective meaning between cells.

Interdigital Between the anatomical digits, i.e., fingers or toes.

Interface dermatitis Interface dermatitis is a histological term describing inflammation at the junction (interface) between the epidermis and dermis. It may be lichenoid or vacuolar.

Interleukin Interleukin means between leukocytes; a cytokine produced by a white blood cell (leukocyte) to act on another white blood cell (leukocyte). There are many different interleukins involved in both innate and adaptive immune responses.

Interstitial Interstitial is an adjective pertaining to the interstitium, the intercellular connective tissue.

Intertrigo Intertrigo is a rash affecting body folds due to friction between adjacent skin sites.

Intracellular Intracellular is an adjective pertaining to the inside of a cell, within a cell.

Intradermal naevus Intradermal naevus, also called a dermal naevus, (American spelling nevus) is a benign melanocytic naevus (mole) located entirely within the dermis.

Intravascular Intravascular is an adjective meaning to be inside (within) a blood vessel or lymphatic vessel.

Intron Intron is a sequence of DNA or RNA that is cut out of the RNA transcript before translation into a protein.

Inverted Structure developing into the skin instead on top.

Ipsilateral Ipsilateral is an adjective pertaining to being on the same side of the body.

Isomorphic phenomenon Isomorphic (eponymous name Koebner) phenomenon is the involvement at a site of skin trauma or injury by a preexisting inflammatory skin condition.

Jaundice Jaundice is the yellowing of skin and sclera due to a buildup of bile pigments in the blood (bilirubinemia). This is usually due to biliary or liver disease.

Junctional naevus Junctional naevus (American spelling nevus) is a benign melanocytic naevus (mole) composed of melanocytes only along the dermoepidermal junction.

Juxta-articular Nearby or to the side of a joint.

Karyotype Karyotype is the number and appearance of chromosomes assessed during mitosis (cell division).

Keloid A keloid is an elevated progressive scar formation without regression.

Keratin Keratin is a family of proteins produced by keratinocytes, and forming the bulk of the epidermis, hair, and nails.

Keratinocyte Keratinocyte is the skin cell that is the major building block of the epidermis. It produces keratin.

Keratoderma Keratoderma is thickening of the skin, typically of the palms and soles. Keratoderma may be diffuse or localized.

Keratohyalin granules Specks within the cells of the stratum granulosum. They are correction precursor substances in the formation of finished keratin.

Keratolytic Keratolytic is an adjective and noun pertaining to the softening or destruction of keratin.

Keratoderma Hyperplasia of the stratum corneum.

Keratosis A keratosis is a horny thickening of the skin.

Kerion A kerion is a nodular inflammatory, pustular lesion, due to a fungus infection, Kerion celsi.

Koebner Koebner was a German dermatologist in the nineteenth century who first described the isomorphic response (in lichen planus or psoriasis) now often known eponymously as the Koebner phenomenon.

Koilocyte Koilocyte is a histological term for a “hollow” vacuolated squamous cell infected with the human papillomavirus.

Lacuna Natural, pathologic or artificially created discontinuity.

Lamella Lamella is a thin layer.

Lamina densa Lamina densa is the middle layer of the basement membrane (zone) between the epidermis and dermis. It is found just below the lamina lucida and is mainly composed of type IV collagen.

Langhans cell Foreign body type of giant cell.

Langerhans cell Langerhans cell is a specialized dendritic cell that presents antigens to the immune system. The Langerhans cell is characterized on electron microscopy by cytoplasmic Birbeck granules.

Lanugo hair Fine hair present on almost all parts of the body; in contrast to terminal hair.

Laser Laser is an acronym for light amplification of stimulated emission of radiation. Many uses have been found for laser devices including as a treatment in dermatology.

Lata Flat or broad.

Latent Latent is an adjective pertaining to latency, being dormant or concealed.

Lateral Lateral is an adjective relating to the side. In anatomy, a lateral location means on or towards the side of a body part.

Lenticular Shape or form of a lentil.

Lentigo Lentigo is a pigmented flat or slightly raised skin lesion with a clearly defined edge.

Lethal Deadly, fatal.

Leukocytoclasis Leukocytoclasis is the breakdown of infiltrating neutrophils in inflammation.

Leukoderma Leukoderma means white skin, specifically white skin due to the loss of skin melanin. Also known as achromia and depigmented skin.

Leukonychia Leukonychia is a completely or partially white nail.

Leukotriene Leukotriene is a family of potent biological pro-inflammatory mediators. These mediators are produced in the body from arachidonic acid by the enzyme 5-lipoxygenase and are divided into groups according to their chemical structure.

Lichenification Lichenification is a chronic thickening of the epidermis with exaggeration of its normal markings, often as a result of scratching or rubbing.

Lichenoid Lichenoid is an adjective meaning to resemble lichen. Clinically lichenoid describes papules or plaques that look stuck on to the skin like lichen on a rock or tree. In histology, however, lichenoid describes a band-like inflammation in the upper dermis.

Linear lesion Linear lesion is a skin change forming a line. A linear lesion may be due to an external cause such as scratching, contact dermatitis, or the Koebner phenomenon activating a pre-existing dermatosis. However, a linear lesion may also be developmental following a Blascko line, a dermatome, or a vascular or lymphatic vessel.

Liquefaction degeneration Disintegration or poor delineation of the basal cell layer of the epidermis.

Livedo Livedo is a mottled, typically bluish, vascular pattern in the skin due to slowed or obstructed vascular flow.

Lotion Lotion is a liquid formulation for topical use. A lotion is usually a simple suspension or solution. After application of a lotion, the liquid phase evaporates leaving the active ingredient on the skin surface.

Lupoid Lupus-like condition, showing red-brown discoloration, usually due to granulomas infiltrate.

Lymphadenopathy Lymphadenopathy is the abnormal enlargement of lymph nodes.

Lysosomal Lysosomal is an adjective pertaining to lysosomes, membrane-bound cytoplasmic organelles in cells that contain hydrolytic enzymes.

Maceration Maceration is the process of softening. In dermatology, maceration describes moist peeling skin such as between the toes after inadequate drying.

Macrophage Macrophage literally means big eater, and is another name for the histiocyte, a monocyte that has settled in the tissues including the skin. The macrophage is an actively migratory and phagocytic antigen-presenting cell, important in type IV hypersensitivity reactions and granuloma formation.

Macroscopic Macroscopic is an adjective meaning large enough to be visible with the naked eye.

Macule A macule is a circumscribed area of skin different in color or texture from its surrounding tissue. A maculopapular rash consists of macules and papules.

Maculopapular Maculopapular is an adjective pertaining to both flat macules and bumpy papules.

Madarosis Madarosis is the loss of either eyebrows, eyelashes, or both.

Magnetic resonance imaging Magnetic resonance imaging (MRI) is a medical imaging technique using a magnetic field, radiowaves, and a computer to produce detailed images. MRI is useful for soft tissue injuries affecting muscles, tendons, or ligaments, for assessing the brain and spinal cord, and for finding tumors. MRI does not use X-rays.

Malaise Malaise is a general feeling of unwellness or sickness.

Malformation Malformation is a congenital abnormality due to faulty development of a body part.

Malodor Malodor is a bad or unpleasant smell.

Marginal Marginal is an adjective pertaining to the margin, being on the edge. In dermatology, the word "marginal" may be used for being on the edge of a lesion or edge of a body part.

Mast cell Mast cell is a granulocytic white blood cell found in the connective tissue. Mast cell granules release histamine and other mediators. The mast cell is particularly important in the immune response to parasitic infections and is also activated in some allergic reactions.

Matrix metalloproteinase Matrix metalloproteinase (MMP) is a family of enzymes within the superfamily of matrixins involved in extracellular matrix regulation, inflammation, scarring, and wound repair. The matrix metalloproteinase family can be divided into two major groups—those that breakdown collagen and those affecting other molecules.

Matrix of nail Matrix of nail is the tissue from which the nail is formed. The dorsal (outer) nail plate is formed from the proximal nail matrix under the nailfold but the ventral (inner) nail plate is formed from the nail bed.

Meatus Passage or tunnel.

Medial Medial is an adjective pertaining to the median, the midline, or middle.

MEK MEK is the acronym for mitogen-activated, extracellular signal-regulated kinase, an enzyme in the MAPK signaling pathway which mediates cell growth and survival.

Melanin Melanin is a family of biological pigments derived from the amino acid tyrosine and produced by melanocytes.

Melanocyte Melanocyte is a dendritic cell found in the basal layer of the epidermis and other sites. The epidermal melanocyte produces melanin to protect the skin from damage due to ultraviolet radiation.

Melanocyte-stimulating hormone Melanocyte-stimulating hormone (MSH) is one of the protein products of the pro-opiomelanocortin gene. There are three forms of MSH: -alpha, -beta, and -gamma, with alpha being the most active in humans. MSH-alpha has many effects including on the pigmentary and inflammatory systems as well as on body weight.

Melanoderma Melanoderma is patchy or diffuse darkening of the skin due to increased melanin.

Melanophage Melanophage is a histiocyte (macrophage) which has ingested melanin granules or fragments.

Melanosome Melanosome is a cytoplasmic organelle involved in the synthesis, storage and transport of melanin, and found in melanocytes.

Merkel cell Merkel cell is a neuroendocrine cell found in the epidermis. The exact function of the Merkel cell is not known but is thought to be involved in mechanoreception as it is associated with a nerve ending, especially in highly tactile sites such as fingertips and lips.

Messenger RNA Messenger RNA (acronym mRNA) is the molecule responsible for carrying genetic information from the DNA (following transcription) to the protein-synthesizing ribosomes for translation.

Metachromasia Changed color different from normal tincture (histology).

Metaplasia Metaplasia is the transformation of one type of cell into another because of a changed environment.

Microabscess Microabscess is a tiny collection of neutrophils, eosinophils, or atypical cells, preferentially in the epidermis.

Microarray Microarray is a laboratory tool used in the analysis of thousands of tiny samples of DNA, RNA, or proteins.

Microbiome Microbiome, also called microbiota, is the collection of microorganisms that normally inhabit an organ or site, e.g., the skin microbiome.

Microvascular Microvascular is an adjective pertaining to the smallest blood vessels, usually capillaries.

Midline Midline is an imaginary line through the middle of a structure such that the two sides are equal.

Milium A milium is a tiny, white cyst containing lamellated keratin.

MRI MRI is the acronym for magnetic resonance imaging; a medical imaging technique using a magnetic field, radiowaves, and a computer to produce detailed images. MRI is useful for soft tissue injuries affecting muscles, tendons, or ligaments, for assessing the brain and spinal cord, and for looking for tumors. MRI does not use X-rays.

MSH MSH is the acronym for melanocyte-stimulating hormone, one of the protein products of the pro-opiomelanocortin gene. There are three forms of MSH: -alpha, -beta, and -gamma, with alpha being the most active in humans. MSH-alpha has many effects including on the pigmentary and inflammatory systems as well as on body weight.

Mitotic index Mitotic index is a count of the number of mitotic figures visible on microscopy of a tissue section, giving an estimate of how fast the cells are dividing.

Moniliform In the shape of a necklace.

Monoclonal Monoclonal is an adjective pertaining to a single clone, a group of identical units derived from an original single cell. Monoclonal cells form from a single cell. Monoclonal antibodies are produced by a single clone of plasma cells and have identical antigen-recognizing sequences.

Monocyte Monocyte is a mononuclear white blood cell made in the bone marrow and found only in the bloodstream. A monocyte becomes a macrophage as it actively migrates through body tissues.

Monogenic Monogenic is an adjective pertaining to a single gene.

Monomorphic Monomorphic is an adjective pertaining to one shape or form, all components having the same or an essentially similar appearance. A monomorphic rash looks the same all over, compared to being dimorphic or polymorphic.

Morbidity Morbidity is the state of being unwell.

Morbilliform Morbilliform is an adjective pertaining to the eruption of measles, measles-like rashes. Typically, a morbilliform rash is generalized and erythematous, with macules or papules.

Morbus Disease, illness.

Morphology Morphology is the structure and form of things, and also the study of the forms of things. In dermatology, the description of an individual skin lesion is the lesion morphology.

Mortality Mortality is the state of dying or death.

Mottled Spotty coloration.

mRNA mRNA is the acronym for messenger RNA, the molecule responsible for carrying genetic information from the DNA (after transcription) to the protein-synthesizing ribosomes for translation.

Mucin Mucin is a normal component of the ground substance surrounding the cells and fibers of the dermis. Mucin is mainly composed of hyaluronic and has a stringy clear appearance.

Mucosa Mucosa, also called mucous membrane, is the moist lining of body cavities and passages that can be exposed to the external environment, e.g., the mucosa of the mouth, nose, eyes, and anogenital area.

Multinucleate Multinucleate is an adjective used in histology to describe having two or more nuclei, e.g., a multinucleate giant cell.

Mutagen Mutagen is a physical or chemical agent that alters or changes genetic material; a mutagen causes a mutation in the DNA or RNA sequence.

Mutation Mutation is a permanent transmissible change in the genetic material, i.e., a gene mutation, which may or may not have any visible effect on the phenotype. Common usage tends to mean a visible effect as in a disease-causing mutation.

Myeloid Myeloid is an adjective pertaining to the bone marrow.

Myxoid Myxoid is an adjective meaning mucus-like, but rarely pertains to mucus itself, e.g., digital myxoid cyst, myxoid degeneration.

Natural killer (NK) cell Natural killer (NK) cell is a cytotoxic T lymphocyte involved in the innate immune system, able to induce programmed cell death (apoptosis) of cancer cells and cells infected with a virus.

Necrobiosis Necrobiosis describes partial degeneration of tissue, less than complete necrosis. It is often used to refer to swelling and degeneration of collagen in granuloma annulare and necrobiosis lipoidica.

Necrosis, necrolysis Necrosis is death and separation of tissue or cells.

Neonatal Neonatal is an adjective pertaining to newborns in the first 4 weeks after birth.

Neuron Neuron, also spelled neuron, is a dendritic nerve cell involved in the conduction of electrical impulses to carry messages to other cells.

Neuropathy Neuropathy is any disease, damage, or dysfunction of the nervous system or nerves.

Neutrophil Neutrophil, also known as a neutrophil leukocyte, polymorph, or neutrophilic polymorphonuclear leukocyte, is the most numerous type of granulocytic white blood cell (leukocyte). It is the first-line of defense in tissue damage and infection.

Nevoid Nevus-like.

Nikolsky sign Nikolsky sign is positive when slight rubbing of the skin results in exfoliation or shearing of the skin's outermost layer.

NK cell NK cell is the acronym for a natural killer cell, a cytotoxic T-lymphocyte involved in the innate immune system to induce programmed cell death (apoptosis).

Node A nodule is a solid mass of the skin which can be observed as an elevation or can be palpated. Usually, more than 1 cm in diameter.

Nodule A nodule is a solid mass of the skin which can be observed as an elevation or can be palpated. Usually, 0.5–1 cm in diameter.

Nosocomial Nosocomial is an adjective pertaining to a hospital, e.g., a nosocomial infection is an infection acquired in hospital.

Notalgia Notalgia means pain in the back, from the Greek "nota" (back) and "algia" (pain). In medicine, notalgia is used to describe pain, tingling, or numbness of the back due to a neurological cause.

NSAID NSAID is an acronym for nonsteroidal anti-inflammatory drug, nonsteroidal anti-inflammatory drug.

Nucleotide Nucleotide is the building block of the nucleic acid chains DNA or RNA. A nucleotide consists of a base (adenine, thymine, guanine, cytosine, or uracil) plus a sugar molecule (ribose or deoxyribose) and phosphate groups(s).

Nummular Nummular is an adjective pertaining to a coin, such as being coin-shaped.

Occipital Occipital is an adjective pertaining to the occiput, the back of the head. In surface anatomy, it is used to describe the back of the head overlying the occipital bone.

Occlusion Occlusion is the process of closing, blocking, or sealing. In medicine, occlusion may relate to a blood vessel, hollow organ or surface.

Oedema Oedema (American spelling edema) is tissue swelling due to excess interstitial fluid.

-oid Means like or in the form of…

Oil drop Oil drop is a nail sign, also called a salmon patch, in psoriasis presenting as an orange or brown streak or spot under the nail plate due to white cells in the nail bed.

Ointment Ointment is a semi-solid formulation for topical use based on lipids (oils) and so tends to have a greasy feel. The lack of water in the formulation means preservatives are rarely required.

Oligo- Little, scanty, slight, small.

Oncogene Oncogene is a gene that codes for a protein that can promote the growth and proliferation of tumor cells.

Onych- or onycho- Related to nail.

Onycholysis Onycholysis is the abnormal lifting of the nail plate from the distal nail bed, presenting as a larger than normal white or yellow area at the end of a nail plate.

Onychorrhexis Onychorrhexis is longitudinal ridging and fissuring of the nail plate typically seen with aging and diffuse nail matrix diseases.

Organelle Organelle is a structurally discrete component of a cell that has a specific function.

Orthokeratosis Orthokeratosis is a histological term for the normal stratum corneum consisting of keratinized cells not containing nuclei.

Pachyonychia Pachyonychia means elephant nail and is a congenital abnormal thickening of nail.

Pagetoid Pagetoid is an adjective used in histology to describe a resemblance to Paget cells, their appearance or behavior. Paget cells are large pale cells seen the epidermis in Paget disease.

Palmar Palmar is an adjective pertaining to the palm of the hand.

Palmoplantar Palmoplantar is an adjective pertaining to the palms and soles.

Palpation Palpation is the process of feeling or touching.

Papilla Papilla is a small nipple-shaped protuberance. There are several types of papilla on the tongue surface.

Papillary dermis Papillary dermis is the upper portion of the dermis just beneath the epidermis. It consists of thin irregularly arranged collagen fibers, thin elastic fibers, and ground substance.

Papilloma A nipple-like mass projecting from the surface of the skin.

For example,

Dermal: A soft flesh-colored elevated tumor with a dermal component, fibroma molle.

Epidermal: Acrochordon *or* papillomatous seborrheic keratosis.

Papillomatous Papillomatous is an adjective pertaining to a papilloma. Clinically, it describes the bumpy elevated surface of a lesion such as a viral wart. Histologically, papillomatous describes irregular surface folding.

Papule A papule is a small solid elevation of the skin, less than 0.5 cm in diameter.

Epidermal papule: A papule composed of localized thickening of the epidermis or *of* the stratum corneum.

Dermal papule: A papule composed of a localized solid thickening of the dermis produced by augmentation of normal structures, deposition of metabolic products, concentrations of cells, or other pathologic changes.

Inflammatory papule: A papule produced by inflammation of the dermis, epidermis, or both.

Papulosquamous lesion: A papule that develops a reactive or degenerative epithelial component resulting in desquamation, which is the loss of epithelial cells or of stratum corneum (scaling).

Wheal (Anglosaxon): An elevated compressible, transitory. white or pink papule, or plaque of dermal edema.

Papulopustule Papulopustule is a skin lesion with both papular and pustular components.

Papulosquamous Papulosquamous is an adjective describing being scaly, raised, and palpable, as in papules and plaques.

Papulovesicle Papulovesicle is a skin lesion with both papular (small bumps) and vesicular (small blisters) components, typically a small bump with a tiny blister on top as seen in an insect bite.

Parakeratosis Parakeratosis is a histological word for an abnormal stratum corneum in which the keratinized cells of the skin surface retain their nuclei.

Paraneoplastic Paraneoplastic is an adjective describing being remote to but associated with a neoplasm. A paraneoplastic symptom or sign indicates the presence of an internal cancer.

Paraproteinaemia Paraproteinaemia (American spelling paraproteinemia) is the presence of a monoclonal immunoglobulin in the blood due to a monoclonal gammopathy.

Paronychia Paronychia literally means around the nail and is an inflammatory process around the edge of a nail.

PASI PASI is the acronym for Psoriasis Area and Severity Index and is used for assessment and monitoring of psoriasis.

Paste Paste is a semi-solid formulation for topical application, comprised mostly of a powder such as zinc oxide. The powder is mixed with water or oil in varying proportions to form either a greasy protective fatty paste that is very stiff, or a drying cooling paste that tends to be soothing. Medicaments may be added to the paste, e.g., dithranol in Lassar paste in the Ingram regime.

Patch A large macule, more than 2 cm in diameter..

Pathergy Pathergy is the development or flare of skin lesions after minor trauma, such as a needle prick, typically seen in Behcet disease and pyoderma gangrenosum.

Pathogen Pathogen is an organism that can cause disease. Examples of a pathogen may include a virus, protozoan, or yeast.

Pathogenesis Pathogenesis is the origin, development, and maintenance of a disease.

Pathognomonic Pathognomonic is an adjective meaning characteristic or distinctive. A pathognomonic symptom or sign is one so distinctive that it can be used to make a diagnosis.

Pathophysiology Pathophysiology is the study of the functional changes in living tissue in a particular medical condition.

PCR PCR is the acronym for polymerase chain reaction. PCR is used for the detection and amplification of specific DNA sequences useful in making a diagnosis and gene sequencing.

Peduncle Peduncle is a stalk-like component of a lesion.

Peptide Peptide is a short chain of amino acids, shorter than a protein.

PET PET is the acronym for positron emission tomography; a nuclear medicine imaging test using a radiotracer to assess tissue metabolism.

Perforating Perforating is a verb and adjective pertaining to perforation, penetration, the making of holes. In dermatology, perforating also describes conditions in which something penetrates through a layer as in a perforating dermatosis.

Perifollicular Perifollicular is an adjective meaning close-to or surrounding a hair follicle(s).

Perineum Perineum in the female is from the anus to the posterior fourchette of the vulva. In the male, it is the area between the anus and scrotum. Common usage has widened use to include the perianal skin, groin folds, and vulva or scrotum.

Periodic acid-Schiff (PAS) stain Useful additional stain to show fungi and natural mucopolysaccharides.

Perioral Perioral is an adjective pertaining to the area close-to and around the mouth.

Periorbital Periorbital is an adjective to describe being around the orbit or the eye.

Periorificial Periorificial is an adjective pertaining to the area close-to or around an orifice such as the mouth, eyes, or anus.

Peripheral Peripheral is an adjective pertaining to the outer edge.

Periungual Periungual is an adjective pertaining to around a fingernail or toenail.

Perivascular Perivascular is an adjective used in histology meaning close-to and around blood vessels.

Permeability Permeability is the property of allowing diffusion, transit or passing through, porosity, e.g., the permeability of a membrane.

Petechia A punctate hemorrhagic spot 1 to 2 mm in diameter.

pH pH is a log scale defining hydrogen ion concentration and hence acidity/alkalinity in a solution. The scale ranges from 0 to 14, with 0 as most acidic and 14 as most alkaline. Water is pH 7, defined as a neutral solution.PhagocytePhagocyte is an immune cell that can surround, kill, and ingest particles such as bacteria and other microorganisms or foreign matter, a process is called phagocytosis. A phagocyte can also boost immune responses. Examples of a phagocyte include a macrophage and neutrophil.

Phagocytosis Phagocytosis is the process by which a cell engulfs and ingests a particle.

Phenotype Measurable features of the organism that are expressed by its genotype in conjunction with environmental factors.

Phlebectasia Phlebectasia is the congenital widening (dilation) of a vein.

Photoaging Photoaging (British spelling photoageing) is an acceleration of the skin changes of aging caused by exposure to ultraviolet radiation especially sunlight.

Photoallergen Photoallergen is a substance that causes an allergic reaction to sunlight after either topical contact or systemic exposure. A photoallergen may be a medication, food, plant, or other chemical.

Photoallergy Photoallergy is a delayed hypersensitivity reaction to a substance after exposure to light. It can be due to topical or systemic contact with a photoallergen or photosensitizer such as a medication, plant, or food.

Photodynamic Photodynamic is an adjective pertaining to the activation or intensification of a reaction by exposure to light in a living system, e.g., photodynamic therapy (PDT) applies a topical photosensitizer to increase the reaction to a laser or light.

Photoprotection Photoprotection is the process of using physical or chemical agents to protect against light, e.g., UPF50+ clothing and SPF50+ sunscreens provide photoprotection.

Photosensitivity Photosensitivity is an unusual increase in the reactivity of the skin to sunlight.

Phototoxicity Phototoxicity is a dose-related chemical-induced sensitivity to light that does not involve an immune reaction.

Pilosebaceous unit Pilosebaceous unit consists of a hair follicle and sebaceous (oil) gland.

Pimple Common homely designation for an ugly papule or pustule.

Pit Pit is a depression, hole, or indentation in a surface. To pit is also a verb, meaning to remove the stone of a fruit.

Pityriasis Pityriasis is an adjective meaning finely scaly and is used to describe a bran-like fine powdery scale.

Plantar Plantar is an adjective pertaining to the sole of the foot.

Plaque An elevated area of skin 1 cm or more in diameter. Plaques may have the same subdivisions as mentioned above under papules.

Plasma Plasma is the fluid component of blood or lymph, i.e., that part of blood or lymph without the cells. Plasma is also a state of matter initially thought to only occur at extremely high temperatures but cold plasma has now been developed for use in medicine, e.g., non-laser plasma skin rejuvenation. Plasma is also an adjective to describe a cell type, i.e., plasma cell, an activated form of B-cell.

Plasma cell Plasma cell is an activated tissue B lymphocyte (B cell) producing immunoglobulin in an immune response.

Pleomorphism Pleomorphism is multiple different forms. It is commonly used in histology to mean wide variability in nuclear or cell morphology which typically indicates malignancy.

Poikiloderma A dermatosis characterized by variegated cutaneous pigmentation, atrophy, and telangiectasia.

Poliosis Poliosis is a patch of depigmented hair.

Polycyclic Polycyclic is an adjective describing many circles, which may be used in dermatology to describe a rash composed of rings or partial ring-shaped lesions.

Polygonal Polygonal is an adjective pertaining to many angles. A polygonal skin lesion has a nongeometric shape.

Polymerase chain reaction Polymerase chain reaction (PCR) is a laboratory tool for detecting and amplifying a specific DNA sequence. It is useful in making a diagnosis by detecting DNA sequences of viruses or bacteria such as HPV in cervical swabs or HSV in skin swabs.

Polymorphism Polymorphism has many forms; in histology, nuclear polymorphism means the cell nuclei are variable in shape or appearance, i.e., many forms of the nucleus; in genetics, a polymorphism is a chromosomal locus with more than two alleles in the general population, i.e., many forms of the gene resulting in many forms of the protein product, i.e., protein polymorphisms; a single nucleotide polymorphism (SNP) may change the pharmacodynamics or pharmacokinetics of a drug and hence the therapeutic response.

Polyploid Polyploid is an adjective describing a cell with more than the normal two sets of chromosomes, typically seen in malignant cells.

Pomade Pomade is a greasy or waxy perfumed ointment or gel usually used to style scalp or facial hair.

Pore Passage or opening (ostium).

Positron emission tomography (PET) Positron emission tomography (PET scan) is a nuclear medicine imaging test used for assessing metabolic activity in tissues. Prior to imaging, a radiotracer is introduced into the body by one of a variety of routes including injection. In dermatology, a PET scan may be used to detect skin cancer metastases or assess response to treatment.

Posterior Posterior is an adjective meaning behind or towards the back. In anatomy, a posterior location means on the back of a body part (dorsal).

Powder Powder is a pulverized solid, for example, talc (a mineral) or corn starch (vegetable).

Predilection Predilection is a preference.

Predisposition Predisposition is the susceptibility to a disease or condition.

Protozoa Protozoa: plural of protozoan; eukaryotic unicellular organisms that can be free-living or parasitic. Malaria and leishmaniasis are examples of diseases caused by protozoa.

Proximal Proximal is an adjective pertaining to proximity, a location or distribution closest to a point of origin or attachment. In anatomy, proximal relates to the center of the body, i.e., A being proximal to B means A is closer to the center of the body than B.

Pruritus Pruritus is an irritating skin sensation which elicits the scratch response.
Syn.: itching

Pseudocyst Pseudocyst is a firm lesion that contains fluid or semi-fluid material but, unlike a true cyst, it is not surrounded by a capsule or wall.

Pseudoepitheliomatous Pseudoepitheliomatous hyperplasia is a histological term for a harmless thickening of all layers of the epidermis that can resemble squamous cell carcinoma.

Pseudohypha Pseudohypha is a branched filament produced by yeast resembling a fungal hypha.

Psoriasiform Psoriasiform is an adjective meaning to resemble psoriasis. Psoriasiform may be used clinically to describe psoriasis-like well-defined scaly skin patches, or histologically to describe regular psoriasis-like acanthosis of the epidermis but lacking the other typical histologic features of psoriasis.

Psychodermatology Psychodermatology is the study of skin conditions associated with, caused by, or triggered by mental conditions. Psychodermatology includes conditions that are primarily psychiatric in origin; others where the skin condition causes a secondary psychiatric issue such as depression or anxiety; skin conditions that flare with stress and therefore require treatment of both the stress and the skin; skin symptoms that are neurological in origin; and skin conditions that are treated with psychotropic medications.

Pterygium Pterygium is a wing of extra tissue. In dermatology, pterygium typically describes an abnormal fold of skin connecting to nail in lichen planus and scleroderma. More commonly, a pterygium affects the eye.

Punch biopsy Punch biopsy is an incisional biopsy of tissue obtained using a biopsy punch tool.

Punctate Pointed or marked with dots.

Purpura Discoloration of the skin or mucosa due to extravasation of blood.

Pustule A visible accumulation of pus in the skin.

Pyknosis Pyknosis is a histological term for the change seen in the nucleus of a cell undergoing apoptosis. It is characterized under the microscope as a shrinking and darkening of the nucleus.

Pyoderma Pyoderma is any purulent skin disease, either bacterial or nonbacterial in origin.

Quotidian Quotidian is an adjective meaning daily. Quotidian malaria is the form of malaria with daily fever spikes.

Rash Rash is an eruption of skin lesions which can be localized or widespread. Rash is also an adjective meaning impetuous or without thought.

Raynaud phenomenon Raynaud phenomenon is a vasospastic response to cold in which fingers or toes turn white and numb and are bluish on rewarming before returning to normal. It may be primary (unknown cause) or secondary to connective tissue diseases.

Reagin IgE or other antibody-like substances in the blood.

Rete ridge Rete ridge is an upward projection of connective tissue between epithelial rete pegs.

Reticular dermis Reticular dermis is the deep part of the dermis, composed of coarse elastic fibers and thick collagen bundles parallel to the skin surface.

Reticulate Reticulate derives from the Latin to mean a small net and is used as an adjective to mean covered by a net or network.

Retinoid Retinoid is an adjective and noun pertaining to a molecule resembling vitamin A, e.g., a retinoid drug. Common usage makes retinoid a noun used for a family of drugs related to vitamin A, e.g., a retinoid (drug).

Rhagade Fissures, cracks, or linear scars in the skin.

Ribonucleic acid (RNA) Ribonucleic acid (RNA) is a molecule involved in the coding, replication, and expression of genes. There are several different types of RNA in a cell including messenger RNA (mRNA), ribosomal RNA, and transfer RNA (tRNA). DNA is transcribed into mRNA by enzymes that read one strand of DNA converting the deoxyribose sugar into ribose and substituting the thymine base (T) for a uracil base (U). Ribosomal RNA and tRNA are involved in translating the mRNA code to amino acids and synthesizing a protein. Some viruses use double-stranded or single-stranded RNA instead of DNA as their genetic material.

Roseola Rose-red macules or patches.

Rupioid Rupioid is an adjective to resemble rupia; rupia comes from the Greek rhypos—filth. However, rupioid is often used in dermatology to describe something as layered to resemble an oyster or limpet shell.

Scale A scale is a flat plate or flake of stratum corneum.

Squama types

1) *Collarette scale:* Describes the fine, peripherally attached and centrally detached scale at the edge of an inflammatory lesion.

Example: *Pityriasis rosea*

2) *Furfuraceous:* Describes fine and loose scales.
3) *lchthyosiform:* Describes large, polygonal scales—as in fish scales.
4) *Psoriasiform* (resembling psoriasis): Describes a silvery, white. parakeratotic, lamellated scale similar to a scale of psoriasis.

Scar A scar is the fibrous tissue replacing normal tissues destroyed by injury or disease.

Syn.: cicatrix

Types:

1) *Atrophic scar:* Papyraceous or cigarette paper scar—describes thin wrinkled scars.
2) *Cribriform scar:* Describes a scar perforated with multiple small apertures.
3) *Hypertrophic scar:* An elevated vascular scar with excessive growth of fibrous tissue.

Scarlatiniform Scarlatiniform is an adjective meaning to resemble the rash of scarlet fever, typically a flat red rash.

Sclerodactyly Sclerodactyly is the thickening and tightness of the skin of the fingers or toes, which can result in spindle-shaped digits.

SCORAD SCORAD is a tool used for SCORing Atopic Dermatitis and is used for assessment and monitoring.

Scratch Superficial mostly linear injury of the epidermis, reaching not deeper than to the papillary dermis.

Sclerosis Sclerosis is an induration or hardening of the skin. It is often due to fibrosis.

Scurf Obsolete term for scales or crusts on the scalp see dandruff.

Scutulum Tiny concave crust.

Seborrhoeic Seborrhoeic (American spelling seborrheic) is an adjective pertaining to seborrhoea or resembling seborrhoea. Use in dermatology does not always involve actual seborrhea, including seborrheic area (where seborrheic glands are common), seborrheic dermatitis (typically involves seborrheic areas), and seborrheic keratosis (which can have a greasy appearance unrelated to seborrheic glands).

Segmental Segmental is an adjective pertaining to a segment, a part or section. A segmental distribution in dermatology describes involvement of one or more dermatomes or Blashko lines.

Self-antigen A self-antigen is part of the person's body that can induce an antibody response in some people.

Sensitisation Sensitisation (American spelling sensitization) refers to the process of becoming sensitised (allergic) to an agent.

Sepsis Sepsis is a bacterial infection causing systemic toxic symptoms such as fever.

Serpentine Serpentine is an adjective pertaining to a serpent (snake); serpentine describes having a curling or winding shape or movement like a snake.

Shave biopsy Shave biopsy is a tissue sample obtained by a slice or cut made parallel to the surface of the surrounding skin. A shave biopsy may remove all or part of a lesion for diagnosis or cure.

Single nucleotide polymorphism (SNP) Single nucleotide polymorphism (SNP) is a single nucleotide substitution in a gene seen commonly in the general population resulting in an allele that may influence disease susceptibility.

Sinus A sinus is a cavity or channel; a channel that permits the escape of pus or fluid.

Soft tissue Soft tissue in the body includes tendons, ligaments, fascia, skin, fibrous tissues, fat, synovial membranes, muscles, nerves, and blood vessels. It does not include the bony skeleton, teeth, nail, or hair.

Somatic Somatic is an adjective pertaining to the body.

Somatic mutation Somatic mutation is a gene mutation that has occurred any time after fertilization and so affects only limited cells, but specifically not the gametes (sperm or ova). A somatic mutation is not inherited or passed on to offspring.

Sonography Sonography, also called ultrasonography, is an imaging technique using echoes of ultrasound pulses to detect areas of different density in body tissues.

Sore Boil, ulcer, or other localized painful lesion of the skin.

Spindle cell Spindle cell is a long thin cell. Many cell types may present as a spindle cell so it is a descriptive term used in histology.

Spongiosis Spongiosis is a histological term for intercellular swelling of the epidermis resembling a sponge.

Spore Spore is a unicellular dormant form of a plant or microorganism resistant to adverse conditions capable of germinating after dispersal in favorable situations. A spore may be fungal, protozoal, or bacterial, among others.

Squama Squama (or squame) is a skin scale.

Squamous cell Squamous cell is a flattened keratinocyte in the outermost layers of the epidermis or mucosa forming the surface scale (squames).

Stasis Stasis means a lack of change, which in medicine can refer to the slowing or cessation of flow or movement. Stasis can be used as a noun as in vascular stasis, meaning a lack of blood flow resulting in pooling of blood, or as an adjective as in stasis dermatitis to refer to the skin rash due to the pooling of blood and lack of flow.

Stratum corneum Stratum corneum is the surface horny layer of the epidermis consisting of stacks of dead keratin-filled cells (keratinocytes) without nuclei.

Stratum granulosum Stratum granulosum is the layer of the epidermis under the stratum corneum and is characterized by flattened cells filled with dark granules containing keratohyaline protein.

Stratum spinosum Stratum spinosum, also called the prickle cell layer, of the epidermis contains increasingly flat keratinocytes as they move upward during maturation towards the surface. Desmosomes are prominent producing the spiny shape.

Stria A streak or band of linear, atrophic, pink, purple, or white lesions of the skin due to changes in connective tissue.

Striate Striate is an adjective pertaining to striations, bands, or stripes.

Subcorneal Subcorneal is an adjective meaning beneath the stratum corneum of the epidermis, or under the cornea of the eye.

Subcutaneous Subcutaneous is an adjective pertaining to under the skin, e.g., subcutaneous fat, subcutaneous injection.

Subcutis Subcutis is the fat layer beneath the dermis. It is also called subcutaneous fat or hypodermis.

Subepidermal Subepidermal is an adjective pertaining to being under or below the epidermis.

Submammary Submammary is an adjective pertaining to under the breast(s).

Subungal Subungual means underneath the nail plate.

Suprabasal Suprabasal is an adjective describing being above the lowest layer. In dermatology, it usually pertains to being just above the basal layer of the epidermis.

Susceptibility Susceptibility is a noun meaning the likelihood of succumbing to an influencing factor, e.g., susceptibility to developing an infection or cancer, antibiotic susceptibility of a bacterial isolate.

Sycosis Sycosis is a chronic pustular folliculitis and perifolliculitis involving the beard area.

Syndrome Syndrome is a group of signs and symptoms that occur together and characterize a particular condition.

Systemic Systemic is an adjective describing involvement of the body system as a whole.

Target lesion Target lesion, also known as an iris lesion, has concentric rings like a dartboard or bull's eye appearance.

Targeted therapy Targeted therapy is a drug or agent that targets a specific protein or gene, e.g., targeted cancer therapy, where the target resides in or on a cancer cell.

Telangiectasia A visible vascular lesion formed by dilation of small cutaneous blood vessels.

Telogen Telogen is the resting phase of the hair cycle. Telogen hairs have a clubbed or bulbous tip and last for several months before falling out (shedding).

Telomere Telomere is the cap on the end of a chromosome that protects the DNA from structural damage. A telomere is composed of proteins and thousands of repeats of the DNA sequence TTAGGG in humans. The telomere is important for accurate DNA replication during cell division. There is gradual loss of telomere length after each cell division until there is insufficient length to allow DNA duplication and the cell becomes senescent.

T lymphocyte (T cell) T lymphocyte, also called a T cell, is a type of immune cell that originates in the bone marrow, matures in the thymus, and circulates around the body. There are several specific types of T lymphocyte.

Temporal Temporal is an adjective pertaining to the temple or to time. In surface anatomy, it describes the part of the side of the head overlying the temporal bone, i.e., the temple. It is also used in medicine to describe events related by time, e.g., a temporal relationship between taking a medication and developing a rash.

Teratogen Teratogen is an agent that can cause birth deformities.

Terminal hair Terminal hair is the thick long hair that normally occurs on the scalp and, after puberty, in the armpits, beard, and pubic area.

Thrombosis Thrombosis is the formation of a blood clot (thrombus) in the heart or blood vessels.

Titre Titre (American spelling titer) is an expression of concentration as the maximum dilution still showing activity.

Topical Topical is an adjective pertaining to a topic. When used in a pharmaceutical sense, it describes an application directly to a surface. Common usage makes it also a noun, e.g., using a topical (agent).

Trachyonychia Trachyonychia is rough nail(s) with excessive longitudinal ridging due to proximal nail matrix damage.

Transdermal patch Transdermal patch is a drug delivery system applied to the skin surface with an adhesive from which a medication is absorbed through the skin into the systemic circulation, e.g., estrogen patches used during the menopause, GTN patches used to treat ischemic heart disease.

Translucent Translucent is an adjective pertaining to translucence, being partially or semi-transparent, e.g., light can pass through a translucent membrane.

Trich- or tricho- Related to hair.

Trophic Trophic is an adjective derived from the Greek for nutrition. In dermatology, trophic is usually applied to skin changes associated with numbness due to neurologic causes, but can also be used for changes due to pressure in vascular insufficiency and malnutrition.

Tumor A tumor is an enlargement of the tissues by normal or pathologic material or cells that form a mass. It may be inflammatory or benign or a malignant new growth of cells or tissue.

Tumor necrosis factor-alpha (TNF- alpha) Tumor necrosis factor-alpha (TNF-alpha) is a pro-inflammatory cytokine predominantly synthesized by macrophages. It can also cause tumor cell necrosis.

Tyrosinase Tyrosinase is the enzyme that catalyzes the first step in the production of melanin and other pigments from the amino acid tyrosine.

Ulcer A skin ulcer is a defect or loss of dermis and epidermis produced by sloughing of necrotic tissue.

Ultrasound Ultrasound is a high-frequency sound wave. Ultrasound is used in ultrasonography to detect areas of different density in a body tissue.

Ultraviolet radiation (UVR) Ultraviolet radiation is that part of the sun's electromagnetic spectrum with a wavelength between 100 nm and 400 nm (i.e., shorter than visible light). Ultraviolet radiation is classified in three parts; UVA (230–400 nm), UVB (290–320 nm), UVC (100–290 nm).

Umbilicated Umbilicated is an adjective pertaining to a central dell, usually seen in a vesicle, papule, or nodule such as molluscum contagiosum or herpes simplex.

Urticaria Urticaria, also called hives, is a family of disorders characterized by transient wheals.

Vacuole Vacuole is a membrane-bound fluid-filled cytoplasmic organelle formed from endoplasmic reticulum. On histology, vacuoles look like empty spaces.

Vacuolization Vacuolization is the process of forming vacuoles, membrane-bound fluid-filled cytoplasmic organelles.

Vegetation A vegetation is a growth of pathologic tissue consisting of multiple closely set papillary masses.

Ventral Ventral is an adjective pertaining to the front. In anatomy, a ventral location means on the belly, anterior surface of the trunk, or flexor surface of a limb.

Venule Venule is the smallest type of vein that connects capillaries to the venous system.

Verruca A verruca is an epidermal tumor caused by a papilloma virus. Verrucous describes a lesion with a warty surface.

Verrucous Verrucous is an adjective pertaining to verruca, a wart. Verrucous means wart-like, having a thickened scaly undulating surface.

Vesicle A vesicle is a circumscribed elevation of the skin less than 0.5 cm in diameter and containing a liquid.

Vellus hair Vellus hair is the short, fine, light-colored hair found over most of the body.

Vertex Vertex is the highest point of the scalp where it changes direction from being horizontal to vertical.

Vesicle Vesicle is a small blister, a circumscribed lesion less than 0.5 cm in diameter that contains liquid (clear, serous, or hemorrhagic).

Vesiculobullous Vesiculobullous is an adjective describing the presence of both small and large blisters (vesicles and bullae).

Vibex A vibex is a narrow linear mark, usually hemorrhage, from scratching.

Violaceous Violaceous is an adjective describing a violet or purple hue.

Viscosity Viscosity is a physical characteristic of a fluid describing the fluidity, thickness.

Volar Volar refers to the hollow of the palm and sole but can also refer to the side of the adjoining skin, such as the fingers and forearm.

Warty Warty is an adjective pertaining to a wart, a wart-like surface.

Well-defined Well-defined is an adjective used to describe having a clear sharp border separating it from its surrounds.

Wheal An elevated white compressible, evanescent area produced by dermal edema. It is often surrounded by a red, axon-mediated flare.

Wood lamp Wood lamp emits long wavelength UVA and is used to examine skin pigment changes (e.g., vitiligo or melasma) and fluorescent infections such as cat ringworm.

Xerosis Xerosis is a name for abnormally dry skin.

Zona Girdle or belt.

Zosteriform Zosteriform is an adjective pertaining to herpes zoster, zoster-like, unilateral and restricted to a dermatome or distribution of a single spinal nerve.

Index

H. Gollnick et al. (eds.), *Dermatology Cyberderm WebBook*,
https://doi.org/10.1007/978-3-031-78491-0

G

H

T

MIX
Papier aus verantwortungsvollen Quellen
Paper from responsible sources
FSC® C105338

If you have any concerns about our products,
you can contact us on
ProductSafety@springernature.com

In case Publisher is established outside the EU,
the EU authorized representative is:
Springer Nature Customer Service Center GmbH
Europaplatz 3, 69115 Heidelberg, Germany

Printed by Libri Plureos GmbH
in Hamburg, Germany